Clinical Pathology

Clinical Pathology

Editor: Cecilia Bryant

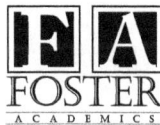

FA FOSTER
ACADEMICS

www.fosteracademics.com

www.fosteracademics.com

FA FOSTER
ACADEMICS

Cataloging-in-Publication Data

Clinical pathology / edited by Cecilia Bryant.
   p. cm.
Includes bibliographical references and index.
ISBN 978-1-63242-775-5
1. Diagnosis, Laboratory. 2. Diagnosis. 3. Pathology. I. Bryant, Cecilia.
RB37 .C55 2019
616.075--dc23

© Foster Academics, 2019

Foster Academics,
118-35 Queens Blvd., Suite 400,
Forest Hills, NY 11375, USA

ISBN 978-1-63242-775-5 (Hardback)

Contents

Preface

The purpose of the book is to provide a glimpse into the dynamics and to present opinions and studies of some of the scientists engaged in the development of new ideas in the field from very different standpoints. This book will prove useful to students and researchers owing to its high content quality.

Clinical pathology is a specialization in medicine, concerned with the laboratory analysis of bodily fluids such as urine and blood, as well as the examination of tissue samples using cultures and automated analyzers to make a diagnosis of diseases. The analysis of such samples is done at macroscopic and microscopic levels. Immunofluorescence, immunocytochemistry, FISH and cytochemistry are also used to aid in the diagnosis. The secondary specialties of clinical pathology include hematopathology, clinical microbiology, chemical pathology, molecular genetics pathology, cytogenetics, etc. There is an evident overlap between clinical pathology and anatomic pathology, which has led to its expansion to molecular diagnostics and proteomics. This book covers in detail some existing theories and innovative concepts revolving around clinical pathology. The various specializations of clinical pathology, along with technological progress that have future implications, are glanced at in this book. With state-of-the-art inputs by acclaimed experts of this field, this book targets students and professionals.

At the end, I would like to appreciate all the efforts made by the authors in completing their chapters professionally. I express my deepest gratitude to all of them for contributing to this book by sharing their valuable works. A special thanks to my family and friends for their constant support in this journey.

Editor

Expression of KOC, S100P, mesothelin and MUC1 in pancreatico-biliary adenocarcinomas: development and utility of a potential diagnostic immunohistochemistry panel

Asif Ali[1*], Victoria Brown[2], Simon Denley[3], Nigel B Jamieson[3], Jennifer P Morton[4], Colin Nixon[4], Janet S Graham[5], Owen J Sansom[4], C Ross Carter[3], Colin J McKay[3], Fraser R Duthie[6] and Karin A Oien[1,6]

Abstract

Background: Pancreatico-biliary adenocarcinomas (PBA) have a poor prognosis. Diagnosis is usually achieved by imaging and/or endoscopy with confirmatory cytology. Cytological interpretation can be difficult especially in the setting of chronic pancreatitis/cholangitis. Immunohistochemistry (IHC) biomarkers could act as an adjunct to cytology to improve the diagnosis. Thus, we performed a meta-analysis and selected KOC, S100P, mesothelin and MUC1 for further validation in PBA resection specimens.

Methods: Tissue microarrays containing tumour and normal cores in a ratio of 3:2, from 99 surgically resected PBA patients, were used for IHC. IHC was performed on an automated platform using antibodies against KOC, S100P, mesothelin and MUC1. Tissue cores were scored for staining intensity and proportion of tissue stained using a Histoscore method (range, 0–300). Sensitivity and specificity for individual biomarkers, as well as biomarker panels, were determined with different cut-offs for positivity and compared by summary receiver operating characteristic (ROC) curve.

Results: The expression of all four biomarkers was high in PBA versus normal ducts, with a mean Histoscore of 150 vs. 0.4 for KOC, 165 vs. 0.3 for S100P, 115 vs. 0.5 for mesothelin and 200 vs. 14 for MUC1 ($p < .0001$ for all comparisons). Five cut-offs were carefully chosen for sensitivity/specificity analysis. Four of these cut-offs, namely 5%, 10% or 20% positive cells and Histoscore 20 were identified using ROC curve analysis and the fifth cut-off was moderate-strong staining intensity. Using 20% positive cells as a cut-off achieved higher sensitivity/specificity values: KOC 84%/100%; S100P 83%/100%; mesothelin 88%/92%; and MUC1 89%/63%. Analysis of a panel of KOC, S100P and mesothelin achieved 100% sensitivity and 99% specificity if at least 2 biomarkers were positive for 10% cut-off; and 100% sensitivity and specificity for 20% cut-off.

Conclusion: A biomarker panel of KOC, S100P and mesothelin with at least 2 biomarkers positive was found to be an optimum panel with both 10% and 20% cut-offs in resection specimens from patients with PBA.

Keywords: Pancreatic cancer, Biomarkers, Immunohistochemistry, Diagnosis

* Correspondence: draliasif7@gmail.com
[1]Wolfson Wohl Cancer Research Centre, Institute of Cancer Sciences, College of Medical Veterinary and Life Sciences, University of Glasgow, Garscube Estate, Switchback Road, Bearsden G61 1QH, UK
Full list of author information is available at the end of the article

Background

Pancreatic ductal adenocarcinoma (PDAC) is the fifth most common cause of cancer death in the UK with a 5-year survival of only 2% [1]. This poor prognosis is partly due to late clinical presentation with advanced disease, when the treatment options are limited and relatively ineffective [2]. Surgical resection is the only curative option but is only available to 15-20% patients with localised disease [3,4]. The remainder with locally advanced and/or metastatic disease are offered palliative chemotherapy, radiotherapy and/or best supportive management [2,3]. Adenocarcinomas of the head of pancreas and extra-hepatic cholangiocarcinomas (CCC) present similarly most often with jaundice, pain or weight loss [5]. Morphological similarities in addition to generally poor prognosis for both diseases enable PDAC to be grouped with extrahepatic CCC to form so-called pancreatico-biliary adenocarcinomas (PBA).

Diagnosis of PBA relies upon a combination of radiological and cytology or pathology findings [6-10]. Confirmatory tissue diagnosis is necessary before chemotherapy or radiotherapy treatment, however a biopsy specimen is not always required for resection when the suspicion of cancer is high; as generally, the resection will provide therapeutic benefit, and substantially delaying surgery to confirm a diagnosis may deny potentially curative treatment [9,11-15].

Endoscopic ultrasound-guided fine needle aspiration (EUS-FNA) is normally used to obtain cytological samples from pancreatic mass lesions, while endoscopic retrograde cholangio-pancreato-graphy (ERCP) biliary brushings are used for cytology collection from strictures of pancreatico-biliary (PB) ducts [16-18]. Cytological analysis requires the distinction of malignant PB epithelial cells from reactive pancreatic and bile duct cells as well as other gastrointestinal contaminants. This task requires tremendous expertise and can be difficult for both quantitative and qualitative reasons [19]. Quantitatively, the cytological sample obtained may be of low cellularity with few, or even no malignant epithelial cells amongst a variety of cell types. Qualitatively, PBA cells can be morphologically similar to reactive PB cells, especially in well-differentiated adenocarcinomas. Chronic reactive changes arising from atrophy or inflammation in pancreatitis or cholangitis are common, and also make diagnosis of adenocarcinoma difficult.

Expressing these issues statistically, the reported sensitivity of EUS-FNA ranges from 78%-95% with specificity reported to be 75-100% [17,18,20-25]. Though the specificity of biliary brush cytology is high, the sensitivity can be low with ranges of 46% to 73% reported [10,16,26,27]. The sensitivity of EUS-FNA cytology decreases to 62% in chronic pancreatitis and to only 50% in cases of chronic pancreatitis with obstructive jaundice [28]. Thus, a tissue diagnosis is not achieved in a significant proportion of PBA cases. Hence, an unmet clinical need exists for the diagnosis of PBA from cytological samples obtained at EUS-FNA and ERCP.

One potential way of improving cytological diagnosis is to use immunohistochemical (IHC) biomarkers as an adjunct to cytology in difficult to diagnose cases. IHC is a technique widely used in diagnostic pathology that enables the observation and localisation of protein expression simultaneously in tissue and cellular compartments [29]. Diagnostic IHC biomarkers have been investigated both as single biomarkers and as part of biomarker panels to improve the diagnosis of PDAC, but to date none has entered into routine clinical practice [30-37]. We performed a meta-analysis of potential PDAC IHC diagnostic biomarkers [38] aiming to generate a list of biomarkers assessed in either surgical or cytology specimens, where PDAC was compared with normal pancreas and/or chronic pancreatitis. Meta-analytical results showed KOC, S100P, mesothelin and MUC1 to be high-ranking candidates. These biomarkers have not entered into routine clinical practice partly because they were investigated in separate studies with relatively small sample sizes and without uniform and clinically appropriate thresholds for positivity.

We sought to investigate the utility of these four candidate biomarkers in the characterisation of PBA, including both PDAC and CCC. CCC has been included because it often enters the clinical and pathological differential diagnosis; and its positive biomarkers are generally shared with PDAC [39-42]. The aim was to identify a clinically useful diagnostic biomarker or panel of biomarkers with a robust cut-off for positivity that could potentially be taken forward for validation in PBA cytology samples.

A biomarker panel of KOC, S100P and mesothelin with at least 2 biomarkers positive was found to be an optimum panel with both 10% and 20% cut-off achieving almost 100% sensitivity and specificity in resection specimens from patients with PBA.

Methods

Tissue Microarrays

Histological sections from tissue microarrays (TMAs) containing samples from 99 surgically resected PBA patients (PDAC = 85, CCC = 14) were used for IHC. All resectional surgery was performed in the West of Scotland Pancreatic Unit, Glasgow Royal Infirmary, UK, during a 10-year period (1st June 1995 to 31st July 2004). Formalin fixed paraffin embedded (FFPE) tumour specimens were archived in the Department of Pathology, Glasgow Royal Infirmary and were used for the construction of TMAs. The construction and use of these TMAs has been previously described [43]. Ethical approval has been granted by the North Glasgow University Hospitals NHS Trust Ethics Committee and by the National Health Service Greater Glasgow and Clyde Ethics Committee. This ethics approval includes the use of archival pathology specimens, where the patients were not given the opportunity to donate their tissue. These TMAs contain five tissue cores (3 tumours and 2 normal) for each patient. Tumour cores are adenocarcinoma cores from PBA patients, whereas normal cores are from adjacent normal pancreatic ducts and acini.

Immunohistochemistry

IHC was performed for KOC, S100P, mesothelin and MUC1 on our TMA cohort, on an automated platform. Details of the antibodies, antibody concentrations and IHC conditions are shown in Table 1.

Scoring of tissue specimens

Stained TMA sections were scanned (Hamamatsu Slide Scanner) and images uploaded in Distiller 2.2 (Leica Biosystems). Microscopic analysis was undertaken blinded to diagnosis or other parameters. IHC staining of all cores was assessed by one author (AA); a second author (KAO) double-scored approximately 15% of cores, in a blinded fashion, as audit. All scores were exported in an Excel spreadsheet from Distiller 2.2 for analysis. A semi-quantitative Histoscore [0 ×% negative cells + 1 ×% weakly stained cells + 2 ×% moderately stained cells + 3 ×% strongly stained cells] was generated for statistical analysis. This Histoscore thus has a range of possible scores between 0 and 300.

Statistics and data analysis

The mean expression of each biomarker in the PBA tumour cores was compared with the mean expression in normal tissue cores. Statistical significance was calculated using the independent sample t-test to generate the p value. The independent sample t test was used rather than the paired sample t test because a full set of matching tumour and normal tissue cores was not available for approximately 5% of patients. This was due to loss of tissue cores during processing, which is expected in a proportion of samples. Sensitivity/specificity analyses were carried out for biomarkers, both individually and in panels of 2–4 biomarkers, and compared. We used two different panel approaches for sensitivity/specificity analysis. One approach assigns the case into the

positive category if the tumour expresses only one biomarker in the panel. The other approach assigns the case into the positive category if the tumour shows staining for at least 2 biomarkers in the panel.

A combined summary receiver operating characteristic (SROC) curve was generated to compare different panels of biomarkers. P value <0.05 was considered statistically significant. SPSS-19 and RevMan-5.1 were used for statistical analysis.

Results

We first performed IHC for each of the four biomarkers on microarrays of normal and tumour tissue from patients with PBA. To fully assess the clinical usefulness of these biomarkers we wanted to analyse the expression of all four biomarkers in PBA versus normal tissue. Moreover, by combining various biomarkers in panels, we hypothesised that we would be able to determine the combination of biomarkers that would deliver the best diagnostic sensitivity and specificity.

Staining characteristics of biomarkers

For each marker assessed in the PB TMAs, IHC staining was seen only in epithelial cells. As expected, KOC expression was observed in the cytoplasm; S100P was expressed in the cytoplasm and nucleus, while mesothelin and MUC1 expression was cytoplasmic and membranous (Figure 1). In general, we observed moderate to strong intensity of staining for KOC, mesothelin, S100P and MUC1 in PBA. Moreover, for all four biomarkers we observed significantly higher expression in tumour versus normal tissue (non-neoplastic ducts or pancreatic acinar tissue). The mean percentage positivity for biomarkers in tumour vs. normal tissue was as follows: for KOC 74% vs. 0.4%; for S100P 75% vs. 0.3%; for mesothelin 75% vs. 4%; and for MUC1 75% vs. 18% (Table 2, p < 0.0001 for all tumour vs. normal comparisons). When scored simply as the percentage of positive staining cells per tumour core, we observed similar results for all four biomarkers in tumour tissue. As shown in Table 2, the mean percentage of positive carcinoma cells in tumour tissue was 74% for KOC, 75% for S100P, 73% for mesothelin and 75% for MUC1.

Table 1 Details of the immunohistochemistry methodology for four antibodies

Antibody	Company	Clone of antibody	Host animal	Antigen retrieval	Antibody dilution	Incubation temperature	Duration of incubation
KOC/IMP3	DAKO	L523S, 69.1	Mouse Monoclonal	HIER* (Citrate buffer PH 6)	1:50	25°C	60 min
S100P	BD Biosciences	16	Mouse monoclonal	Proteinase K (10 minutes)	1:100	25°C	60 min
Mesothelin	Novocastra	5B2	Mouse monoclonal	HIER (Citrate buffer PH 6)	1:20	25°C	60 min
MUC1	Novocastra	MA695	Mouse monoclonal	HIER (Citrate buffer PH 6)	1:200	25°C	60 min

*HIER= Heat Induced epitope retrieval.

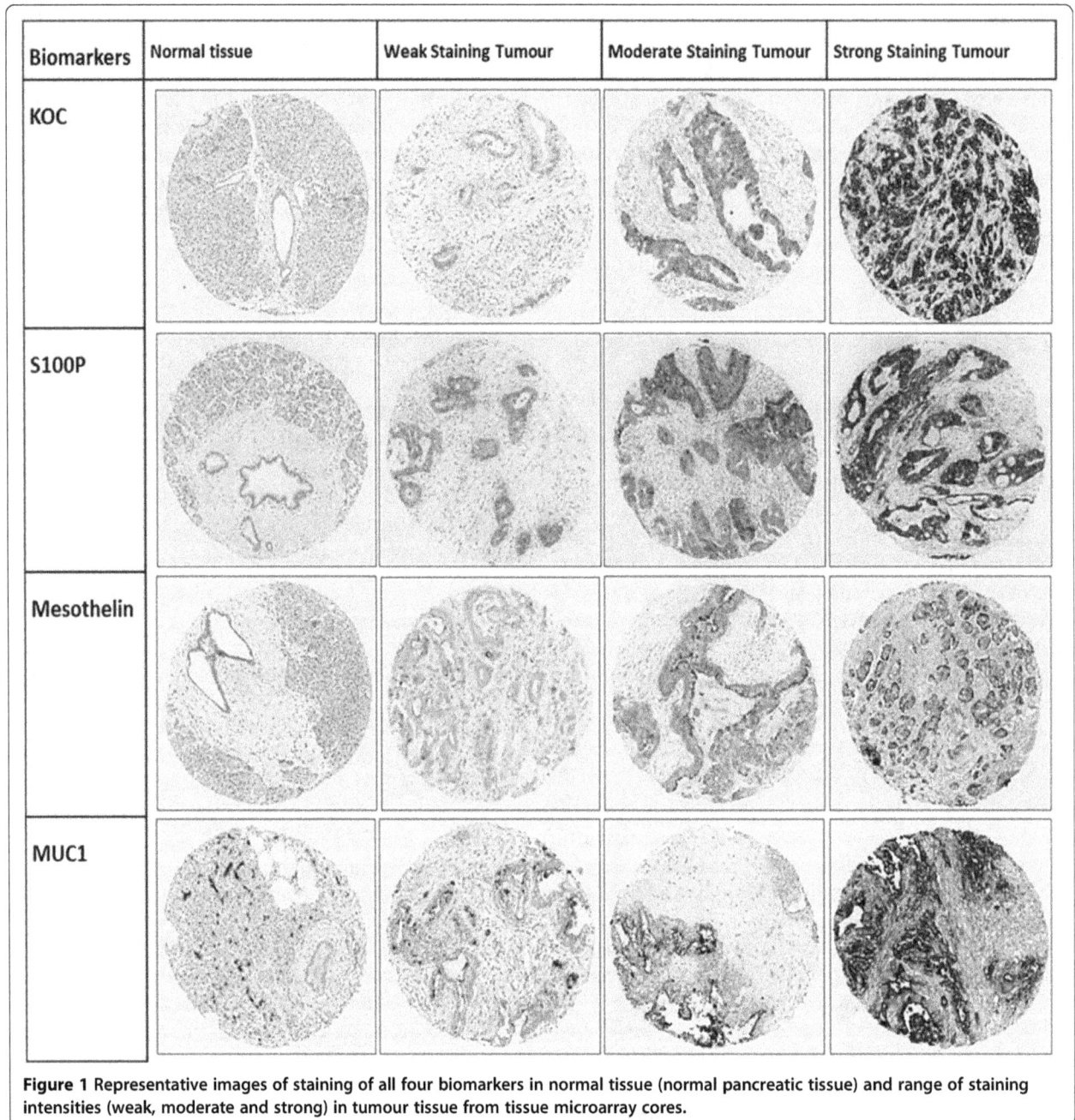

Figure 1 Representative images of staining of all four biomarkers in normal tissue (normal pancreatic tissue) and range of staining intensities (weak, moderate and strong) in tumour tissue from tissue microarray cores.

By employing a Histoscore scoring method, which takes into account both the extent of expression across the tissue core, and the staining intensity, we were able more to perform a more comprehensive analysis of our biomarkers. Utilizing this method to score the degree and intensity of staining revealed variance of expression of the different biomarkers. As shown in Table 2, the mean tumour tissue versus mean normal tissue Histoscore for MUC1 was 193 vs. 48, while for S100P, KOC and mesothelin, the mean tumour tissue versus mean normal tissue Histoscores were 165 vs. 0.3, 150 vs. 0.5 and 115 vs. 4 respectively.

Although one biomarker, MUC1, was expressed in normal tissue as evidenced by the mean percentage positivity of 16% of normal cells in normal tissues, the expression of the other three biomarkers was very low in normal tissue (Table 2). Furthermore, there were no significant differences in biomarker expression between normal ducts only and normal ducts and acini together (see Additional file 1). Thus, IHC staining using these markers could greatly facilitate interpretation of cytology samples.

Biomarkers expression was also assessed in PDAC compared to CCC as shown in Additional file 2. The expression of all four biomarkers is similar in PDAC and

Table 2 Summary statistics of KOC, S100P, mesothelin and MUC1 expression on a per core basis comparing pancreatico-biliary adenocarcinomas with normal tissue

Biomarkers		Pancreaticobiliary adenocarcinoma	Normal tissue	P value
KOC				
*Positivity**	Mean	74%	0.4%	<0.0001
	Median	100%	0%	
Histoscore	Mean	150	0.5	<0.0001
	Median	180	0	
S100P				
Positivity	Mean	75%	0.3%	<0.0001
	Median	100%	0%	
Histoscore	Mean	165	0.3	<0.0001
	Median	180	0	
Mesothelin				
Positivity	Mean	73%	4%	<0.0001
	Median	90%	0%	
Histoscore	Mean	115	4	<0.0001
	Median	110	0	
MUC1				
Positivity	Mean	75%	18%	<0.0001
	Median	90%	10%	
Histoscore	Mean	193	48	<0.0001
	Median	200	30	

Note: *Positivity (percentage of positive cells with any staining intensity in tumour and normal tissue); P value (shows the statistical significance of the difference in expression of a biomarker in tumour vs. normal tissue); Positivity range (0–100), Histoscore range (0–300).

CCC and thus there is no statistically significant difference in the mean expression of biomarkers between these two tumour types (p > 0.05, independent sample t test). Therefore, for sensitivity and specificity analyses PDAC and CCC were grouped as PBA.

Sensitivity and specificity analysis
Establishing cut-offs from ROC curve analysis
The sensitivity and specificity of these four biomarkers were evaluated using five cut-offs (thresholds) for positivity as follows: 5% positive cells of any staining intensity; 10% positive cells of any staining intensity; 20% positive cells of any staining intensity; moderate or strong staining of any cells; and Histoscore ≥20. Three of these cut-offs were based on percentage of positive cells and identified by ROC curve analysis. The sensitivity of each biomarker was plotted against 1 – specificity, and ROC curves with coordinates were generated for all four biomarkers (Figure 2). The area under the curve was 0.93 (0.88-0.97, 95% CI) for KOC, 0.92 (0.85-0.99, 95% CI) for S100P, 0.95 (0.92-0.99, 95% CI) for mesothelin, and 0.87 (0.81-0.93, 95% CI) for MUC1. Based on

percentage of positive cells in the tumour compared with normal cores, ROC curve analysis allowed us to assess potential cut-offs, from 5% positive cells to 95% positive cells, with their corresponding sensitivity and specificity values for all four biomarkers (Figure 2 and Additional file 3). Three best cut-offs; 5%; 10% or 20% of positive cells of any staining intensity were selected based on their sensitivity and specificity values.

The fourth cut-off was based on moderate to strong staining intensity (+2/+3 staining) in any of the cells. This was selected as moderate to strong staining was expected to be easily interpreted by pathologists. Interestingly, cases with +2/+3 staining for all four biomarkers have more than 20% cells positive for each of the four biomarkers. Indeed patients with +2/+3 staining have only 5 cases with less than 50% of cells positive for MUC1, 2 cases in which KOC was expressed in fewer than 50% of cells, and only 1 case each for mesothelin and S100P staining with less than 50% positivity.

The fifth cut-off was based on a Histoscore value of 20 (HS20), and was selected from ROC curve analysis (see Additional file 4).

Sensitivity and specificity of candidate biomarkers
The sensitivities and specificities of all four biomarkers were calculated using these five cut-offs, as shown in Figure 3. KOC expression appears to show reasonably high sensitivity and specificity for all cut-offs except for the cut-off based on +2/+3 staining, which resulted in low sensitivity of only 67%. The 20% positive cells cut-off achieves marginally better sensitivity (84%) and specificity (100%) values compared with other cut-offs for KOC (Figure 3A). S100P appears to have similar sensitivity and specificity values for all five cut-offs with the 20% cut-off again achieving better combination of specificity and sensitivity, with values of 83% sensitivity and 100% specificity (Figure 3B).

Applying the five cuts-offs to the analysis of mesothelin expression resulted in significantly different sensitivity and specificity values, however, the best combination was again achieved using the 20% cut-off, with 88% sensitivity and 92% specificity (Figure 3C). Although the sensitivity of MUC1 as biomarker is high across all cut-offs, its specificity is unacceptably low for all cut-offs, with a range of 18%-63% compromising the diagnostic accuracy of MUC1 (Figure 3D).

Sensitivity and specificity analysis using biomarker panels
We next wanted to assess the sensitivity and specificity achieved using panels of biomarkers. The 10% and 20% cut-offs were selected for this investigation, based on their diagnostic performance.

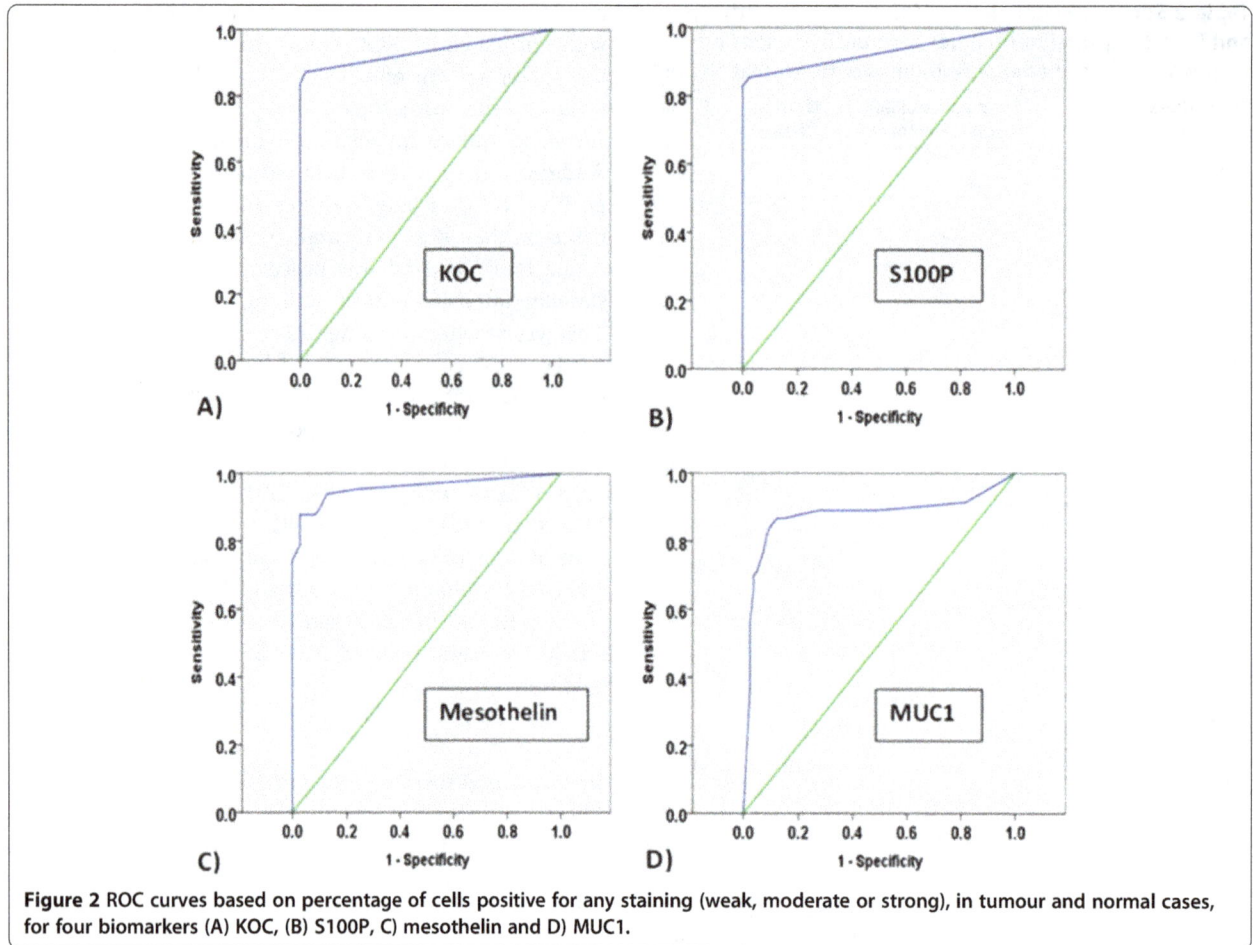

Figure 2 ROC curves based on percentage of cells positive for any staining (weak, moderate or strong), in tumour and normal cases, for four biomarkers (A) KOC, (B) S100P, C) mesothelin and D) MUC1.

Analysis based on one positive biomarker in a panel

We first assessed the sensitivity and specificity achieved when one biomarker in a panel is positive, using four different panels (Table 3). These panels were: a panel comprising all four biomarkers; a panel of three biomarkers (KOC, S100P and mesothelin); and two panels of two biomarkers (KOC and mesothelin, KOC and S100P). As expected, a panel of all four biomarkers achieved very low specificity of 40% and 65% respectively for 10% and 20% cut-offs, due to the low specificity of MUC1 as a biomarker. A panel of KOC, S100P and mesothelin achieved sensitivity/specificity of 100%/88% for the 10% cut-off and 99%/94% for the 20% cut-off. A panel of KOC and mesothelin achieved sensitivity/specificity of 97%/87% and 96%/93% for the 10% cut-off and 20% cut-offs, respectively. Finally, a panel of KOC and S100P achieved sensitivity/specificity of 98%/96% for the 10% cut-off and 99%/99% for the 20% cut-off.

These panels were compared by combined SROC curve, using both the 10% cut-off (Figure 4A) and 20% cut-offs (Figure 4B). The combined SROC curve shows that a panel of KOC and S100P is superior to the other panels for both 10% and 20% cut-offs.

Analysis based on two or more positive biomarkers in a panel

Finally, one biomarker panel comprising KOC, S100P and mesothelin was tested for sensitivity and specificity when at least 2 biomarkers in the panel are positive. This panel achieved almost 100% sensitivity/specificity for both 10% and 20% cut-offs (Table 3). Taken together, our results show that this panel could be used to improve diagnosis of PBA in difficult to diagnose cases.

Discussion

Four potentially diagnostic biomarkers, KOC, S100P, mesothelin and MUC1, were investigated in a relatively large cohort of PB patients (n = 99). The expression levels of KOC, S100P and mesothelin were high in tumour tissue compared with normal tissue. The diagnostic accuracy (sensitivity and specificity) of KOC and S100P individually was greater than that of mesothelin and MUC1. A panel of KOC, S100P and mesothelin with at least 2 biomarkers positive achieved almost perfect diagnostic accuracy in the differentiation of carcinoma from normal tissue.

IHC biomarkers have previously been investigated in surgical and cytological cohorts but none is yet routinely used

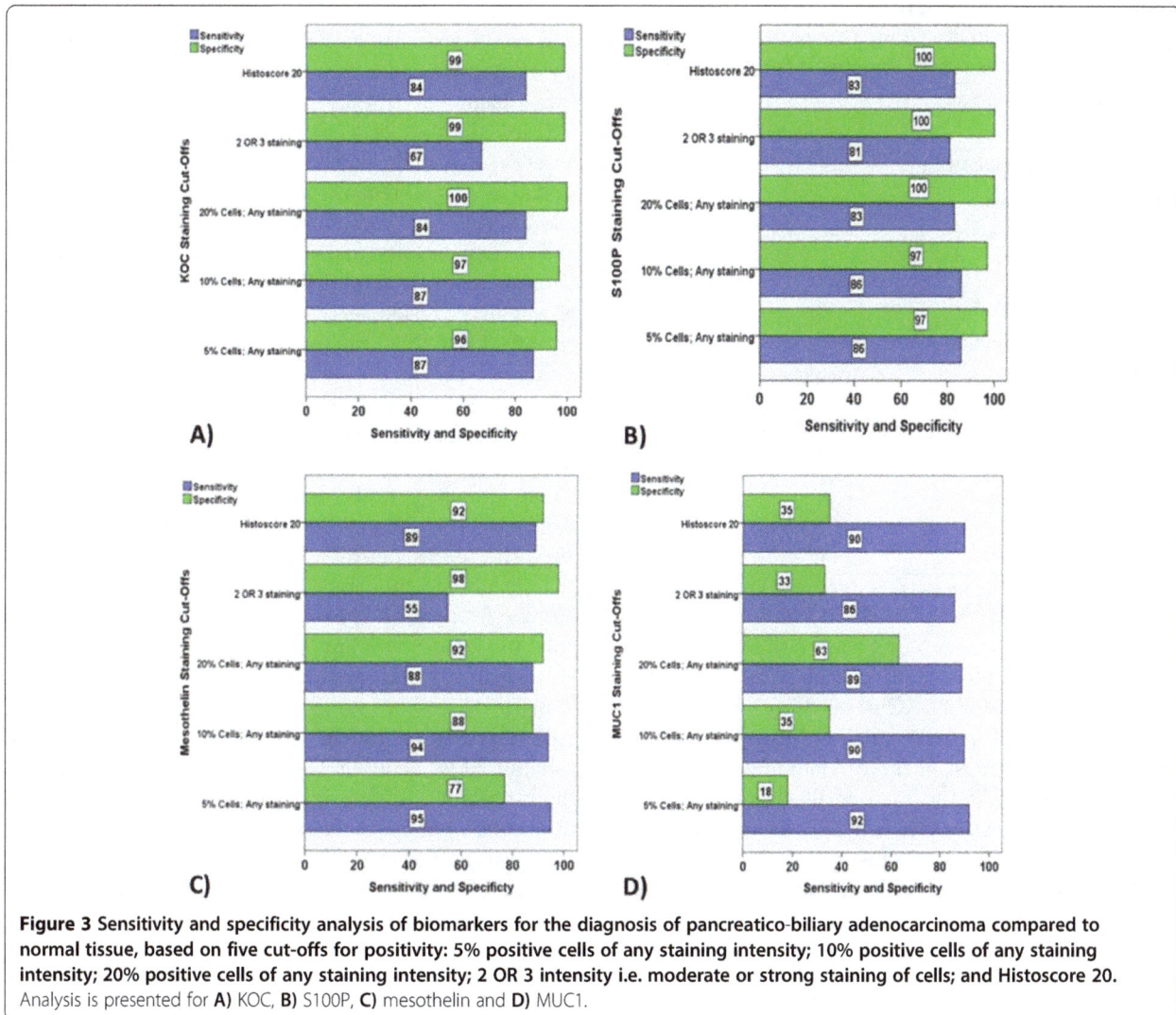

Figure 3 Sensitivity and specificity analysis of biomarkers for the diagnosis of pancreatico-biliary adenocarcinoma compared to normal tissue, based on five cut-offs for positivity: 5% positive cells of any staining intensity; 10% positive cells of any staining intensity; 20% positive cells of any staining intensity; 2 OR 3 intensity i.e. moderate or strong staining of cells; and Histoscore 20. Analysis is presented for **A)** KOC, **B)** S100P, **C)** mesothelin and **D)** MUC1.

for improving the diagnosis of PBA [35-37,41,44-46]. There are six significant reasons delaying the clinical translation of diagnostic biomarkers in PBA and other cancers. These reasons and our approach to address them are outlined below.

Firstly, a plethora of research exists on diagnostic IHC biomarkers coming from the bench assessed in pilot studies. There are many excellent papers but fewer validation studies for biomarkers that have shown promising results. Clearly, validation is important for future clinical application. Therefore, we performed a meta-analysis on diagnostic IHC biomarkers for PDAC [38], to review, quantify and assess the performance of already existing biomarkers and to try and identify superior candidate biomarkers.

The biomarkers derived from the meta-analysis in PDAC were applied in our study to both PDAC and CCC samples. Separate meta-analysis was not performed for CCC, because there are relatively few published

papers on biomarkers in CCC (approximately 20-fold fewer than for PDAC; PubMed search in June 2014, unpublished data). However, those papers which are available for CCC suggest that the biomarker expression profile is similar to PDAC. To our knowledge, all of the known positive biomarkers for PDAC (versus corresponding normal tissue), including MUC1, P53, CK17, mesothelin, fascin, MUC4, 14-3-3σ and prostate stem cell antigen, show similar IHC expression in CCC (versus corresponding normal tissue) [39-42].

For these reasons, we focused on PDAC for the identification of potential diagnostic biomarkers then tested the resulting candidates in TMAs containing tissue from both PDAC and CCC using IHC. From our meta-analysis, we selected KOC [36,37,44,47], S100P [32,35,48], mesothelin [30,49,50] and MUC1 [31,40,51] for investigation.

We found that expression of these biomarkers was similar in PDAC and CCC (Additional File 2): our results therefore supporting the previous literature [39-42].

Table 3 Panels of biomarkers used for analysis of specificity and sensitivity, using 10% positive cells and 20% positive cells as cut-off thresholds for positivity

10% positive cells as cut-off

Panels	Sensitivity	Specificity
KOC, S100P, Mesothelin, MUC1	100%	40%
KOC, S100P, Mesothelin	100%	88%
KOC, Mesothelin	97%	87%
KOC, S100P	98%	96%
KOC, S100P, Mesothelin*	100%	99%

20% positive cells as cut-off

Panels	Sensitivity	Specificity
KOC, S100P, Mesothelin, MUC1	100%	65%
KOC, S100P, Mesothelin	99%	94%
KOC, Mesothelin	96%	93%
KOC, S100P	99%	99%
KOC, S100P, Mesothelin*	100%	100%

Note: *At least 2 biomarkers required to be positive in this panel. In the rest of the panels only one biomarker was required to be positive in a panel.

Second, the sample size for studies investigating diagnostic biomarkers for PDAC is relatively small (median sample size, n = 48 from 57 articles). Moreover, matched normal tissue for most of the carcinoma case is not always available, leading to even smaller sample sizes for calculating biomarker specificity. Therefore, statistical power is relatively low and subsequently potentially useful biomarkers may be ignored. Our relatively larger

sample size of 99 PBA cases (n = 99 adenocarcinomas and n = 99 matched normal tissue for each case; total n = 198) provided a solid platform for investigating these diagnostic IHC biomarkers.

Third, the lack of a standardised scoring system and absence of a uniform cut-off (threshold) for the interpretation of IHC remains problematic. Thus, researchers use a variety of traditional and novel scoring systems and diverse cut-offs, making the adoption of scoring systems and cut-offs potentially challenging for the pathologists [30,35,37,41,46,49,52-54]. We systematically chose cut-offs from ROC curve analysis to fully explore the diagnostic potential of all four biomarkers. These cut-offs provide an opportunity for the pathologists to select the best threshold that is more clinically applicable and has the potential to be routinely used in pathology. Three of these cut-offs are based on proportion of positive cells (5%, 10% and 20%) with staining of any intensity. The fourth cut-off is based on any proportion of cells exhibiting moderate and strong staining intensity, and the fifth cut-off is based on a Histoscore of 20. Notably, the 20% cut-off and Histoscore 20 provide reasonable sensitivity and specificity values for PBA diagnosis. A higher Histoscore value could potentially lead to more false negatives in tumour cases, therefore, a low cut-off value of 20 was chosen. Clearly, this cut-off will remove the probability of false negative and should increase the diagnostic confidence of pathologists for higher Histoscore values. For example, a Histoscore value of 200 for a biomarker in a suspicious case might help the

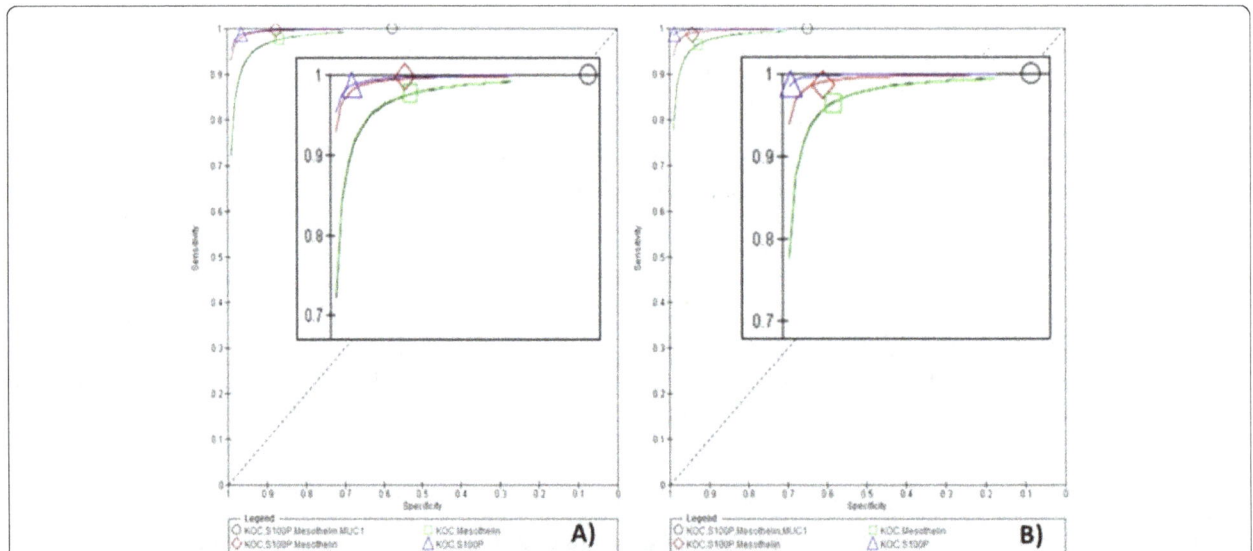

Figure 4 *Combined Summary ROC curves for 10% (A) and 20% (B) cut-offs if only one biomarker was required to be positive in a panel. Four panels of biomarkers were compared. Panel 1 - KOC, S100P, Mesothelin and MUC1; Panel 2 - KOC, S100P, Mesothelin; Panel 3 - KOC, S100P; Panel 4 - KOC, Mesothelin. *Summary ROC curves plot sensitivity against specificity and draw a summary line depicting combined sensitivity and specificity of a panel. Combined Summary ROC curves compare different panels to show the most "accurate" panel. The summary line at the top left corner shows the biomarker which is most accurate compared to others lying lower and further to the right. This enables the most accurate panel to be identified.

pathologist to diagnose a tumour with confidence and with a much higher specificity.

Fourth, most of the IHC diagnostic biomarkers have been investigated individually [32,46,47,55,56], with few studies reporting the utility of biomarker panels [30,36]. We carefully selected candidate biomarkers reported in different studies (KOC, mesothelin, S100P and MUC1) for investigation in a single experimental setting. Investigation of these biomarkers in a single cohort gave us the opportunity to compare biomarkers, and then further explore their diagnostic accuracy in a panel. Expectation from an ideal diagnostic biomarker is its ability to identify the diseased population (sensitivity) and exclude the normal population (specificity) in 100% cases. However, no single biomarker is 100% perfect; therefore these biomarkers were investigated in various combinations, to select an optimum panel for potential clinical application. For example, the individual sensitivity/specificity of KOC and S100P at a cut-off of 20% positive cells was 84%/100% and 83%/100% respectively. However, using a panel of KOC and S100P improved sensitivity to 99% without compromising the specificity (99%).

Furthermore, using a panel of KOC, S100P and mesothelin with at least 2 positive biomarkers achieved almost 100% sensitivity and specificity for both 10% and 20% cut-offs. This approach would assign a patient into the tumour positive category if 2 or more biomarkers are positive, possibly giving more assurance to the pathologist before assigning patient into positive category. Moreover, a combination of KOC, S100P and mesothelin antibodies should stain all major cellular compartments (cell membrane, nucleus and cytoplasm). Clinically, a cytology sample comprises a mixed population of cells and this panel will stain malignant cells more intensely making the interpretation of IHC convenient for the pathologist. The possible additional advantage of KOC is that it is not expressed in the contaminating gastrointestinal epithelial cells that are usually present in cytological samples [44,57]. Our data also confirm the lack of expression of KOC in normal duodenum. Taken together, our results reinforce the reported sensitivity/specificity values for KOC, S100P and mesothelin [30,35,37,57] and further explores their utility as a panel.

The fifth reason is that different research groups use different IHC experimental conditions, primary antibodies, clones, dilutions and manual/automated platforms that could potentially lead to a diverse range of sensitivity and specificity values for biomarkers [30,45,54,58-60]. We thoroughly searched the literature for IHC parameters for KOC, S100P, mesothelin and MUC1. Those IHC parameters that achieved superior diagnostic accuracy were selected and further optimised in our histology laboratory before staining our cohort.

Finally, an important requirement for biomarker translation to the clinic is independent validation with the aim of improving already existing diagnosis. Purposeful validation in surgical and cytological tissue from PBA cohorts and subsequent prospective clinical study on cytological samples is deficient. Therefore, as an important step for potential clinical translation we investigated KOC, S100P, mesothelin and MUC1 in a surgical cohort of PBA patients with promising results for KOC, S100P and mesothelin as a biomarker panel.

The next step forward is to possibly investigate these biomarkers in a retrospective and then in a prospective cohort of cytology samples. This manuscript systematically attempted to answer all six major reasons hindering the clinical translation of diagnostic IHC biomarkers for pancreatic cancer. It also provides future direction and work packages to be performed before these diagnostic biomarkers can be used in day-to-day pathology practice.

Conclusions

Our results demonstrate that a biomarker panel of KOC, S100P and mesothelin is capable of categorising PB malignancy with high diagnostic accuracy in resection specimens. We plan to investigate this panel in archival cytological samples. As an adjunct to cytology, this panel has the potential to augment the categorisation for challenging diagnostic cases in routine clinical practice.To our knowledge, this is the first study of PB literature that identified cut-offs systematically for diagnostic purposes and used stringent panels to identify an optimum biomarker panel.

Additional files

Additional file 1: Summary statistics of KOC, S100P, mesothelin and MUC1 expression on a per core basis comparing pancreatico-biliary adenocarcinomas with normal ducts and normal ducts & acini together.

Additional file 2: Summary statistics of KOC, S100P, mesothelin and MUC1 expression on a per core basis comparing pancreatic ductal adenocarcinoma with cholangiocarcinoma.

Additional file 3: Cut-offs resulting from ROC curve analysis based on the percentage of positive cells of any staining intensity (weak, moderate or strong) in tumour and normal cases for four biomarkers KOC, S100P, mesothelin and MUC1.

Additional file 4: ROC curves based on histoscores, in tumour and normal cases, for four biomarkers A) KOC, B) S100P, C) mesothelin and D) MUC1.

Abbreviations
PDAC: Pancreatic ductal adenocarcinoma; PBA: Pancreatico-biliary adenocarcinomas; ERCP: Endoscopic retrograde cholangio-pancreato-graphy; EUS-FNA: Endoscopic ultrasound-guided fine needle aspiration; IHC: immunohistochemistry; ROC curve: receiver operating characteristic curve; TMA: tissue microarrays; SROC: summary receiver operating characteristic.

Competing interests
The authors declare that they have no competing interests.

Authors' contributions

KAO, AA, FRD and VB participated in the conception and study design. AA, VB, SD carried out data collection. AA, VB and CN carried out immunostaining. AA, NBJ, JPM, JSG and KAO contributed in data analysis and interpretation. NBJ, JPM, OJS, CRC, CJM, FRD, JSG, AA, KAO were involved in manuscript preparation and provided their critical comments from surgical, pathological and scientific perspectives. All authors have read and approved the final manuscript.

Acknowledgements

We thank Clare Orange and Roderick Ferrier for their technical assistance.

Author details

[1]Wolfson Wohl Cancer Research Centre, Institute of Cancer Sciences, College of Medical Veterinary and Life Sciences, University of Glasgow, Garscube Estate, Switchback Road, Bearsden G61 1QH, UK. [2]Pathology Laboratory, Forth Valley Royal Hospital, Stirling Road, Larbert FK5 4WR, UK. [3]West of Scotland Pancreatic Unit and Glasgow Royal Infirmary, Alexandra Parade, Glasgow G31 2ER, UK. [4]Beatson Institute for Cancer Research, Glasgow G61 1BD, UK. [5]Medical Oncology, Beatson West of Scotland Cancer Centre, Glasgow G12 0YN, UK. [6]Department of Pathology, Southern General Hospital, Greater Glasgow & Clyde NHS, Glasgow G51 4TF, UK.

References

1. Cancer Research UK. London: *News and Resources [cited 2012April24]. Pancreatic cancer statistics- Key facts*. Available from: http://info. cancerresearchuk.org/cancerstats/keyfacts/pancreatic-cancer/.
2. Hidalgo M: **Pancreatic cancer.** *N Engl J Med* 2010, **362**(17):1605–1617.
3. Ferrone CR, Pieretti-Vanmarcke R, Bloom JP, Zheng H, Szymonifka J, Wargo JA, Thayer SP, Lauwers GY, Deshpande V, Mino-Kenudson M, Fernández-del Castillo C, Lillemoe KD, Warshaw AL: **Pancreatic ductal adenocarcinoma: long-term survival does not equal cure.** *Surgery* 2012, **152**(3 Suppl 1):S43–S49.
4. Richter A, Niedergethmann M, Sturm JW, Lorenz D, Post S, Trede M: **Long-term results of partial pancreaticoduodenectomy for ductal adenocarcinoma of the pancreatic head: 25-year experience.** *World J Surg* 2003, **27**(3):324–329.
5. Woo SM, Ryu JK, Lee SH, Yoo JW, Park JK, Kim YT, Jang JY, Kim SW, Kang GH, Yoon YB: **Recurrence and prognostic factors of ampullary carcinoma after radical resection: comparison with distal extrahepatic cholangiocarcinoma.** *Ann Surg Oncol* 2007, **14**(11):3195–3201.
6. Bond-Smith G, Banga N, Hammond TM, Imber CJ: **Pancreatic adenocarcinoma.** *Br Med J* 2012, **344**:e2476.
7. Dabizzi E, Assef MS, Raimondo M: **Diagnostic management of pancreatic cancer.** *Cancer* 2011, **3**(1):494–509.
8. Karmazanovsky G, Fedorov V, Kubyshkin V, Kotchatkov A: **Pancreatic head cancer: accuracy of CT in determination of resectability.** *Abdom Imaging* 2005, **30**(4):488–500.
9. Miura F, Takada T, Amano H, Yoshida M, Furui S, Takeshita K: **Diagnosis of pancreatic cancer.** *HPB* 2006, **8**(5):337–342.
10. Van Beers BE: **Diagnosis of cholangiocarcinoma.** *HPB* 2008, **10**(2):87–93.
11. Adler D, Max Schmidt C, Al-Haddad M, Barthel JS, Ljung BM, Merchant NB, Romagnuolo J, Shaaban AM, Simeone D, Bishop Pitman M, Field A, Layfield LJ: **Clinical evaluation, imaging studies, indications for cytologic study, and preprocedural requirements for duct brushing studies and pancreatic FNA: the Papanicolaou Society of Cytopathology recommendations for pancreatic and biliary cytology.** *Diagn Cytopathol* 2014, **42**(4):325–332.
12. Chang KJ: **State of the art lecture: endoscopic ultrasound (EUS) and FNA in pancreatico-biliary tumors.** *Endoscopy* 2006, **38**(Suppl 1):S56–S60.
13. Iqbal S, Friedel D, Gupta M, Ogden L, Stavropoulos SN: **Endoscopic-ultrasound-guided fine-needle aspiration and the role of the cytopathologist in solid pancreatic lesion diagnosis.** *Pathol Res Int* 2012, **2012**:317167.
14. Kudo T, Kawakami H, Kuwatani M, Eto K, Kawahata S, Abe Y, Onodera M, Ehira N, Yamato H, Haba S, Kawakubo K, Sakamoto N: **Influence of the safety and diagnostic accuracy of preoperative endoscopic ultrasound-guided fine-needle aspiration for resectable pancreatic cancer on clinical performance.** *World J Gastroenterol* 2014, **20**(13):3620–3627.
15. Raut CP, Grau AM, Staerkel GA, Kaw M, Tamm EP, Wolff RA, Vauthey JN, Lee JE, Pisters PW, Evans DB: **Diagnostic accuracy of endoscopic ultrasound-guided fine-needle aspiration in patients with presumed pancreatic cancer.** *J Gastrointest Surg* 2003, **7**(1):118–126. discussion 127–118.
16. Stewart CJ, Mills PR, Carter R, O'Donohue J, Fullarton G, Imrie CW, Murray WR: **Brush cytology in the assessment of pancreatico-biliary strictures: a review of 406 cases.** *J Clin Pathol* 2001, **54**(6):449–455.
17. Wakatsuki T, Irisawa A, Bhutani MS, Hikichi T, Shibukawa G, Takagi T, Yamamoto G, Takahashi Y, Yamada Y, Watanabe K, Obara K, Suzuki T, Sato Y: **Comparative study of diagnostic value of cytologic sampling by endoscopic ultrasonography-guided fine-needle aspiration and that by endoscopic retrograde pancreatography for the management of pancreatic mass without biliary stricture.** *J Gastroenterol Hepatol* 2005, **20**(11):1707–1711.
18. Yoshinaga S, Suzuki H, Oda I, Saito Y: **Role of endoscopic ultrasound-guided fine needle aspiration (EUS-FNA) for diagnosis of solid pancreatic masses.** *Dig Endosc* 2011, **23**(Suppl 1):29–33.
19. Harewood GC, Wiersema LM, Halling AC, Keeney GL, Salamao DR, Wiersema MJ: **Influence of EUS training and pathology interpretation on accuracy of EUS-guided fine needle aspiration of pancreatic masses.** *Gastrointest Endosc* 2002, **55**(6):669–673.
20. Agarwal B, Abu-Hamda E, Molke KL, Correa AM, Ho L: **Endoscopic ultrasound-guided fine needle aspiration and multidetector spiral CT in the diagnosis of pancreatic cancer.** *Am J Gastroenterol* 2004, **99**(5):844–850.
21. Eloubeidi MA, Chen VK, Eltoum IA, Jhala D, Chhieng DC, Jhala N, Vickers SM, Wilcox CM: **Endoscopic ultrasound-guided fine needle aspiration biopsy of patients with suspected pancreatic cancer: diagnostic accuracy and acute and 30-day complications.** *Am J Gastroenterol* 2003, **98**(12):2663–2668.
22. Horwhat JD, Paulson EK, McGrath K, Branch MS, Baillie J, Tyler D, Pappas T, Enns R, Robuck G, Stiffler H, Jowell P: **A randomized comparison of EUS-guided FNA versus CT or US-guided FNA for the evaluation of pancreatic mass lesions.** *Gastrointest Endosc* 2006, **63**(7):966–975.
23. Hwang CY, Lee SS, Song TJ, Moon SH, Lee D, Park do H, Seo DW, Lee SK, Kim MH: **Endoscopic ultrasound guided fine needle aspiration biopsy in diagnosis of pancreatic and peripancreatic lesions: a single center experience in Korea.** *Gut Liver* 2009, **3**(2):116–121.
24. Touchefeu Y, Le Rhun M, Coron E, Alamdari A, Heymann MF, Mosnier JF, Matysiak T, Galmiche JP: **Endoscopic ultrasound-guided fine-needle aspiration for the diagnosis of solid pancreatic masses: the impact on patient-management strategy.** *Aliment Pharmacol Ther* 2009, **30**(10):1070–1077.
25. Varadarajulu S, Tamhane A, Eloubeidi MA: **Yield of EUS-guided FNA of pancreatic masses in the presence or the absence of chronic pancreatitis.** *Gastrointest Endosc* 2005, **62**(5):728–736. quiz 751, 753.
26. Bellizzi AM, Stelow EB: **Pancreatic cytopathology: a practical approach and review.** *Arch Pathol Lab Med* 2009, **133**(3):388–404.
27. Logrono R, Kurtycz DF, Molina CP, Trivedi VA, Wong JY, Block KP: **Analysis of false-negative diagnoses on endoscopic brush cytology of biliary and pancreatic duct strictures: the experience at 2 university hospitals.** *Arch Pathol Lab Med* 2000, **124**(3):387–392.
28. Krishna NB, Mehra M, Reddy AV, Agarwal B: **EUS/EUS-FNA for suspected pancreatic cancer: influence of chronic pancreatitis and clinical presentation with or without obstructive jaundice on performance characteristics.** *Gastrointest Endosc* 2009, **70**(1):70–79.
29. Taylor CR: **Standardization in immunohistochemistry: the role of antigen retrieval in molecular morphology.** *Biotech Histochem* 2006, **81**(1):3–12.
30. Agarwal B, Ludwig OJ, Collins BT, Cortese C: **Immunostaining as an adjunct to cytology for diagnosis of pancreatic adenocarcinoma.** *Clin Gastroenterol Hepatol* 2008, **6**(12):1425–1431.
31. Chhieng DC, Benson E, Eltoum I, Eloubeidi MA, Jhala N, Jhala D, Siegal GP, Grizzle WE, Manne U: **MUC1 and MUC2 expression in pancreatic ductal carcinoma obtained by fine-needle aspiration.** *Cancer* 2003, **99**(6):365–371.
32. Deng H, Shi J, Wilkerson M, Meschter S, Dupree W, Lin F: **Usefulness of S100P in diagnosis of adenocarcinoma of pancreas on fine-needle aspiration biopsy specimens.** *Am J Clin Pathol* 2008, **129**(1):81–88.
33. Giorgadze TA, Peterman H, Baloch ZW, Furth EE, Pasha T, Shiina N, Zhang PJ, Gupta PK: **Diagnostic utility of mucin profile in fine-needle aspiration specimens of the pancreas: an immunohistochemical study with surgical pathology correlation.** *Cancer* 2006, **108**(3):186–197.
34. Jhala N, Jhala D, Vickers SM, Eltoum I, Batra SK, Manne U, Eloubeidi M, Jones JJ, Grizzle WE: **Biomarkers in Diagnosis of pancreatic carcinoma in fine-needle aspirates.** *Am J Clin Pathol* 2006, **126**(4):572–579.

35. Kosarac O, Takei H, Zhai QJ, Schwartz MR, Mody DR: **S100P and XIAP expression in pancreatic ductal adenocarcinoma: potential novel biomarkers as a diagnostic adjunct to fine needle aspiration cytology.** *Acta Cytol* 2011, **55**(2):142–148.

36. Ligato S, Zhao H, Mandich D, Cartun RW: **KOC (K homology domain containing protein overexpressed in cancer) and S100A4-protein immunoreactivity improves the diagnostic sensitivity of biliary brushing cytology for diagnosing pancreaticobiliary malignancies.** *Diagn Cytopathol* 2008, **36**(8):561–567.

37. Toll AD, Witkiewicz AK, Bibbo M: **Expression of K homology domain containing protein (KOC) in pancreatic cytology with corresponding histology.** *Acta Cytol* 2009, **53**(2):123–129.

38. Ali A, Ul-Haq Z, Mohamed M, MacKay DF, Duthie F, Oien K: **Abstract 1142: systematic review and meta-analysis of immunohistochemical diagnostic markers for pancreatic ductal adenocarcinoma.** *Cancer Res* 2013, **73**(8 Supplement):1142.

39. Argani P, Shaukat A, Kaushal M, Wilentz RE, Su GH, Sohn TA, Yeo CJ, Cameron JL, Kern SE, Hruban RH: **Differing rates of loss of DPC4 expression and of p53 overexpression among carcinomas of the proximal and distal bile ducts.** *Cancer* 2001, **91**(7):1332–1341.

40. Chu PG, Schwarz RE, Lau SK, Yen Y, Weiss LM: **Immunohistochemical staining in the diagnosis of pancreatobiliary and ampulla of Vater adenocarcinoma: application of CDX2, CK17, MUC1, and MUC2.** *Am J Surg Pathol* 2005, **29**(3):359–367.

41. Hassan R, Laszik ZG, Lerner M, Raffeld M, Postier R, Brackett D: **Mesothelin is overexpressed in pancreaticobiliary adenocarcinomas but not in normal pancreas and chronic pancreatitis.** *Am J Clin Pathol* 2005, **124**(6):838–845.

42. Swierczynski SL, Maitra A, Abraham SC, Iacobuzio-Donahue CA, Ashfaq R, Cameron JL, Schulick RD, Yeo CJ, Rahman A, Hinkle DA, Hruban RH, Argani P: **Analysis of novel tumor markers in pancreatic and biliary carcinomas using tissue microarrays.** *Hum Pathol* 2004, **35**(3):357–366.

43. Denley SM, Jamieson NB, McCall P, Oien KA, Morton JP, Carter CR, Edwards J, McKay CJ: **Activation of the IL-6R/Jak/stat pathway is associated with a poor outcome in resected pancreatic ductal adenocarcinoma.** *J Gastrointest Surg* 2013, **17**(5):887–898.

44. Yantiss RK, Cosar E, Fischer AH: **Use of IMP3 in identification of carcinoma in fine needle aspiration biopsies of pancreas.** *Acta Cytol* 2008, **52**(2):133–138.

45. Lim YJ, Lee JK, Jang WY, Song SY, Lee KT, Paik SW, Rhee JC: **Prognostic significance of maspin in pancreatic ductal adenocarcinoma.** *Kor J Intern Med* 2004, **19**(1):15–18.

46. Maass N, Hojo T, Ueding M, Luttges J, Kloppel G, Jonat W, Nagasaki K: **Expression of the tumor suppressor gene Maspin in human pancreatic cancers.** *Clin Cancer Res* 2001, **7**(4):812–817.

47. Yantiss RK, Woda BA, Fanger GR, Kalos M, Whalen GF, Tada H, Andersen DK, Rock KL, Dresser K: **KOC (K homology domain containing protein overexpressed in cancer): a novel molecular marker that distinguishes between benign and malignant lesions of the pancreas.** *Am J Surg Pathol* 2005, **29**(2):188–195.

48. Lin F, Shi J, Liu H, Hull ME, Dupree W, Prichard JW, Brown RE, Zhang J, Wang HL, Schuerch C: **Diagnostic utility of S100P and von Hippel-Lindau gene product (pVHL) in pancreatic adenocarcinoma - With implication of their roles in early tumorigenesis.** *Am J Surg Pathol* 2008, **32**(1):78–91.

49. Argani P, Iacobuzio-Donahue C, Ryu B, Rosty C, Goggins M, Wilentz RE, Murugesan SR, Leach SD, Jaffee E, Yeo CJ, Cameron JL, Kern SE, Hruban RH: **Mesothelin is overexpressed in the vast majority of ductal adenocarcinomas of the pancreas: Identification of a new pancreatic cancer marker by serial analysis of gene expression (SAGE).** *Clin Cancer Res* 2001, **7**(12):3862–3868.

50. McCarthy DM, Maitra A, Argani P, Rader AE, Faigel DO, Van Heek NT, Hruban RH, Wilentz RE: **Novel markers of pancreatic adenocarcinoma in fine-needle aspiration: mesothelin and prostate stem cell antigen labeling increases accuracy in cytologically borderline cases.** *Appl Immunohistochem Mol Morphol* 2003, **11**(3):238–243.

51. Wang Y, Gao J, Li Z, Jin Z, Gong Y, Man X: **Diagnostic value of mucins (MUC1, MUC2 and MUC5AC) expression profile in endoscopic ultrasound-guided fine-needle aspiration specimens of the pancreas.** *Int J Cancer* 2007, **121**(12):2716–2722.

52. Awadallah NS, Shroyer KR, Langer DA, Torkko KC, Chen YK, Bentz JS, Papkoff J, Liu W, Nash SR, Shah RJ: **Detection of B7-H4 and p53 in pancreatic cancer: potential role as a cytological diagnostic adjunct.** *Pancreas* 2008, **36**(2):200–206.

53. Boltze C, Schneider-Stock R, Aust G, Mawrin C, Dralle H, Roessner A, Hoang-Vu C: **CD97, CD95 and Fas-L clearly discriminate between chronic pancreatitis and pancreatic ductal adenocarcinoma in perioperative evaluation of cryocut sections.** *Pathol Int* 2002, **52**(2):83–88.

54. Cao D, Zhang Q, Wu LSF, Salaria SN, Winter JW, Hruban RH, Goggins MS, Abbruzzese JL, Maitra A, Ho L: **Prognostic significance of maspin in pancreatic ductal adenocarcinoma: tissue microarray analysis of 223 surgically resected cases.** *Mod Pathol* 2007, **20**(5):570–578.

55. Baruch AC, Wang H, Staerkel GA, Evans DB, Hwang RF, Krishnamurthy S: **Immunocytochemical study of the expression of mesothelin in fine-needle aspiration biopsy specimens of pancreatic adenocarcinoma.** *Diagn Cytopathol* 2007, **35**(3):143–147.

56. Swartz MJ, Batra SK, Varshney GC, Hollingsworth MA, Yeo CJ, Cameron JL, Wilentz RE, Hruban RH, Argani P: **MUC4 expression increases progressively in pancreatic intraepithelial neoplasia.** *Am J Clin Pathol* 2002, **117**(5):791–796.

57. Zhao H, Mandich D, Cartun RW, Ligato S: **Expression of K homology domain containing protein overexpressed in cancer in pancreatic FNA for diagnosing adenocarcinoma of pancreas.** *Diagn Cytopathol* 2007, **35**(11):700–704.

58. Argani P, Rosty C, Reiter RE, Wilentz RE, Murugesan SR, Leach SD, Ryu B, Skinner HG, Goggins M, Jaffee EM, Yeo CJ, Cameron JL, Kern SE, Hruban RH: **Discovery of new markers of cancer through serial analysis of gene expression: prostate stem cell antigen is overexpressed in pancreatic adenocarcinoma.** *Cancer Res* 2001, **61**(11):4320–4324.

59. Bhardwaj A, Marsh WL Jr, Nash JW, Barbacioru CC, Jones S, Frankel WL: **Double immunohistochemical staining with MUC4/p53 is useful in the distinction of pancreatic adenocarcinoma from chronic pancreatitis: a tissue microarray-based study.** *Arch Pathol Lab Med* 2007, **131**(4):556–562.

60. Ordonez NG: **Application of mesothelin immunostaining in tumor diagnosis.** *Am J Surg Pathol* 2003, **27**(11):1418–1428.

2

Comparing gene expression data from formalin-fixed, paraffin embedded tissues and qPCR with that from snap-frozen tissue and microarrays for modeling outcomes of patients with ovarian carcinoma

William H. Bradley[1*], Kevin Eng[2,4], Min Le[3], A. Craig Mackinnon[3], Christina Kendziorski[2] and Janet S. Rader[1]

Abstract

Background: Previously, we have used clinical and gene expression data from The Cancer Genome Atlas (TCGA) to model a pathway-based index predicting outcomes in ovarian carcinoma. This data were obtained from snap-frozen tissue measured with the Affymetrix U133 platform. In the current study, we correlate the data used to model with data derived from TaqMan qPCR both snap frozen and paraffin embedded (FFPE) samples.

Methods: To compare the effect of preservation methods on gene expression measured by qPCR, we assessed 18 patient and tumor sample matched snap-frozen and FFPE ovarian carcinoma samples. To compare gene measurement technologies, we correlated qPCR data from 10 patients with tumor sample matched snap-frozen ovarian carcinoma samples with the microarray data from TCGA. We normalized results to the average expression of three housekeeping genes. We scaled and centered the data for comparison to the Affymetrix output.

Results: For the 18 specimens, gene expression data obtained from snap-frozen tissue correlated highly with that from FFPE samples in our TaqMan assay (r > 0.82). For the 10 duplicate TCGA specimens, the reported microarray data correlated well (r = 0.6) with our qPCR data, and ranges of expression along pathways were similar.

Conclusions: Gene expression data obtained by qPCR from FFPE serous ovarian carcinoma samples can be used to assess in the pathway-based predictive model. The normalization procedures described control variations in expression, and the range calculated along a specific pathway can be interpreted for a patient's risk profile.

Background

Using gene expression and clinical data from The Cancer Genome Atlas (TCGA), we previously developed a model that predicts variations in response of high-grade serous ovarian cancer to cytotoxic chemotherapies. In that publication [1], we described a method for reducing the list of genes needed to predict clinical outcomes to fewer than 100. We selected those genes from more than 10,000 possibilities by identifying genes within a core group of 12 cancer pathways [2, 3] whose variation in expression had the greatest effect on disease progression. Predictions of response to specific chemotherapeutic agents were suggested by the cumulative levels of gene expression among the 91 genes selected from the 12 pathways. Three of the pathways did not have genes identified, leaving 9 core pathways informative. We defined the predictions made by gene expression within these pathways as the Patient-Specific Risk Profile (PSRP).

Gene expression levels reported by Affymetrix microarrays and qPCR may differ significantly, creating potential difficulties for models developed on one platform and utilized in the other [4]. For example, measurements of reference RNAs from commercial sets of ~1000 genes

* Correspondence: wbradley@mcw.edu
[1]Department of Obstetrics and Gynecology, Medical College of Wisconsin, 8701 Watertown Plank Road, Milwaukee, WI 53226, USA
Full list of author information is available at the end of the article

from human brain, liver, and lung showed correlations (r) ranging from 0.45 to 0.75 when TaqMan measurements were compared with Applied Biosystems and Agilent microarray technologies [5]. The MicroArray Quality Control (MAQC) project showed correlations of r = ≥0.9 between Affymetrix and TaqMan data [6], but those measurements and correlations were made with reference RNA from a large gene set, undirected by model building or clinical practice. Moreover, the technology used to measure expression may have a greater or lesser influence on output, depending on how the genes of interest are selected. A predictive model that features only highly differentially expressed genes may more easily translate from microarray to qPCR than a model not based on large changes in expression [7]. A requirement of highly differentiated genes may not represent the biology of the disease, and the modeling we have done includes lower expressed genes in the set.

TCGA derives gene expression by placing RNA from snap-frozen tissue on an Affymetrix U133 Array platform [8]. To migrate to a more clinically functional platform, we evaluated the reliability of gene expression inputs derived by using qPCR to analyze formalin-fixed, paraffin-embedded tumor samples. Because FFPE blocks are readily available from primary debulking surgery, whereas snap-frozen tissue is not, this modified approach increases the number of patients who can potentially benefit from this profiling technique.

Two factors could significantly affect the clinical utility of our profiles when FFPE tissue samples are used: (i) differences in tissue preservation techniques altering the RNA quality and expression detection between snap-frozen and FFPE and (ii) gene expression levels differing due to alterations in technology between Affymetrix Microarray and TaqMan qPCR. Although either or both changes could have a major effect on predictive capability, the effect might be modified depending on the number of genes measured or the ways the data are analyzed for prediction. For example, the impact of variance in expression measurements could be ameliorated by aggregating multiple data points when using multiple genes for prediction [9].

In this study, we compared gene expression measurements for individual genes selected by our PSRP 91 gene assay (gene by gene) and for those same genes aggregated into the pathways of our model (pathway by pathway). We derived correlations between snap-frozen and FFPE tissue preparations and between Affymetrix U133 Microarrays and TaqMan qPCR. In addition, we used techniques for normalizing qPCR gene expression that allows us to directly compare qPCR assays with the TCGA microarray data. The result is that our PSRP 91 model developed from snap-frozen tissue on an Affymetrix platform can be tested using a qPCR outputs and FFPE specimens.

Methods
Study subjects
To compare tissue preservation methods, we measured gene expression from 18 patients who had both snap-frozen ovarian carcinoma samples in the Medical College of Wisconsin (MCW) gynecologic tissue bank and a case-matched FFPE sample archived by the Department of Pathology. All samples were taken during debulking surgery of patients diagnosed with Stage IIIC or IV, grade 3 serous ovarian carcinoma. Tissue samples were taken to pathology immediately after extirpation. Once assessed by a pathologist, the portion acquired for tissue banking was excised, and snap frozen in the pathology lab. The remainder was fixed in formalin and processed per standard pathology protocol. Prior to analysis, the tissues had been stored as FFPE blocks or snap frozen sections for up to 3 years. The pathology for each MCW patient was reviewed with hematoxylin and eosin (H&E) to confirm both the diagnosis and a tumor content of at least 75 % [8]. Approval from the Institutional Review Board (IRB) of the Human Research Protection Office and Medical College of Wisconsin was obtained, and all patients signed an informed consent for tissue banking.

To compare two methods of assaying gene expression, we used TCGA identification numbers to identify 10 snap-frozen tumor samples submitted to the TCGA from the tissue bank at Washington University in St. Louis. Approval from the institutional Human Research Protection Office was obtained. For each patient's sample, TCGA had reported gene expression and annotated pathology. All of these samples were from patients with Stage IIIC, grade 3 serous ovarian carcinoma, and microarray analysis had been performed by TCGA. A qPCR expression level of the 91 genes was measured in the 10 snap frozen samples.

Gene list
The genes whose expression we assayed were selected from a gene set constituting the 9 core pathways described previously [1]. 91 genes were chosen from our previously published PSRP results. Analysis was performed according to the 9 core pathways as well as a revised six-gene set representing the neurotrophin pathway, making a total of 10 pathways available for analysis (Additional file 1: Table S1). The subsets of genes used to define a pathway's expression are listed in the Supplement as well (Additional file 1: Table S2). We used the housekeeping genes glyceraldehyde 3-phosphate dehydrogenase (GAPDH), hypoxanthine phosphoribosyltransferase 1 (HPRT1), and beta-D-glucuronidase (GUSB) to normalize gene expression.

RNA isolation, cDNA, and qPCR
RNA from the snap-frozen tissue samples was extracted using an RNAqueous Kit from Life Technologies

(Carlsbad, CA, USA). RNA from FFPE blocks was extracted using a RecoverAll™ Total Nucleic Acid Isolation Kit, also from Life Technologies. All RNAs were treated with Ambion TURBO DNase. RNA concentrations were determined with a Qubit™ RNA Assay Kit (Carlsbad, CA, USA), and integrity was checked on an Experion Automated Electrophoresis Station (Hercules, CA, USA).

All reagents used in cDNA synthesis and qPCR were obtained from Applied Biosystems (Carlsbad, CA, USA). RNA concentration was adjusted to 40 ng/μl for the reverse transcription reaction. cDNA synthesis was carried out with a High-Capacity cDNA Reverse Transcription Kit. About 200 ng of RNA was used in a final 10-μl RT reaction. The TaqMan® Array Plates 96 Plus were custom-made to include TaqMan Gene Expression Assays of 91 target genes and the three endogenous control genes. Best Coverage probes from Applied Biosystems were used to target the genes of interest. The assays of 91 target genes and 3 housekeeping genes were pooled at 0.2X concentration for the PreAmp reaction. cDNAs (2 μl) were preamplified in a 20-μl reaction for 10 cycles, using TaqMan PreAmp Master Mix and pooled assays. The reaction products were diluted 5-fold with 1X TE and mixed with 500 μl of TaqMan Fast Advanced Master Mix. Water was added to give a final mixture volume of 1 ml. A 10 μl aliquot of the assay mixture was added to each well of the TaqMan Gene Expression Assay Plate, and amplification was carried out on a 7500 Fast Real Time PCR System. Genes that were not detected within 34 cycles (Ct > 34) were considered unexpressed for the purpose of our evaluation.

Normalization of affymetrix and TaqMan data

TCGA derives gene expression by extracting RNA from snap-frozen tissue and aggregating data from three different array platforms (Affymetrix U133a 2.0, Digital Gene Expression from Illumina, and a custom high-density Agilent array). We evaluated the Affymetrix results only as these were the most complete reported and had fully accessible probe information.

To compare gene expression across the two technologies (Affymetrix Microarray and TaqMan qPCR) we used the following normalization techniques for data output. For the Affymetrix data, we took the Robust Multi-array Average (RMA; Affymetrix) for each gene, and then normalized to the average of the endogenous housekeeping genes GAPDH, HPRT1 and GUSB.

For TaqMan qPCR, we used two techniques to normalize gene measurements. First, we used the average of the cycles from the same three housekeeping genes as the control within the array. We then subtracted the number of cycles of a target gene from the average of the housekeeping genes. Reported Ct values of

34 or greater were considered to be unidentified or unexpressed genes. This method is demonstrated in Fig. 1 was used to correlate gene expression levels for each of the 91 genes measured by the two different technologies – Affymetrix and TaqMan.

TaqMan qPCR-based expression levels passed through a quality control step and were normalized using housekeeping genes. Reported Ct values of 34 or greater were considered to be unexpressed and therefore were not considered in the analysis of a given pathway on a subject-by-subject basis. The average of the housekeeping genes GAPDH, HPRT1 and GUSB served as an endogenous control for the assay. Noting that large Ct values imply less gene sample expression, we subtracted each probe's ΔCt value from the control to obtain a Ct score that rises with expression consistent with the array-based expression measurement.

Calibration and PSRP 91 gene computation

Each TaqMan qPCR assay is normalized so it requires no control outside of its own assay. However there are technology-specific differences between the Affymetrix and TaqMan probes. We accounted for this in a calibration step: In deriving the array-based measurements we relied on mean zero, standard deviation one (scaled and centered) values for constructing the risk indexes that comprise the Patient-Specific Risk Profile (PSRP)[1]. We also normalized the TaqMan qPCR expression values by scaling and centering using the observed probe average and standard deviation (Additional file 1: Table S3). Thus a new sample can be normalized and calibrated and the PSRP 91 gene indexes can be computed.

Statistical methods

For each sample, we used Pearson and Spearman's rank correlation to compare measurements. The curves for each patient's 91 gene expression measurements are provided in Fig. 1. We used a locally weighted scatterplot smoothing (LOWESS) to obtain a summary of the relationship between gene expression derived by one technology and that derived by the other.

Results
RNA quality metrics and dropped genes

The quality of the RNA derived from the snap-frozen tissues was uniformly high with a RNA quality indicator (RQI) of >7 for 20 of the 28 specimens. The remaining 8 specimens were all 6.2 or greater, except a single outlier with a RQI of 2.9. The FFPE samples had predictably low RQI levels ranging from 1.9 to 3.1. The range of storage time of the tissue samples did not correla te with RQI for the FFPE samples. TaqMan probes for *WNT16*, *WNT3*, and *DNTT* had ΔCt of >34 and were considered unexpressed in most assays (84 %

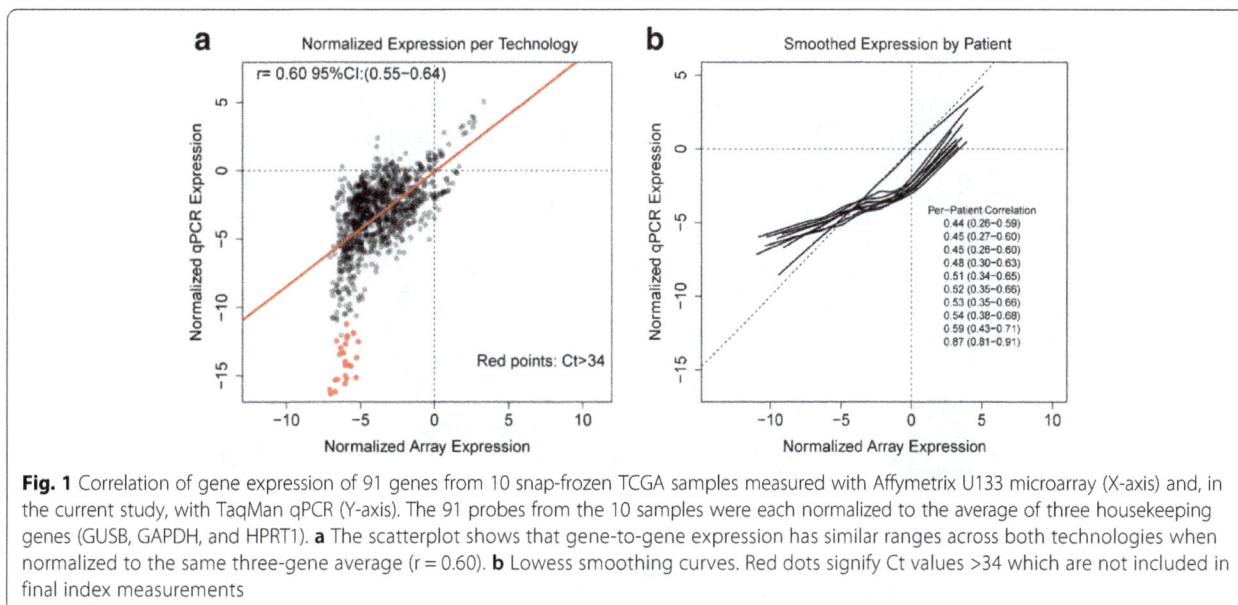

Fig. 1 Correlation of gene expression of 91 genes from 10 snap-frozen TCGA samples measured with Affymetrix U133 microarray (X-axis) and, in the current study, with TaqMan qPCR (Y-axis). The 91 probes from the 10 samples were each normalized to the average of three housekeeping genes (GUSB, GAPDH, and HPRT1). **a** The scatterplot shows that gene-to-gene expression has similar ranges across both technologies when normalized to the same three-gene average (r = 0.60). **b** Lowess smoothing curves. Red dots signify Ct values >34 which are not included in final index measurements

unexpressed, 94 % unexpressed, and 100 % unexpressed respectively); *PLA2G2D* and *CACNG1* were not expressed in 37 % and 46 % of assays respectively, and 15 other probes were not expressed at least once in 68 total TaqMan assays (Additional file 1: Table S4). These findings are consistent with the data showing that these were among the lowest expressing genes in TCGA samples. Samples with low RQI levels still exhibited reportable gene expression levels. Probes considered unexpressed (Ct >34) were removed from samples on a per-assay basis and were not included in the denominator for the index calculation.

Gene-to-gene comparison of expression levels measured by Affymetrix microarrays and TaqMan qPCR

From TCGA, we obtained gene expression levels in snap-frozen ovarian cancer samples from patients treated at Washington University (St. Louis, MO). To evaluate the concordance of expression measured by array-based probes and qPCR-based probes we acquired ovarian carcinoma samples extracted from the same patient and case, using TCGA numbers for identification. When the microarray and qPCR outputs were plotted against each other and matched gene for gene across the patients, the overall correlation was r = 0.60 (Fig. 1). The plotted slope confirms that the two techniques gave equivalent expression levels and that higher expression of a target gene resulted in a higher number (arbitrary value) on the y-axis. Taking the 10 specimens individually and performing a per-patient smooth estimate of the output (Fig. 1) showed a consistent correlation across the various genes measured. Using housekeeping genes to normalize expression of both technologies also demonstrated that the expression levels of the 91 genes of interest were similar across the two measurement platforms.

Validating TaqMan assay profiles between matched paraffin-embedded and snap frozen samples

To gauge whether our PSRP 91 gene TaqMan qPCR assay provides equivalent expression measurements from both snap-frozen and paraffin-embedded samples, we measured gene expression in the tumor-matched samples of the 18 patients at the Medical College of Wisconsin who had tumor tissue preserved by both snap- freezing and the standard FFPE. The expression outputs were correlated for each gene between the two preservation techniques for each patient. Intra-patient gene expression was higher than any inter-patient gene expression (Fig. 2). Eight of the patients are highlighted in Fig. 2, and the degree of correlation across genes is noted. The correlation between preservation techniques was excellent: > = 0.82 per pair of matched samples. The range of correlation among the 18 sample sets was from 0.82 to 0.96 when comparing snap frozen to FFPE samples. A qPCR was repeated on a second cut from the snap frozen specimens, and the correlation ranged from 0.84 to 0.97 for the 18 samples demonstrating a high level of reproducibility.

Distribution of pathway expression from 18 FFPE samples measured with qPCR and mapped to the TCGA cohort

Plotting the distribution of Affymetrix pathway expression for patients from the TCGA gave a normal curve. Samples measured by qPCR (noted with red ticks in Fig. 3) centered under these normal curves. Figure 3 shows the TCGA-generated expression distribution for each pathway. The distribution of each of the 18 samples we measured by qPCR falls within the normal curves, and does not appear biased when we observe their position under the Affymetrix-generated

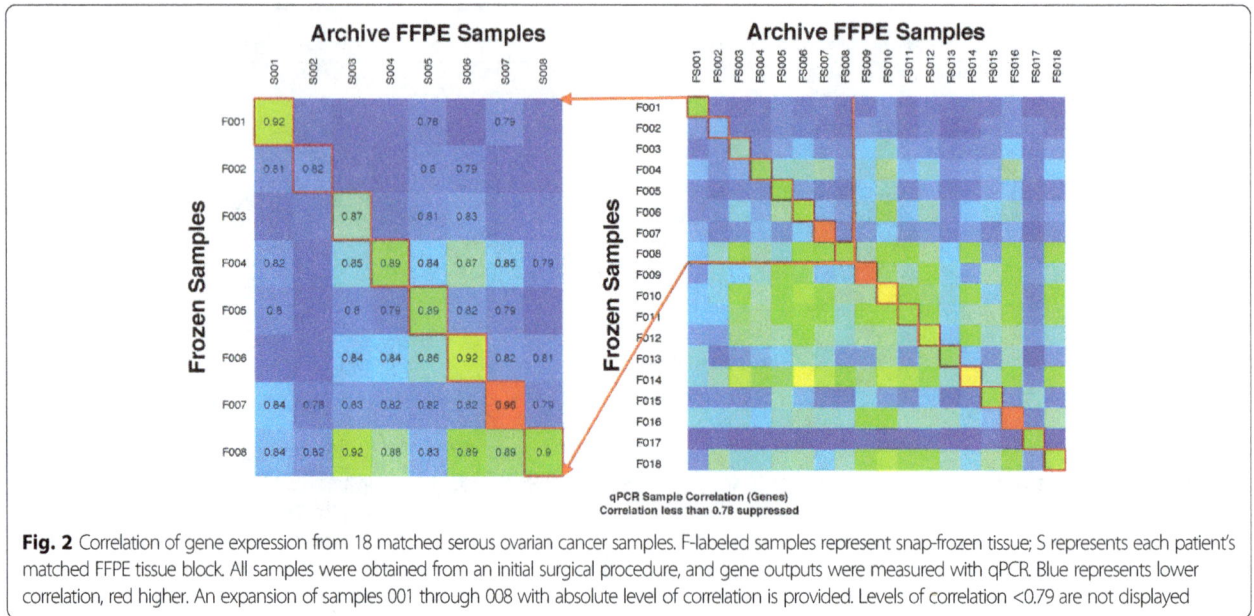

Fig. 2 Correlation of gene expression from 18 matched serous ovarian cancer samples. F-labeled samples represent snap-frozen tissue; S represents each patient's matched FFPE tissue block. All samples were obtained from an initial surgical procedure, and gene outputs were measured with qPCR. Blue represents lower correlation, red higher. An expansion of samples 001 through 008 with absolute level of correlation is provided. Levels of correlation <0.79 are not displayed

curves for each of the 10 pathways. The PSRP 91 gene assay utilizes gene expression aggregated within a pathway to stratify outcomes. Distribution of these aggregations is not biased by changes in technology or preservation.

Discussion

This manuscript demonstrates the feasibility of comparing measurements of gene expression used to model clinical outcomes in ovarian cancers from alternative technology and tissue preservation. We demonstrated

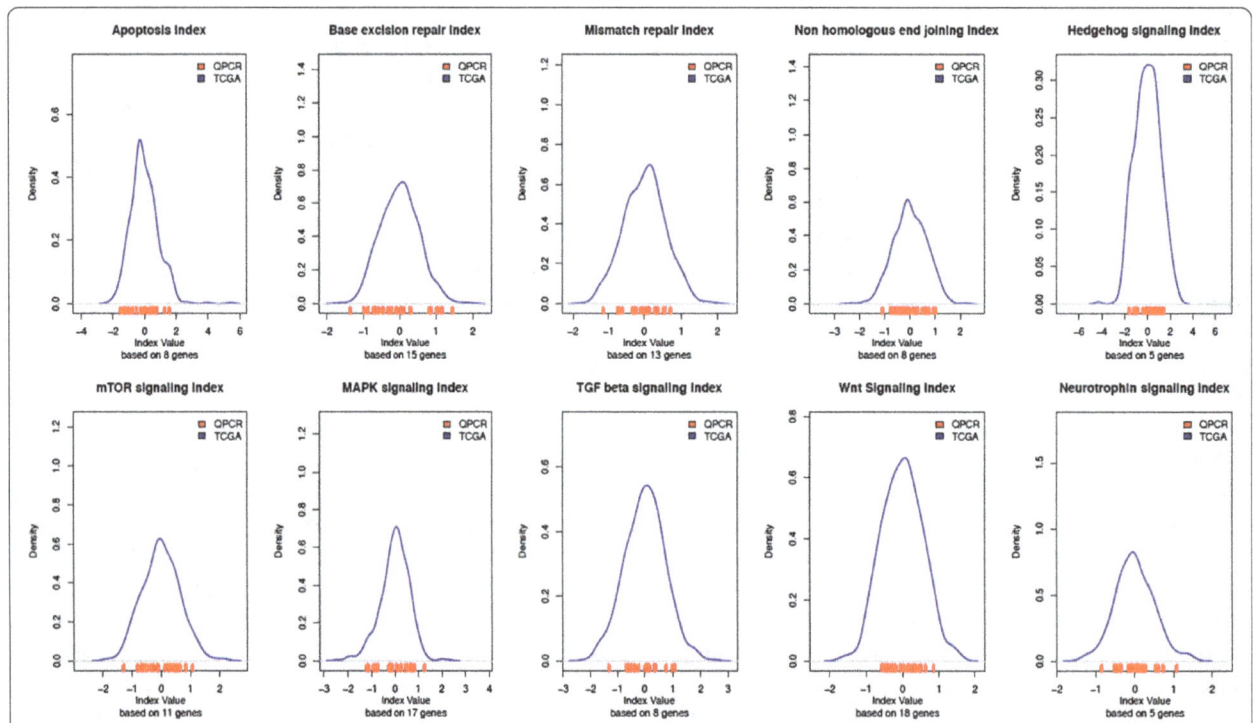

Fig. 3 Range of gene expression measured from the selected pathways. The bell curve represents the distribution of expression across the entire TCGA cohort, using Affymetrix array. The red ticks on the x-axis represent gene expression levels aggregated within a pathway from the 18 patients whose FFPE samples were measured using qPCR. The range of expression can be normalized across the Affymetrix and TaqMan qPCR platforms. Patient samples measured with qPCR have a range of expression that does not appear biased within the normal curve

that qPCR outputs of high-grade serous ovarian carcinoma specimens were nearly identical whether tissue was preserved by snap freezing or fixed with formalin and embedded in a paraffin block. This work was driven by the discovery of a gene panel that is predictive of ovarian cancer patient survival and response to therapy. The correlations described here will enable us to better test our modeling in archived FFPE tissue samples.

A similar correlation between fresh-freezing and FFPE has been observed with breast cancer samples, but a cDNA-mediated annealing, selection, extension, and ligation (DASL) platform was used for gene measurement [10]. That correlation was observed across an unselected whole genome assay when the data was median centered, a technique similar to ours. Interestingly, these authors noted a high level of concordance between tissue types when they applied a selected predictive model that used 291 genes. When ovarian tissue gene expression in 240 FFPE samples was measured using DASL, the correlation was 0.618 to gene signatures described by Tothill and a TCGA working group [9], a high enough level to allow for preservation of the predictive value of the gene sets. Our predictive technique relies less on direct gene-to-gene comparison, as a group of genes is evaluated within a pathway. However, we observed a similar gene-to-gene correlation for our selected set ($r = 0.60$). A second qPCR run of the snap frozen samples against the FFPE demonstrated that the measurements were stable.

Large variations in expression have been noted to provide confidence in cross-technological measurements. Fedorowicz found correlation between fresh- frozen and FFPE ovarian cancer samples, but that study was confined to the top 100 differentially expressed genes [7]. In contrast, our PSRP 91 gene TaqMan assay did not require genes to have high levels of differential. Although we observed lower expression genes drop out occasionally (e.g., 16 % of the WNT16 assays), this did not seem to offer significant changes at the level of pathway expression. The degree this drop out effects the overall prediction capacity of the model needs further clarification.

We used a combination of two techniques to normalize gene expression across the two technological platforms. First, we averaged housekeeping genes and simply subtracted the result from the target gene in both technologies. Second, we used the scale and center technique that is commonly used in Affymetrix analyses. To ensure the expression levels of the TaqMan data were on the same scale as those from the TCGA Affymetrix data, TaqMan qPCR outputs were centered and scaled. After that normalization they showed comparable ranges of expression.

Variations in expression levels reported from this study are within previously described tolerances [11–14], and the range of differences over an entire pathways appears to have a potentially small or negligible effect on predictive power. Thus, our method for applying the Patient-Specific Risk Profile that was derived with snap-frozen tissue and large-scale Affymetrix microarrays can be effectively applied to a limited gene set measured by qPCR, using RNA extracted from FFPE tissues. Our PSRP 91 gene assay uses measurements aggregated within a cellular pathway, with unbiased selection techniques. This allows poorly expressed genes to be weighted as much as highly expressed genes in the predictive model.

Our work was limited by the small sample size of the snap-frozen tissues we obtained to compare to outputs provided by TCGA. Moreover, we did not measure gene expression in samples preserved for more than 3 years when we compared the FFPE blocks to the snap-frozen samples. The inability to detect expression changes as FFPE blocks age has been a concern in prior reports, but improved techniques and choices in housekeeping genes appear to have reduced its potential impact [15]. Variations in pathologic processing and the ischemia in the tissue sample may be a source of noise in the FFPE gene measurements. Thus far, our assessment of RQI showed lower quality for these specimens, which is expected. This did not seem to effect the quality of measurement for a plurality of the genes assayed. Fixation for snap frozen and FFPE samples occurred simultaneously after surgical removal. Another concern is intra-tumor heterogeneity in duplicate patient samples. Variation in a single patient's tumor profiling has been identified by groups measuring expression arrays from multiple tumor sites. Our comparisons were from the same tumor excised at the same time, but variation in location may affect the correlation of the two tumor sites [16]. The loss of detection of some lower expressing genes in the qPCR (e.g., WNT16) is a concern for future modeling. Alternative technologies may need to be considered depending on the weighted importance of specific genes.

In summary, this study validated the use of FFPE tissue and qPCR—instead of snap-frozen tissue and microarrays—to obtain gene expression data for core cellular pathways. This supports the use these tissue samples when predictive modeling of ovarian cancer was done in larger data sets such as the TCGA. The variation in expression noted between our different samples does not appear to significantly distort expected outputs, leading us to believe that a model derived from expression reported using one approach could be used with a more convenient and "real world" approach when evaluating clinical samples. Our assay will be tested in a recurrent disease setting to more definitively evaluate predictive capacity prospectively.

Conclusion

This study offers evidence that a predictor model based on a large data set generated from Affymetrix microarray and snap frozen ovarian carcinoma samples can be applied to paraffin embedded clinical samples from a local pathology lab. Our predictive model used a "pathway" approach, and we observed that these local samples had pathway measurements across 10 separate pathways that fell within expected ranges. Normalization with scaling and centering was used for this in the qPCR data generated.

Abbreviations

TCGA: The Cancer Genome Atlas; qPCR: Quantitative real-time reverse transcription polymerase chain reaction; FFPE: Formalin fixed, paraffin embedded; PSRP: Patient specific risk profile; MAQC: Microarray quality control; GAPDH: Glyceraldehyde 3-phosphate dehydrogenase; HPRT1: Hypoxanthine phosphoribosyltransferase 1; GUSB: beta-D-glucuronidase; LOWESS: Locally weighted scatterplot smoothing; DASL: cDNA-mediated Annealing, Selection, extension, and Ligation.

Competing interests

The authors declare that we have no competing interests

Authors' contributions

WB conceived the study, collected the tissue samples, and drafted the manuscript. KE ran statistical correlations. ML ran tissue microarrays and quality control. AM evaluated tumor density and quality of tissue samples, supervised tissue control, and microarrays. CK reviewed the statistical correlations. JR helped conceive the study and draft the manuscript. All authors read and approved the final manuscript.

Authors' information

Not applicable.

Acknowledgements

David G. Mutch, MD generously provided tissue samples from Washington University. The results published here are in part based upon data generated by the TCGA research network: http://cancergenome.nih.gov/.

Funding

Support and funding was received by the Froedtert Foundation, the Women's Health Research Program, Falk Medical Trust, The Heitz Foundation, and National Center for Research Resources and the National Center for Advancing Translational Sciences, National Institutes of Health, through Grant Numbers 8UL1TR000055 and GM102756. Its contents are solely the responsibility of the authors and do not necessarily represent the official views of the NIH.

Author details

[1]Department of Obstetrics and Gynecology, Medical College of Wisconsin, 8701 Watertown Plank Road, Milwaukee, WI 53226, USA. [2]Department of Biostatistics and Medical Informatics, University of Wisconsin-Madison, Madison, WI 53792, USA. [3]Department of Pathology, Medical College of Wisconsin, Milwaukee, WI 53226, USA. [4]Current Address: Department of Biostatistics and Bioinformatics, Roswell Park Cancer Institute, Buffalo, NY, USA.

References

1. Eng KH, Wang S, Bradley WH, Rader JS, Kendziorski C. Pathway index models for construction of patient-specific risk profiles. Stat Med. 2013; 32(9):1524-1535
2. Jones D. Pathways to cancer therapy. Nat Rev Drug Discov. 2008;7:875–6.
3. Jones S, Zhang X, Parsons DW, Lin JC, Leary RJ, Angenendt P, et al. Core signaling pathways in human pancreatic cancers revealed by global genomic analyses. Science. 2008;321:1801–6.
4. Irizarry RA, Warren D, Spencer F, Kim IF, Biswal S, Frank BC, et al. Multiple-laboratory comparison of microarray platforms. Nat Methods. 2005;2:345–50.
5. Wang Y, Barbacioru C, Hyland F, Xiao W, Hunkapiller KL, Blake J, et al. Large scale real-time PCR validation on gene expression measurements from two commercial long-oligonucleotide microarrays. BMC Genomics. 2006;7:59.
6. Consortium M, Shi L, Reid LH, Jones WD, Shippy R, Warrington JA, et al. The MicroArray Quality Control (MAQC) project shows inter- and intraplatform reproducibility of gene expression measurements. Nat Biotechnol. 2006;24:1151–61.
7. Fedorowicz G, Guerrero S, Wu TD, Modrusan Z. Microarray analysis of RNA extracted from formalin-fixed, paraffin-embedded and matched fresh-frozen ovarian adenocarcinomas. BMC Med Genomics. 2009;2:23.
8. Cancer Genome Atlas Research Network. Integrated genomic analyses of ovarian carcinoma. Nature. 2011;474: 609–15.
9. Sfakianos GP, Iversen ES, Whitaker R, Akushevich L, Schildkraut JM, Murphy SK, et al. Validation of ovarian cancer gene expression signatures for survival and subtype in formalin fixed paraffin embedded tissues. Gynecol Oncol. 2013;129:159–64.
10. Mittempergher L, de Ronde JJ, Nieuwland M, Kerkhoven RM, Simon I, Rutgers EJ, et al. Gene expression profiles from formalin fixed paraffin embedded breast cancer tissue are largely comparable to fresh frozen matched tissue. PLoS One. 2011;6:e17163.
11. Farragher SM, Tanney A, Kennedy RD, Paul HD. RNA expression analysis from formalin fixed paraffin embedded tissues. Histochem Cell Biol. 2008;130:435–45.
12. Arikawa E, Sun Y, Wang J, Zhou Q, Ning B, Dial SL, et al. Cross-platform comparison of SYBR Green real-time PCR with TaqMan PCR, microarrays and other gene expression measurement technologies evaluated in the MicroArray Quality Control (MAQC) study. BMC Genomics. 2008;9:328.
13. Shi L, Jones WD, Jensen RV, Harris SC, Perkins RG, Goodsaid FM, et al. The balance of reproducibility, sensitivity, and specificity of lists of differentially expressed genes in microarray studies. BMC Bioinformatics. 2008;9 Suppl 9:S10.
14. Canales RD, Luo Y, Willey JC, Austermiller B, Barbacioru CC, Boysen C, et al. Evaluation of DNA microarray results with quantitative gene expression platforms. Nat Biotechnol. 2006;24:1115–22.
15. Walter RF, Mairinger FD, Wohlschlaeger J, Worm K, Ting S, Vollbrecht C, et al. FFPE tissue as a feasible source for gene expression analysis–a comparison of three reference genes and one tumor marker. Pathol Res Pract. 2013;209:784–9.
16. Gerlinger M, Rowan AJ, Horswell S, Larkin J, Endesfelder D, Gronroos E, et al. Intratumor heterogeneity and branched evolution revealed by multiregion sequencing. N Engl J Med. 2012;366:883–92.

3

Prognostic value of the MicroRNA regulators Dicer and Drosha in non-small-cell lung cancer: co-expression of Drosha and miR-126 predicts poor survival

Kenneth Lønvik[1,2]*, Sveinung W Sørbye[1], Marit N Nilsen[2] and Ruth H Paulssen[3]

Abstract

Background: Dicer and Drosha are important enzymes for processing microRNAs. Recent studies have exhibited possible links between expression of different miRNAs, levels of miRNA processing enzymes, and cancer prognosis. We have investigated the prognostic impact of Dicer and Drosha and their correlation with miR-126 expression in a large cohort of non-small cell lung cancer (NSCLC) patients. We aimed to find patient groups within the cohort that might have an advantage of receiving adjunctive therapies.

Methods: Dicer expression in the cytoplasm and Drosha expression in the nucleus were evaluated by manual immunohistochemistry of tissue microarrays (TMAs), including tumor tissue samples from 335 patients with resected stages I to IIIA NSCLC. In addition, *in situ* hybridizations of TMAs for visualization of miR-126 were performed. Kaplan–Meier analysis was performed, and the log-rank test via SPSS v.22 was used for estimating significance levels.

Results: In patients with normal performance status (ECOG = 0, n = 197), high Dicer expression entailed a significantly better prognosis than low Dicer expression (P = 0.024). Dicer had no significant prognostic value in patients with reduced performance status (ECOG = 1–2, n = 138). High Drosha expression was significantly correlated with high levels of the microRNA 126 (miR-126) (P = 0.004). Drosha/miR-126 co-expression had a significant negative impact on the disease-specific survival (DSS) rate (P < 0.001). Multivariate analyses revealed that the interaction Dicer*Histology (P = 0.049) and Drosha/miR-126 co-expression (P = 0.033) were independent prognostic factors.

Conclusions: In NSCLC patients with normal performance status, Dicer is a positive prognostic factor. The importance of Drosha as a prognostic factor in our material seems to be related to miR-126 and possibly other microRNAs.

Keywords: NSCLC, Dicer, Drosha, microRNA, miR-126, Immunohistochemistry

Background

Lung cancer is a heterogeneous disease and a leading cause of cancer-related death in most developed countries. Although there have been advances in treatment over the past few years, the 5-year disease-specific survival (DSS) rate is still < 15%. Therefore, it is important to investigate possible prognostic factors among the survivors in order to gain a better understanding of NSCLC malignancy and to develop treatment options for different NSCLC patient subgroups [1].

Recently, an increasing number of reports have implicated a role for miRNAs in lung cancer progression [2,3]. MicroRNAs are potential targets for treating NSCLC carcinomas [4], and research has focused on the diagnostic and prognostic potential of different microRNAs (miRNAs or miRs) in NSCLC. It is believed that miRNA expression is important in NSCLC development [5,6]. Expression profiling of miRNAs in normal and diseased lung tissues have revealed unique expression patterns, and

---

* Correspondence: kentosj@gmail.com
[1]Department of Clinical Pathology, University Hospital of Northern Norway, N-9038 Tromsø, Norway
[2]Department of Medical Biology, Tromsø, Norway
Full list of author information is available at the end of the article

a number of miRNAs have been characterized as tumor suppressor genes or oncogenes [7-13].

Several studies have identified miR-126 as a novel prognostic marker for predicting the overall survival rate of patients with some types of cancer [14,15]. MiR-126 has been found to be expressed predominantly by endothelial cells, thereby influencing angiogenesis [16,17] by downregulation of VEGF-A expression through the interaction with the 3'-untranslated region [18]. An independent and tissue-specific prognostic impact of miR-126 has been demonstrated in NSCLC, where co-expression of miR-126 with vascular endothelial growth factor-A (VEGF-A) predicts poor survival [19]. Other research has implied that mir-126 inhibits tumor cell growth, and its expression level correlates with poor survival of NSCLC patients [7]. The expression and roles of miR-126 might be different in various malignancies where miR-126 is downregulated, thereby acting as potential tumor suppressor [19-22].

Understanding the biogenesis of miRNAs has caught the interest of many researchers, and several papers have been published that focus on the enzymes necessary for synthesizing miRNAs [23-25]. MicroRNAs are generated in a two-step processing pathway mediated by two major enzymes, Dicer and Drosha, both of which belong to the class of RNase III endonucleases. The intranuclear miRNA processing enzyme Drosha and the extranuclear microRNA-processing enzyme Dicer play pivotal roles in miRNA maturation. Drosha is part of a multiprotein complex that mediates the nuclear processing of the primary miRNAs into stem-loop precursors (pre-miRNA). In the cytoplasm, the pre-miRNA is cleaved by Dicer into mature nucleotide miRNA. In the biogenesis of the majority of miRNAs, both Dicer and Drosha are necessary factors, together with several other proteins involved in the miRNA processing machinery [23,26]. Dicer and Drosha seem to have a prognostic impact, and both have been found to be differentially expressed in various cancer tissue types when compared to normal tissue [27-32].

The Eastern Cooperative Oncology Group (ECOG) performance status [33] provides scales and criteria for assessing how a patient's disease is progressing and helps to determine appropriate treatment options and prognosis. Many studies include patients with an ECOG performance status grade of 0 and 1 only. Patients in these groups are either, fully active and able to carry on all pre-disease performance without restrictions, or are restricted in physically strenuous activity and able to carry out work of a light or sedentary nature. In this study we have also included NSCLC patients with an ECOG grade of 0–2 that are capable of all self-care but unable to carry out any work activities and have more than 50% of waking hours. Cancer patients with an ECOG grade of

3–4 have reduced survival regardless of other clinical and pathological variables.

Although several studies have been performed on different cancer types in order to elucidate and decipher the roles of Dicer and Drosha in carcinogenesis and their potential impact on prognosis, the contribution of Dicer and Drosha on miR-126 expression in NSCLC has not been addressed. Therefore, this study investigates the possible prognostic value of the expression of the miRNA regulators Dicer and Drosha on miR-126 processing in a NSCLC patient cohort.

Methods
Ethics statement
The study was approved by The National Data Inspection Board, The Regional Committee for Research Ethics (REK Nord). The Regional Committee for Research Ethics specifically waived the need for consent, since this is a retrospective study with more than half of patients deceased.

Patients and clinical samples
The study examined primary tumor tissues from anonymized patients diagnosed with NSCLC pathologic stage I to IIIA within the period from 1990 to 2004 at the University Hospital of North Norway (UNN) and Nordland Central Hospital (NLCH). During this period adjuvant chemotherapy had not yet been introduced in Norway. Thus, 371 patients were considered as potential candidates for this study, of which 36 patients were excluded due to (i) chemotherapy or radiotherapy prior to surgery (n = 10), (ii) other malignancy within five years prior to NSCLC diagnosis (n = 13), and (iii) inadequate paraffin-embedded fixed tissues (n = 13). The analysis was, therefore, left with 335 patients with complete medical records and adequate paraffin-embedded tissues. All prognostic clinicopathologic variables as predictors for DSS in 335 NSCLC patients are summarized in Additional file 1: Table S1 and were reported in a previous study [19].

The NSCLC patients included in this study have an ECOG rating of 0, 1, or 2, where normal performance status is equal to 0 and reduced performance status is 1 or 2. NSCLC patients are rated from 0–5, but only patients with ratings from 0–2 are eligible for surgery. The rating system has been explained in detail in previous publications [33] and http://www.ecog.org/general/perf_-stat.html.

All tumor tissues were selected at primary surgery of previous non-treated lung cancer patients and the follow-up started directly after surgery. The last follow-up data included was from November 30, 2008. The median follow-up for survivors was 86 (range 48–216) months. The tumors were staged according to the new 7th edition of TNM classification in Lung Cancer and histologically subtyped and graded according to the World Health Organization's guidelines [34,35].

Immunohistochemistry (IHC)

All lung cancer cases were histologically reviewed by two experienced pathologists (Samer Al-Saad and Khalid Al-Shibli), and the most representative areas of viable tumor cells (neoplastic epithelial cells) were carefully selected. Within these areas, four cores from each patient were randomly sampled and assembled in TMA (tissue microarray) blocks. The detailed methodology has been reported previously [36]. As controls served samples of normal lung tissue localized distant from the primary tumor, and normal lung tissue samples from 20 patients without any cancer diagnosis (see Additional file 2: Figure S1). Multiple 4 μm sections were cut with a Microm microtome (HM355S) and analyzed via immunohistochemistry with regard to the miRNA regulators Dicer and Drosha.

Specific antibodies for Dicer (13D6-ChIP grade, ab14601) and Drosha (ab85027) (both Abcam, Cambridge, UK) have been validated in-house by the manufacturer for IHC analysis on paraffin-embedded material prior to use. Sections were deparaffinized with xylene and rehydrated through graded ethanol series (Drosha) or by using Ventana reagents for automatic staining of Dicer (Ventana BenchMark XT, Ventana Medical Systems Inc.). Manual antigen retrieval (for Drosha) was performed by placing the specimens in a 10 mM Tris–HCl/1 mM EDTA buffer, with pH 9.0, and subsequent microwave heating for 20 - minutes at 450 W. Automatic antigen retrieval (for Dicer) (Ventana Benchmark XT) was performed by heating the sections for 30 minutes in a Tris-based buffer (CC1 mild). Staining was performed with a detection reagent containing a secondary antibody plus an avidin-biotin enzyme complex (manual procedure), or a polymer of secondary antibodies conjugated with an enzyme (Ventana). Primary antibodies were diluted at 1:20 (Dicer) and 1:100 (Drosha) or incubated overnight at room temperature (Drosha) and for 32 minutes at 37°C (Dicer). Diaminobenzidine (DAB) was used to visualize the antigens. The detection system in the Ventana XT was the ultraView DAB. Finally, counterstaining was performed with hematoxylin and by mounting the slides. In negative control slides, the primary antibody was replaced with the primary antibody diluent, and for positive staining controls, we used breast carcinoma samples (data not shown).

In Situ Hybridization (ISH)

The *in situ* hybridization method was adapted from [37] and performed with minor adjustments due to different batches of labelled probes. *In situ* hybridizations of TMA sections for visualization of miR-126 were essentially performed in accordance with recent research [19].

Scoring of IHC

The IHC-stained TMA slides were scanned with the ARIOL imaging system (Genetix, San Jose, CA) as follows: The slides were loaded in the automated loader (Applied Imaging SL 50) and TMA slides were scanned at low (1.25 x) and high resolutions (20 x) by using the Olympus BX 61 microscope with an automated platform. Representative and viable tissue sections were scored manually and semi-quantitatively for cytoplasmic staining (Dicer) and for staining the tumor cell nuclei (Drosha) via a computer screen. The average staining intensity of the majority of cells was scored as 0 = negative, 1 = weak, 2 = intermediate, and 3 = strong (see Figures 1 and 2), as described previously [36]. In case of disagreement (score variance > 1), the slides were re-examined and an agreement was reached by the observers. In most cores there was a mixture of stromal cells and tumor cells. By morphological criteria only tumor cells were scored for staining intensity.

All samples were anonymized and independently scored by an experienced pathologist and a technician (S.W.S. and K.L.). When scoring the samples, the observers were blind to the scores of the other observer and to the outcome. The mean score for each case was calculated from all four cores by both examiners. High expression of both Dicer and Drosha in neoplastic tumor cells was defined as a mean score ≥ 2. This cut-off value was selected to find the two groups with the largest possible difference in survival. It is hereby noted that the results might be depended on the choice of the cut-off value. However, for miR-126 we used the same cut-off value and the same scoring system as previously described in detail [19,38].

Inter-observer variability

An inter-observer scoring agreement was tested for both Dicer and Drosha, and the agreement was robust ($r = 0.92$, $P < 0.001$).

Statistical methods

In brief, statistical analyses were conducted with the statistical package SPSS (Chicago, IL), version 22. The Chi-square test and Fisher's exact test were used to examine the association between Dicer and Drosha expressions and various clinicopathological parameters. The IHC scores from each observer were compared for inter-observer reliability by use of a two-way random effect model with absolute agreement definition. The intraclass correlation coefficient (reliability coefficient) was obtained from these results. The Kaplan–Meier method was used to plot DSS according to expression levels, and statistical significance between survival curves was assessed by the log-rank test. DSS was determined from the date of surgery to the time of death from lung cancer. The multivariate analysis was conducted with the Cox

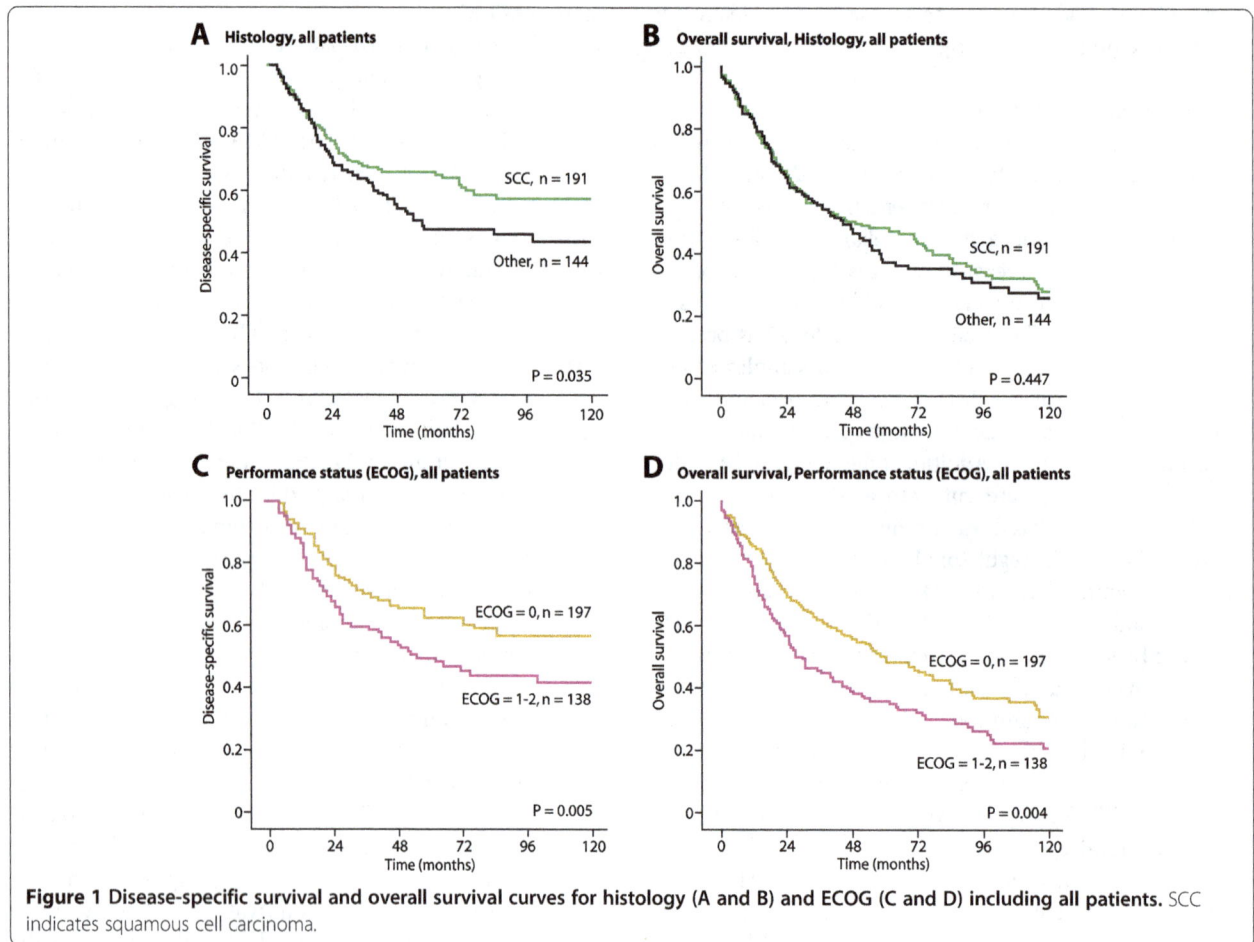

Figure 1 Disease-specific survival and overall survival curves for histology (A and B) and ECOG (C and D) including all patients. SCC indicates squamous cell carcinoma.

proportional hazards model. Only those variables of significant value from the univariate analysis were entered into the Cox regression analysis. Differences in expression of Dicer, Drosha, and miR-126 as continuous variables by histology are analyzed using ANOVA. The significance level employed was $P < 0.05$.

Results

Overall NSCLC patient group characteristics

The NSCLC patient cohort comprised 253 males (75%) and 82 females (25%), (Additional file 1: Table S1). The follow-up time was up to 250 months (20 years). During follow-up, 236 (70%) patients died, 137 (40%) from lung cancer and 99 (30%) from other reasons (data not shown). The 5- year DSS was 56% for males and 63% for females (Additional file 1: Table S1). On a continuous scale (0–3), the mean expression of Dicer, Drosha, and miR-126 in all patients was 1.18, 1.41, and 1.14, respectively. Patients with squamous cell carcinoma had significantly higher expression of Dicer and miR-126 than patients with adenocarcinoma (Additional file 1: Table S2). Using ≤ 2.0 as a cut-off of expression (Additional file 2: Figure S1), about 70–80% of the patients had low expression and 20–30% of

the patients had high expression of Dicer, Drosha, and miR-126 (data not shown).

Performance status (ECOG), disease-specific survival (DSS), and overall survival (OS) in NSCLC patient groups—Univariate analyses

WHO performance status (ECOG, $P = 0.013$), histology ($P = 0.028$), tumor differentiation ($P < 0.001$), surgical procedure ($P < 0.004$), pathological stage ($P < 0.001$), tumor status ($P < 0.001$), nodal status ($P < 0.001$), and vascular infiltration ($P < 0.001$) were all significant indicators for DSS in univariate analyses (Additional file 1: Table S1 and [19]).

Patients with squamous cell carcinoma had significantly longer DSS than lung cancer patients with other histology ($P = 0.035$, Figure 1A). However, there were no significant differences regarding overall survival between patients with squamous cell carcinoma compared to patients with other histology ($P = 0.447$, Figure 1B). Patients with normal performance status (ECOG = 0) had significantly longer DSS and overall survival than patients with reduced performance status (ECOG = 1–2), $P = 0.005$ (Figure 1C) and $P = 0.004$ (Figure 1D).

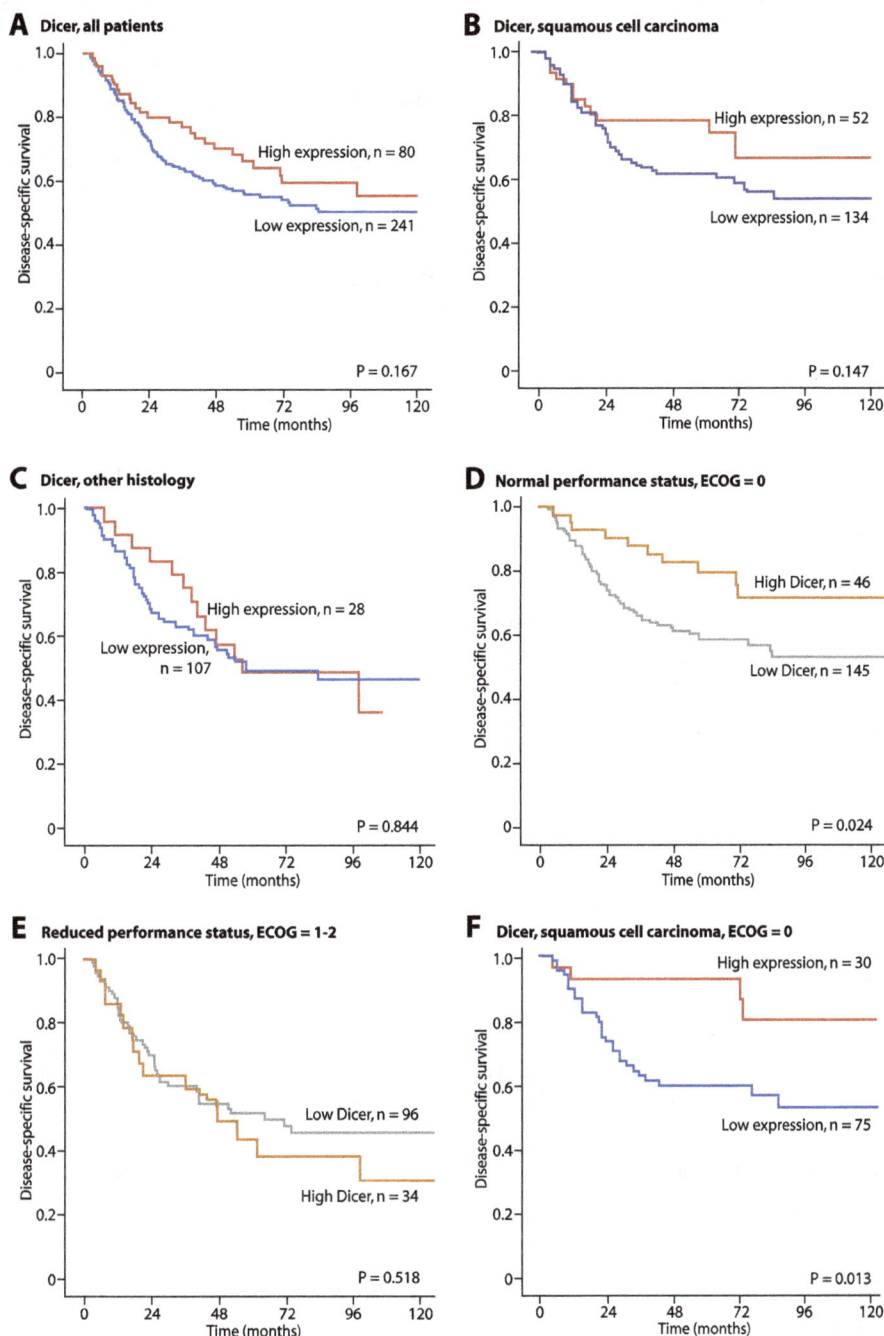

Figure 2 Disease-specific survival curves for high and low expression of Dicer in NSCLC patients (n = 321) (A), in patients with squamous cell carcinoma (n = 186) (B), in patients with other histology (n = 135) (C), in patients with normal performance status (ECOG = 0, n = 191) (D), in patients with reduced performance status (ECOG = 1–2, n =140) (E), and in patients with squamous cell carcinoma with normal performance status (ECOG = 0, n = 105) (F).

Dicer and Drosha expressions and correlations

Dicer was expressed in the cytoplasm of most neoplastic tumor cells, and slight staining was observed in the nucleus of some cells as well (Additional file 2: Figure S2). Thirty-five patients (10.4%) scored negative on all four cores. Drosha was primarily expressed in the nucleus, but some staining was observed in the cytoplasm (Additional file 2: Figure S3). We found 14 patients (4.2%) that scored negative on all four sample cores. Inflammatory cells, pneumocytes, and fibroblasts showed greater variability in expressing both Dicer and Drosha when compared to tumor cells. A significant, but low correlation between Dicer expression in cytoplasm and Drosha expression in the nucleus of neoplastic tumor cells (r = 0.473, P < 0.001) was observed (Additional file 2: Figure S4).

The expression of Dicer (P = 0.008) and miR-126 (P = 0.020) was different in the tumor subgroups (see Additional file 1: Table S2). Expression of Dicer was not correlated with DSS when all patients were analyzed in one group (P = 0.167, Figure 2A). The expression of Dicer was of not

correlated with DSS in patients with squamous cell carcinoma (P = 0.147, Figure 2B) or other histologies (P = 0,844, Figure 2C). However, in patients with normal performance status (ECOG = 0), high expression of Dicer was significantly correlated with longer DSS (P = 0.024,) (Figure 2D), but no differences in patients with reduced performance status (ECOG = 1–2) were observed (P = 0.518, Figure 2E). In

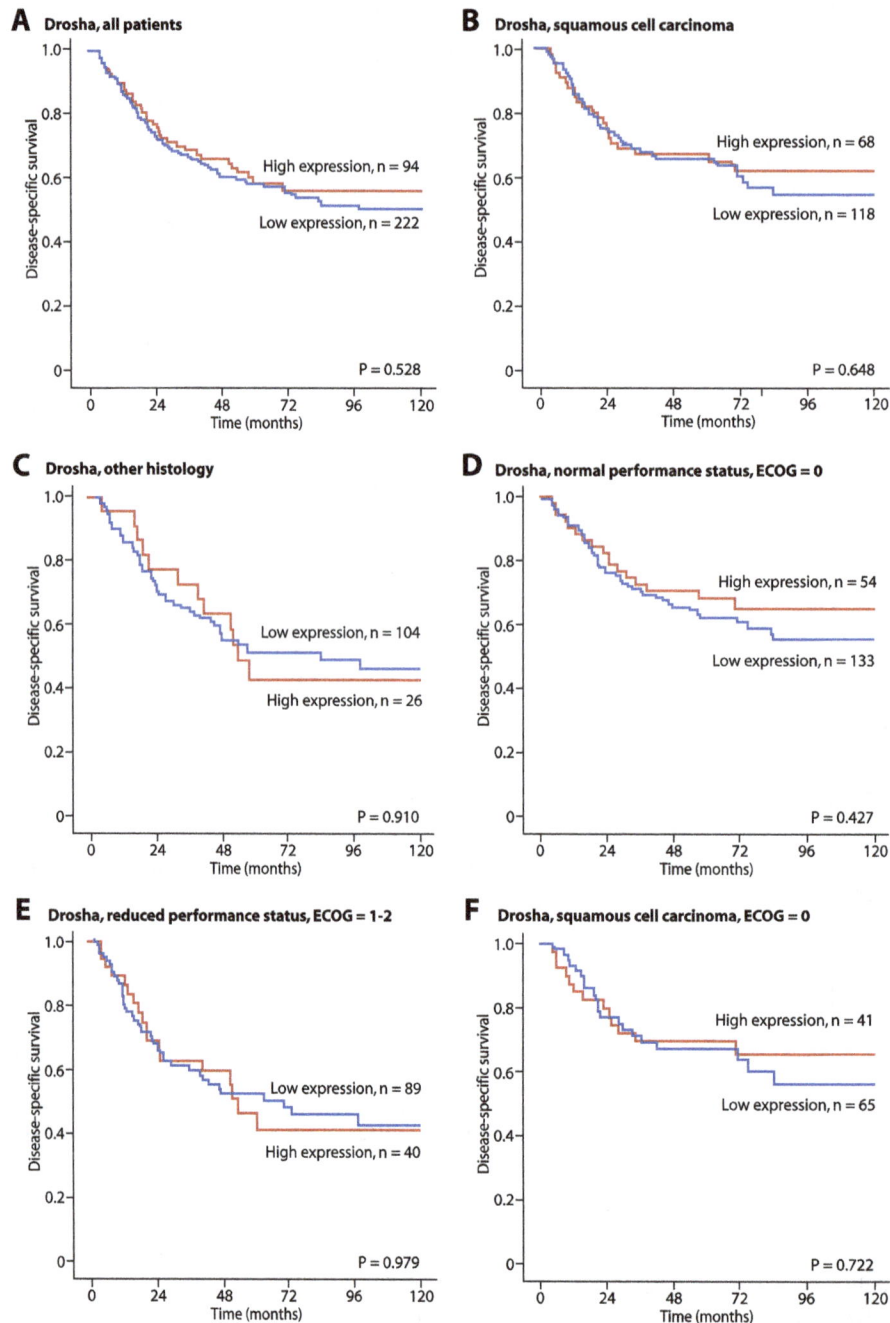

Figure 3 Disease-specific survival curves for high and low expression of Drosha in NSCLC patients (n = 316) (A), in patients with squamous cell carcinoma (n = 186) (B), in patients with other histology (n = 130) (C), in patients with normal performance status (ECOG = 0, n = 187) (D), in patients with reduced performance status (ECOG = 1–2, n = 129) (E), and in patients with squamous cell carcinoma with normal performance status (ECOG = 0, n = 116) (F).

patients with both squamous cell carcinoma and normal performance status (ECOG = 0), high expression of Dicer was significantly correlated with long DSS (P = 0.013, Figure 2F). Expression of Drosha was not correlated with DSS for any subgroups of histology and performance status (Figure 3A– F).

When combining expression of Drosha and miR-126, the subgroup of patients with both high Drosha and high miR-126 expression had significantly shorter DSS (P < 0.001) (Figure 4A) and overall survival (P = 0.001, Figure 4B).

Multivariate cox proportional hazard analysis

Tumor status (T-stage, P = 0.002), nodal status (N-stage, P < 0.001), performance status (0.003), vascular infiltration (P = 0.016), interaction of Dicer with histology (Dicer*Histology, P = 0.049), and Drosha/miR-126 co-expression (P = 0.033) were independently significantly correlated with DSS (Table 1). In the subgroup of patients with both squamous cell carcinoma and normal performance status (ECOG = 0, n = 107), tumor status (P = 0.021), nodal status (P = 0.001), vascular infiltration (P = 0.011), and expression of Dicer (P = 0.031), but not tumor differentiation (P = 0.587), were independently correlated with DSS (Table 2).

When Dicer and Drosha are analyzed on a continuous scale (0–3) instead of two groups of expression (high and low), none of them correlated with DSS in the total patient material (Additional file 1: Table S3). To identify other relevant factors regarding expression of Dicer, the expression was tested by histology, performance status, tumor differentiation, tumor status, nodal status, and vascular infiltration. High expression was found in SCC (P = 0.012) and in tumors with vascular infiltration (P = 0.035, Additional file 1: Table S4). The Dicer interaction with histology was highly significant (P = 0.005, Additional

file 1: Table S5). This was not the case for Dicer interaction with ECOG (Additional file 1: Table S6) and Dicer interaction with vascular infiltration (Additional file 1: Table S7). The proportionality of hazards was tested graphically and the results are depicted in Additional file 2: Figure S5.

Co-expression of Drosha and miR-126

For co-expression analyses, we used miR-126 data obtained by ISH of TMAs from a previously published study [19] demonstrating that high miR-126 expression is an independent negative prognostic factor in the total patient cohort. As illustrated in Figure 4, a univariate analysis found that the co-expression of Drosha and miR-126 had a significant impact on DSS, with 5-year survival rates of 58% (patients with low Drosha and low miR-126 expression), 61% (low Drosha and high miR-126 expression), 74% (high Drosha and low miR-126 expression), and 17% (high Drosha and high miR-126 expression) (p < 0.001). In a multivariate analysis, these co-expressions were independent prognostic indicators for DSS (p = 0.016). For patients with high Drosha/high miR-126, the HR was 2.1 (1.1–4.0 at 95% CI, p < 0.001) compared to patients with high Drosha/low miR-126 (Table 1).

Discussion

In this large-scale study comprising primary tumors from 335 patients, we investigated the prognostic impact of the miRNA regulators Dicer and Drosha in NSCLC. The observed expression of the nuclear enzyme Drosha and the cytoplasmic enzyme Dicer correlated positively with each other, suggesting their mutual dependence in the miRNA-regulatory pathway in NSCLC. Reduced Dicer and Drosha expression has been reported in various cancers, and based on previous publications on

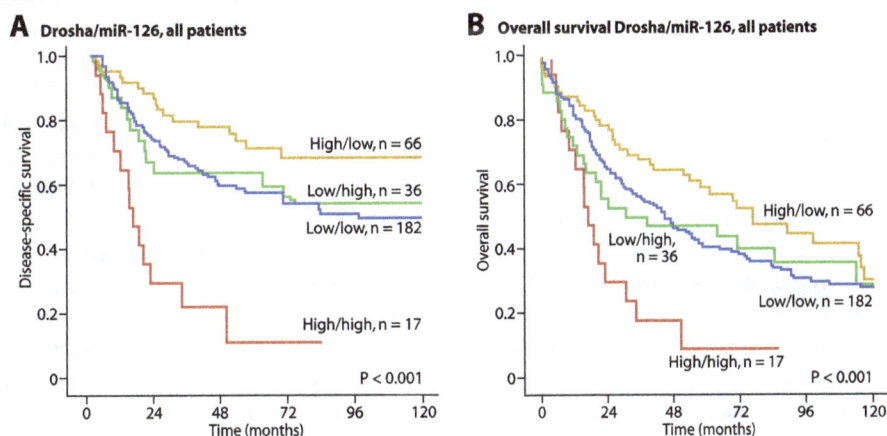

Figure 4 Disease-specific survival (A) and overall survival (B) curves for co-expression of Drosha and miR-126 in the total patient material (n = 301).

Table 1 Cox regression analysis summarizing significant independent prognostic factors

Factor	HR	95% CI	P
Tumor status			0.002*
1	1.00		
2	1.54	0.91 – 2.59	0.108
3	2.73	1.53 – 4.90	0.001
Nodal status			<0.001*
0	1.00		
1	1.98	1.27 – 3.08	0.003
2	3.13	1.80 – 5.46	<0.001
Histology			
SCC	1.00		
Other NSCLC	0.99	0.500 – 1.98	0.986
Differentiation			0.094*
Poor	1.00		
Moderate	0.70	0.46 – 1.05	0.083
Well	0.56	0.29 – 1.10	0.095
Performance status			
ECOG = 0	1.00		
ECOG = 1-2	1.80	1.23 – 2.64	0.003
Vascular infiltration			
No	1.00		
Yes	1.82	1.12 – 2.98	0.016
Dicer**	0.87	0.65 – 1.16	0.333
Dicer*Histology***	1.27	1.00 – 1.61	0.049
Drosha / miR-126			0.033*
Low / Low	1.00		
Low / High	1.13	0.62 – 2.05	0.696
High / Low	0.63	0.37 – 1.07	0.089
High / High	1.96	1.04 – 3.69	0.037

*Overall significance as a prognostic factor.
**B = −0.141.
***B = 0.240.
Dicer*Histology = the interaction between Dicer and Histology.
HR: Hazard ration; CI: confidence interval.

Table 2 Cox regression analysis summarizing significant independent prognostic factors in patients with squamous cell carcinoma and normal performance status (ECOG = 0), n = 107

Factor	HR	95% CI	P
Tumor status			0.021*
1	1.00		
2	2.52	0.82 – 7.79	0.108
3	5.11	1.54 – 16.89	0.008
Nodal status			0.001*
0	1.00		
1	2.11	1.21 – 2.89	0.045
2	20.06	3.70 – >99	0.001
Differentiation			0.587*
Poor	1.00		
Moderate	0.64	0.26 – 1.56	0.328
Well	0.72	0.23 – 2.26	0.578
Vascular infiltration			
No	1.00		
Yes	3.10	1.29 – 7.42	0.011
Dicer			
Low	1.00		
High	0.30	0.10 – 0.90	0.031

*Overall significance as a prognostic factor.
HR: Hazard ratio; CI: confidence interval.

biological properties [33]. This might explain why Dicer expression had no impact on survival in this group of patients, and might also explain the differences of Dicer impact compared with other NSCLC studies, where ECOG performance is rarely mentioned. Our results clearly show that low Dicer expression is a significant negative prognostic marker in patients with normal performance status ECOG = 0 (Figure 2D). This patient group might therefore have an advantage in receiving adjunctive treatment. In addition, for patients with normal ECOG performance status, the low expression of Dicer was positively correlated with better survival rates in the patient group with squamous cell carcinoma (see Figure 2F), whereas Dicer expression had no prognostic impact on other histological subgroups (data not shown).

Dicer, Drosha, and miRNAs are involved in cell growth and differentiation, implying an impact on tumorigenesis [39]. Various studies focusing on Dicer and/or Drosha have confirmed this theory and revealed that these two regulators of the miRNA processing pathway play either a positive or a negative role in tumor transformation. There is evidence that reduced Dicer expression is associated with poor prognosis in NSCLC [28]. However, in vitro experiments showed that silencing of Dicer and

NSCLC [28,29], there was an expectation that both Dicer and Drosha would have a positive prognostic impact on DSS, where reduced Dicer and Drosha expression would entail a poorer prognosis compared to higher expressions. Our results found no significant association between the miRNA regulators and DSS (Figure 2A). Dicer is usually reported as a more powerful prognosticator for survival than Drosha [27,28]. Stratified by ECOG, Dicer expression turned out to be significant for patients with normal performance status (ECOG = 0) only (Figure 2D). In general, patients with reduced performance status (ECOG = 1–4) have a more advanced disease and poor prognosis, independent of the tumor's

Drosha decreases angiogenesis [24]. In our study, we found that increased expression of Dicer correlates with better prognosis. Neuroblastoma and leukemia are two other examples where low levels of Dicer and Drosha are significant predictive factors for poor outcomes [27,40]. In other types of cancer, the importance of Dicer and Drosha might be the opposite. A recent study by Faber et al. using TMA technology and a scoring system like the one described here, found evidence that Dicer is a negative prognosticator for DSS in colorectal cancer [41]. Clearly, the functions of Dicer and Drosha are not fully understood in cancer development, and their functions appear to vary between different cancer types [42-44].

In most cancers, the majority of all miRNAs are down-regulated, suggesting that most miRNAs have tumor suppressive effects [44]. Regulation of miRNA biogenesis is a complex process involving a myriad of different enzymes and proteins, where Dicer and Drosha are two key regulators necessary for the processing of most functional, mature miRNAs. We previously described the prognostic impact of miR-126 in NSCLC [19], where the co-expression of miR-126 and VEGF-A was a strong predictor for poor survival. We know that VEGF-A is a potent angiogenesis promoter, and miR-126 has been linked to angiogenesis in several other studies [11,45,46]. Interestingly, we found that the co-expression of Drosha and miR-126 also predicts poor survival, which is even more significant than the co-expression of miR-126 and VEGF-A reported previously [19]. Although not significant (p = 0.06), the combination of high Drosha and low miR-126 was the most favorable in relation to DSS (see Table 1), suggesting that Drosha in itself is not a good prognostic marker for overall survival in NSCLC, which is consistent with our univariate analyses (see Figure 3A). We tested the co-expressions of both Dicer and Drosha, in combination with the miRNAs miR-126 and miR-155 [47] in all 335 patients, and miR122a and let-7a in 40 randomly selected patients (data not shown). These tests demonstrated that the only combination with impact on DSS was the Drosha and miR-126 combination (see Figure 4). The significance of Drosha, as well as Dicer, in driving angiogenesis *in vitro* has been reported previously [24]. However, *in vivo* experiments showed that only Dicer reduces angiogenesis [48]. Our results imply that Drosha in itself is not a good prognostic marker in NSCLC, and that the effect of Drosha might be influenced by different miRNAs involved in tumor angiogenesis.

In addition, Dicer-independent, and probably Drosha-independent maturing of miRNAs is possible, suggesting alternative pathways and different roles for Dicer and Drosha in various cancers [49,50]. As an example, miR-451 is processed by Ago, without the need for Dicer [51]. Several studies have also shown that knockdown of Dicer and Drosha

only reduces a subset of miRNAs, implying alternative pathways for miRNA synthesis [49-51]. Further studies are clearly needed to investigate these possibilities.

Conclusion
The immunohistochemical approach reveals the varying presence of Dicer and Drosha in NSCLC tumors, and these two enzymes may be important in NSCLC development. Our research points to Dicer as an important factor in regard to DSS in patients with normal ECOG, and implies that Drosha in combination with miR-126 and possibly other angiogenesis-related miRNAs, is a strong and important prognosticator for DSS in NSCLC. The Dicer and Drosha expression status in various histologic subtypes of lung cancer and at different stages of lung cancer development might explain abnormalities in miR profiles of NSCLC. Additional studies are needed, since optimized treatment of NSCLC requires better identification of high-risk patients who will benefit from adjuvant therapy.

Additional files

Additional file 1: Table S1. Prognostic Clinicopathologic Variables as Predictors for Disease-Specific Survival in 335 NSCLC Patients (Univariate Analyses; Log-rank Test) adapted from [19]. **Table S2.** Expression of Dicer, Drosha and miR-126 by histology. **Table S3.** Cox regression analysis summarizing significant independent prognostic factors in the total patient material with Dicer and Drosha as covariates on a continuous scale. **Table S4.** Expression of Dicer by histology, performance status, tumor differentiation, tumor status, nodal status and vascular infiltration. **Table S5.** Cox regression analysis summarizing significant independent prognostic factors exploring Dicer interaction with histology. **Table S6.** Cox regression analysis summarizing significant independent prognostic factors exploring Dicer interaction with ECOG. **Table S7.** Cox regression analysis summarizing significant independent prognostic factors exploring Dicer interaction with vascular infiltration.

Additional file 2: Figure S1. Normal lung tissue. **Figure S2.** Immunohistochemical (IHC) staining of Dicer in NSCLC tissues, representing (A) negative staining, (B) weak staining, (C) intermediate staining, and (D) strong staining. Dicer is found primarily in cytoplasm, see brown staining. **Figure S3.** Immunohistochemical (IHC) staining of Drosha in NSCLC tissues, representing (A) negative staining, (B) weak staining, (C) intermediate staining, and (D) strong staining. Drosha is primarily found in the nuclei, see brown staining. **Figure S4.** Correlation between Dicer and Drosha expression in the total patient material. **Figure S5.** Proportionality of the hazards.

Competing interests
The authors declare that they have no competing interests.

Authors' contributions
KL participated in the study design, contributed to the clinical demographic database, did the statistical analyses and drafted the manuscript. SWS contributed to the clinical demographic database, performed the scoring, and performed the statistical analyses. MNH carried out the IHC. RHP supervised and participated in the study design, result interpretation and writing of the manuscript. All authors have read and approved the final manuscript.

Acknowledgements
This study was supported by the Northern Norway Regional Health Authority (Helse Nord RHF). We are grateful to pathologists Samer Al-Saad, at the Department of Pathology at the University Hospital of North Norway (UNN), and Khalid-Al-Shibli,

Nordland Central Hospital in Bodø, Norway, for histological evaluations of patient tissue samples.

Author details
[1]Department of Clinical Pathology, University Hospital of Northern Norway, N-9038 Tromsø, Norway. [2]Department of Medical Biology, Tromsø, Norway. [3]Department of Clinical Medicine, UiT – The Arctic University of Norway, N-9037 Tromsø, Norway.

References
1. Jemal A, Siegel R, Xu J, Ward E: Cancer Statistics 2010. *CA Cancer J Clin* 2010, **60**(4):277–300.
2. Zhang W-C, Liu J, Xu X, Wang G: The role of microRNAs in lung cancer progression. *Med Oncol* 2013, **30**:675–683.
3. Saito M, Schetter AJ, Mollerup S, Kohno T, Skaug V, Bowman ED, Mathé EA, Takenoshita S, Yokota J, Haugen A, Harris CC: The association of microRNA expression with prognosis and progression in early-stage, non-small cell lung adenocarcinoma: a retrospective analysis of three cohorts. *Clin Cancer Res* 2011, **17**:1875–1882.
4. Malleter M, Jacquot C, Rousseau B, Tomasoni C, Juge M, Pineau A, Sakanian V, Roussakis C: miRNAs, a potential target in the treatment of Non-Small-Cell Lung Carcinomas. *Gene* 2012, **506**:355–359.
5. Raponi M, Dossey L, Jatkoe T, Wu X, Chen G, Fan H, Beer DG: MicroRNA classifiers for predicting prognosis of squamous cell lung cancer. *Cancer Res* 2009, **69**:5776–5783.
6. Lin PY, Lu SL, Yang PC: MicroRNAs in lung cancer. *Br J Cancer* 2010, **103**:1144–1148.
7. Yang J, Lan H, Huang X, Liu B, Tong Y: MicroRNA-126 inhibits tumor cell growth and its expression level correlates with poor survival in non-small cell lung cancer patients. *PLoS One* 2012, **7**:e42978.
8. Wang R, Wang ZX, Yang JS, Pan X, De W, Chen LB: MicroRNA-451 functions as a tumor suppressor in human non-small cell lung cancer by targeting ras-related protein 14 (RAB14). *Oncogene* 2011, **30**:2644–2658.
9. Jang JS, Jeon HS, Sun Z, Aubry MC, Tang H, Park CH, Rakhshan F, Schutz DA, Kolbert CP, Lupu R, Park JY, Harris CC, Yang P, Jen J: Increased mir-708 expression in NSCLC and its association with poor survival in lung adenocarcinoma from never smokers. *Clin Cancer Res* 2012, **18**:3658–3667.
10. Ma L, Huang Y, Zhu W, Zhou S, Zhou J, Zeng F, Lin X, Zhang Y, Yu J: An integrated analysis of miRNA and mRNA expressions in non-small cell lung cancers. *PLoS One* 2011, **6**:e26502.
11. Dønnem T, Fenton CG, Lønvik K, Berg T, Eklo K, Andersen S, Stenvold H, Al-Shibli K, Al-Saad S, Bremnes R, Busund LT: MicroRNA signatures in tumor tissue related to angiogenesis in non-small cell lung cancer. *PLoS One* 2012, **7**:e29671.
12. Tan X, Qin W, Zhang L, Hang J, Li B, Zhang C, Wan J, Zhou F, Shao K, Sun Y, Wu J, Zhang X, Qui B, Li N, Shi S, Feng X, Zhao S, Wang Z, Zhao X, Chen Z, Mitchelson K, Cheng J, Guo Y, He J: A 5-microRNA signature for lung squamous cell carcinoma diagnosis and hsa-miR-31 for prognosis. *Clin Cancer Res* 2011, **17**:6802–6811.
13. Boeri M, Verri C, Conte D, Roz L, Modena P, Facchinetti F, Calabrò E, Croce CM, Pastorino U, Sozzi G: MicroRNA signatures in tissues and plasma predict development and prognosis of computed tomography detected lung cancer. *Proc Natl Acad Sci U S A* 2011, **108**:3713–3718.
14. Tavazoie SF, Alarcon C, Oskarsson T, Padua D, Wang Q, Bos PD, Gerald WL, Massagué J: Endogenous human microRNAs that suppress breast cancer metastasis. *Nature* 2008, **451**:147–152.
15. Ebrahimi F, Gopalan V, Smith RA, Lam AK-Y: miR-126 in human cancers: Clinical roles and current perspectives. *Exp Mol Pathol* 2014, **96**:98–107.
16. Cho WC, Chow AS, Au JS: Restoration of tumor-repressor hsa-miR-145 inhibits cancer cell growth in lung adenocarcinoma patients with epidermal growth factor receptor mutation. *Eur J Cancer* 2008, **45**:22197–22206.
17. Agudo J, Ruzo A, Tung N, Salmon H, Leboeuf M, Hashimoto D, Becker C, Garrett-Sinha LA, Baccarini A, Merad M, Brown BD: The miR-216-VEGFR2 axis controls the innate response to pathogen-associated nucleic acids. *Nature Immunol* 2014, **15**:54–62.
18. Zhu X, Li L, Hui L, Chen H, Wang X, Shen H, Xu W: miR-126 enhances the sensitivity of non-small cell lung cancer cells to anticancer agents by targeting vascular endothelial growth factor A. *Acta Biochim Biophys Sin* 2012, **44**:519–526.
19. Dønnem T, Lonvik K, Eklo K, Berg T, Sorbye SW, Al-Shibli K, Al-Saad S, Andersen S, Stenvold H, Bremnes R, Busund LT: Independent and tissue-specific prognostic impact of miR-126 in non-small cell lung cancer. *Cancer* 2011, **117**:3193–3200.
20. Chen H, Miao R, Fan J, Han Z, Wu J, Qui G, Tang H, Peng Z: Decreased expression of mir-126 correlates with metastatic recurrence of hepatocellular carcinoma. *Clin Exp Metastasis* 2013, **30**:651–658.
21. Tomasetti M, Staffolani S, Nocchi L, Neuzil J, Strafella E, Manzella N, Mariotti L, Bracci M, Valentino M, Amati M, Santarelli L: Clinical significance of circulating mir-126 quantification in malignant mesothelioma patients. *Clin Biochem* 2012, **45**:575–581.
22. Meister J, Schmidt MHH: miR-126 and miR-126*: New players in Cancer. *Sci World J* 2010, **10**:2090–2100.
23. Davis BN, Hata A: Regulation of microRNA biogenesis: a myriad of mechanisms. *Cell Commun Signal* 2009, **7**:18.
24. Suarez Y, Fernandez-Hernando C, Yu J, Gerber SA, Harrison KD, Pober JS, Iruela-Arispe ML, Merkenschlager M, Sessa WC: Dicer-dependent endothelial microRNAs are necessary for postnatal angiogenesis. *Proc Natl Acad Sci U S A* 2008, **105**:14082–14087.
25. Yang JS, Lai EC: Alternative miRNA biogenesis pathways and the interpretation of core miRNA pathway mutants. *Mol Cell* 2011, **43**:892–903.
26. Macrae IJ, Zhou K, Li F, Repic A, Brooks AN, Cande WZ, Adams PD, Doudna JA: Structural basis for double-stranded RNA processing by Dicer. *Science* 2006, **311**:834–838.
27. Lin RJ, Lin YC, Chen J, Kuo HH, Chen YY, Diccianni MB, London WB, Chang CH, Yu AL: MicroRNA signature and expression of dicer and drosha can predict prognosis and delineate risk groups in neuroblastoma. *Cancer Res* 2010, **70**:7841–7850.
28. Karube Y, Tanaka H, Osada H, Tomida S, Tatematsu Y, Yanagisawa K, Yatabe Y, Takamizawa J, Miyoshi S, Mitsudomi T, Takahashi T: Reduced expression of Dicer associated with poor prognosis in lung cancer patients. *Cancer Sci* 2005, **96**(2):111–115.
29. Merritt WM, Lin YG, Han LY, Kamat AA, Spannuth WA, Schmandt R, Urbauer D, Pennachio LA, Cheng JF, Nick AM, Deavers MT, Mourad-Zeidan A, Wang H, Mueller P, Lenburg ME, Gray JW, Mok S, Birrer MJ, Lopez-Berestein G, Coleman RL, Bar-Eli M, Sood AK: Dicer, Drosha and outcomes in patients with ovarian cancer. *N Engl J Med* 2008, **359**:2641–2650.
30. Grelier G, Voirin N, Ay AS, Cox DG, Chabaud S, Treilleux I, Léon-Goddard S, Rimokh R, Mikaelian I, Venoux C, Puisieux A, Lasset C, Moyret-Lalle C: Prognostic value of Dicer expression in human breast cancers and association with the mesenchymal phenotype. *Br J Cancer* 2009, **101**:673–683.
31. Chiosea S, Jelezcova E, Chandran U, Luo J, Mantha G, Sobol RW, Dacic S: Overexpression of Dicer in precursor lesions of lung adenocarcinoma. *Cancer Res* 2007, **67**:2345–2350.
32. Guo X, Liao Q, Chen P, Li X, Xiong W, Ma J, Li X, Luo Z, Tang H, Deng M, Zheng Y, Wang R, Zhang W, Li G: The microRNA-processing enzymes: Drosha and Dicer can predict prognosis of nasopharyngeal carcinoma. *J Cancer Res Clin Oncol* 2012, **138**:49–56.
33. Oken MM, Creech RH, Tormey DC, Horton J, Davis TE, McFadden ET, Carbone PP: Toxicity and response criteria of the Eastern Cooperative Oncology Group. *Am J Clin Oncol* 1982, **5**:649–655.
34. Goldstraw P: The 7th Edition of TNM in Lung Cancer: what now? *J Thorac Oncol* 2009, **4**:671–673.
35. World Health Organization: *Histological Typing of Lung and Pleural Tumours.* 3rd edition. Geneva, Switzerland: Springer-Verlag; 1999.
36. Sørbye SW, Kilvær TK, Valkow A, Dønnem T, Smeland E, Al-Shibli K, Bremnes RM, Busund LT: Prognostic impact of Jab1, p16, p21, p62, ki67 and Skp2 in soft tissue sarcomas. *PLoS One* 2012, **7**:e47068.
37. Nuovo GJ, Elton TS, Nana-Sinkam P, Volinia S, Croce CM, Schmittgen TD: A methodology for the combined in situ analyses of the precursor and mature forms of microRNAs and correlation with their putative targets. *Nat Protoc* 2009, **4**:107–115.
38. Dønnem T, Al-Saad S, Al-Shibli K, Delghandi MP, Persson M, Nilsen MN, Busund LT, Bremnes RM: Inverse prognostic impact of angiogenic marker expression in tumor cells versus stromal cells in non small cell lung cancer. *Clin Cancer Res* 2007, **13**:6649–6657.
39. Davis-Dusenbery BN, Hata A: MicroRNA in cancer: the involvement of aberrant microRNA biogenesis regulatory pathways. *Genes Cancer* 2011, **1**:1100–1114.

40. Zhu DX, Fan L, Lu RN, Fang C, Shen WY, Zou ZJ, Wang YH, Zhu HY, Miao KR, Liu P, Xu W, Li JY: **Downregulated dicer expression predicts poor prognosis in chronic lymphocytic leukemia.** *Cancer Sci* 2012, **103**:875–881.

41. Faber C, Horst D, Hlubek F, Kirchner T: **Overexpression of dicer predicts poor survival in colorectal cancer.** *Eur J Cancer* 2011, **47**:1414–1419.

42. Shu G-S, Yang Z-L, Liu D-C: **Immounohistochemical study of Dicer and Drosha expression in the benign and malignant lesions of gallbladder and their clinicopathological significances.** *Pathol Res Pract* 2012, **208**:392–397.

43. Vaksman O, Hetland TE, Trope CG, Reich R, Davidson B: **Argonaute, Dicer, and Drosha are up-regulated along tumor progression in serious ovarian carcinoma.** *Hum Pathol* 2012, **43**:2062–2069.

44. Sassen S, Miska EA, Caldas C: **MicroRNA – implications for cancer.** *Virchows Arch* 2008, **451**:1–10.

45. Anand S, Cheresh DA: **MicroRNA-mediated regulation of the angiogenic switch.** *Curr Opin Hematol* 2011, **18**:171–176.

46. Chen CC, Zhou SH: **Mesenchymal stem cells overexpressing miR-126 enhance ischemic angiogenesis via the AKT/ERK-related pathway.** *Cardiol J* 2011, **18**:675–681.

47. Dønnem T, Eklo K, Berg T, Sørbye SW, Lønvik K, Al-Saad S, Al-Shibli K, Stenvold H, Bremnes RM, Busund LT: **Prognostic Impact of MiR-155 in non-small Cell Lung cancer evaluated by in Situ Hybridization.** *J Transl Med* 2011, **9**:6.

48. Kuehlbacher A, Ubrich C, Zeiher AM, Dimmler S: **Role of Dicer and Drosha for endothelial microRNA expression and angiogenesis.** *Circ Res* 2011, **101**:59–69.

49. Palermo EI, de Campos SG, Campos M, Nogueira de Souza N, Guerreiro IDC, Carvalho AL, Marques MMC: **Mechanisms and role of microRNA deregulation in cancer onset and progression.** *Gen Mol Biol* 2011, **34**:363–370.

50. Farazi TA, Spitzer JI, Morozow P, Tusch T: **miRNAs in human cancer.** *J Pathol* 2011, **223**:102–115.

51. Cheloufi S, Dos Santos CO, Chong MM, Hannon GJ: **A dicer-independent miRNA biogenesis pathway that requires Ago catalysis.** *Nature* 2010, **465**:584–589.

4

Tumor-specific expression of HMG-CoA reductase in a population-based cohort of breast cancer patients

Emma Gustbée[1], Helga Tryggvadottir[1,2], Andrea Markkula[1], Maria Simonsson[1], Björn Nodin[1], Karin Jirström[1], Carsten Rose[3], Christian Ingvar[4], Signe Borgquist[1,2] and Helena Jernström[1*]

Abstract

Background: The mevalonate pathway synthetizes cholesterol, steroid hormones, and non-steriod isoprenoids necessary for cell survival. 3-Hydroxy-3-methylglutaryl-coenzyme A reductase (HMGCR) is the rate-limiting enzyme of the mevalonate pathway and the target for statin treatment. HMGCR expression in breast tumors has recently been proposed to hold prognostic and treatment-predictive information. This study aimed to investigate whether HMGCR expression in breast cancer patients was associated with patient and tumor characteristics and disease-free survival (DFS).

Methods: A population-based cohort of primary breast cancer patients in Lund, Sweden was assembled between October 2002 and June 2012 enrolling 1,116 patients. Tumor tissue microarrays were constructed and stained with a polyclonal HMGCR antibody (Cat. No HPA008338, Atlas Antibodies AB, Stockholm, Sweden, diluted 1:100) to assess the HMGCR expression in tumor tissue from 885 patients. HMGCR expression was analyzed in relation to patient- and tumor characteristics and disease-free survival (DFS) with last follow-up June 30th 2014.

Results: Moderate/strong HMGCR expression was associated with less axillary lymph node involvement, lower histological grade, estrogen and progesterone receptor positivity, HER2 negativity, and older patient age at diagnosis compared to weak or no HMGCR expression. Patients were followed for up to 11 years. The median follow-up time was 5.0 years for the 739 patients who were alive and still at risk at the last follow-up. HMGCR expression was not associated with DFS.

Conclusion: In this study, HMGCR expression was associated with less aggressive tumor characteristics. However, no association between HMGCR expression and DFS was observed. Longer follow-up may be needed to evaluate HMGCR as prognostic or predictive marker in breast cancer.

Keywords: Breast cancer, HMG-CoA reductase, Tumor characteristics, Treatment, Early breast cancer events, Prognosis

Introduction

New prognostic and treatment-predictive markers are needed to improve treatment decisions and consequently prognosis and treatment response in breast cancer patients. Recent data suggest that the enzyme 3-hydroxy-3-methylglutaryl-coenzyme A reductase (HMGCR), which is inhibited by statins that are commonly used as a cholesterol-lowering treatment, may be associated with breast tumor characteristics, prognosis and treatment response [1–3]. HMGCR is the rate-limiting enzyme in the mevalonate pathway [4]. The mevalonate pathway produces cholesterol, steroid hormones, and non-steroid isoprenoids, which are necessary for cell survival [5]. Previous studies demonstrated that HMGCR inhibitors (e.g., statins) exert anti-carcinogenic effects by inducing apoptosis and inhibiting inflammation [6], proliferation and migration [7–9]. HMGCR inhibitors can also inhibit angiogenesis [10]. Whether statins also reduce the risk of

* Correspondence: helena.jernstrom@med.lu.se
[1]Division of Oncology and Pathology, Department of Clinical Sciences, Lund, Lund University, Barngatan 2B, SE 22185 Lund, Sweden
Full list of author information is available at the end of the article

cancer remains debated [11–17]. HMGCR is differentially expressed among breast cancers, as well as between normal epithelial cells and tumor cells, with higher expression in the tumor cells. This difference is presumably caused by resistance against the feedback system of the mevalonate pathway [18]. Several studies examined the relationship between tumor-specific HMGCR expression and other tumor characteristics [1, 2]. In previous studies, stronger expression of HMGCR was associated with a less aggressive tumor profile, such as a low histological grade, a small tumor size, estrogen receptor (ER) positivity, and low proliferation [1, 2]. One study reported that patients with HMGCR-positive tumors exhibited longer recurrence-free survival, which was more pronounced in patients with ER-positive tumors [2]. Another study observed longer recurrence-free survival in patients treated with tamoxifen who had HMGCR-positive and ER-positive tumors compared to patients who had ER-positive and HMGCR-negative tumors, indicating that HMGCR may predict tamoxifen response [3].

Hypothesis and aim

We hypothesized that stronger HMGCR expression was associated with markers of good prognosis and prolonged disease-free survival (DFS), as well as a better response to tamoxifen, in this population-based unselected cohort of primary breast cancer patients. The aims of the study were to investigate whether HMGCR expression in breast cancer was associated with patient and tumor characteristics, prognosis and treatment response.

Materials and methods
Patients

Women diagnosed with a primary breast cancer at Skåne University Hospital in Lund, Sweden between October 2002 and June 2012 were invited to take part in an ongoing prospective cohort study: the Breast Cancer (BC) Blood study. During the inclusion period, 1,116 patients were included in the study and followed-up until June 30th, 2014. Patients with a previous breast cancer diagnosis or another cancer diagnosis during the previous ten years were not included. The aim was to study factors that could affect prognosis or treatment response and to identify new markers that may help better tailor adjuvant therapy to individual breast cancer patients. The study was approved by Lund University Ethics Committee (Dnr LU75-02, LU37-08, LU658-09, LU58-12, and LU379-12). All patients signed a written informed consent. The study adhered to the REMARK criteria [19].

All patients completed questionnaires preoperatively. Post-operative questionnaires were completed after 3–6 months, 7–9 months, and 1, 2, 3, 5, 7, 9 and 11 years. The questionnaires included questions concerning medication intake during the last week, lifestyle, and reproductive

factors. Medications were coded according to the Anatomic Therapeutic Chemical (ATC) classification system codes [20]. Patients who reported smoking during the last week or smoking at parties were considered current smokers. Coffee consumption was categorized as 0–1 or 2+ cups/day, as previously described [21]. A research nurse obtained body measurements, including, height, weight, waist and hip circumferences, and breast volumes, at the pre-operative visit. Breast volume was measured as previously described [22, 23].

Tumor characteristics were acquired from the patients' pathology reports. The estrogen receptor (ER) and progesterone receptor (PgR) expression were analyzed in the Department of Pathology at Skåne University Hospital in Lund, Sweden. Until December 2009, immunohistochemistry was performed using the Dako LSAB kit system (Dako, Glostrup, Denmark) and the M7047 (ER) and M3569 (PgR) antibodies (DAKO) [24, 25]. From 2010 onwards, the ER (SP1) and PgR (1E2) antibodies from Ventana Medical Systems (Ventana, AZ, USA) were used in combination with a Ventana Benchmark Ultra instrument (Ventana Medical Systems) [26]. Tumors with more than 10 % positive nuclear staining were considered ER-positive or PgR-positive according to current Swedish clinical guidelines. Histological type was classified into ductal, lobular and 'other' types. Ten tumors had a mixed ductal and lobular histology and were classified as 'other'. Since the tumors were not routinely analyzed for HER2 amplification until November 2005, patients included in the study prior to that time were excluded from analyses that included HER2 status.

Information on type of surgery, treatment, and breast cancer related events was obtained from patient charts and the regional tumor registry. The date of death was collected from the Swedish Population Registry. Patients who had received preoperative treatment (n = 51) and patients with cancer *in situ* (n = 39) were excluded from the analyses, leaving 1,026 preoperatively untreated patients with invasive breast cancer as the study population (Fig. 1).

Tissue microarray construction

Tumor tissue was available from 992 of the 1,026 patients. Tissue microarrays (TMAs) for the tumors were constructed by sampling 1 mm duplicate cores from representative, non-necrotic tumor regions from the donating formalin-fixed paraffin-embedded tumor tissue block from surgical resection, using a semi-automated tissue array device (Beecher Instruments, Sun Prairie, WI, USA).

Immunohistochemistry

An automatic PT-link system (DAKO, Glostrup, Denmark) was used to deparaffinize and pretreat 4 µm TMA-sections for HMGCR staining. HMGCR staining was performed

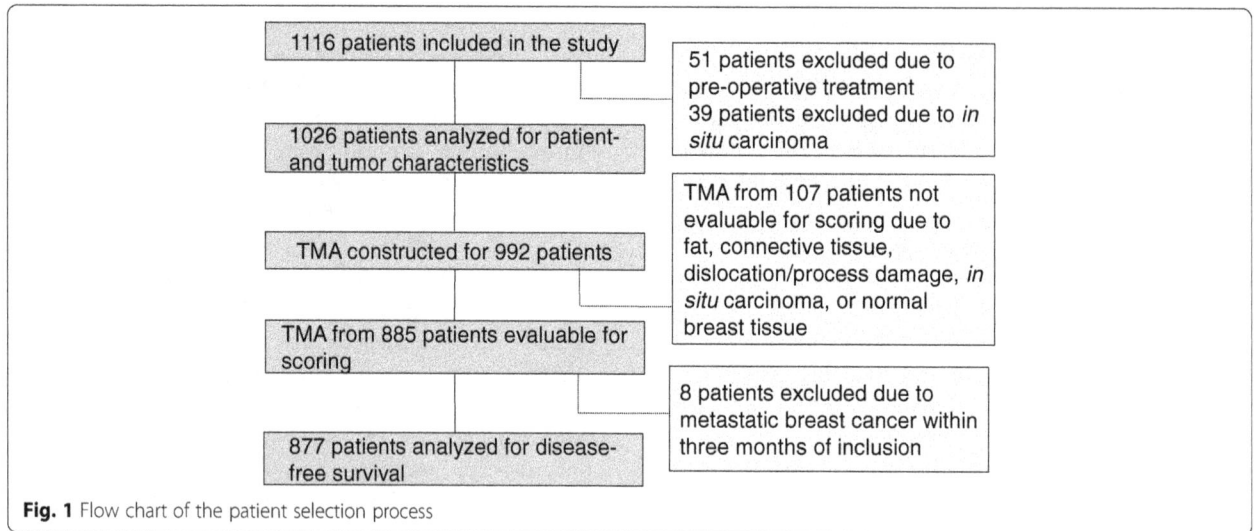

Fig. 1 Flow chart of the patient selection process

using an Autostainer Plus, according to the manufacturer's instructions (DAKO). The staining procedure employed an HMGCR antibody (Cat. No HPA008338, Atlas Antibodies AB, Stockholm, Sweden) (diluted 1:100) and an EnVision FLEX high-pH kit. HMGCR expression could be evaluated in tumors from 885/992 patients. In 57 cases, the TMA-cores contained non-representative tissue, in 27 cases, the cores were damaged or lost during processing, and in 23 cases, the cores could not be evaluated due to a combination of the reasons mentioned above. HMGCR expression was evaluated based on the staining intensity in the cytoplasm (i.e., negative = 0, weak = 1, moderate = 2, and strong = 3), as shown in Fig. 2, and based on the fraction of HMGCR-positive cells (0 % = 0, 1-10 % = 1, 11-50 % = 2, 51-100 % = 3). Two investigators, who were blinded to the patient data and clinical outcome, evaluated all samples simultaneously (EG, HT). When the two investigators could not reach a consensus, a senior investigator (SB) was consulted and a consensus was reached. The HMGCR expression differed between the duplicate cores for 109 patients. In all cases but one, the intensity only differed by one step. Discordant cores were reevaluated jointly to obtain a pooled score based on the intensity represented in the majority of cancer cells. When one core was classified as negative and the other core was classified as positive, the pooled score was classified as positive. Only 22 tumors showed strong intensity of HMGCR expression, and this group was combined with tumors expressing HMGCR with a moderate intensity (n = 195). A total of 28 of the 1,026 patients had bilateral tumors; tissue from both tumors was available for 15 patients. Scoring of both bilateral tumors was possible for 10 of these patients. For the three cases where the intensity differed, the highest intensity was used. In most cases (94.9 %) for which the staining was positive in any cell, HMGCR

was expressed in the majority of the cells (51-100 %). Therefore, the fraction of HMGCR-positive cells was excluded from further analyses.

Statistics

The statistical analyses were performed using SPSS Statistics 19 (IBM, Chicago, IL, USA). Patient and tumor characteristics were analyzed in relation to HMGCR expression. The Chi-square and Linear-by-Linear tests were used for categorical variables. The Kruskal-Wallis and Jonckheere-Terpstra tests were used for continuous variables because some of these variables were not normally distributed. Tumor characteristics in relation to HMGCR tumor expression were also analyzed with linear regression and adjusted for age as a continuous variable. The DFS was calculated from the date of inclusion until the first breast cancer related event (i.e., local or regional recurrence, contralateral breast cancer, or distant metastasis); in cases with no breast cancer related events, DFS was calculated using the last study follow-up or death before July 1st, 2014. Non-breast cancer-related death was censored at the time of death. Patients with distant metastases detected earlier than three months after inclusion were excluded from the survival analyses (n = 8). Univariable survival analyses were calculated using Log-Rank tests. Cox proportional hazard regression was used for multivariable testing, with adjustments for invasive tumor size (>20 mm or muscular or skin involvement), axillary lymph node involvement, histological grade (III), ER and PgR status (positive/negative), age <50 years (yes/no), current preoperative smoking (yes/no), and body mass index (BMI) <25 kg/m^2 (yes/no) [27]. All statistical tests were two-tailed. P-values < 0.05 were regarded as statistically significant. Nominal P-values were presented without adjustment for multiple testing.

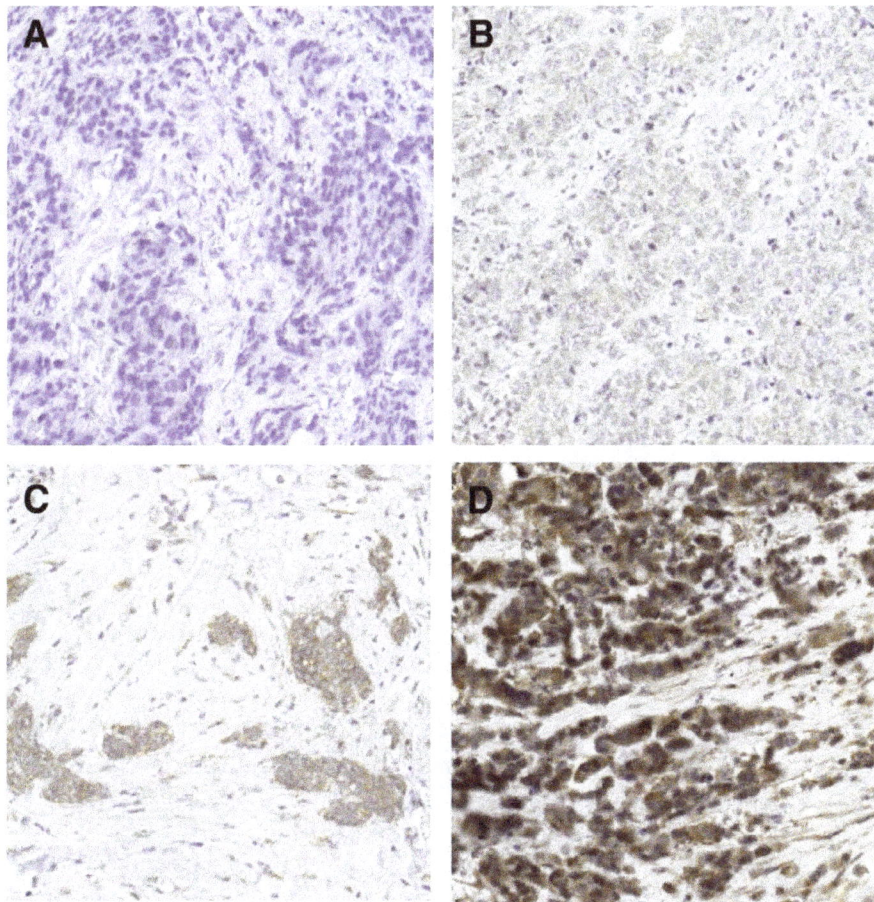

Fig. 2 Examples of HMGCR expression, representing no staining (**a**), and weak (**b**), moderate (**c**), and strong (**d**) expression. The original magnification before scale-down was 20x for each example

Results

Patient characteristics and HMGCR expression

The patient characteristics are presented in relation to the HMGCR expression (Table 1). Of the 885 cases evaluable for scoring, the intensity of HMGCR expression was negative in 113 cases (12.8 %), weak in 555 cases (62.7 %), and moderate/strong in 217 (24.5 %) cases. Patients of all ages were included (range 24–99 years). The median age at inclusion in the study was 61.1 years (interquartile range 52.1 to 68.1). Patients younger than 50 years at inclusion were significantly taller, had a lower BMI, and had smaller waist and hip circumferences, waist-to-hip ratios, and breast volumes than older patients ($P \leq 0.001$ for all comparisons); however, these patients had a weight similar to that of older patients. The final surgery performed included partial mastectomy in 531 cases (60 %) and modified radical mastectomy in 354 cases (40 %). Postoperative radiotherapy was given to 559 patients (63.2 %) and 226 patients (25.5 %) received adjuvant chemotherapy. As adjuvant endocrine therapy, tamoxifen treatment was prescribed to 466 patients (52.7 %) and 302 patients (34.1 %) were

treated with aromatase inhibitors. As of November 2005, 55 patients (8.6 %) had received adjuvant treatment with trastuzumab (n = 640). Patients often received more than one type of treatment.

Patients with tumors that expressed moderate/strong HMGCR were significantly older than patients in the other HMGCR intensity groups at inclusion. Patients with tumors that expressed weak HMGCR were significantly taller than patients in the other HMGCR intensity groups. No other significant associations were observed between patient characteristics and HMGCR expression. The results remained essentially the same when excluding patients who reported statin usage preoperatively (n = 99).

HMGCR expression and established tumor characteristics

Table 2 displays the tumor characteristics in relation to HMGCR expression. Tumor size was not associated with HMGCR expression. Tumors that expressed moderate/strong HMGCR were of significantly lower histological grade, were more frequently ER-positive, PgR-positive, and HER2-negative, and were less likely to show axillary lymph

Table 1 Association of HMGCR expression with patient characteristics

	All patients median (IQR) or %	Missing	Patients with evaluable TMA	HMGCR expression-Intensity median (IQR) or %			
				No staining = 0	Weak = 1	Moderate/Strong = 2/3	P-value
n=	1026		885	113	555	217	
Age at inclusion, yrs	61.1 (52.1-68.1)	0	60.9 (52.2-67.9)	61.2 (53.7-69.2)	60.1 (51.6-67.4)	64.3 (53.9-69.4)	0.004^c
Body mass index (BMI), (kg/m-2)	25.1 (22.5-28.3)	28	25.2 (22.5-28.4)	25.7 (23.2-28.7)	25.0 (22.4-28.3)	25.3 (22.5-29.0)	0.39^c
Height (cm)	165 (162–170)	26	165 (162–170)	164 (160–169)	166 (162–170)	165 (161–169)	0.03^c
Weight (kg)	69 (62–78)	26	69 (62–78)	70 (62–79)	69 (62–78)	69 (61–80)	0.91^c
Waist-Hip-Ratio	0.86 (0.81-0.9)	38	0.86 (0.81-0.90)	0.86 (0.81-0.92)	0.85 (0.80-0.90)	0.86 (0.81-0.90)	0.32^c
Waist (cm)	87 (79–97)	38	87 (80–97)	89 (82–97)	87 (79–97)	89 (80–98)	0.24^c
Hip (cm)	102 (97–109)	38	102 (97–109)	104 (99–109)	102 (97–109)	102 (96–111)	0.57^c
Breast volume (ml)	1000 (650–1500)	161	1000 (650–1550)	1000 (700–1550)	950 (640–1500)	1000 (656–1600)	0.28^c
Age at menarche, yrs	13 (12–14)	7	13 (12–14)	13 (13–14)	13 (12–14)	13 (12–14)	0.68^c
Nulliparous	124 (12.1 %)	1	109 (12.3 %)	17 (15.0 %)	67 (12.1 %)	25 (11.5 %)	0.41^d
Parity	2 (1–3)	1	2 (1–3)	2 (1–3)	2 (1–3)	2 (1–2)	0.46^c
Age at first child, years*	25 (22–28)	6	24 (22–28)	24 (21–27)	25 (21–28)	25 (22–29)	0.09^b
Ever use of HRT	449 (43.9 %)	3	386 (43.8 %)	55 (48.7 %)	231 (41.8 %)	100 (43.8 %)	0.28^a
Ever oral contraceptives	726 (70.8 %)	1	625 (70.7 %)	82 (72.6 %)	394 (71.1 %)	149 (68.7 %)	0.42^d
Current smoker	210 (20.5 %)	2	177 (20.0 %)	26 (23.0 %)	111 (20.1 %)	40 (18.4 %)	0.34^d
Coffee, 2+ cups per day	832 (81.4 %)	4	708 (80.4 %)	89 (78.8 %)	448 (81.3 %)	171 (78.8 %)	0.66^a
Alcohol abstainer	107 (10.5 %)	7	96 (10.9 %)	15 (13.3 %)	56 (10.1 %)	25 (11.6 %)	0.58^a

*Among Parous women, IQR = Inter quartile range ^{a}Chi-Square, ^{b}Jonckheere-Terpstra, ^{c}Kruskal-Wallis, ^{d}Linear-by-linear

node involvement compared to patients whose tumors had weak or no HMGCR expression. Histological type was not associated with HMGCR expression. HER2 amplification was more common among patients with HMGCR-negative tumors. These associations remained significant after adjustment for age. The results remained essentially the same after exclusion of patients with preoperative statin usage. Ki67 was only available for 365 patients (41.2 %) and was not further analyzed.

Risk of early breast cancer related events

Patients were followed for up to 11 years. The median follow-up time was 5.0 years (interquartile range 3.0-7.2 years) for the 739 patients who were alive and still at risk at the last follow-up. The total number of patients with a breast cancer related event during follow-up was 104, of whom 68 patients were diagnosed with distant metastases. Of these 104 patients with a breast cancer related event, 53 patients subsequently died during follow-up. An additional 34 patients died without a prior recorded breast cancer related event. No significant association was observed between HMGCR expression and DFS either in univariable (Log-Rank $P_{trend} = 0.42$) (Fig. 3) or or multivariable models (Table 3). Likewise, no difference in DFS was observed between patients with any HMGCR expression and patients with HMGCR-negative tumors (Log-Rank $P_{trend} = 0.90$). In

addition, no significant association was observed between HMGCR expression and distant metastasis-free survival (Log-Rank $P_{trend} = 0.44$), or overall survival (Log-Rank $P_{trend} = 0.87$). The results remained essentially the same in analyses restricted to patients with ER-positive tumors. Further stratification according to ER status, treatment (e.g., tamoxifen, aromatase inhibitors, radiotherapy, or chemotherapy), age or BMI failed to yield any significant associations between HMGCR expression and DFS in either univariable or multivariable models. The results remained essentially the same when excluding preoperative statin users. Similarly, the results did not differ when three patients with *in situ* breast cancer related events were excluded.

Discussion

The main finding of this study was that moderate/strong HMGCR expression was significantly associated with several indolent tumor characteristics, including lower histological grade, ER and PgR positivity, HER2 negativity, and less axillary lymph node involvement. These findings are largely consistent with a previous study that reported an association between stronger HMGCR expression and small tumor size, low histological grade, low Ki67, and ER expression [1]. However, in the present study, no association was observed between tumor size and HMGCR expression, and Ki67 was not included in

Table 2 Association of HMGCR expression with tumor characteristics

	All patients median (IQR) or %	Missing	Patients with evaluable TMA	HMGCR expression-Intensity median (IQR) or %			
				No staining = 0	Weak = 1	Moderate/Strong = 2/3	P-value
n=	1026		885	113	555	217	
pT		0					0.77[a]
1	740 (72.1 %)		631 (71.3 %)	77 (68.1 %)	404 (72.8 %)	150 (69.1 %)	
2	269 (26.2 %)		238 (26.9 %)	34 (30.1 %)	140 (25.2 %)	64 (29.5 %)	
3	15 (1.5 %)		14 (1.6 %)	2 (1.8 %)	9 (1.6 %)	31 (1.4 %)	
4	2 (0.2 %)		2 (0.2 %)	0 (0 %)	2 (0.4 %)	0 (0 %)	
Axillary node involvement		2					0.020[b]
0	627 (61.2 %)		532 (60.2 %)	60 (53.1 %)	330 (59.6 %)	142 (65.7 %)	
1-3	306 (29.9 %)		270 (30.6 %)	37 (32.7 %)	177 (31.9 %)	56 (25.9 %)	
4+	91 (8.9 %)		81 (9.2 %)	16 (14.2 %)	47 (8.5 %)	18 (8.3 %)	
Histological grade		1					0.013[b]
I	252 (24.6 %)		203 (22.9 %)	20 (17.7 %)	126 (22.7 %)	57 (26.3 %)	
II	511 (49.9 %)		443 (50.1 %)	54 (47.8 %)	278 (50.1 %)	111 (51.2 %)	
III	262 (25.6 %)		239 (27.0 %)	39 (34.5 %)	151 (27.2 %)	49 (22.6 %)	
Histological type		1					0.512[a]
Mainly ductal	836 (81.6 %)		737 (83.4 %)	96 (85.0 %)	467 (84.3 %)	174 (80.2 %)	
Mainly lobular	121 (11.8 %)		97 (11.0 %)	11 (9.7 %)	55 (9.9 %)	31 (14.3 %)	
Other or mixed	66 (6.4 %)		50 (5.7 %)	6 (5.3 %)	32 (5.8 %)	12 (5.5 %)	
Hormone receptor status		2					
ER+	896 (87.5 %)		771 (87.2 %)	84 (74.3 %)	484 (87.4 %)	203 (93.5 %)	<0.0001[b]
PgR+	726 (70.9 %)		627 (70.9 %)	70 (61.9 %)	389 (70.2 %)	168 (77.4 %)	0.003[b]
HER 2 amplification*		59					0.009[b]
HER 2 positive	86 (11.7 %)		71 (11.1 %)	13 (21.0 %)	46 (11.2 %)	12 (7.2 %)	
HER 2 negative	601 (81.4 %)		527 (82.3 %)	47 (75.8 %)	340 (82.7 %)	140 (83.8 %)	

*Patients younger than 70 years of age and included as of November 2005 [a]Chi-Square, [b]Linear-by-linear

the analyses as this marker was not routinely analyzed until March 2009 [28].

Patients with tumors that expressed moderate/strong HMGCR were significantly older at the time of inclusion in the present study, and only one of the patients with strong HMGCR staining was less than 50 years of age. This finding is consistent with another study that studied premenopausal patients and reported no tumors with strong expression of this marker [3]. ER-positive tumors are more common in postmenopausal patients than in premenopausal patients [29]. In the present study, moderate/strong HMGCR expression was associated with ER positivity, indicating that there might be an association between age, HMGCR expression and ER-positive tumors. This association may be linked to 27-hydroxycholesterol (27HC), which is a primary cholesterol metabolite and a selective estrogen receptor modulator (SERM) exerting ER agonistic effects, as recently shown in a study of murine models [30, 31]. The study demonstrated how conversion of cholesterol to 27HC was necessary for effects on ER-positive breast cancer cells and how the actions of 27HC

on tumor growth were dependent on ER. Those findings shed light on how 27HC may promote cancer growth and serve as the link between hypercholesterolemia and ER-positive breast cancer in postmenopausal women.

Normal cells can obtain cellular cholesterol in two ways; either via receptor-mediated uptake (low-density-lipoprotein receptor) or by synthesizing cholesterol through the mevalonate pathway and the activity of HMGCR. The normal cellular response to low intracellular cholesterol levels is to increase HMGCR activity to maintain an intact mevalonate pathway. However, tumor cells that fail to respond to this feed-back loop might have lost the checkpoint controls that maintain an intact pathway or may have a deregulated pathway [1, 32]. This dysregulation of the mevalonate pathway and HMGCR activity can contribute to the transformation involved in oncogenesis and may be essential for the metabolic transformation of tumor cells, at least in some cancers [32]. Therefore, potential biomarkers within the mevalonate pathway that could predict the response to statin treatment are of interest.

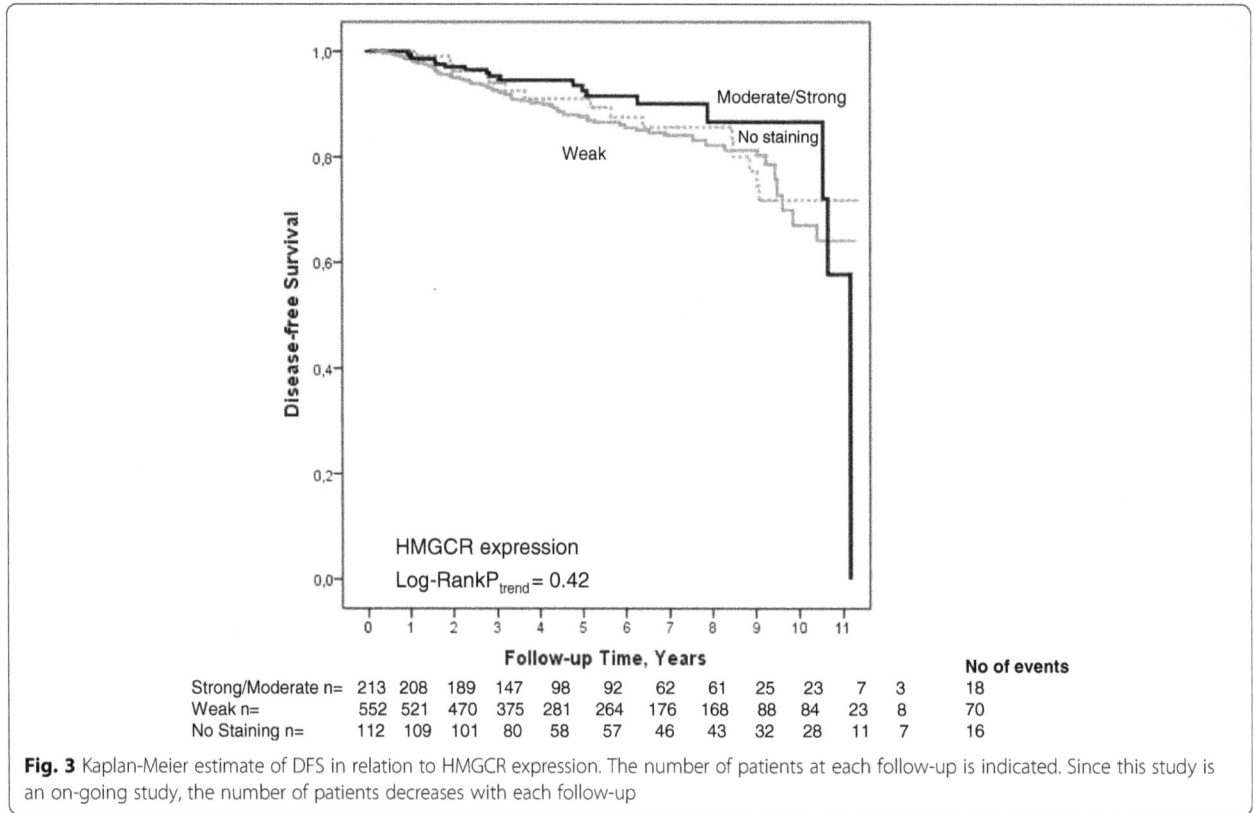

Fig. 3 Kaplan-Meier estimate of DFS in relation to HMGCR expression. The number of patients at each follow-up is indicated. Since this study is an on-going study, the number of patients decreases with each follow-up

A previous study has reported that ER-negative breast cancer is less likely to arise among statin users and that ER-negative cell lines are more sensitive to statin inhibition than ER-positive cell lines [33]. In the present study, tumors that were negative for both ER and HMGCR had a higher histological grade significantly more often than tumors that were positive for these markers (data not shown). This association may reflect an inability of less differentiated cancer cells to maintain an intact mevalonate pathway. It was previously proposed that

some cancer cells could be statin-sensitive and unable to maintain adequate levels of mevalonate end products when exposed to statins, resulting in apoptosis [32]. In contrast, statin-insensitive tumor cells demonstrate a feedback response similar to that of normal cells, in which HMGCR is up-regulated; this response may protect these cells from the anticancer effects of statins [32]. It is possible that well-differentiated cancer cells but not less differentiated cancer cells are capable of initiating this response. Further studies are needed to explain the role of HMGCR in breast cancer.

Table 3 Multivariable analysis of risk for breast cancer related events in relation to HMGCR status in all patients

	HR	95 % CI Lower	Upper
HMGCR no staining	1.000		
HMGCR weak expression	1.389	0.792	2.436
HMGCR moderate/strong expression	1.103	0.548	2.218
Invasive tumor size ≥ 21 mm or muscular/skin involvement	2.041	1.329	3.133
Axillary nodal involvement	1.427	0.946	2.153
Histological grade III	1.292	0.789	2.115
ER status	0.596	0.316	1.125
PgR status	0.740	0.448	1.223
Age ≥ 50 years	0.647	0.416	1.005
BMI ≥ 25 kg/m^2	1.305	0.867	1.966
Preoperative smoker	1.289	0.811	2.050

No significant association was observed between HMGCR expression and DFS in the present study. Two previous studies reported associations between recurrence-free survival and HMGCR expression [2, 3]. However, the median follow-up time of the present study was only 5.0 years, compared to median follow-up times of 10.7 years [2] and 13.9 years [3] in the previous studies. Moderate/strong HMGCR expression was strongly associated with ER-positive tumors. ER-positive tumors are known to relapse later than ER-negative tumors; because 87.5 % of the patients in the present study had ER-positive tumors, a longer follow-up time may be needed [34].

HMGCR expression was negative in 12.8 % of the cases in this study. The percentage of tumors with negative staining varied between 18 % and 52.7 % of cases in previous studies [1–3, 35]. However, these studies had fewer tumors that stained for HMGCR. In addition, one study included only premenopausal patients [3], which may have affected the results because HMGCR was significantly associated with age in the present study. Although the intensity varied between studies, the finding in the current study that HMGCR is expressed in the majority of the cells when present is consistent with other studies [2, 3].

HMGCR is differentially expressed and often overexpressed in tumor cells [18] and high expression appears to be associated with less aggressive tumor characteristics [1, 2]. Previous studies reported that HMGCR expression was a good prognostic marker [2, 3]. A previous window-of-opportunity study demonstrated that patients who were treated with statins for two weeks pre-operatively exhibited increased expression of HMGCR in the tumor and a reduced proliferation rate of Ki67 [35]. The increase of HMGCR expression that occurs after statin treatment indicate that statins affected the tumor either directly through inhibition of HMGCR and the mevalonate pathway within the tumor or indirectly through lowered circulating levels of cholesterol and in both cases, a negative feed-back loop resulting in elevated intratumoral HMGCR levels [32]. Associations of HMGCR expression with more favorable tumor characteristics and a prolonged survival have also been demonstrated in patients with other types of cancer such as colorectal cancer [36].

Some limitations of this study should be considered. One weakness of the present study may be that HMGCR expression was evaluated on TMAs rather than in whole slide tumor tissue sections. However, a previous study stained five whole slide tumor tissue sections for HMGCR and this marker was homogeneously expressed in all of the sections [1]. Therefore, we believe that the HMGCR results obtained from TMAs are representative. The BC-blood study is an ongoing, population-based prospective study, which limits the risk for recall bias. The most common reason that patients did not participate in the present study was the lack of available research nurses. A previous study demonstrated that the patients who did not participate had patient and tumor characteristics similar to those who did participate [28]. This similarity makes the findings generalizable for breast cancer patients at Skåne University Hospital in Lund, Sweden. The patients were never asked about ethnicity. However, the majority of the patients were ethnic Swedes. To the authors' knowledge, the variation of HMGCR expression in cancer cells among different ethnic groups has not been investigated previously.

In conclusion, high HMGCR expression appears to be associated with less aggressive tumor characteristics in this population-based cohort of unselected primary breast cancer patients. Despite this finding, no association between HMGCR expression and short-term DFS was observed. Since previous studies had longer follow-up times, their findings can be neither confirmed nor rejected. Further studies and a prolonged follow-up time are needed to evaluate HMGCR as a prognostic and treatment-predictive marker.

Abbreviations
ATC: Anatomic Therapeutic Chemical; BMI: Body mass index; DFS: Disease-free survival; ER: Estrogen receptor; HER2: Human epidermal growth factor 2; HMGCR: 3-hydroxy-3-methylglutaryl-coenzyme A reductase; 27-OHC: 27-hydroxycholesterol; PgR: Progesterone receptor; REMARK: Recommendations for tumour MARKer prognostic studies; TMA: Tissue micro array.

Competing interests
The authors declare that they have no competing interests.

Authors' contributions
EG and HT performed the immunohistochemical evaluation. EG performed the statistical analyses and drafted the manuscript. HT has been involved in analysis and interpretation of data, and in revising the manuscript critically. AM and MS have been involved in acquisition of data and have revised the manuscript. BN constructed TMAs, carried out the IHC staining, and assisted with the immunohistochemical evaluation. KJ evaluated all tumors prior to TMA construction and revised the manuscript critically for important intellectual content. CI and CR have been involved in conception and design of the study and have revised the manuscript. SB was involved in conception and design of the study, performed immunohistochemical re-evaluation of selected cases, analysis and interpretation of data and revising the manuscript critically for important intellectual content. HJ has been involved in acquisition of data, in conception and design of the study, analysis and interpretation of data, in drafting the manuscript, and has revised the manuscript critically for important intellectual content. All authors have read and approved the final version of the manuscript.

Acknowledgments
This work was supported by grants from The Swedish Cancer Society (CAN 2011/497), the Swedish Research Council (K2012-54X-22027-01-3) (PI H Jernström), the Medical Faculty at Lund University, the Mrs. Berta Kamprad Foundation, the Gunnar Nilsson Foundation, the Swedish Breast Cancer Group (BRO), the South Swedish Health Care Region (Region Skåne ALF), Konung Gustaf V:s Jubileumsfond, the Lund Hospital Fund, the RATHER consortium (http://www.ratherproject.com/) and the Seventh Framework programme. The funding sources had no involvement in the collection, analysis and interpretation of data; in the writing of the report; or in the decision to submit the article for publication.
We thank our research nurses Maj-Britt Hedenblad, Karin Henriksson, Anette Möller, Monika Meszaros, Anette Ahlin Gullers, Anita Schmidt Casslén, Helén Thell, Linda Ågren, and Jessica Åkesson. We thank Erika Bågeman, Maria Hietala, and Maria Henningson for data entry, Elise Nilsson for TMA construction, and Kristina Lövgren and Catarina Blennow for sectioning.

Author details
[1]Division of Oncology and Pathology, Department of Clinical Sciences, Lund, Lund University, Barngatan 2B, SE 22185 Lund, Sweden. [2]Department of Oncology, Skåne University Hospital, Lund, Sweden. [3]CREATE Health and Department of Immunotechnology, Lund University, Medicon Village, Building 406, Lund, Sweden. [4]Department of Clinical Sciences, Division of Surgery, Lund, Lund University, Lund, Sweden and Skåne University Hospital, Lund, Sweden.

References

1. Borgquist S, Djerbi S, Ponten F, Anagnostaki L, Goldman M, Gaber A, et al. HMG-CoA reductase expression in breast cancer is associated with a less aggressive phenotype and influenced by anthropometric factors. Int J Cancer. 2008;123:1146–53.

2. Borgquist S, Jögi A, Ponten F, Rydén L, Brennan DJ, Jirström K. Prognostic impact of tumour-specific HMG-CoA reductase expression in primary breast cancer. Breast Cancer Res. 2008;10:R79.

3. Brennan DJ, Laursen H, O'Connor DP, Borgquist S, Uhlen M, Gallagher WM, et al. Tumor-specific HMG-CoA reductase expression in primary premenopausal breast cancer predicts response to tamoxifen. Breast Cancer Res. 2011;13:R12.

4. Goldstein JL, Brown MS. Regulation of the mevalonate pathway. Nature. 1990;343:425–30.

5. Mo H, Elson CE. Studies of the isoprenoid-mediated inhibition of mevalonate synthesis applied to cancer chemotherapy and chemoprevention. Exp Biol Med. 2004;229:567–85.

6. Jain MK, Ridker PM. Anti-inflammatory effects of statins: clinical evidence and basic mechanisms. Nat Rev Drug Discov. 2005;4:977–87.

7. Campbell MJ, Esserman LJ, Zhou Y, Shoemaker M, Lobo M, Borman E, et al. Breast cancer growth prevention by statins. Cancer Res. 2006;66:8707–14.

8. Wejde J, Blegen H, Larsson O. Requirement for mevalonate in the control of proliferation of human breast cancer cells. Anticancer Res. 1992;12:317–24.

9. Wong WW, Dimitroulakos J, Minden MD, Penn LZ. HMG-CoA reductase inhibitors and the malignant cell: the statin family of drugs as triggers of tumor-specific apoptosis. Leukemia. 2002;16:508–19.

10. Dulak J, Jozkowicz A. Anti-angiogenic and anti-inflammatory effects of statins: relevance to anti-cancer therapy. Curr Cancer Drug Targets. 2005;5:579–94.

11. Friis S, Poulsen AH, Johnsen SP, McLaughlin JK, Fryzek JP, Dalton SO, et al. Cancer risk among statin users: a population-based cohort study. Int J Cancer. 2005;114:643–7.

12. Strandberg TE, Pyorala K, Cook TJ, Wilhelmsen L, Faergeman O, Thorgeirsson G, et al. Mortality and incidence of cancer during 10-year follow-up of the Scandinavian Simvastatin Survival Study (4S). Lancet. 2004;364:771–7.

13. Beck P, Wysowski DK, Downey W, Butler-Jones D. Statin use and the risk of breast cancer. J Clin Epidemiol. 2003;56:280–5.

14. Boudreau DM, Yu O, Miglioretti DL, Buist DS, Heckbert SR, Daling JR. Statin use and breast cancer risk in a large population-based setting. Cancer Epidemiol Biomarkers Prev. 2007;16:416–21.

15. Desai P, Chlebowski R, Cauley JA, Manson JE, Wu C, Martin LW, et al. Prospective analysis of association between statin use and breast cancer risk in the women's health initiative. Cancer Epidemiol Biomarkers Prev. 2013;22:1868–76.

16. Kaye JA, Jick H. Statin use and cancer risk in the General Practice Research Database. Br J Cancer. 2004;90:635–7.

17. Nielsen SF, Nordestgaard BG, Bojesen SE. Statin use and reduced cancer-related mortality. N Engl J Med. 2012;367:1792–802.

18. Elson CE, Peffley DM, Hentosh P, Mo H. Isoprenoid-mediated inhibition of mevalonate synthesis: potential application to cancer. Exp Biol Med. 1999;221:294–311.

19. McShane LM, Altman DG, Sauerbrei W, Taube SE, Gion M, Clark GM. REporting recommendations for tumor MARKer prognostic studies (REMARK). Breast Cancer Res Treat. 2006;100:229–35.

20. Markkula A, Hietala M, Henningson M, Ingvar C, Rose C, Jernstrom H. Clinical profiles predict early nonadherence to adjuvant endocrine treatment in a prospective breast cancer cohort. Cancer Prev Res. 2012;5:735–45.

21. Simonsson M, Söderlind V, Henningson M, Hjertberg M, Rose C, Ingvar C, et al. Coffee prevents early events in tamoxifen-treated breast cancer patients and modulates hormone receptor status. Cancer Causes Control. 2013;24:929–40.

22. Ringberg A, Bågeman E, Rose C, Ingvar C, Jernström H. Of cup and bra size: reply to a prospective study of breast size and premenopausal breast cancer incidence. Int J Cancer. 2006;119:2242–3. author reply 2244.

23. Markkula A, Bromee A, Henningson M, Hietala M, Ringberg A, Ingvar C, et al. Given breast cancer, does breast size matter? Data from a prospective breast cancer cohort. Cancer Causes Control. 2012;23:1307–16.

24. Bågeman E, Ingvar C, Rose C, Jernström H. Coffee consumption and CYP1A2*1 F genotype modify age at breast cancer diagnosis and estrogen receptor status. Cancer Epidemiol Biomarkers Prev. 2008;17:895–901.

25. Jernström H, Bågeman E, Rose C, Jönsson PE, Ingvar C. CYP2C8 and CYP2C9 polymorphisms in relation to tumour characteristics and early breast cancer related events among 652 breast cancer patients. Br J Cancer. 2009;101:1817–23.

26. Simonsson M, Markkula A, Bendahl PO, Rose C, Ingvar C, Jernström H. Pre- and postoperative alcohol consumption in breast cancer patients: impact on early events. SpringerPlus. 2014;3:261.

27. World Health Organization. BMI Classification. 2006. http://apps.who.int/bmi/index.jsp?introPage = intro_3.html Access date March 24, 2014

28. Lundin KB, Henningson M, Hietala M, Ingvar C, Rose C, Jernström H. Androgen receptor genotypes predict response to endocrine treatment in breast cancer patients. Br J Cancer. 2011;105:1676–83.

29. Rose DP, Vona-Davis L. Interaction between menopausal status and obesity in affecting breast cancer risk. Maturitas. 2010;66:33–8.

30. Nelson ER, Wardell SE, Jasper JS, Park S, Suchindran S, Howe MK, et al. 27-Hydroxycholesterol links hypercholesterolemia and breast cancer pathophysiology. Science. 2013;342:1094–8.

31. Warner M, Gustafsson JA. On estrogen, cholesterol metabolism, and breast cancer. N Engl J Med. 2014;370:572–3.

32. Clendening JW, Penn LZ. Targeting tumor cell metabolism with statins. Oncogene. 2012;31:4967–78.

33. Kumar AS, Benz CC, Shim V, Minami CA, Moore DH, Esserman LJ. Estrogen receptor-negative breast cancer is less likely to arise among lipophilic statin users. Cancer Epidemiol Biomarkers Prev. 2008;17:1028–33.

34. Osborne CK, Yochmowitz MG, Knight 3rd WA, McGuire WL. The value of estrogen and progesterone receptors in the treatment of breast cancer. Cancer. 1980;46:2884–8.

35. Bjarnadottir O, Romero Q, Bendahl PO, Jirström K, Rydén L, Loman N, et al. Targeting HMG-CoA reductase with statins in a window-of-opportunity breast cancer trial. Breast Cancer Res Treat. 2013;138:499–508.

36. Bengtsson E, Nerjovaj P, Wangefjord S, Nodin B, Eberhard J, Uhlen M, et al. HMG-CoA reductase expression in primary colorectal cancer correlates with favourable clinicopathological characteristics and an improved clinical outcome. Diagn Pathol. 2014;9:78.

5

Impact of add-on laboratory testing at an academic medical center: a five year retrospective study

Louis S. Nelson[1], Scott R. Davis[1], Robert M. Humble[1], Jeff Kulhavy[1], Dean R. Aman[2] and Matthew D. Krasowski[1*]

Abstract

Background: Clinical laboratories frequently receive orders to perform additional tests on existing specimens ('add-ons'). Previous studies have examined add-on ordering patterns over short periods of time. The objective of this study was to analyze add-on ordering patterns over an extended time period. We also analyzed the impact of a robotic specimen archival/retrieval system on add-on testing procedure and manual effort.

Methods: In this retrospective study at an academic medical center, electronic health records from were searched to obtain all add-on orders that were placed in the time period of May 2, 2009 to December 31, 2014.

Results: During the time period of retrospective study, 880,359 add-on tests were ordered on 96,244 different patients. Add-on testing comprised 3.3 % of total test volumes. There were 443,411 unique ordering instances, leading to an average of 1.99 add-on tests per instance. Some patients had multiple episodes of add-on test orders at different points in time, leading to an average of 9.15 add-on tests per patient. The majority of add-on orders were for chemistry tests (78.8 % of total add-ons) with the next most frequent being hematology and coagulation tests (11.2 % of total add-ons). Inpatient orders accounted for 66.8 % of total add-on orders, while the emergency department and outpatient clinics had 14.8 % and 18.4 % of total add-on orders, respectively. The majority of add-ons were placed within 8 hours (87.3 %) and nearly all by 24 hours (96.8 %). Nearly 100 % of add-on orders within the emergency department were placed within 8 hours. The introduction of a robotic specimen archival/retrieval unit saved an average of 2.75 minutes of laboratory staff manual time per unique add-on order. This translates to 24.1 hours/day less manual effort in dealing with add-on orders.

Conclusion: Our study reflects the previous literature in showing that add-on orders significantly impact the workload of the clinical laboratory. The majority of add-on orders are clinical chemistry tests, and most add-on orders occur within 24 hours of original specimen collection. Robotic specimen archival/retrieval units can reduce manual effort in the clinical laboratory associated with add-on orders.

Keywords: Clinical chemistry tests, Clinical laboratory information services, Clinical laboratory services, Hematology, Laboratory automation, Robotics

* Correspondence: mkrasows@healthcare.uiowa.edu
[1]Department of Pathology, University of Iowa Hospitals and Clinics, Iowa City, IA 52242, USA
Full list of author information is available at the end of the article

Background

Clinical laboratories frequently receive orders to perform additional tests on existing specimens ('add-ons'). Melanson et al. in 2004 was the first published report analyzing the operational impact of add-on testing, demonstrating patterns of misutilization (e.g., failure to follow laboratory testing algorithms in institutional chest pain protocols) in a significant fraction of add-on orders [1]. A follow-up study in 2006 compared add-on testing between two academic hospitals, showing similarities in add-on ordering patterns and proposing strategies to improve the process [2]. There have been several other studies on add-on test ordering, each analyzing less than one month of add-on orders [3–5].

In this study at an academic medical center, we retrospectively analyzed add-on testing data over a five and a half year period (May 2009- Dec 2014). This allowed for the analysis of add-on ordering trends over a much longer period of time than in previous studies. Also, during this time period, the core clinical laboratory of the institution introduced a robotic archival specimen retrieval system that changed the add-on testing procedure. We analyzed the impact of this unit on add-on testing procedure and manual workload.

Methods

Institutional setting

The study was approved by the University of Iowa Institutional Review Board as a retrospective study covering the time period from May 2, 2009- December 31, 2014. In this large retrospective study, there was waiver of informed consent and authorization approved by the Institutional Review Board for all subjects. The institution in this study is the University of Iowa Hospitals and Clinics (UIHC), a 730 bed academic medical center that includes an emergency department (ED) with level one trauma capability, adult and pediatric inpatient floors, and multiple intensive care units (ICUs; neonatal, pediatric, medical, cardiovascular, and neurologic/surgical). Outpatient services are located at the main medical campus in Iowa City, IA, as well as at a multispecialty outpatient facility located three miles away. Smaller primary care clinics are located throughout the local region. A core clinical laboratory within the Department of Pathology provides clinical chemistry and hematopathology testing. Two critical care laboratories (one located near the main operating rooms and another embedded within the neonatal ICU) perform blood gas and activated clotting time testing. There are also separate clinical laboratories for anatomic pathology, blood center, and microbiology/molecular pathology located within the main medical campus.

Hospital and laboratory informatics

The electronic health record (EHR) for UIHC was Epic (Epic Systems, Inc, Madison, WI). Computerized provider order entry (CPOE) is available in Epic to licensed independent providers. Add-on orders can be placed within the EHR by CPOE or by calling the laboratory. Throughout the period of retrospective study, providers were directed, when feasible, to place orders within the EHR and limit the number of verbal orders requiring laboratory-initiated testing orders. In general, chemistry and hematology tests are all orderable individually. However, there are some panels built in Epic: basic metabolic panel with total calcium (BMP; sodium, chloride, carbon dioxide, potassium, blood urea nitrogen, creatinine, glucose, total calcium), electrolyte panel (sodium, chloride, carbon dioxide, potassium), complete blood count (CBC; white blood cell count, hemoglobin, hematocrit, red blood cell count, platelet count), and lipid panel (total cholesterol, high-density lipoprotein, triglycerides, calculated low-density lipoprotein). For the purposes of analysis in this manuscript, panels were broken apart into individual tests except where described otherwise. Categories of testing were also defined (Table 1) to provide better comparison to other published studies on add-on testing [1, 2, 5].

The laboratory information system (LIS) for all UIHC pathology laboratories until August 2, 2014 was Cerner (Kansas City, MO, USA) "Classic", currently version 015. On August 2, 2014, the clinical pathology laboratories switched to Epic Beaker as the LIS, retaining Cerner as the LIS for anatomic pathology, blood center, and some parts of hematopathology and molecular pathology. The switch to Epic Beaker allowed for accurate capture of the timing of add-on orders relative to when the original specimen was received in the laboratory. During this nearly 5 month period (August 2 to December 31, 2014), there were 56,389 add-on orders with complete time data.

Laboratory instrumentation and add-on testing procedures

The instrumentation and informatics within the core laboratory of UIHC has been described in detail in previous reports [6, 7]. Throughout the time period of retrospective analysis, the main chemistry instrumentation in the core laboratory was from Roche Diagnostics (Indianapolis, IN, USA). Front-end automation was provided by a Modular Pre-Analytic (MPA)-7 unit. In February 2014, the core laboratory went live with a Roche Diagnostics P701 automated archival/retrieval system. This system changed the add-on process (Fig. 1). Originally, specimens were placed into archival racks by the instrument flexible sample sorters. The most recent racks were kept near the instruments. The racks were then archived manually to a set of refrigerators for storage for 3 to 5 days (dependent on available refrigerator space and number of specimens). The P701 automated the sample storage and retrieval process (Fig. 1b), eliminating manual steps.

The manual effort involved from the moment the add-on is printed into the laboratory to the time the sample is

Table 1 Abbreviations for assay categories

Abbreviation	Full Name	Test(s) Included
A1C	Hemoglobin A1C	Hemoglobin A1C
ANEMIA	Anemia Testing	Iron, total iron-binding capacity, ferritin, folate, vitamin B_{12}
BILD	Bilirubin, Direct	Direct (conjugated) bilirubin
BMP	Basic Metabolic Panel	Sodium, potassium, chloride, carbon dioxide, blood urea nitrogen, creatinine, glucose, and calcium
CARDIAC	Cardiac Markers	Creatine kinase-MB, troponin T, N-terminal B-type natriuretic peptide
CBC	Complete Blood Count	White blood cell count, red blood cell count, hemoglobin, hematocrit, platelet count
CRP	C-Reactive Protein	C-Reactive Protein
DIFF	Differential	White blood cell differential
ENDO	Endocrinology Testing	Thyroid-stimulating hormone, thyroxine (T_4) – total and free, triiodothyronine (T_3) – total and free, cortisol, testosterone, and 25-hydroxyvitamin D
ESR	Erythrocyte Sedimentation Rate	Erythrocyte sedimentation rate
GASES	Blood Gas Analyzer Laboratory Studies[a]	Lactic acid, potassium, glucose, hemoglobin, hematocrit, sodium, chloride, ionized calcium, pO_2, pCO_2, oxygen saturation, methemoglobin, carboxyhemoglobin
HAPT	Haptoglobin	Haptoglobin
HEPC	Hepatitis C Antibody	Hepatitis C antibody
HBSG	Hepatitis B Surface Antigen	Hepatitis B surface antigen
LFP	Liver Function Panel	Albumin, alkaline phosphatase, total bilirubin, total protein, alanine aminotransferase, aspartate aminotransferase, and γ-glutamyltranspeptidase
LDH	Lactate Dehydrogenase	Lactate dehydrogenase
REFERENCE	Reference Laboratory Testing	All testing referred to external reference laboratory
OSMO	Osmolality	Serum and urine osmolality
PO4MG	Phosphorus and Magnesium	Phosphorus, magnesium
PREALB	Prealbumin	Prealbumin
PT/INR	Prothrombin Time/INR	Prothrombin time/International normalized ratio
PTT	Partial Thromboplastin Time	Partial thromboplastin time
RETIC	Reticulocytes	Reticulocytes
TAP	Toxic Alcohol Panel	Sodium, glucose, blood urea nitrogen, osmolality, ethanol
URIC	Uric Acid	Uric acid

[a]These are studies using whole blood and not plasma or serum

loaded on the proper analyzer averaged approximately 3.5 minutes prior to introduction of the P701 (composed in large part in retrieving specimens from racks near instruments or in the refrigerators), and 45 seconds once the P701 was implemented. In the prior system of manual archiving and retrieval, instances where samples were archived improperly could significantly delay the process.

Results

Timing trends in add-on testing

In the time period of retrospective study (May 2, 2009 to December 31, 2014), there were a total of 880,359 add-on orders at UIHC. This comprised 3.3 % of the total laboratory test volume performed within the clinical laboratories. The total number of add-on orders increased every year from 2009 to 2013 and then decreased slightly in 2014 (Fig. 2a, b). Fig. 2c shows the variation of add-on orders by month. The inpatient population had the majority of add-on orders (66.8 %), while the ED and outpatient clinics accounted for 14.8 % and 18.4 % of add-on orders, respectively.

Capture of the exact timing of add-on orders relative to initial specimen collect was only possible with the new LIS (August 2, 2014 – December 31, 2014; complete data available on 56,389 add-on orders). Fig. 3a plots the timing of add-on orders, showing the percentage within periods of time. The majority of add-ons were placed within 8 hours (87.3 %) and nearly all by 24 hours (96.8 %). The timing of ordering varied by patient location. Add-on orders placed for patients in the ED were generally closer to original specimen collect time as compared to inpatient units and outpatient clinics. Nearly 100 % of add-on orders within

A

B

Fig. 1 Add-on Testing Procedure. **a** Layout of the core laboratory prior to the automated specimen archival/retrieval unit. Add-on orders generate a print-out in the core laboratory with the testing information and patient demographics (1). A laboratory assistant reviews the print-out. If an add-on can be performed, the assistant prints an additional label with test information to a designated area of the laboratory (e.g., chemistry, 2a, or hematology, 2b) depending on the add-on order. A technologist enters in accession number into the computer program that tracks the archival rack and position for the specimen. Then technologist retrieves the specimen from the archival rack (3a or 3b) or from the refrigerator. The technologist loads specimen on proper analyzer (4a, 4b). **b** Layout of the core laboratory after the automated specimen archival/retrieval unit. Similar to above, add-on orders generate a print-out in the core laboratory that is reviewed by laboratory assistant (1). If an add-on can be performed, the assistant then uses a computer program to request the specimen be retrieved from the archiver (1). The archiver then locates the specimen and dispenses it (2). The assistant retrieves the specimen from archiver and loads specimen on to proper analyzer (3a or 3b)

Fig. 2 Add-on Order Volumes. **a** Yearly add-on testing volumes from 2009 – 2014. The data in 2009 is normalized to an entire year based on order volume from May 2, 2009 to end of that calendar year. **b** Monthly add-on testing volumes spanning 2009 – 2014. **c** Add-on test volumes per month

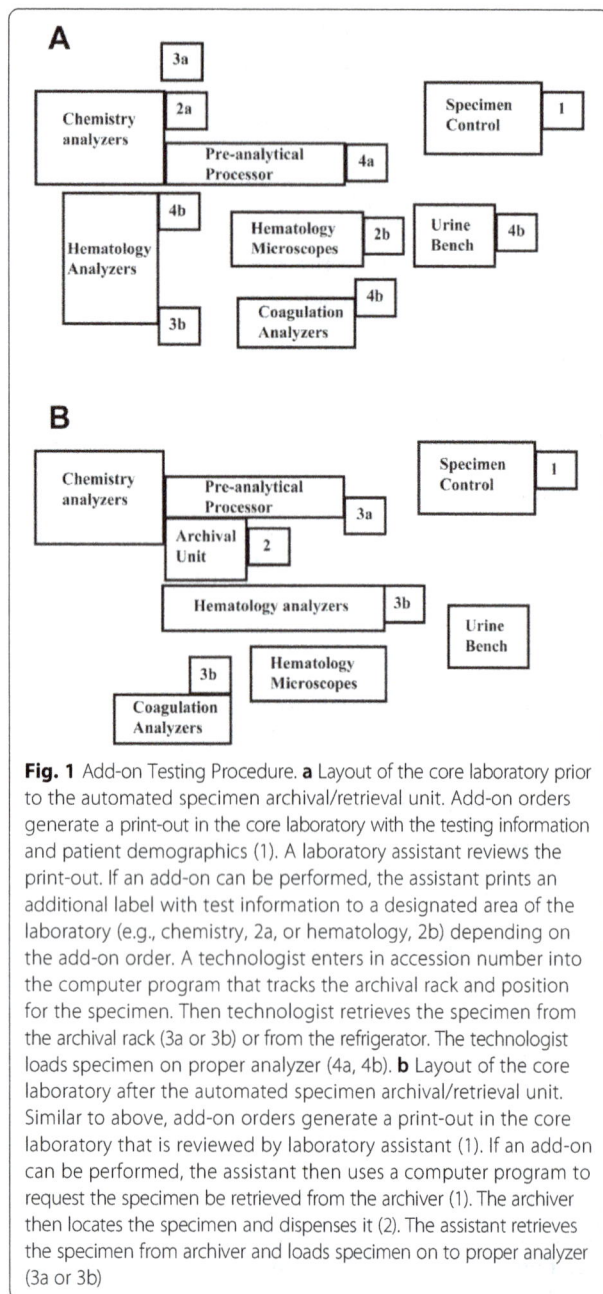

the ED were placed within 8 hours. Timing of add-on orders for inpatient units and outpatient clinics were similar, except that there was a longer tail of add-on orders placed 24 hours or more later than original specimen collect in the outpatient population (Fig. 3a).

The peak times for add-on order placement were between 08:00 – 12:00, with 47.8 % of add-ons ordered between 07:00 and 13:00 (Fig. 3b). Add-on orders were more frequent during weekdays, with Saturdays and Sundays only accounting for slightly more than 20 % of total add-on volume (Fig. 3c).

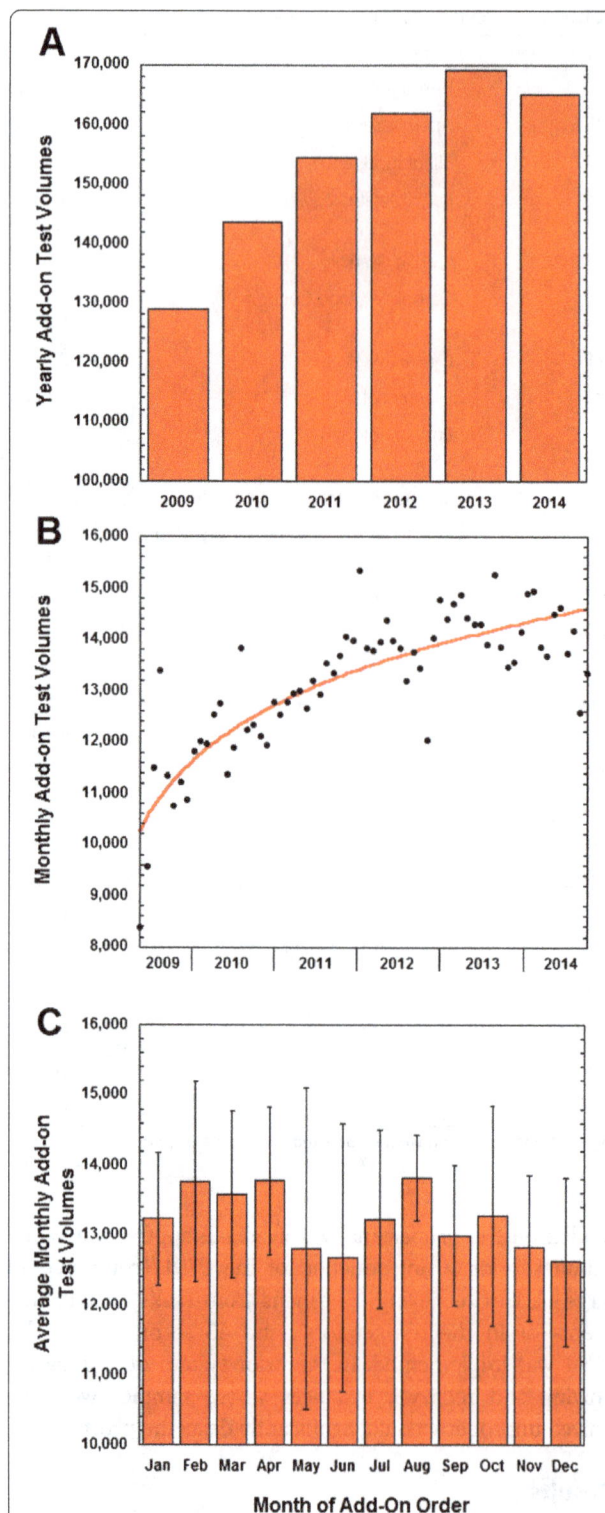

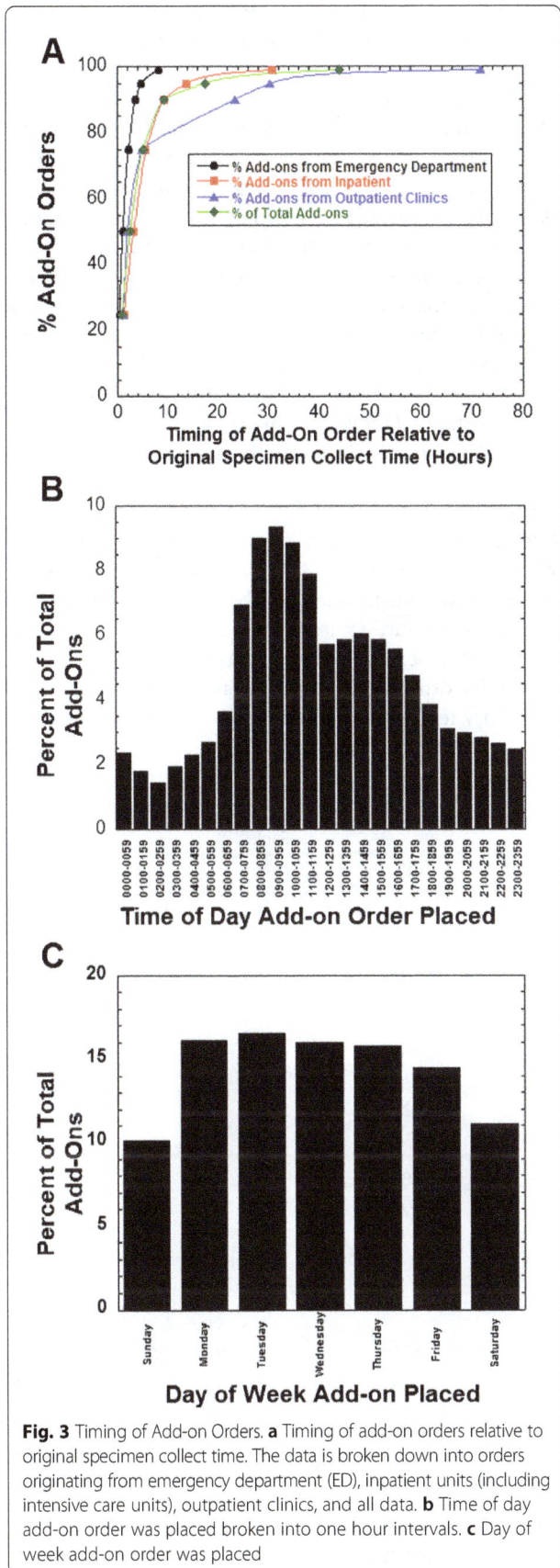

Fig. 3 Timing of Add-on Orders. **a** Timing of add-on orders relative to original specimen collect time. The data is broken down into orders originating from emergency department (ED), inpatient units (including intensive care units), outpatient clinics, and all data. **b** Time of day add-on order was placed broken into one hour intervals. **c** Day of week add-on order was placed

Distribution of add-on testing by category of testing

Figure 4 shows a breakdown of add-on testing by category of testing. The majority of the add-on tests were chemistry tests (78.8 % of total add-on orders comprising 3.3 % of overall chemistry test volumes), with the most frequent being within the following categories (all percentages are of the total overall add-on orders): LFP (25.6 %), BMP (11.7 %), MGPO4 (7.0 %), Cardiac (4.6 %), and Anemia (3.2 %). Hematology and coagulation tests were the next most frequent areas of add-on testing. The most frequent hematology and coagulation add-ons were in the following categories (all percentages are of the total overall add-on orders): CBC (2.70 %), Diff (2.19 %), PTT (1.19 %), PT/INR (1.71 %), and ESR (0.85 %). Within the critical care laboratories, the most frequent add-on orders were the following tests performed on blood gas analyzers using whole blood specimens: lactic acid (0.97 %), potassium (0.78 %), glucose (0.62 %), hemoglobin/hematocrit (0.49 %), and sodium (0.49 %). Urinalysis-related tests accounted for less than 1 % of total add-ons. For the critical care laboratory tests, in most cases the parameters had already been determined as part of a cartridge of testing on the blood gas analyzers; results were suppressed from reporting to the LIS if not ordered by the provider. Thus, the add-on order for these tests required only that staff perform the computer steps necessary to release the previously unordered test from the instrument to the LIS.

Table 2 summarizes the most frequent add-on orders broken down into categories of testing. LFP, BMP, MGPO4, ENDO, and CARDIAC ranked in the top ten

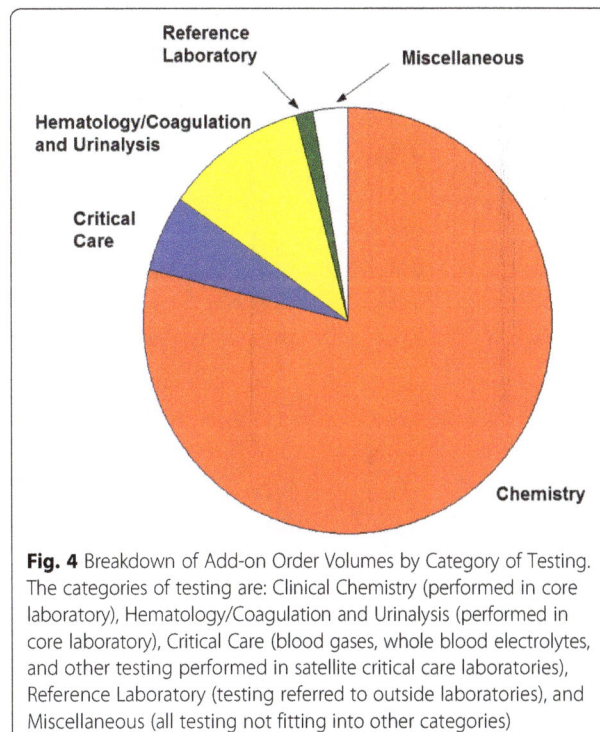

Fig. 4 Breakdown of Add-on Order Volumes by Category of Testing. The categories of testing are: Clinical Chemistry (performed in core laboratory), Hematology/Coagulation and Urinalysis (performed in core laboratory), Critical Care (blood gases, whole blood electrolytes, and other testing performed in satellite critical care laboratories), Reference Laboratory (testing referred to outside laboratories), and Miscellaneous (all testing not fitting into other categories)

most frequent add-on orders overall and also individually for inpatient units, ED, and outpatient clinics. Not surprisingly, GASES were an infrequent add-on order in the outpatient clinics but were the fourth most common overall add-on order. A1C was more frequently added-on in the outpatient clinics than from the ED or inpatient units. Table 3 lists the most frequent individual tests added-on. The top five most frequent individual add-on tests were magnesium (4.0 %), albumin (3.8 %), alanine aminotransferase (3.8 %), aspartate aminotransferase (3.8 %), and total bilirubin (3.7 %). Table 3 also lists the percentage of times each individual test was ordered as an add-on. For six of the tests (amylase, creatine kinase, hemoglobin A1C, lactate dehydrogenase, lipase, troponin T), over 10 % of orders for that particular test were placed as add-ons.

Reference laboratory testing comprised only 1.4 % of total add-ons, with no single test accounting for more than 0.05 % of total add-ons (Table 4). There were 618 different reference laboratory tests available in the EHR test menu that were ordered at least once as an add-on in the time period of retrospective study. This included 193 orders of "Miscellaneous Test", an order option in the EHR for reference laboratory testing not built in the EHR test menu. Our analysis does not capture attempts

to order reference laboratory testing that could not be completed due to lack of suitable existing specimen.

Workload impact of add-on testing

Table 5 summarizes the workload of add-on testing over the period of retrospective study. Of the 880,359 add-on orders, there were 443,411 unique ordering instances, leading to an average of 1.99 add-on tests per instance. Some patients had multiple episodes of add-on test orders at different points in time (e.g., during different days of a multi-day inpatient encounter), leading to an average of 9.15 add-on tests per patient. The introduction of the robotic specimen archival/retrieval unit saved an average of 2.75 mins of laboratory staff manual time per unique ordering instance (Table 5). This translates to 24.1 hr/day less manual effort in dealing with add-on orders.

Discussion

Add-on testing can occupy a significant amount of clinical laboratory resources [1, 3–5]. The main challenges are storage of specimens and the labor involved in retrieving specimens for further testing [1, 5]. Add-on testing can theoretically serve a useful purpose in allowing for thoughtful ordering of additional testing based on initial laboratory test results or other clinical data. On the other

Table 2 Most frequently ordered add-on test categories by ordering location

Test Category	Inpatient Unit %	Rank	Emergency Department %	Rank	Outpatient Clinics %	Rank	All Locations %	Rank
LFP	28.79 %	1	29.86 %	1	16.91 %	1	26.76 %	1
BMP	12.00 %	2	10.14 %	2	15.12 %	2	12.30 %	2
MGPO4	7.41 %	4	4.02 %	4	2.87 %	5	6.08 %	3
GASES	8.41 %	3	2.51 %	9	0.10 %	19	6.01 %	4
ENDO	3.30 %	6	3.09 %	6	8.81 %	3	4.28 %	5
CARDIAC	4.19 %	5	7.25 %	3	2.09%	7	4.25 %	6
ANEMIA	2.66 %	7	0.78 %	18	6.67 %	4	3.12 %	7
DIFF	2.40 %	8	1.73 %	15	1.78 %	9	2.19 %	8
CBC	2.24 %	9	1.83 %	14	2.00 %	8	2.14 %	9
PT/INR	1.43 %	12	3.57 %	5	0.88 %	13	1.65 %	10
LIPASE	1.49 %	11	3.01 %	8	0.77 %	15	1.58 %	11
A1C	1.33 %	14	0.95 %	17	2.52 %	6	1.49 %	12
CRP	1.29 %	15	2.22 %	10	1.39 %	11	1.45 %	13
LDH	1.50 %	10	0.64 %	19	1.43 %	10	1.36 %	14
AMYLASE	1.37 %	13	2.02 %	12	0.68 %	16	1.34 %	15
PTT	0.97 %	16	3.03 %	7	0.19 %	17	1.13 %	16
ESR	0.61 %	18	2.00 %	13	0.78 %	13	0.85 %	17
BILD	0.94 %	17	0.59 %	20	0.92 %	12	0.85 %	18
D-DIMER	0.24 %	19	2.07 %	11	0.11 %	18	0.48 %	19
TAP	0.16 %	20	1.61 %	16	0.03 %	20	0.35 %	20
Total	82.7 %		82.9 %		66.1 %		79.7 %	

Table 3 Most frequently ordered individual add-on tests

Test	% of Total Add-on Orders	% of Times Test Ordered as Add-on (vs. Routine)
Magnesium	4.0	5.9
Albumin	3.8	6.5
Alanine aminotransferase	3.8	5.4
Aspartate aminotransferase	3.8	5.5
Bilirubin, total	3.7	6.4
Alkaline phosphatase	3.4	5.8
Gamma-glutamyltransferase	3.2	4.7
Total protein	3.1	6.3
Phosphorus	3.0	6.9
Troponin T	2.2	14.5
Complete blood count	2.1	1.5
Automated white blood cell differential	2.1	2.3
Creatinine	1.7	1.1
Potassium	1.6	1.1
Thyroid stimulating hormone with reflex to free thyroxine	1.6	9.6
Lipase	1.6	15.9
Hemoglobin A1C	1.5	10.2
Prothrombin time/International normalized ratio	1.5	1.8
Basic metabolic panel with calcium	1.5	1.1
C-Reactive protein	1.4	8.1
Lactic acid dehydrogenase	1.4	10.7
Creatine kinase, total	1.3	22.7
Amylase	1.3	15.3
Blood urea nitrogen	1.3	0.9
Calcium, total	1.2	1.3

Table 4 Most frequently ordered reference laboratory add-on tests

Test	% of Total Add-on Orders
Helicobacter pylori antibody, IgG	0.050 %
Mitochondrial M2 antibodies	0.049 %
Hepatitis C virus quantitative PCR	0.033 %
IgG subclasses	0.022 %
Miscellaneous test[a]	0.019 %
Vitamin D, 1,25-dihydroxy	0.018 %
Aldosterone, serum	0.017 %
Alpha-1-antitrypsin, phenotyping	0.013 %
Lyme disease antibodies, IgG and IgM	0.013 %
Histoplasma antigen, urine	0.013 %

[a]Covers any test ordered that is not on list of laboratory tests built in electronic medical record

Table 5 Summary of add-on tests

Total number of add-ons	880,359
Unique ordering instances[1]	443,411
Number of patients	96,244
Average number of add-on tests per unique ordering instance	1.99
Average number of add-on tests per patient[2]	9.15
Estimated hours per day of manual effort for add-on testing prior to introduction of robotic archival storage/retrieval unit	30.7
Estimated hours per day of manual effort for add-on testing with use of robotic archival storage/retrieval unit	6.6

[1]These are unique add-on orders at a specific time
[2]This includes all add-on tests per each patient, which may span multiple unique ordering instances

hand, add-on testing can also be a result of disorganized ordering practices (e.g., neglecting to order essential laboratory testing upfront) or even misutilization of testing, as has been shown in previous studies [1, 2]. Our analysis does not capture attempts at add-on testing that could not be completed due to lack of existing specimens or add-on testing that was duplicate to previously ordered testing (e.g., hemoglobin/hematocrit placed as add-on when CBC already performed). We have analyzed duplicate testing as an example of misutilization in a previous study [6].

The results of this study are similar to previous studies in showing that the majority of add-ons are clinical chemistry tests [2, 4, 5]. As with previous studies, LFP, BMP, MGPO4, and CARDIAC were in the top tier of ordered add-on tests. Hematology and coagulation testing only accounted for 11.2 % of total add-ons; however, add-ons comprised 5.6 % of the overall hematology/coagulation test volumes. Four common tests (CBC, DIFF, PT/INR, and PT) accounted for over two-thirds of the hematology and coagulation add-on tests.

In the present study, the 5.86 % percent of add-ons for the critical care laboratories posed the least manual effort because in most cases the parameters had already been determined but were suppressed from reporting to the LIS if not ordered by the provider. Therefore, most critical care laboratory add-ons only needed to be sent from instrument to LIS rather than having to locate the sample and analyze it again (assuming specimen would even be viable at that point). Reference laboratory add-ons were only a small fraction of total add-ons but spanned a wide variety of tests. No single reference laboratory test exceeded 0.05 % of total add-ons. These results are comparable to previous studies [2, 5]. Add-on requests for reference laboratory tests not built in the LIS or EHR may entail extra work in first determining the specimen requirements for the requested test and then checking if pre-existing specimens can be used.

Similar to previous studies, our study shows a high fraction of add-ons ordered within eight hours of original specimen collect time [1, 2, 5]. The ED tended to order add-ons more quickly compared to inpatient units and outpatient clinics. Only a small fraction of add-on orders were placed more than 24 hours after original specimen collection. Less than 1 % of total add-ons occurred more than 48 hours after specimen collection. Outpatient clinics accounted for the majority of add-on orders submitted more than 24 hours after original specimen collection, a finding similar to a previous study [5].

Depending on workload, add-on orders can entail substantial manual effort from clinical laboratory staff [1, 2, 4, 5]. In our study, add-ons comprised 3.3 % of overall test volume, a figure that is very close to one previous study [4] and higher than another study [1]. Some laboratories, including ours, have implemented robotic specimen archival/retrieval units. As we have shown, the estimated impact of this type of unit on manual time can be substantial, with an estimated reduction of 24.1 hrs/day of manual add-on processing time in handling add-on order requests. However, the timing of add-on orders suggests that improvements on this design may include a combination of short-term/rapidly accessible and longer-term/less accessible specimen storage. Storage of specimens in a rapidly accessible buffer (e.g., very close to the chemistry analyzers) for a limited period of time (e.g., between 8 and 24 hours) would capture the majority of add-on orders. After this time period, specimens can be archived for longer-term storage in a space more distant from the instruments. At that point, turnaround time is likely less important.

The main limitations of our study are that the analysis is retrospective and confined to an academic medical center. The results may not generalize to other hospital or clinic settings. Nevertheless, it is hoped that the results described here provide useful to other institutions attempting to manage the challenges of add-on testing.

Conclusions
Add-on orders significantly impact the workload of the clinical laboratory. In this study at an academic medical center, the majority of add-on orders were clinical chemistry tests, and most add-on orders occur within 24 hours of original specimen collection. Robotic specimen archival/retrieval units can reduce manual effort in the clinical laboratory associated with add-on orders.

Abbreviations
A1C: Hemoglobin A1C; BILD: Direct bilirubin; BMP: Basic metabolic panel; CBC: Complete blood count; CPOE: Computerized provider order entry; CRP: C-reactive protein; DIFF: White blood count differential; ED: Emergency department; EHR: Electronic health record; ESR: Erythrocyte sedimentation rate; HAPT: Haptoglobin; HBSG: Hepatitis B surface antigen; HEPC: Hepatitis C antibody; ICU: Intensive care unit; LDH: Lactate dehydrogenase; LFP: Liver function panel; LIS: Laboratory information system; OSMO: Serum/plasma osmolality; PO4MG: Phosphorus and magnesium; PREALB: Prealbumin; PT/INR: Prothrombin time/international normalized ratio; PTT: Partial thromboplastin time; TAP: Toxic alcohol panel; UIHC: University of Iowa Hospitals and Clinics; URIC: Uric acid.

Competing interests
The authors declare that they have no competing interests.

Authors' contributions
LSN and MDK were involved in the study concept and design, analysis and interpretation of the data, drafting and revisions of the manuscript. SRD, RMH, and JK assisted with data analysis and interpretation. DRA helped with extraction and analysis of data from the laboratory information system. All authors have read and approved the final manuscript.

Acknowledgements
MDK thanks the Department of Pathology (Dr. Nitin Karandikar, Department Executive Officer) for providing research funding.

Author details
[1]Department of Pathology, University of Iowa Hospitals and Clinics, Iowa City, IA 52242, USA. [2]Hospital Computing Information Services, University of Iowa Hospitals and Clinics, Iowa City, IA 52242, USA.

References

1. Melanson SF, Hsieh B, Flood JG, Lewandrowski KB. Evaluation of add-on testing in the clinical chemistry laboratory of a large academic medical center: operational considerations. Arch Pathol Lab Med. 2004;128(8):885–9.
2. Melanson S, Flood J, Lewandrowski K. Add-on testing the clinical laboratory: observations from two large academic medical centers. Lab Med. 2006;37(11):675–8.
3. Kim JY, Kamis IK, Singh B, Batra S, Dixon RH, Dighe AS. Implementation of computerized add-on testing for hospitalized patients in a large academic medical center. Clin Chem Lab Med. 2011;49(5):845–50.
4. Loh TP, Saw S, Sethi SK. Clinical value of add-on chemistry in a large tertiary care teaching hospital. Lab Med. 2012;43(3):82–5.
5. Naumova NN, Schappert J, Kaplan LA. Patterns of add-on tests for hospitalized and for private patient populations. Arch Pathol Lab Med. 2007;131(12):1794–9.
6. Krasowski MD, Chudzik D, Dolezal A, Steussy B, Gailey MP, Koch B, et al. Promoting improved utilization of laboratory testing through changes in an electronic medical record: experience at an academic medical center. BMC Med Inform Decis Mak. 2015;15:11.
7. Krasowski MD, Davis SR, Drees D, Morris C, Kulhavy J, Crone C, et al. Autoverification in a core clinical chemistry laboratory at an academic medical center. J Pathol Inform. 2014;5:13.

6

Characterisation and prognostic value of tertiary lymphoid structures in oral squamous cell carcinoma

Anna M Wirsing[1], Oddveig G Rikardsen[1,2], Sonja E Steigen[1,3], Lars Uhlin-Hansen[1,3] and Elin Hadler-Olsen[1*]

Abstract

Background: Oral squamous cell carcinomas are often heavily infiltrated by immune cells. The organization of B-cells, follicular dendritic cells, T-cells and high-endothelial venules into structures termed tertiary lymphoid structures have been detected in various types of cancer, where their presence is found to predict favourable outcome. The purpose of the present study was to evaluate the incidence of tertiary lymphoid structures in oral squamous cell carcinomas, and if present, analyse whether they were associated with clinical outcome.

Methods: Tumour samples from 80 patients with oral squamous cell carcinoma were immunohistochemically stained for B-cells, follicular dendritic cells, T-cells, germinal centre B-cells and high-endothelial venules. Some samples were sectioned at multiple levels to assess whether the presence of tertiary lymphoid structures varied within the tumour.

Results: Tumour-associated tertiary lymphoid structures were detected in 21 % of the tumours and were associated with lower disease-specific death. The presence of tertiary lymphoid structures varied within different levels of a tissue block.

Conclusions: Tertiary lymphoid structure formation was found to be a positive prognostic factor for patients with oral squamous cell carcinoma. Increased knowledge about tertiary lymphoid structure formation in oral squamous cell carcinoma might help to develop and guide immune-modulatory cancer treatments.

Keywords: Oral squamous cell carcinoma, Prognostic factor, Tertiary lymphoid structure, B-cell, High-endothelial venule, Follicular dendritic cell, Germinal centre

Background

Oral squamous cell carcinomas (OSCCs) are tumours known to metastasize to lymph nodes at an early stage of their development [1]. Despite current improvements in clinical management of this cancer type, mortality and morbidity rates of OSCC patients have remained high over the last decades, with an average 5-year survival rate of about 50% [2,3]. The TNM staging of the tumour, and especially the presence and extent of lymph node metastasis (N stage), have considerable prognostic importance for patients with OSCC [4] and are used to guide treatment strategies. However, tumours of the same clinical stage may respond differently to the same treatment and may also have distinct clinical outcomes [5].

Considerable interest has been devoted to the complex interplay between tumour cells and host-immune response, and especially to how infiltrating immune cells might affect the clinical outcome of cancer patients. Anti-tumour functions of tumour-infiltrating lymphocytes (TILs), particularly of T-cells, have been observed in numerous types of cancer [6]. Accumulating evidence indicates that infiltrating immune cells may also be involved in the development and progression of oral cancer, where they have shown both favourable and detrimental effects [7]. It is well established that immune cells infiltrating to sites of chronic inflammation organize themselves both anatomically and functionally similar to secondary lymphoid organs (SLOs), a phenomenon called tertiary lymphoid structure (TLS) formation [8]. Similar to lymphoid follicles, TLSs typically comprise aggregates of B-cells in a meshwork of follicular dendritic cells (FDCs) that are then surrounded by T-cells as well as specialized blood vessels

* Correspondence: elin.hadler-olsen@uit.no
[1]Department of Medical Biology, Faculty of Health Sciences, University of Tromsø, Tromsø 9037, Norway
Full list of author information is available at the end of the article

referred to as high-endothelial venules (HEVs) [9]. HEVs express the lymphoid chemokine peripheral node addressin (PNAd), which binds to L-Selectin on naive lymphocytes and thus promote lymphocyte recruitment to sites of chronic inflammation [10]. Furthermore, a complex interplay between different lymphotoxin- and chemokine-induced signalling pathways is required for the initiation of TLS formation [9]. In contrast to lymph nodes, TLSs are not encapsulated, resulting in constitutive, direct antigenic stimulation from their surrounding microenvironment [11]. Lymphatic vessels have also been found in association with TLSs, but their functional interplay is not yet fully clarified [12]. The presence of ongoing germinal centre (GC) reactions in B-cell clusters of ectopic lymphoid structures has been reported, indicating that adaptive immunity can be triggered at sites different from SLOs [11]. In autoimmune disorders, formation of ectopic lymphoid tissue is associated with disease progression [11], whereas TLS development in breast, ovarian, non-small-cell lung, renal and colorectal cancer is reported to be associated with a favourable prognosis [13-23].

The aim of the present study was to evaluate the incidence of TLSs in OSCCs, and if present, analyse whether they were associated with clinical outcome. The study included tissue samples and clinical data from 80 patients diagnosed with OSCCs between 1986 and 2002 at the Diagnostic Clinic – Clinical Pathology, University Hospital of North Norway (UNN). The presence of TLSs was determined based on immunohistochemical staining patterns of B-cells, FDCs, GC B-cells, T-cells and HEVs. We established that the presence of TLSs is a positive prognostic factor for patients with OSCC. Understanding and interpreting TLS formation in OSCC might help to implement and guide immunotherapeutic interventions. In terms of individual clinical management, reliable prognostic markers together with targeted anti-cancer therapies might improve the consistently low survival rates in patients with oral cancer.

Methods
Patients
The study broadly follows the REMARK recommendations for tumour marker prognostic studies [24]. Eighty patients with histologically verified primary SCC of the oral cavity in the period 1986–2002 were selected from the archives of the Diagnostic Clinic – Clinical Pathology, UNN. The last day of follow-up was January 1st, 2012. The specimens were formalin-fixed, paraffin-embedded tumour resections or biopsies from the mobile tongue, floor of the mouth, buccal mucosa, gingiva and soft and hard palate. We excluded specimens from the base of the tongue and the tonsils – sites naturally rich in lymphatic tissue. Patients with a history of former head and neck cancer were also excluded from the study. Clinical data, including tumour

staging according to the TNM-classification and treatment modalities, were retrieved from the patients' hospital files, pathology reports and the Statistics of Norway, Cause of Death Registry, and are listed in Table 1. Information on the HPV status determined by p16 immunohistochemical staining was obtained from the Diagnostic Clinic – Clinical Pathology, UNN, and is also presented in Table 1. In addition to the patient samples, formalin-fixed, paraffin-embedded normal oral tissue was used as control. The study was approved by the Regional Committee for Medical and Health Research Ethics, Northern Norway (REK-number 22/2007), which also gave the permission to access patient files containing the clinical data. All clinical data were kept anonymous.

Immunohistochemistry
Four-micrometer-thick sections of formalin-fixed, paraffin-embedded tissue of patients with OSCC on Superfrost Plus slides were subjected to immunohistochemical staining. From patients where several tumour-containing paraffin-blocks were available, a block with representative material, based on H/E staining, was chosen without specific evaluation of the inflammatory infiltrate. Before staining, all specimens were incubated overnight at 60°C, deparaffinised in xylene, rehydrated in graded alcohol baths and subjected to heat-induced antigen retrieval in 0.01 M sodium citrate buffer at pH 6.0. Prior to antibody incubation, inherent peroxidase activity in the tissue was blocked with 3% H_2O_2 (Ventana Medical Systems, France or Dako Glostrup, Denmark). The following primary antibodies were used: Mouse anti-CD20, clone L26; Mouse anti-CD21, clone 2G9; Mouse anti-bcl-6, clone GI191E/A8; Mouse anit-CD34, clone QBEnd/10; Rabbit anti-CD3, clone 2GV6 (all from Ventana Medical Systems, France); Mouse anti-Podoplanin, clone D2-40 (Dako, Glostrup, Denmark) and Rat anti-PNAd, clone MECA-79, (Biolegend, San Diego). Dilutions and incubation times are listed in Table 2. Except for the PNAd antibody, all immunohistochemical stainings were done in the automated slide stainer Ventana Benchmark, XT (Ventana) at the Diagnostic Clinic – Clinical Pathology, UNN, which is accredited according to the ISO/IEC 15189 standard for the respective stainings, using the same protocols, positive and negative controls as in the clinical routines. For these automated stainings, a cocktail of HRP labelled goat anti-mouse IgG/IgM and mouse anti-rabbit secondary antibodies together with diaminobenzidine from the Ventana UltraView Universal DAB Detection Kit (#760-500, Ventana) were applied for visualization.

Manual staining with the PNAd primary antibody was performed as previously described [25], using HRP-labelled goat anti-rat light chain secondary antibody (#AP202P, Millipore, Temecula, CA) and diaminobenzidine (Dako EnVision + System-Horseradish Peroxidase,

Table 1 Comparison of clinicopathological variables between 80 OSCC patients with and without TLSs using Pearson's Chi-square test

	TLS-negative (N = 63) (no. (%))	TLS-positive (N = 17) (no. (%))	P-value
Gender			
Male	35 (55.6)	11 (64.7)	0.498
Female	28 (44.4)	6 (35.3)	
Age at diagnosis, years			
Mean	63.19	63.71	0.178
0-59	23 (36.5)	6 (35.3)	0.926
≥ 60	40 (63.5)	11 (64.7)	
Smoking history			
Never smoker	14 (22.2)	4 (23.5)	
Former smoker	10 (15.9)	1 (5.9)	0.722
Current smoker	34 (54.0)	11 (64.7)	
Unknown	5 (7.9)	1 (5.9)	
Alcohol consumption			
Never	12 (19.0)	1 (5.9)	
≤ 1 times weekly	24 (38.1)	6 (35.3)	0.114
> 1 times weekly or daily	17 (27.0)	3 (17.6)	
Unknown	10 (15.9)	7 (41.2)	
Tumour site			
Mobile tongue	29 (46.0)	9 (52.9)	
Floor of mouth	17 (27.0)	5 (29.4)	
Soft palate	1 (1.6)	0 (0.0)	0.956
Buccal mucosa	7 (11.1)	1 (5.9)	
Alveolar ridge	8 (12.7)	2 (11.8)	
Unknown	1 (1.6)	0 (0.0)	
Tumour differentiation			
Well	20 (31.7)	10 (58.8)	
Moderate	39 (61.9)	5 (29.4)	0.058
Poor	4 (6.3)	2 (11.8)	
T stage			
T1	23 (36.5)	6 (35.3)	
T2	18 (28.6)	9 (52.9)	0.187
T3, T4	21 (33.3)	2 (11.8)	
Unknown	1 (1.6)	0 (0.0)	
N stage			
N0	41 (65.1)	13 (76.5)	0.670
N+	17 (27.0)	3 (17.6)	
Unknown	5 (7.9)	1 (5.9)	
M stage			
M0	57 (90.5)	17 (100.0)	
M+	1 (1.6)	0 (0.0)	0.417
Unknown	5 (7.9)	0 (0.0)	
Treatment			
Surgery local +/− neck resection	7 (11.1)	2(11.8)	
Surgery and radiotherapy	41 (65.1)	12 (70.6)	
Radiotherapy +/− chemotherapy	8 (12.7)	3 (17.6)	0.700
None or palliative	5 (7.9)	0 (0.0)	
Unknown	2 (3.2)	0 (0.0)	
HPV/p16			
Negative	52 (82.5)	16 (94.1)	
Positive	5 (7.9)	1 (5.9)	0.386
Unknown	6 (9.5)	0 (0.0)	

Dako) for detection. Counterstaining was done with Harris hematoxylin (Sigma-Aldrich, St. Louis, MO). Finally, the sections were dehydrated in graded alcohol and xylene baths, and mounted with Histokit (Chemiteknikk, Oslo, Norway). Negative controls were treated identically but with the primary antibodies replaced by the antibody diluting solution. Formalin-fixed, paraffin-embedded human lymph nodes served as positive controls for the PNAd staining. Negative control sections never showed any staining, whereas the positive control sections (lymph nodes) always showed positive staining confined to the cells that were supposed to be positive (data not shown). The specificity of the PNAd antibody was evaluated on consecutive sections from six different OSCC samples and three samples of normal oral mucosa. These OSCC and normal tissue sections were assessed for

Table 2 Antibodies for immunohistochemistry

Antibody	Dilution	Incubation time
Mouse anti-CD20, clone L26, Ventana Medical Systems, France	Pre-diluted	16 min
Mouse anti-CD21, clone 2G9, Ventana	Pre-diluted	32 min
Mouse anti-bcl-6, clone GI191E/A8, Ventana	Pre-diluted	40 min
Mouse anti-Podoplanin, clone D2-40, Dako, Glostrup, Denmark	1:25	32 min
Mouse anit-CD34, clone QBEnd/10, Ventana	Pre-diluted	32 min
Rabbit anti-CD3, clone 2GV6, Ventana	Pre-diluted	16 min
Rat anti-PNAd, clone MECA-79, Biolegend, San Diego	1:25	30 min
Goat anti-rat light chain antibody, #AP202P, Millipore, Temecula, CA	1:250	30 min

overlapping immunohistochemical staining for the PNAd antibody, the blood vessel marker CD34 and the lymphatic endothelial cell marker D2-40. In the OSCC samples, sporadic CD34+ blood vessels were to a minor degree positive for PNAd, whereas no D2-40+ lymphatic vessels were positive, indicating a high degree of antibody specificity. No HEV staining was seen in the three samples from normal oral mucosa.

Immunohistochemical evaluation

Eighty patients were included in the study. In 25 of the patients, the presence of TLSs was evaluated at a single level in the tumour tissue block. In 45 of the patients – randomly chosen from the 80 patients – TLS formation was evaluated at two discrete levels at about 100 μm distance in the tissue block. Additionally, tumour tissue blocks from 10 of the patients – nine of them negative for TLSs in the superficial level – were cut down completely and presence of TLSs was evaluated at 100 μm distance throughout the tumour sample.

We used a two-step method for TLS detection. First, the tissue sections were immunohistochemically stained for the pan B-cell marker CD20 and assigned to three different groups based on their staining pattern: obvious B-cell aggregates, indistinct aggregates of B-cells and no or scattered B-cells. Second, staining for the FDC marker CD21, the T-cell marker CD3 and the HEV marker PNAd was performed on consecutive sections of those with obvious and indistinct B-cell aggregates. For FDC evaluation, areas with clusters of B-cells were examined at high-power magnification (400×). All tumours that had one or several accumulations of B-cells containing CD21 positive FDCs were defined as TLS-positive. All TLSs also contained HEVs and T-cells. The TLS-positive tumours were further subdivided into classical and non-classical TLSs. A classical TLS was defined as a B-cell aggregate containing a continuous FDC meshwork, and a non-classical TLS as a B-cell aggregate with a more diffuse distribution of the FDCs. Sections from seven of the TLS-positive tumours were stained with BCL-6 to verify the presence of GC B-cells in B-cell clusters of TLSs.

Statistical analysis

All statistical analyses were performed with the SPSS software version 22.0 for Windows (IBM, Armonk, NY). The association between various clinicopathological variables was examined by the Pearson's Chi-square test. Disease-specific death (DSD) and disease-specific survival (DSS) curves were estimated in univariate analyses and by Kaplan Meier method. The log-rank test was used to evaluate significant differences between the groups of patients. Variables that were statistically significant in the univariate analysis were entered into multivariate Cox

regression analyses to identify independent prognostic factors in the presence of other variables. Validity of the proportionality assumption was verified by plotting log-minus-log plots. P-values less than 0.05 were considered statistically significant.

Results
Presence of TLSs in OSCC

TLSs are highly organized structures that typically appear as clusters of B-cells containing FDCs. These clusters are then surrounded by T-cells and HEVs as shown schematically in Figure 1. We investigated the presence of TLSs in tumour specimens from 80 patients with OSCCs using immunohistochemistry. Sections with distinct or more diffuse B-cell aggregates were considered likely to have TLSs, and their consecutive sections were stained for FDCs, T-cells and HEVs, whereas sections without B-cell aggregates were not further analysed. At the first level assessed, TLSs were found in 13 of the 80 specimens. Eleven of these TLSs were found in sections with distinct B-cell aggregates, and only two in sections with diffuse B-cell aggregates. Pictures of a classical TLS are shown in Figure 2. One more TLS-positive tumour was identified by staining for TLSs at an additional level about 100 μm deeper in the tissue blocks from 45 of the patients. Three additional TLS-positive tumours were detected by assessing the whole tissue sample from 10 patients. These three TLS-positive tumours showed TLSs at multiple levels. Altogether, TLSs were found in 17 (21 %) of the 80 patients included in the study. The maximum number of TLSs in a single section was four, but usually not more than two TLSs were detected in each of the positive sections. The TLSs were mainly found in the peri-tumoural stroma within 0.5 mm distance from the tumour front, in lymphocyte-rich subepithelial areas.

Within the B-cell aggregates, FDCs were found in either of two patterns: distinct meshworks (Figure 3A) or diffuse accumulations (Figure 3B) of CD21 positive cells. Only B-cell aggregates with contiguous FDC meshworks showed distinct accumulations of BCL6+ GC B-cells (Figure 3C) and are here referred to as *classical TLSs*. In the B-cell aggregates with diffuse accumulations of FDCs, GC B-cells were either absent (Figure 3D) or dispersed throughout the follicle, and these are here referred to as *non-classical TLSs*. Sometimes both classical and non-classical TLSs were found in the same section. Analyses of multiple tissue levels showed that some TLSs classified as non-classical on one tissue level presented a classical pattern on another tissue level and vice versa.

Clinicopathological characteristics and prognostic value of TLSs

Clinicopathological data of the patients were analysed for correlation with the presence of TLSs, and the

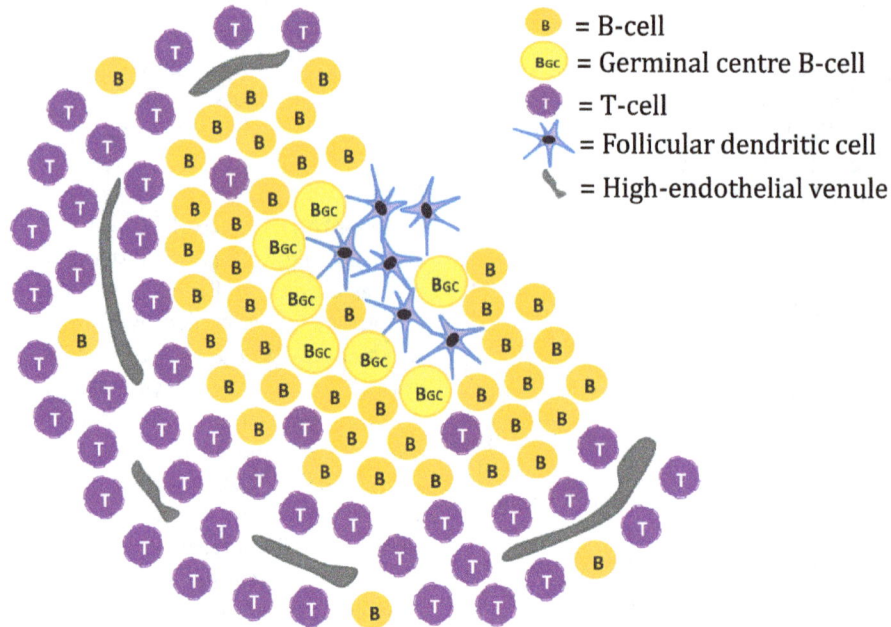

Figure 1 Schematic model of tertiary lymphoid structures. Specialized cell populations arrange themselves into distinct patterns forming a classical tertiary lymphoid structure (TLS).

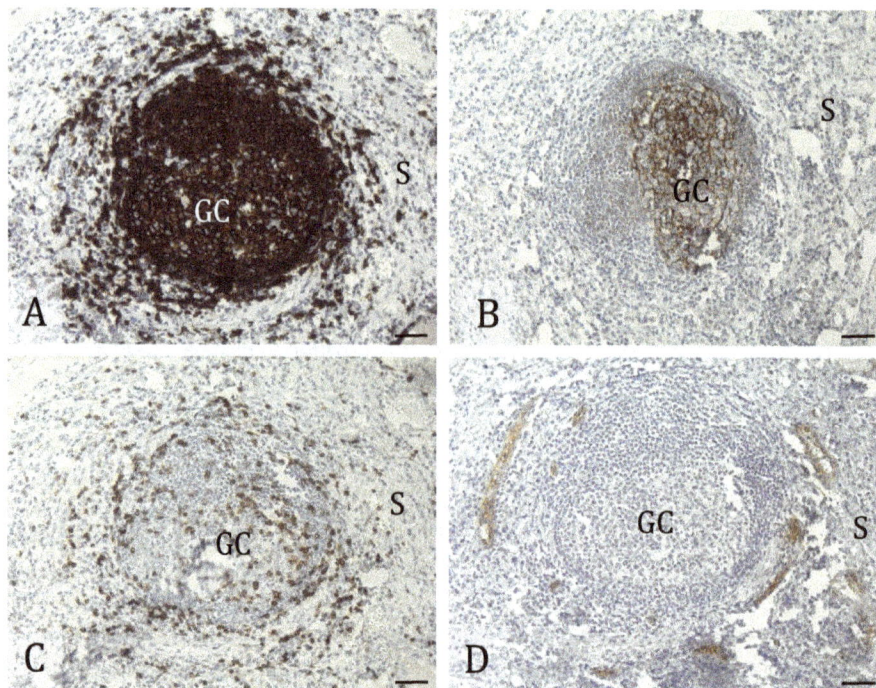

Figure 2 Tertiary lymphoid structures in oral squamous cell carcinoma. The pictures show representative immunohistochemical stainings on consecutive sections of the same oral squamous cell carcinoma (OSCC) tissue sample for detection of classical tertiary lymphoid structures (TLSs). A section that presents clusters of CD20+ B-cells **(A)** typically shows organized accumulations of follicular dendritic cells (FDCs) in a consecutive section stained for CD21 **(B)**. T-cell areas within and around the B-cell follicle are found by staining another consecutive section for CD3 **(C)**. High-endothelial venules (HEVs) adjacent to the B-cell follicle are detected when staining a consecutive section for PNAd, as shown in **(D)**. CD20+, CD21+ and CD3+ cells as well as PNAd + vessels are stained brown, and cell nuclei are stained blue by hematoxylin. Germinal centres are labelled "GC" and stroma surrounding the TLS is labelled "S" in the micrographs. Scale bars indicate 40 μm.

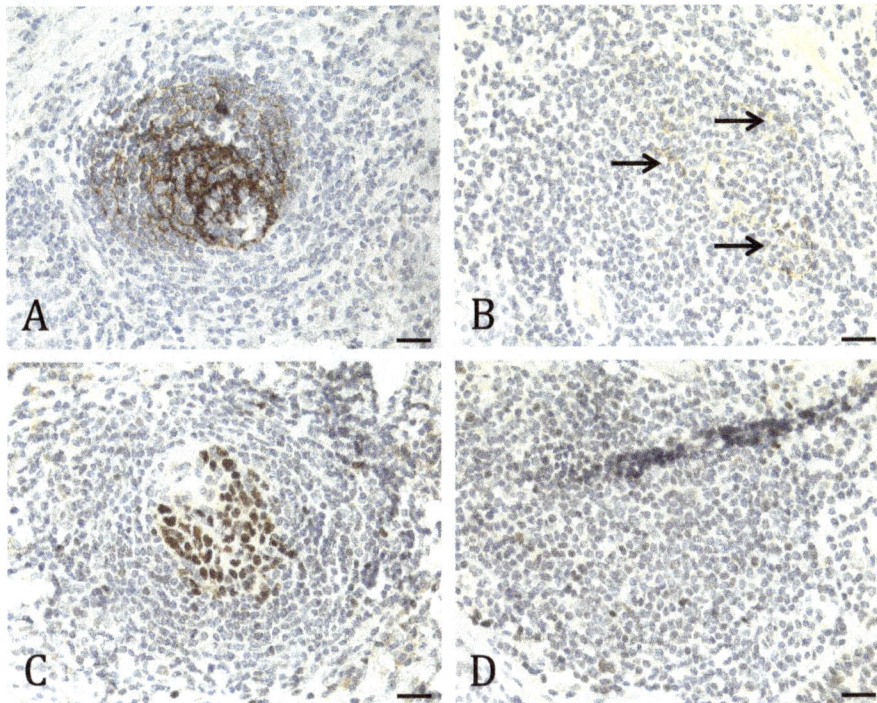

Figure 3 Classical and non-classical tertiary lymphoid structures. The pictures show representative immunohistochemical stainings on consecutive sections of two different oral squamous cell carcinoma (OSCC) tissue samples (A/C *vs.* B/D) for detection of classical (A/C) and non-classical (B/D) tertiary lymphoid structures (TLSs). B-cell follicles of classical TLSs normally comprise contiguous meshworks of CD21+ follicular dendritic cells (FDCs), as indicated in **(A)**, and show distinct accumulations of germinal centre (GC) B-cells when staining a consecutive section for BCL6, as presented in **(C)**. B-cell follicles of non-classical TLSs usually contain scattered FDCs, as shown in **(B**; arrows), and lack GC B-cells on a consecutive section stained for BCL6 **(D)**. In some cases, non-classical TLSs also show abnormal GCs with BCL6+ cells dispersed throughout the follicle (data not shown). CD21+ and BCL6+ cells are stained brown, and cell nuclei are stained blue by hematoxylin. Scale bars indicate 40 μm.

results are presented in Table 1. Although not statistically significant, the majority of TLSs were found in patients with well-differentiated tumours. Further, there were more TLSs in T1 and T2 tumours compared to T3/T4 tumours. TLSs showed no statistically significant association with the other variables examined. The prognostic value of various clinicopathological variables in OSCC was investigated in univariate analysis using the log-rank test (Table 3). Based on the assessment of one tissue level, TLS-positive tumours indicated a trend toward improved survival. When the assessment of TLSs was based on multiple tissue levels, a significant association between the presence of TLSs and favourable outcome in OSSC patients was found, as shown in Figure 4. As patients presented various TLS subtypes (either classical, non-classical or both classical and non-classical), we analysed whether the TLS subtype influenced 5-year DSD. As presented in Additional file 1: Table S1, there was a tendency towards lower 5-year DSD for all patients with TLSs, regardless of the subtype. However, the differences were not statistically significant. Presence of classical TLSs alone or in combination with non-classical TLSs seemed to be associated with better prognosis compared to the presence of only non-classical

TLSs, but again, no statistical significant difference between the subtypes was found (P = 0.304; data not shown). Furthermore, our results also confirmed the prognostic value of the T, N and M stages. The variables that showed statistically significant association with DSD in the univariate analyses (T, N stage and TLS) were entered into multivariate Cox regression analyses. The M status was excluded from multivariate analyses as there was only one M + patient. Proportional hazards assumptions were satisfied for multivariate analyses as shown by parallel curves for different categories of prognostic variables on log-minus-log plots (Additional file 1: Figure S1). In multivariate analyses, only the T status remained independently associated with disease-specific death (P < 0.001, Table 4).

Discussion

In the present study, we have demonstrated TLSs in OSCC by immunohistochemical analyses. To the best of our knowledge, this is the first report of TLSs in OSCCs. TLSs were found in 16% of the patients when a single level of the tumour was assessed, and in 21% of the patients when multiple levels of the tumours were analysed. This is a rather low occurrence compared to what

Table 3 Clinicopathologic variables as predictors for 5-year disease-specific death in univariate analysis for 80 patients with OSCC

	Patients (N = 80) (no. (%))	5-Year death (%)	P-value
Gender			
Male	46 (57.5)	37.0	0.403
Female	34 (42.5)	29.4	
Age at diagnosis, years			
0-59	29 (36.3)	31.0	0.637
≥ 60	51 (63.8)	35.3	
Smoking history			
Never smoker	18 (22.5)	27.8	
Former smoker	11 (13.8)	27.3	0.897
Current smoker	45 (56.3)	37.3	
Unknown	6 (7.5)	33.3	
Alcohol consumption			
Never	13 (16.3)	23.1	
≤ 1 times weekly	30 (37.5)	33.3	0.633
> 1 times weekly or daily	20 (25.0)	35.0	
Unknown	17 (21.3)	41.2	
Tumour site			
Mobile tongue	38 (47.5)	21.1	
Floor of mouth	22 (27.5)	40.9	0.074
All others*	20 (25.0)	50.0	
Tumour differentiation			
Well	30 (37.5)	26.7	
Moderate	44 (55.0)	36.4	0.296
Poor	6 (7.5)	50.0	
T stage**			
T1	29 (36.7)	20.7	
T2	27 (34.2)	11.1	<0.001
T3, T4	23 (29.1)	78.3	
N stage			
N0	54 (67.5)	22.2	
N+	20 (25.0)	70.0	<0.001
Unknown	6 (7.5)	16.7	
M stage			
M0	74 (92.5)	33.8	
M+	1 (1.3)	100.0	0.021
Unknown	5 (6.3)	20.0	
HPV/p16			
Negative	68 (85.0)	35.3	
Positive	6 (7.5)	16.7	0.720
Unknown	6 (7.5)	33.3	
TLS single level			

Table 3 Clinicopathologic variables as predictors for 5-year disease-specific death in univariate analysis for 80 patients with OSCC (Continued)

Negative	67 (83.8)	37.3	0.156
Positive	13 (16.3)	15.4	
TLS multiple level			
Negative	63 (78.8)	39.7	0.039
Positive	17 (21.3)	11.8	

P-values were calculated using the log-rank test.
*For univariate survival analysis, the tumour sites were grouped into three categories.
**Only 79 patients were analysed because the unknown case was taken out from the calculations.

has previously been reported in colorectal cancer and lung cancer, suggesting that the occurrence of TLSs varies among different types of tumours [14,19,26]. When assessed at a single level, presence of TLSs was not a significant predictor of survival. However, when analysed at multiple levels, their presence in the tumour was a positive prognostic factor. This indicates that the prognostic value of TLSs depends on the type of analysis, probably due to their rather infrequent occurrence and tumour heterogeneity. In multivariate analyses, only T stage turned out to be an independent prognostic factor. TLS status, however, performed better than N stage, which is recognized as one of the best prognostic factors in OSCCs [4]. In the TLS-positive tumours, either single or multiple TLSs were found in the same tissue section. In some of the TLSs, GC B-cells and FDC meshworks were

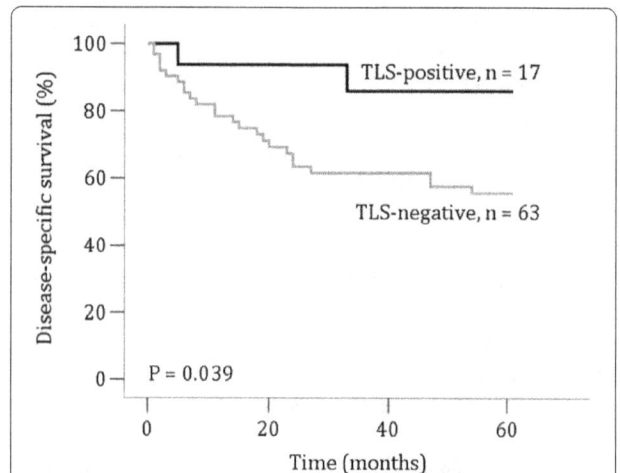

Figure 4 Results from multiple level analysis: Kaplan Meier analysis of 5-year disease-specific survival for 80 patients with oral squamous cell carcinoma with and without tertiary lymphoid structures. The presence of tertiary lymphoid structures (TLSs) is associated with improved survival in patients with oral squamous cell carcinoma (OSCC) (P = 0.039). The Kaplan-Meier curve shows a 5-year disease-specific survival rate of 88.2% for TLS-positive patients and 60.3% for TLS-negative patients. The P-value was calculated using the log-rank test.

Table 4 Results from multiple level analysis: multivariate analysis of 5-year disease-specific death according to Cox's proportional hazards model*

Variable	Hazard ratio	95% C.I.	P-value
T stage	—	—	< 0.001
T stage (1) (T1 [n = 29] v. T2 [n = 27])	0.538	0.134 - 2.151	0.381
T stage (2) (T1 [n = 29] v. T3/T4 [n = 23])	7.237	2.814 - 18.612	< 0.001
N stage	—	—	0.359
N stage (1) (N0 [n = 54] v. N + [n = 20])	1.820	0.742 - 4.461	0.191
N stage (2) (N0 [n = 54] v. unknown [n = 5])	2.342	0.290 - 18.900	0.424
TLS (negative [n = 62] v. positive [n = 17])	2.409	0.556 - 10.448	0.240

*Only 79 patients were analysed because the case with unknown T stage was taken out from the calculations.

observed, providing evidence that the TLSs comprised all cells needed to generate a functional immune response. We called lymphoid structures with defined FDC meshworks and GCs *classical TLSs*, as this phenotype has been mostly described for TLSs in literature. Besides the classical TLSs, we also found TLSs with diffuse accumulations of FDCs and scattered or absent GC B-cells that we termed *non-classical TLSs*. It remains elusive whether non-classical TLSs have the same immunological properties as classical TLSs. Immunohistochemistry on multiple tissue planes of the same tumour showed in some cases that classical and non-classical phenotypes corresponded to the same ectopic lymphoid structure. This implies that the two different patterns may be artefacts of the methodical approach of TLS detection. This is also supported by the fact that both classical and non-classical TLSs were found on the same tissue plane. Moreover, patients with TLSs showed prolonged survival regardless of TLS subtype, indicating that none of the TLS subtypes alone are particularly associated with survival. However, we found a trend towards better prognosis for patients with classical TLSs or with both classical and non-classical TLSs compared to patients with non-classical TLSs only. This indicates that, in some cases, non-classical TLSs could also represent immature follicles that may later develop into classical TLSs with full immunogenic properties. Previous studies have already reported the presence of fully and not fully mature TLSs in cancer and other inflammatory diseases [27].

Many questions about TLS development in oral cancer remain to be elucidated. Ectopic lymphoid formation is a common feature in chronically inflamed tissues and has been found in a number of different diseases at various anatomical sites [11]. After the switch from acute to chronic inflammation, gradual accumulation of lymphocytes as well as promotion of lymphangiogenesis and transformation of blood vessels into lymphocyte-guiding HEVs has been observed [28]. In oral cancer, chronically inflamed tissue precedes most of the tumours [29], providing favourable sites for TLS formation. In our OSCC samples, the TLSs were mainly located in the subepithelial lymphocytic infiltrate close to the tumour front. It would be of great interest to find out why the chronic infiltrate sometimes organizes into these structures. Disclosing the mechanisms that regulate TLS development may give important information on how to improve immune-modulating cancer therapy. Lymphoid neogenesis has been most extensively studied in autoimmune disorders such as rheumatoid arthritis, Sjögrens' syndrome and Hashimoto's thyroiditis, where TLSs might contribute to disease progression [11]. In some ectopic GCs, B-cells producing antibodies against self-antigens have been recognized, but data are still sparse [28]. In OSCC, it is not yet clear which antigenic targets the lymphocytes might react to and whether auto-antigens play a role in the induction of TLSs. In terms of viral agents that are linked to human tumours, human papillomavirus (HPV) has become a topic of interest during the last years. While HPV is a known risk factor for oropharyngeal cancer, it probably plays only a minor role in cancers arising in the oral cavity [30]. In the present study, there was no correlation between HPV-status and TLS formation. Although the antigenic stimuli directing TLS formation in OSSC are unknown, it seems likely that the immune-modulating factors that promote TLS development derive from the cancer cells rather than from autoimmunity or infection. Our results show that TLSs are most likely to form in well-differentiated tumours. It has been proposed that tumour growth might be related to stem and amplifying cell patterns, and that dedifferentiation may play a role in the origin of cancer stem cells (CSCs) in OSCC [31]. CSCs are a minority of malignant cells that are thought to be able to attenuate host anti-tumour immune responses [32]. Thus, one could speculate that dedifferentiation makes the tumour cells less antigenic and thereby elicits a milder inflammatory reaction with lower induction of TLSs. Previous studies on lymphoid neogenesis have revealed that clearance of the inflammation-inducing antigen or clinical therapy are able to cause a complete remission of the ectopic lymphoid structure [9]. This might be advantageous in autoimmune diseases to stop aggravation of the disease. However, as TLSs are thought to be conducive for patient survival in OSCC, characterization of stimulating agents might be used therapeutically to promote TLS formation by presentation of the causative agent. Investigation of circulating lymphocytes in blood samples of OSCC patients may provide new insights into the involvement of the host immune reaction in TLS development. A long-lasting chronic inflammation, as in larger tumours, could promote TLS development. In the present study, however, more TLSs were found in smaller tumours, clearly indicating that TLS formation can also take place in the early phases of tumour growth.

Conclusion

We found TLS formation to be a positive prognostic factor for patients with OSSC when tumours were analysed at multiple levels. Thus, patients with TLS-positive tumours might benefit from more restrictive treatment while a closer follow-up and more aggressive therapy should be considered for patients with TLS-negative tumours. However, before we can envisage TLSs as prognostic factors in individual clinical management of OSCC patients, larger studies on ectopic lymphoid structures are needed. Our study shows that correct assessment of TLS by immunohistochemistry requires careful analyses. When assessing CD20 B-cell staining, both dense and more diffuse aggregates of B-cells should be considered as putative TLSs. We found however, that about a third of the TLS-positive patients were missed when analysing only one level in the tissue block. This may be due to the fact that we selected blocks with representative tumour material rather than the tumour blocks with most intense inflammation. By selecting differently, the chance of discovering TLSs on a single tissue level might have increased. PCR-based approaches, such as combining analyses of a combination of mature FDC markers, HEV markers and TLS associated chemokines such as CCL19, CCL21 and CXCL13 [21], could also decrease the chance of missing TLS-positive tumours. Furthermore, analyses of TLS associated chemokines in serum from cancer patients could be a possible indicator of TLS formation.

The future trend in clinical cancer management points to personalized treatment. The use of biomarkers to guide treatment decisions along with development of immunotherapy may benefit the patient. Thus, understanding TLS formation in OSCC might help to guide targeted anti-cancer therapies and improve the dismal survival rates of patients with oral cancer.

Abbreviations

OSCCs: Oral squamous cell carcinomas; TILs: Tumour-infiltrating lymphocytes; SLO: Secondary lymphoid organ; TLS: Tertiary lymphoid structure; FDCs: Follicular dendritic cells; HEV: High-endothelial venule; PNAd: Peripheral node addressin; GC: Germinal centre; CSC: Cancer stem cell.

Competing interests

The authors declare that they have no competing interest.

Authors' contributions

AW carried out the manual immunohistochemical staining, participated in interpretation and scoring of the immunohistochrmical stainings and the statistical analyses and drafted the manuscript. OR retrieved the clinical information from patient journals, participated in the statistical analyses and critically reviewed the manuscript. SES participated in interpretations of the immunohistochemical stainings and the statistical analyses, and critically reviewed the manuscript. LUH participated in design of the study and in interpretations of the immunohistochemical stainings, and critically reviewed the manuscript. EHO participated in design of the study, scoring of the immunohistocehemical stainings and helped to draft the manuscript. All authors read and approved the final manuscript.

Acknowledgments

This work was supported by grants from The Norwegian Cancer Society, The North Norwegian Regional Health Authorities and The Erna and Olav Aakre Foundation for Cancer Research. We are also grateful for advice from Dr. Kristin A. Fenton, Dr. Elin Mortensen and M.Sc. Stine Figenshou at the Department of medical Biology, UiT, and for excellent technical help from Anne-Lise Klodiussen at the Diagnostic Clinic - Clinical Pathology, UNN and Bente Mortensen and Marit Nina Nilsen at the Department of Medical Biology, UiT. We also thank Dr. Gunbjørg Svineng and M.Sc. Maarten Beerepoot for advice and critical revision of the manuscript.

Author details

[1]Department of Medical Biology, Faculty of Health Sciences, University of Tromsø, Tromsø 9037, Norway. [2]Department of Otorhinolaryngology, University Hospital of North Norway, Tromsø 9038, Norway. [3]Diagnostic Clinic – Clinical Pathology, University Hospital of North Norway, Tromsø 9038, Norway.

References

1. Barnes L: **Pathology And Genetics Of Head And Neck Tumours.** vol. 9th edition. Lyon: IARC Press; 2005.
2. Funk GF, Karnell LH, Robinson RA, Zhen WK, Trask DK, Hoffman HT: **Presentation, treatment, and outcome of oral cavity cancer: a National Cancer Data Base report.** *Head Neck* 2002, **24**(2):165–180.
3. Massano J, Regateiro FS, Januário G, Ferreira A: **Oral squamous cell carcinoma: Review of prognostic and predictive factors.** *Oral Surg Oral Med Oral Pathol Oral Radiol Endodontol* 2006, **102**(1):67–76.
4. Woolgar JA: **Histopathological prognosticators in oral and oropharyngeal squamous cell carcinoma.** *Oral Oncol* 2006, **42**(3):229–239.
5. Shah NG, Trivedi TI, Tankshali RA, Goswami JV, Jetly DH, Shukla SN, Shah PM, Verma RJ: **Prognostic significance of molecular markers in oral squamous cell carcinoma: a multivariate analysis.** *Head Neck* 2009, **31**(12):1544–1556.
6. Fridman WH, Pagès F, Sautès-Fridman C, Galon J: **The immune contexture in human tumours: impact on clinical outcome.** *Nat Rev Cancer* 2012, **12**(4):298–306.
7. Freiser ME, Serafini P, Weed DT: **The immune system and head and neck squamous cell carcinoma: from carcinogenesis to new therapeutic opportunities.** *Immunol Res* 2013, **57**(1–3):52–69.
8. Mebius RE: **Organogenesis of lymphoid tissues.** *Nat Rev Immunol* 2003, **3**(4):292–303.
9. Drayton DL, Liao S, Mounzer RH, Ruddle NH: **Lymphoid organ development: from ontogeny to neogenesis.** *Nat Immunol* 2006, **7**(4):344–353.
10. Martinet L, Garrido I, Girard J-P: **Tumor high endothelial venules (HEVs) predict lymphocyte infiltration and favorable prognosis in breast cancer.** *Oncolmmunol* 2012, **1**(5):61–60.
11. Aloisi F, Pujol-Borrell R: **Lymphoid neogenesis in chronic inflammatory diseases.** *Nat Rev Immunol* 2006, **6**(3):205–217.
12. Stranford S, Ruddle NH: **Follicular dendritic cells, conduits, lymphatic vessels, and high endothelial venules in tertiary lymphoid organs: parallels with lymph node stroma.** *Front Immunol* 2012, **3**:article 350.

13. Coppola D, Nebozhyn M, Khalil F, Dai H, Yeatman T, Loboda A, Mule JJ: **Unique ectopic lymph node-like structures present in human primary colorectal carcinoma are identified by immune gene array profiling.** *Am J Pathol* 2011, **179**(1):37–45.

14. Dieu-Nosjean MC, Antoine M, Danel C, Heudes D, Wislez M, Poulot V, Rabbe N, Laurans L, Tartour E, de Chaisemartin L, Lebecque S, Fridman WH, Cadranel J: **Long-term survival for patients with non-small-cell lung cancer with intratumoral lymphoid structures.** *J Clin Oncol* 2008, **26**(27):4410–4417.

15. Remark R, Alifano M, Cremer I, Lupo A, Dieu-Nosjean MC, Riquet M, Crozet L, Ouakrim H, Goc J, Cazes A, Fléjou JF, Gibault L, Verkarre V, Régnard JF, Pagès ON, Oudard S, Mlecnik B, Sautès-Fridmaan C, Fridman WH, Damotte D: **Characteristics and clinical impacts of the immune environments in colorectal and renal cell carcinoma lung metastases: influence of tumor origin.** *Clin Cancer Res* 2013, **19**(15):4079–4091.

16. Nelson BH: **CD20+ B cells: the other tumor-infiltrating lymphocytes.** *J Immunol* 2010, **185**(9):4977–4982.

17. Nzula S, Going JJ, Stott DI: **Antigen-driven clonal proliferation, somatic hypermutation, and selection of B lymphocytes infiltrating human ductal breast carcinomas.** *Cancer Res* 2003, **63**(12):3275–3280.

18. Ogino S, Nosho K, Irahara N, Meyerhardt JA, Baba Y, Shima K, Glickman JN, Ferrone CR, Mino-Kenudson M, Tanaka N, Dranaoff G, Giovannucci EL, Fuchs CS: **Lymphocytic reaction to colorectal cancer is associated with longer survival, independent of lymph node count, microsatellite instability, and CpG island methylator phenotype.** *Clin Cancer Res* 2009, **15**(20):6412–6420.

19. Di Caro G, Bergomas F, Grizzi F, Doni A, Bianchi P, Malesci A, Laghi L, Allavena P, Mantovani A, Marchesi F: **Occurrence of tertiary lymphoid tissue is associated with T-cell infiltration and predicts better prognosis in early-stage colorectal cancers.** *Clin Cancer Res* 2014, **20**(8):2147–2158.

20. Goc J, Germain C, Vo-Bourgais TK, Lupo A, Klein C, Knockaert S, de Chaise-martin L, Ouakrim H, Becht E, Alifano M, Validire P, Remark R, Hammond SA, Cremer I, Damotte D, Fridman WH, Sautès-Fridman C, Dieu-Nosjean MC: **Dendritic cells in tumor-associated tertiary lymphoid structures signal a Th1 cytotoxic immune contexture and license the positive prognostic value of infiltrating CD8+ T cells.** *Cancer Res* 2014, **74**(3):705–715.

21. Goc J, Fridman WH, Sautes-Fridman C, Dieu-Nosjean MC: **Characteristics of tertiary lymphoid structures in primary cancers.** *Oncoimmunol* 2013, **2**(12):e26836.

22. Germain C, Gnjatic S, Tamzalit F, Knockaert S, Remark R, Goc J, Lepelley A, Becht E, Katsahian S, Bizouard G, Validire P, Damotte D, Alifano M, Magdeleinat P, Cremer I, Teillaud JL, Fridman WH, Sautès-Fridman C, Dieu-Nosjean MC: **Presence of B cells in tertiary lymphoid structures is associated with a protective immunity in patients with lung cancer.** *Am J Respir Crit Care Med* 2014, **189**(7):832–844.

23. Bergomas F, Grizzi F, Doni A, Pesce S, Laghi L, Allavena P, Mantovani A, Marchesi F: **Tertiary intratumor lymphoid tissue in colo-rectal cancer.** *Cancers* 2011, **4**(1):1–10.

24. McShane LM, Altman DG, Sauerbrei W, Taube SE, Gion M, Clark GM: **REporting recommendations for tumour MARKer prognostic studies (REMARK).** *Br J Cancer* 2005, **93**(4):387–391.

25. Hadler-Olsen E, Wetting HL, Rikardsen O, Steigen SE, Kanapathippillai P, Grénman R, Winberg J-O, Svineng G, Uhlin-Hansen L: **Stromal impact on tumor growth and lymphangiogenesis in human carcinoma xenografts.** *Virchows Arch* 2010, **457**(6):677–692.

26. Fridman WH, Dieu-Nosjean MC, Pages F, Cremer I, Damotte D, Sautes-Fridman C, Galon J: **The immune microenvironment of human tumors: general significance and clinical impact.** *Cancer Microenvironment* 2013, **6**(2):117–122.

27. Page G, Lebecque S, Miossec P: **Anatomic localization of immature and mature dendritic cells in an ectopic lymphoid organ: correlation with selective chemokine expression in rheumatoid synovium.** *J Immunol* 2002, **168**(10):5333–5341.

28. Neyt K, Perros F, van Geurts Kessel CH, Hammad H, Lambrecht BN: **Tertiary lymphoid organs in infection and autoimmunity.** *Trends Immunol* 2012, **33**(6):297–305.

29. Lu S-L, Reh D, Li AG, Woods J, Corless CL, Kulesz-Martin M, Wang X-J: **Overexpression of transforming growth factor β1 in head and neck epithelia results in inflammation, angiogenesis, and epithelial hyperproliferation.** *Cancer Res* 2004, **64**(13):4405–4410.

30. Chaturvedi AK, Anderson WF, Lortet-Tieulent J, Curado MP, Ferlay J, Franceschi S, Rosenberg PS, Bray F, Gillison ML: **Worldwide trends in incidence rates for oral cavity and oropharyngeal cancers.** *J Clin Oncol* 2013, **31**(36):4550–4559.

31. Costea D, Tsinkalovsky O, Vintermyr O, Johannessen A, Mackenzie I: **Cancer stem cells–new and potentially important targets for the therapy of oral squamous cell carcinoma.** *Oral Dis* 2006, **12**(5):443–454.

32. Schatton T, Frank MH: **Antitumor immunity and cancer stem cells.** *Ann N Y Acad Sci* 2009, **1176**(1):154–169.

7

Comparison of targeted next-generation sequencing and Sanger sequencing for the detection of *PIK3CA* mutations in breast cancer

Ruza Arsenic[*], Denise Treue, Annika Lehmann, Michael Hummel, Manfred Dietel, Carsten Denkert and Jan Budczies

Abstract

Background: Phosphatidylinositol-4,5-bisphosphate 3-kinase, catalytic subunit alpha, *PIK3CA*, is one of the most frequently mutated genes in breast cancer, and the mutation status of *PIK3CA* has clinical relevance related to response to therapy.
The aim of our study was to investigate the mutation status of PIK3CA gene and to evaluate the concordance between NGS and SGS for the most important hotspot regions in exon 9 and 20, to investigate additional hotspots outside of these exons using NGS, and to correlate the *PIK3CA* mutation status with the clinicopathological characteristics of the cohort.

Methods: In the current study, next-generation sequencing (NGS) and Sanger Sequencing (SGS) was used for the mutational analysis of *PIK3CA* in 186 breast carcinomas.

Results: Altogether, 64 tumors had *PIK3CA* mutations, 55 of these mutations occurred in exons 9 and 20. Out of these 55 mutations, 52 could also be detected by Sanger sequencing resulting in a concordance of 98.4 % between the two sequencing methods. The three mutations missed by SGS had low variant frequencies below 10 %. Additionally, 4.8 % of the tumors had mutations in exons 1, 4, 7, and 13 of *PIK3CA* that were not detected by SGS. *PIK3CA* mutation status was significantly associated with hormone receptor-positivity, HER2-negativity, tumor grade, and lymph node involvement. However, there was no statistically significant association between the *PIK3CA* mutation status and overall survival.

Conclusions: Based on our study, NGS is recommended as follows: 1) for correctly assessing the mutation status of *PIK3CA* in breast cancer, especially for cases with low tumor content, 2) for the detection of subclonal mutations, and 3) for simultaneous mutation detection in multiple exons.

Keywords: Next-generation sequencing, Breast cancer, Sanger sequencing, *PIK3CA*

Background

Historically, Sanger sequencing (SGS) has been the gold standard for detecting DNA mutations. However, SGS has limitations due to its restricted sensitivity and its inability to perform parallel investigation of multiple targets. Furthermore, somatic cancer mutations can be difficult to detect using SGS without performing microdissections because tumors are heterogeneous and often mixed with normal tissue. Recent progress in massive parallel sequencing, termed next-generation sequencing (NGS), has increased the speed and efficiency of mutation testing in molecular pathology [1–9]. NGS allows for the detection of a broad spectrum of mutations, including single nucleotide substitutions, small insertions and deletions, large genomic duplications and deletions, and rare variations [9].

Targeted NGS, which involves the targeted enrichment of a set of DNA regions, is used for the parallel sequencing of amplicons derived from multiplex polymerase chain reaction (PCR) or other amplicon-based

* Correspondence: ruza.arsenic@charite.de
Institute of Pathology, Charité University Hospital Berlin, Berlin, Germany

enrichment approaches, such as hybridization capture. When the amplicon size is kept small (e.g., <175 bp) in the design of the sequencing panel, NGS is also applicable to formalin-fixed tissue samples. Moreover, targeted NGS is more cost efficient than SGS [10]. This high-throughput technology is currently used with several platforms, including the Genome Analyzer/HiSeq/MiSeq (Illumina Solexa), the SOLiD System (Thermo Fisher Scientific), the Ion PGM/Ion Proton (Thermo Fisher Scientific), and the HeliScope Sequencer (Helicos BioSciences) [11, 12].

NGS can be used to detect both somatic and germline mutations in the cancer genome. The somatic genetic changes can be classified as either driver or passenger mutations. The former contribute to tumor development [13, 14], while the latter do not directly contribute to tumor development and may be the product of genomic instability within the tumor. Although SGS and PCR are routinely used to identify clinically relevant mutations and select the best treatment for patients, these techniques are insensitive to changes occurring at an allele frequency lower than 20 %, apart from real-time PCR, which could reach higher sensitivity [15, 16].

However, the more sensitive and cost-effective multiplex NGS testing platforms provide comprehensive genomic information, and thus allow for the implementation of targeted therapies and improved treatment decisions [17]. *TP53* and *PIK3CA* are the most frequently mutated genes in breast cancer (BC), both being mutated in about one-third of all primary breast carcinomas [18, 19]. In recent years, several studies identified the clinical relevance of *PIK3CA* mutations in terms of decreasing the benefits of anti-HER2 therapies and poly-chemotherapies in patients with *PIK3CA* mutations [20–22] . In the present study, we investigated the *PIK3CA* status of 186 primary BC patients from the Berlin area using targeted NGS and SGS. Recent studies have analyzed mutations in hot spots (i.e., exon 9 and 20) and only a few studies have analyzed mutations in other exons [23] Consequently, our aims were to evaluate the concordance between NGS and SGS for the most important hotspot regions in exon 9 and 20, to investigate additional hotspots outside of these exons using NGS, and to correlate the *PIK3CA* mutation status with the clinicopathological characteristics of the cohort.

Methods

Patient cohort and histopathological evaluation
Tissue samples were collected from 186 patients with a diagnosis of primary BC at the Department of Pathology, University Hospital Charité and the Breast Cancer Center at the DRK Klinikum Koepenick in Berlin, Germany. The median follow-up time was 38 months. Data on tumor histology and tumor grade were evaluated at the time of primary diagnosis and extracted from pathology reports. Tumors were graded according to the Bloom-Richardson

grading system modified by Elston and Ellis [24]. HER2 status was determined by immunohistochemistry (IHC) using the Dako HercepTest kit (Dako, Carpinteria, CA, USA). Chromatic in situ hybridization (CISH) was also performed on samples with a HER2 score of 2+. The estrogen receptor (ER) monoclonal antibody clone SP1 (NeoMarkers, Fremont, CA, USA) was used to identify the ER status, and the progesterone receptor (PR) status was determined with the PR monoclonal antibody PgR 636 (Dako, Wiesentheid, Germany). Only nuclear labeling was scored as positive. Negative ER and PR status was defined as positivity in <1 % of tumor cells according to ASCO/CAP guidelines [25]. HER2 negativity (HER2-) was defined as the absence of membranous staining or weak, discontinuous membranous staining. Cases with moderate membranous staining in >10 % of the tumor cells were examined by CISH according to ASCO/CAP guidelines [26]. A proliferation index was not available for all samples. Representative tumor samples containing at least 30 % tumor cells were selected for molecular studies.

Sample cohort and clinical parameters
Median patient age at the time of diagnosis was 65 years, with a range of 34–95 years.

A total of 149 patients (80.1 %) had ductal carcinoma and 20 (10.7 %) had lobular carcinoma. Seventeen patients (9.1 %) had carcinoma of another histological type, such as mucinous ductal carcinoma with squamous differentiation, mixed-ductal and lobular carcinoma, medullary carcinoma, or invasive papillary adenocarcinoma. None of the patients received any medical treatment related to BC before surgery. After diagnosis, most (93 %) of the hormone receptor-positive (HR+) cases were administered hormonal therapy alone or in combination with other therapies according to relevant guidelines.

Ethics approval
Patients provided written informed consent for use of their biomaterial samples in biomarker studies. Consent was obtained using the standardized informed consent forms of the participating institutions. The project and consent process was approved by the ethics board of the Charité Hospital, Berlin (reference number EA1/139/05, last amendment 2013).

DNA extraction, PCR, and *PIK3CA* semiconductor next-generation sequencing
Briefly, 10 consecutive 10-μm thick sections were prepared. The first section was stained with hematoxylin/eosin and the tumor area was marked by a pathologist. The corresponding area was manually microdissected from each of the consecutive unstained sections and transferred to 180 μl of lysis buffer (QIAamp® DNA Mini

Kit, Qiagen, Venlo, Niederlande) for 10 min at 95 °C. Enzymatic lysis was carried out with 20 µl of Proteinase K for 1 h at 56 °C. Subsequent DNA preparation was performed according to the manufacturer's instructions, and the DNA was eluted in 80 µl of elution buffer. Total nucleic acid concentrations were measured with a Qubit fluorometer HS DNA Assay (Life Technologies, Carlsbad, CA, USA) and a TaqMan RNase P Detection Reagents Kit (Life Technologies). Ten nanograms of genomic DNA were utilized for the library preparation. The final library was quantified using an Ion AmpliSeq Library Kit 2.0 (Life Technologies). The samples were 8-fold multiplexed and amplified on Ion Spheres Particles using the Ion One-Touch™ 200 Template Kit v2 DL (Life Technologies). After library enrichment and quality control on a Qubit instrument (Ion Sphere Quality Control Kit, Life Technologies), the samples were sequenced using the Ion 318 chip v2 according to the standard protocol of the chip manufacturer.

A customized sequencing panel consisting of 154 amplicons from 48 genes was designed using the Ion AmpliSeq Designer to cover the most frequent somatic mutations found in BC. The panel included six amplicons located in *PIK3CA* exons 1, 4, 7, 9, 13, and 20. The genomic positions and primer sequences can be found in the well plate data sheet generated by the Ion AmpliSeq Designer (Additional file 1: Table S1). Only samples with at least 30 % tumor cells within the dissected area were included in the study.

Base calling and alignment to the human genome (hg19) were executed with the Torrent Suite Software 4.0.3. The mean coverages (minimum – maximum) of the amplicons were 4128 bp (1315–22668 bp) for exon 1, 5237 bp (1962–25371 bp) for exon 4, 2044 bp (347–12066 bp) for exon 7, 3588 bp (278–20808 bp) for exon 9, 3742 bp (1386–20063 bp) for exon 13, and 1552 bp (438–9901 bp) for exon 20. Variant calling was executed using the Torrent Variant Caller 4.2 and the low stringency somatic variant calling protocol. Only non-synonymous nucleotide exchanges were considered for the analysis of single nucleotide polymorphisms.

Sanger sequencing primers and sequencing parameters

Primers were designed using the Primer Design Tool from NCBI. The primers were as follows:

exon 9 forward 5′-
GGGAAAAATATGACAAAGAAAGC-3′,
exon 9 reverse 5′-GAGATCAGCCAAATTCAGTT-3′,
exon 20 part 1 forward 5′-
CATTTGCTCCAAACTGACCA-3′,
exon 20 part 1 reverse 5′-
TgTgCATCATTCATTTgTTTCA-3′,

exon 20 part 2 forward 5′-
TTGATGACATTGCATACATTCG-3′,
and exon 20 part 2 reverse 5′-
GGTCTTTGCCTGCTGAGAGT-3′.

The sequencing reactions were loaded on the 3730xl DNA Analyzer from Hitachi (Applied Biosystems). Sequence traces from tumor DNA samples were aligned to the genomic reference sequence and analyzed using Seq-Pilot software (Applied Biosystems).

Statistical evaluation

Statistical analyses were conducted using the SPSS 19 statistical software (SPSS Inc., Chicago, IL, USA) and the statistical language R (Foundation for Statistical Computing, Vienna, Austria). Significance of associations between *PIK3CA* status and age, ER/PR status, tumor stage, and histological grade were assessed using a Fisher's exact test, a chi-squared test, and a chi-squared test for trends. Overall survival was analyzed using the Kaplan-Meier method and the log-rank test. All tests were two-tailed, and results were considered significant when $p < 0.05$. Barplots and beeswarm plots were produced using the R package graphics and beeswarm [27, 28].

Results

Prevalence of different types of *PIK3CA* mutations using NGS

Using NGS to sequence the *PIK3CA* gene in each of the 186 tissue samples identified a total of 64 tumors with exon mutations (34.4 %), which agreed with the 36 % *PIK3CA* mutation rate in BC reported by the Cancer Genome Atlas (TCGA) [18, 19]. As shown in Fig. 1, the mutations were distributed as follows: exon 20 (34 cases; 18.3 %), exon 9 (19 cases; 10.2 %), and other exons (1, 4, 7, or 13) (9 cases; 4.8 %). In very few samples (2 cases; 1.1 %), we found mutations in two exons. The majority of mutations were base pair substitutions (60 cases, 93.8 %). Additionally, we detected deletions (4 cases, 6.3 %). Sixty of the tumors (93.7 %) had a single mutation in the *PIK3CA* gene, while three tumors had two mutations in the *PIK3CA* gene. The most frequent mutations were p.H1047R (31 cases, 48.4 %), p.E545K (11 cases, 17.2 %), and p.E542K (6 cases, 9.4 %) (Table 1).

Three mutations, p.N347T, p.G451_D454del, and p.L456V, were not described in any of the studies reported in COSMIC (http://cancer.sanger.ac.uk/cancergenome/ projects/cosmic), TCGA [18, 19], or any other large genomic database [29, 30]. Thus, they are being described for the first time in our study. Additionally, a single nucleotide polymorphism (rs3729674) (NC_000003.11:g. 178917005A > G) was found in 33 cases. Out of a total of 55 mutations in exons 9 and 20 that were detected using NGS, 49 were also detected by SGS. By resequencing

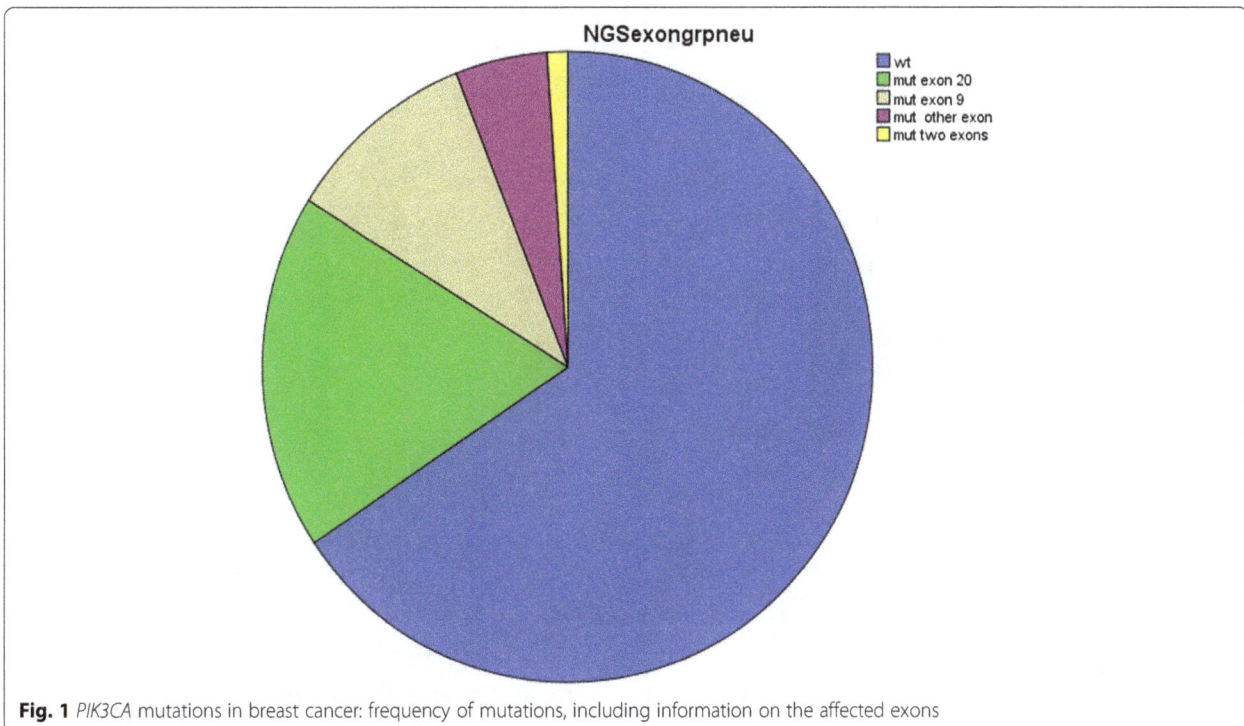

Fig. 1 *PIK3CA* mutations in breast cancer: frequency of mutations, including information on the affected exons

discrepant cases using SGS, we found an additional three cases with mutations with small peak heights that could be detected by analyzing the electropherograms manually. A comparison of the NGS and SGS results is shown in Fig. 2. The three mutations in exon 9 and exon 20 that were missed by SGS had low variant frequencies of 4 % (twice) and 7 %.

PIK3CA mutations and clinical characteristics

PIK3CA mutations were analyzed for correlation with several clinicopathological parameters at the time of the diagnosis: age, tumor size, tumor grade, nodal status, HR status, HER2 expression, and histological subtype (Table 2). *PIK3CA* mutations were most frequently found in HR+, HER2- ($p = 0.002$), and well-differentiated (G1; $p < 0.001$) cases (Fig. 3a and b). Furthermore, there was a statistically significant difference between cases with

different nodal statuses; there were more cases with *PIK3CA* mutations in the N1 group ($p = 0.042$). We found no statistically significant correlation between mutation status and age, tumor size, or histological tumor type.

When we compared mutations in the other exons (1, 4, 7, and 13) with the clinicopathological parameters, we found a trend toward enrichment of the mutations in lower grade tumors, but this trend did not reach statistical significance ($p = 0.104$). There was no statistically significant difference between *PIK3CA* mutation status in these other exons and cases that were HR+, HR-, HER2+, or HER2-. Also, we could not detect differences in nodal status, tumor size, or age.

An overall survival analysis was performed on 184 patients with available follow-up data. In this group, no statistically significant association was found between long-term survival and the *PIK3CA* mutation status

Table 1 Hotspots of *PIK3CA* mutations in breast cancer

Exon	Mutation	Number	Frequency (%)	Total number
1	R108del, R109del	1, 2	1.6, 3.1	3
4	N345K, N347T (new), D350N	3,1,1	4.7, 1.6, 1.6	5
7	G451_D454del (new), p.L456V (new)	1,1	1.6, 1.6	2
9	E542K, E545K, Q546K, Q546R	6, 11, 1, 1	9.4, 17.2	19
13	E726K	2	3,1	2
20	D1029H, N1044K, H1047L, H1047R, G1049R	1, 1, 3, 31, 1	1.6, 1.6, 48.4, 4.7, 1.6	37
		total: 68		

Using semiconductor NGS, we identified a total of 68 non-silent mutations in 186 breast cancer samples (34.4 %). The most frequent aberrations were p.H1047R, p.E545K, and p.E542K

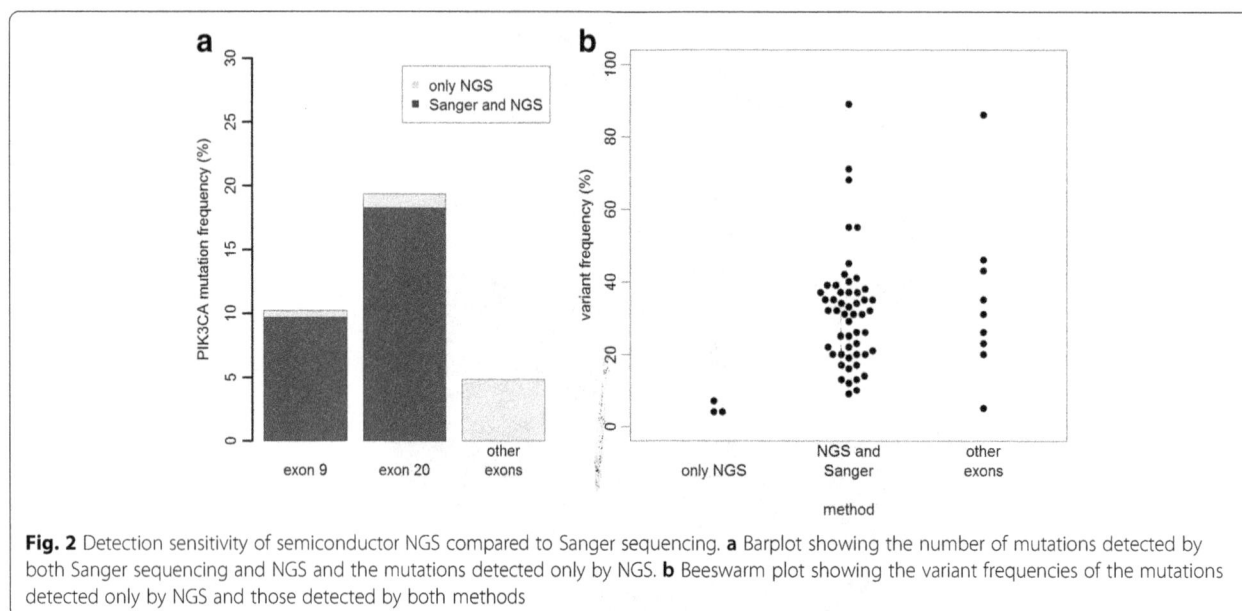

Fig. 2 Detection sensitivity of semiconductor NGS compared to Sanger sequencing. **a** Barplot showing the number of mutations detected by both Sanger sequencing and NGS and the mutations detected only by NGS. **b** Beeswarm plot showing the variant frequencies of the mutations detected only by NGS and those detected by both methods

(Fig. 4a). There was also no difference in overall survival related to the mutational status of different *PIK3CA* exons (Fig. 4b).

Discussion

The precise identification of genomic alterations is crucial for personalized cancer therapy. Molecular testing for mutations in cancer susceptibility genes is mainly performed using SGS of individual exons after PCR. The detection threshold of SGS requires an allele frequency of approximately 20 % [31], but BC tissue is heterogeneous, consisting of tumor, stromal, and inflammatory cells, leading to a varying proportion of tumor cells ranging from 20-95 % [32]. Therefore, we speculated that a significant proportion of *PIK3CA* mutations are missed by SGS. There are studies available from other organ systems, including the lung, which report a higher detection rate of mutations using NGS rather than SGS [33, 34]. In general, the detection sensitivity of NGS reported in previous studies ranges from 94–99.9 % [35–39], which is above the sensitivity of Sanger Sequencing. Accordingly, the aim of the present study was to use NGS for the analysis of *PIK3CA* mutations to determine whether additional changes could be identified that might lead to better correlation of the clinicopathological characteristics of breast tumors with *PIK3CA* mutations. We also sought to evaluate the prognostic significance of *PIK3CA* mutation status as previously reported by several authors [40–44]. To this end, we compared the performance of NGS and SGS in the same cohort of patients, and identified *PIK3CA* mutations in 34.4 % of breast tumors using NGS, which is in agreement with the mutation rate reported in TCGA [45].

Overall, we were able to report a good degree of concordance between the two sequencing methods. Only three mutations that were detected by NGS could not be found by SGS due to low variant frequencies below 10 %. Nevertheless, this finding indicates that NGS is more sensitive than SGS, particularly for the detection of low frequency mutations. This has also been reported in previous studies. Rohlin et al. [46] showed that Sanger-based sequencing techniques have problems picking out "minority" gene sequences (mutations below 15 %). Meanwhile, Walsch et al. performed a study on 300 high-risk BC families that screened for mutations in hotspots, and found previously undetected changes in 52 probands [47]. These results clearly support the use of targeted sequencing because it is more sensitive than SGS when it comes to identifying low frequency mutations. Our study, which is the first to compare NGS and SGS for sequencing the *PIK3CA* gene in BC, adds support for this viewpoint. Additionally, the results of our study showed that ~5 % of the mutations were in other exons, and the best and most cost-effective method for detecting these mutations was to use parallel sequencing or targeted NGS. Due to the low mutation rate in these other exons (1, 4, 7, and 13) and a lack of statistical significance when correlated with clinicopathological data, we abstained from validating these mutations by SGS. The clinical relevance of *PIK3CA* mutations outside exon 9 and 20 should be further investigated in future studies.

The *PIK3CA* mutations detected by NGS in our study clustered in two previously reported "hotspot" regions in exons 9 and 20, with most of the mutations clustering in exon 20, which is in agreement with the SGS results reported in our previous study [48]. The consequences of

Table 2 Correlation of *PIK3CA* mutation status with the clinicopathological characteristics of breast cancer

Clinicopathological parameters	Mutated (%)	Wild type (%)	P
All Tumor Cases	64 (34.4)	122 (65.6)	NS
Histological Type			NS
Ductal/Other Carcinoma	53 (32.5)	110 (67.5)	
Lobular Carcinoma	11 (47.8)	12 (52.2)	
Tumor Stage			NS
T1	13 (30.2)	28 (65.1)	
T2	37 (34.9)	69 (65.1)	
T3	9 (42.9)	12 (57.1)	
T4	5 (41.7)	7 (58.3)	
Node Status			0.042
N0	25 (27.8)	65 (72.2)	
N+	37 (42.5)	50 (57.5)	
Tumor Grade			<0.001
G1	16 (80.0)	4 (20.0)	
G2	35 (36.5)	61 (63.5)	
G3	13 (18.8)	56 (81.2)	
Hormone Receptor Status			0.002
HR+	58 (40.3)	86 (59.7)	
HR-	6 (14.3)	36 (85.7)	
HER2 Status			0.032
HER2+	3 (13.6)	19 (86.4)	
HER2-	61 (37.2)	103 (62.8)	
Age			NS
<50 years	6 (26.1)	17 (73.9)	
>50 years	58 (35.6)	105 (64.4)	
Molecular Type			0.003
HR+/HER2-	57 (42.5)	77 (57.5)	
HR+/HER2+	1 (10.0)	9 (90.0)	
HR-/HER2+	2 (16.7)	10 (83.3)	
HR-/HER2-	4 (13.3)	26 (86.7)	

The mutation frequency, as determined by NGS, decreased with increasing tumor grade: 85 % for G1, 37 % for G2, and 20 % for G3. *PIK3CA* mutations were more frequently detected (42 %) in HR+ breast cancer than in HR- breast cancer (14 %). *PIK3CA* mutations were more frequently detected in HER2- breast cancer (38 %) than in HER2+ breast cancer (14 %)

each mutation on the function and regulation of *PIK3CA* requires further consideration. The three novel mutation detected in our study are located in the C2 domain of the PIK3CA gene. The C2 is often involved in phospholipid membrane binding, consequently it is possible that these mutations lead to increased membrane binding, as extensively discussed in the study by Ikenoue at al. [49]. In the study by Gymnopoulos at al, the authors showed that the mutants in C2 domain increase basic positive surface charge of that domain and may therefore mediate improved recruitment of p110α to the cell membrane,

making lipid kinase activity independent of signals transmitted through the regulatory subunit, p85 [50]. One of these three mutations, p.L456V is predicted to be probably damaging with a score of 0.988 (sensitivity: 0.27; specificity: 0.99) when analyzed with polyPhen-2 prediction programe.

The goal of our previous study was to analyse only exon 9 and 20 mutations, hence we could not detect these three mutations in this study.

We also noted the presence of multiple mutations in four cases, which has not been reported previously. The significance of these double mutants is unknown, but it is possible that these tumors are multiclonal, and a second hit was required to provide a selective growth advantage if the first mutation was a less potent activator of the kinase.

We found that *PIK3CA* was most frequently mutated in cases that were HR+ and HER2-, which agrees with previously published data [51, 52]. We found significantly more *PIK3CA* mutations in G1 tumors suggesting that theses mutations occur early in BC development, which has also been shown in other studies [53]. Additionally, *PIK3CA* mutations were highly correlated with lymph node status (N+), which is one of the clinical markers associated with patient survival and response to therapy [54, 55]. The finding that *PIK3CA* mutations are more commonly found in HR+ tumors may point to differences in pathogenesis and disease progression between HR+ and HR- tumors. Furthermore, the correlation between *PIK3CA* mutations and lymph node metastasis suggests that activation of the PI3K/Akt pathway may increase the invasion of cancer cells into the lymph nodes. This is supported by the fact that PIP3 regulates cell mobility [56].

There is controversy regarding the prognostic significance of *PIK3CA* mutations. Cizkova et al. [57] described more favorable metastasis-free survival in patients with *PIK3CA* mutations, but Jensen et al. [22] and Baselga et al. [58] reported reduced survival rates and worse outcomes. The largest published study evaluated the *PIK3CA* genotype in 687 tumor samples from patients enrolled in a prospective phase III clinical trial. Those with *PIK3CA* mutations had a better prognosis for the first three years compared to those carrying wild type *PIK3CA* alleles, but this difference disappeared with a longer follow-up [59,60]. In our study, there was no significant association between *PIK3CA* mutational status and overall survival, indicating that an activated *PIK3CA* pathway alone is not a prognostic factor for BC.

An interesting finding by Fu at al. showed that *PIK3CA*-activating mutations are associated with better outcomes in ER+ patients receiving endocrine therapy [61]. This agrees with the observation that *PIK3CA* mutations are more frequent in luminal A tumors compared

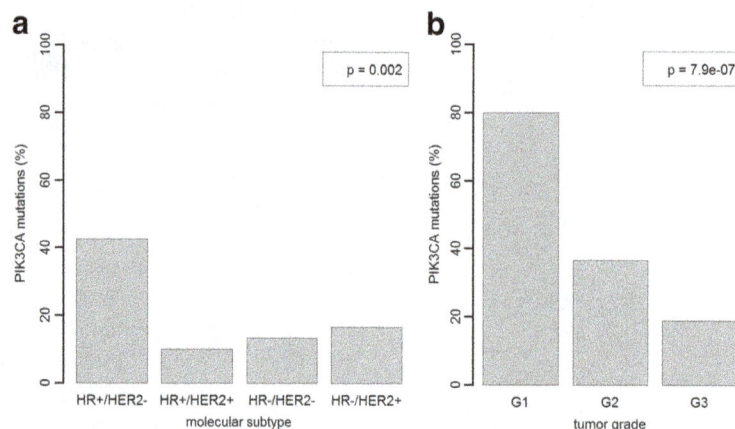

Fig. 3 Strong association of *PIK3CA* status with molecular subtype and tumor grade in breast cancer. **a** *PIK3CA* mutations were more frequent in HR+/HER2- breast cancer (40 %) compared with the other subtypes (11 %-20 %). **b** The mutation frequency decreased with increasing tumor grade: 80 % in G1, 36 % in G2, and 19 % in G3

with luminal B tumors (e.g., 45 % vs. 29 % in the TCGA cohort) [45]. In contrast, in HER2+ BC, several reports show that *PIK3CA* mutations predict adverse outcomes after treatment with trastuzumab [20, 21]. As such, the impact of *PIK3CA* mutations on the clinical outcome of BC seems to vary with the background of other genomic alterations such as HER2 status.

PIK3CA mutations also appear to have a significant interest in the prediction of response to targeted therapies, as many drugs specifically targeting PI3K or other effectors of the PI3K/AKT pathway are intended to be administered only to patients with tumor bearing a mutation of *PIK3CA*, which makes the somatic mutations detection more and more important [62].

In summary, our results show that NGS is more sensitive than SGS for detecting *PIK3CA* mutations in BC samples, and that *PIK3CA* mutations are significantly related to HR and HER2 expression status and tumor grade. Further studies are needed to systematically explore the functional relevance of *PIK3CA* mutations and the contribution of PIK3CA mediated activation of the downstream and upstream signaling pathways in breast tumor development and progression.

Conclusions

1. This is the first paper in which NGS and SGS were compared sequencing PIK3CA gene in breast cancer.

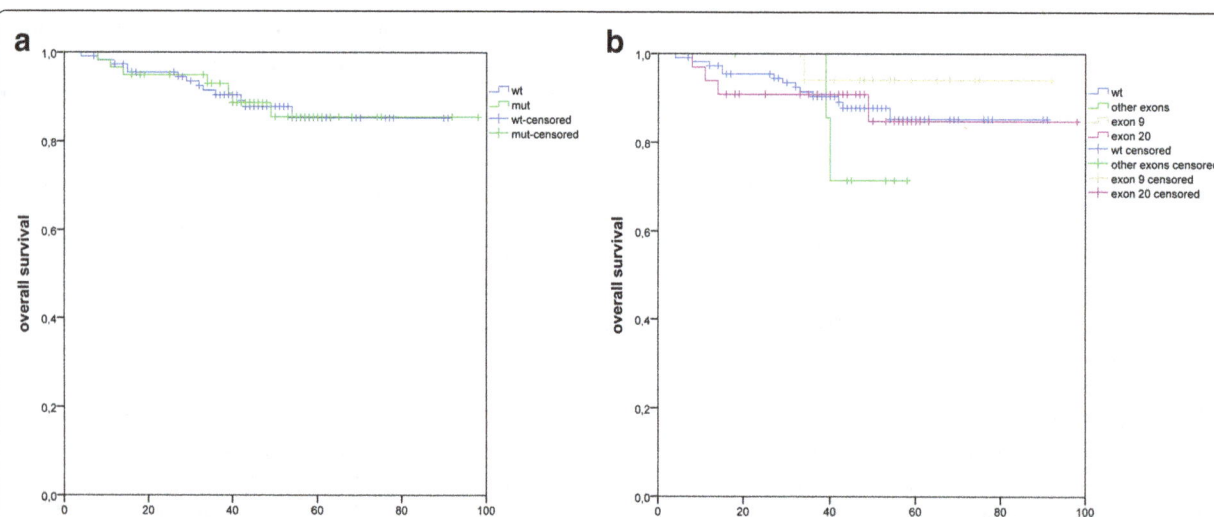

Fig. 4 Correlation of overall survival with the *PIK3CA* mutation status in breast cancer. **a** Kaplan-Meier analysis comparing patients with mutated *PIK3CA* (green line) and wild type *PIK3CA* (blue line) did not reveal a statistically significant difference in survival. **b** Kaplan-Meier analysis of the *PIK3CA* mutation status stratified for the affected exon did not reveal a statistically significant difference in survival, but there was a trend toward better survival for the cases with a mutation in exon 9. Exon 9 mutation ($p = 0.39$) vs. exon 20 mutation ($p = 0.41$) vs. other exon mutations ($p = 0.16$)

2. We found overall a good concordance between the two methods (98,4 %), but better sensitivity of NGS when it comes to identifying low frequency mutations(<10 %).

3. *PIK3CA* mutation status in breast cancer correlated strongly with HR+ and HER2-, and N1 + .

Competing interests

The authors declare that they have no competing interests.

Authors' contributions

Each of the authors contributed to the manuscript. AR and JB wrote the manuscript and performed the analysis. JB performed the statistics. AL, DT, MH, CD and MD corrected the manuscript. All authors are responsible for the overall content of the manuscript. All authors read and approved the final manuscript.

Acknowledgments

We would like to thank Ines Koch for the excellent technical assistance.

References

1. Chan M, Ji SM, Yeo ZH, Gan L, Yap E, Yap, YS et al. Development of a next-generation sequencing method for BRCA mutation screening a comparison between a high-throughput and a benchtop platform. J Mol Diagn. 2012; 14(6):602–12.
2. Chou LS, Liu CS-J, Boese B, Zhan X, Mao R. DNA Sequence Capture and Enrichment by Microarray Followed by Next-Generation Sequencing for Targeted Resequencing: Neurofibromatosis Type 1 Gene as a Model. Clin Chem. 2010;56(1):62–72.
3. De Leeneer, KHellemans J, De Schrijver J, Baetens M, Poppe B., Van Criekinge W, et al. Massive parallel amplicon sequencing of the breast cancer genes BRCA1 and BRCA2: opportunities, challenges, and limitations. Hum Mutat. 2011;32(3):335–44.
4. Goossens D, Moens LN, Nelis E, Lenaerts AS, Glassee W, Kalbe A, et al. Simultaneous mutation and copy number variation (CNV) detection by multiplex PCR-based GS-FLX sequencing. Hum Mutat. 2009;30(3):472–6.
5. Hernan I, Borràs E, de Sousa Dias M, Gamundi MJ, Mañé B, Llort G, et al. Detection of genomic variations in BRCA1 and BRCA2 genes by long-range PCR and next-generation sequencing. J Mol Diagn. 2012;14(3):286–93.
6. Mamanova L, Coffey AJ, Scott CE, Kozarewa I, Turner EH, Kumar A, et al. Target-enrichment strategies for next-generation sequencing. Nat Methods. 2010;7(2):111–8.
7. Ozcelik H, Shi X, Chang MC, Tram E, Vlasschaert M, Di Nicola N, et al. Long-range PCR and next-generation sequencing of BRCA1 and BRCA2 in breast cancer. J Mol Diagn. 2012;14(5):467–75.
8. Pritchard CC, Smith C, Salipante SJ, Lee MK, Thornton AM, Nord AS, et al. ColoSeq provides comprehensive lynch and polyposis syndrome mutational analysis using massively parallel sequencing. J Mol Diagn. 2012;14(4):357–66.
9. Walsh T, Lee MK, Casadei S, Thornton AM, Stray SM, Pennil C, et al. Detection of inherited mutations for breast and ovarian cancer using genomic capture and massively parallel sequencing. Proc Natl Acad Sci U S A. 2010;107(28):12629–33.
10. Walsh T, Casadei S, Lee MK, Pennil CC, Nord AS, Thornton AM, et al. Mutations in 12 genes for inherited ovarian, fallopian tube, and peritoneal carcinoma identified by massively parallel sequencing. Proc Natl Acad Sci U S A. 2011;108(44):18032–7.
11. Rothberg JM, Hinz W, Rearick TM, Schultz J, Mileski W, Davey M, et al. An integrated semiconductor device enabling non-optical genome sequencing. Nature. 2011;475(7356):348–52.
12. Voelkerding KV, Dames SA, Durtschi JD. Next-generation sequencing: from basic research to diagnostics. Clin Chem. 2009;55(4):641–58.
13. Hanahan D, Weinberg RA. The hallmarks of cancer. Cell. 2000;100(1):57–70.
14. Hanahan D, Weinberg RA. Hallmarks of cancer: the next generation. Cell. 2011;144(5):646–74.
15. MacConaill LE. Existing and emerging technologies for tumor genomic profiling. J Clin Oncol. 2013;31(15):1815–24.
16. Bustin SA. Absolute quantification of mRNA using real-time reverse transcription polymerase chain reaction assays. J Mol Endocrinol. 2000;25(2): 169–93.
17. Meyerson M, Gabriel S, Getz G. Advances in understanding cancer genomes through second-generation sequencing. Nat Rev Genet. 2010; 11(10):685–96.
18. Forbes SA, Bindal N, Bamford S, Cole C, Kok CY, Beare D, et al. COSMIC: mining complete cancer genomes in the Catalogue of Somatic Mutations in Cancer. Nucleic Acids Res. 2011;39(Database issue):D945–50.
19. Robbins DE, Grüneberg A, Deus HF, Tanik MM, Almeida SJ. A self-updating road map of The Cancer Genome Atlas. Bioinformatics. 2013;29(10):1333–40.
20. Chandarlapaty S, Sakr RA, Giri D, Patil S, Heguy A, Morrow M, et al. Frequent mutational activation of the PI3K-AKT pathway in trastuzumab-resistant breast cancer. Clin Cancer Res. 2012;18(24):6784–91.
21. Cizkova M, Cizkova M, Dujaric ME, Lehmann-Che J, Scott V, Tembo O, et al. Outcome impact of PIK3CA mutations in HER2-positive breast cancer patients treated with trastuzumab. Br J Cancer. 2013;108(9):1807–9.
22. Jensen JD, Knoop A, Laenkholm AV, Grauslund M, Jensen MB, Santoni-Rugiu E, et al. PIK3CA mutations, PTEN, and pHER2 expression and impact on outcome in HER2-positive early-stage breast cancer patients treated with adjuvant chemotherapy and trastuzumab. Ann Oncol. 2012;23(8):2034–42.
23. Bai X, Zhang E, Ye H, Nandakumar V, Wang Z, Chen L, et al. PIK3CA and TP53 gene mutations in human breast cancer tumors frequently detected by ion torrent DNA sequencing. PLoS One. 2014;9(6):e99306.
24. Frierson Jr HF, Wolber RA, Berean KW, Franquemont DW, Gaffey MJ, Boyd JC, et al. Interobserver reproducibility of the Nottingham modification of the Bloom and Richardson histologic grading scheme for infiltrating ductal carcinoma. Am J Clin Pathol. 1995;103(2):195–8.
25. Hammond ME, Hayes DF, Dowsett M, Allred DC, Hagerty KL, Badve S, et al. American Society of Clinical Oncology/College of American Pathologists guideline recommendations for immunohistochemical testing of estrogen and progesterone receptors in breast cancer. Arch Pathol Lab Med. 2010; 134(6):907–22.
26. Wolff AC, Hammond ME, Hicks DG, Dowsett M, McShane LM, Allison KH, et al. Recommendations for human epidermal growth factor receptor 2 testing in breast cancer: American Society of Clinical Oncology/College of American Pathologists clinical practice guideline update. Arch Pathol Lab Med. 2014;138(2):241–56.
27. A.E. beeswarm: The bee swarm plot, an alternative to stripchart. R package version 0.1.6. 2013. http://CRAN.R-project.org/package=beeswarm.
28. R.C.T. R: A language and environment for statistical computing. R Foundation for Statistical Computing, Vienna, Austria. 2014. URL http://www.R-project.org/.
29. Cerami E, Gao J, Dogrusoz U, Gross BE, Sumer SO, Aksoy BA, et al. The cBio cancer genomics portal: an open platform for exploring multidimensional cancer genomics data. Cancer Discov. 2012;2(5):401–4.
30. Fokkema IF, Taschner PE, Schaafsma GC, Celli J, Laros JF, den Dunnen JT, et al. LOVD v. 2.0: the next generation in gene variant databases. Hum Mutat. 2011;32(5):557–63.
31. Kohlmann A, Klein HU, Weissmann S, Bresolin S, Chaplin T, Cuppens H, et al. The Interlaboratory RObustness of Next-generation sequencing (IRON) study: a deep sequencing investigation of TET2, CBL and KRAS mutations by an international consortium involving 10 laboratories. Leukemia. 2011; 25(12):1840–8.
32. Cleator SJ, Powles TJ, Dexter T, Fulford L, Mackay A, Smith IE, et al. The effect of the stromal component of breast tumours on prediction of clinical outcome using gene expression microarray analysis. Breast Cancer Res. 2006;8(3):R32.
33. Buttitta F, Felicioni L, Del Grammastro M, Filice G, Di Lorito A, Malatesta S, et al. Effective assessment of egfr mutation status in bronchoalveolar lavage and pleural fluids by next-generation sequencing. Clin Cancer Res. 2013; 19(3):691–8.
34. Moskalev EA, Stöhr R, Rieker R, Hebele S, Fuchs F, Sirbu H, et al. Increased detection rates of EGFR and KRAS mutations in NSCLC specimens with low tumour cell content by 454 deep sequencing. Virchows Arch. 2013;462(4): 409–19.

35. Chin ELH, C da Silva, M Hegde. Assessment of clinical analytical sensitivity and specificity of next-generation sequencing for detection of simple and complex mutations. BMC Genet. 2013;14:14-6

36. Guan YF, Hu H, Peng Y, Gong Y, Yi Y, Shao L, et al. Detection of inherited mutations for hereditary cancer using target enrichment and next generation sequencing. Fam Cancer. 2015;14(1):9–18.

37. Hadd AG, Houghton J, Choudhary A, Sah S, Chen L, Marko AC, et al. Targeted, high-depth, next-generation sequencing of cancer genes in formalin-fixed, paraffin-embedded and fine-needle aspiration tumor specimens. J Mol Diagn. 2013;15(2):234–47.

38. Lin MT, Mosier SI, Thiess M, Beierel KF, Debeljak M, Tseng LH, et al. Clinical Validation of KRAS, BRAF, and EGFR mutation detection using next-generation sequencing. Am J Clin Pathol. 2014;141(6):856–66.

39. Nijman IJ, van Montfrans JM, Hoogstraat M, Boes ML, van de Corput L, Renner ED, et al. Targeted next-generation sequencing: a novel diagnostic tool for primary immunodeficiencies. J Allergy Clin Immunol. 2014;133(2):529–34.

40. Barbareschi M, Buttitta F, Felicioni L, Cotrupi S, Barassi F, Del Grammastro M, et al. Different prognostic roles of mutations in the helical and kinase domains of the PIK3CA gene in breast carcinomas. Clin Cancer Res. 2007; 13(20):6064–9.

41. Lai YL, Mau BL, Cheng WH, Chen HM, Chiu HH, Tzen CY. et al. PIK3CA exon 20 mutation is independently associated with a poor prognosis in breast cancer patients. Ann Surg Oncol. 2008;15(4):1064–9.

42. Li SY, Rong M, Grieu F, Iacopetta B. PIK3CA mutations in breast cancer are associated with poor outcome. Breast Cancer Res Treat. 2006;96(1):91–5.

43. Mangone FR, Bobrovnitchaia IG, Salaorni S, Manuli E, Nagai MA.PIK3CA exon 20 mutations are associated with poor prognosis in breast cancer patients. Clinics (Sao Paulo). 2012;67(11):1285–90.

44. Saal LH, Holm K, Maurer M, Memeo L, Su T, Wang X, et al. PIK3CA mutations correlate with hormone receptors, node metastasis, and ERBB2, and are mutually exclusive with PTEN loss in human breast carcinoma. Cancer Res. 2005;65(7):2554–9.

45. Koboldt DC, Fulton RS, McLellan, MD, Schmidt H, Kalicki-Veizer J, McMichael, JF, et al. Comprehensive molecular portraits of human breast tumours. Nature. 2012;490(7418):61–70.

46. Rohlin A, Wernersson J, Engwall Y, Wiklund L, Bjoerk J, Nordling M, et al. Parallel sequencing used in detection of mosaic mutations: comparison with four diagnostic DNA screening techniques. Hum Mutat. 2009;30(6): 1012–20.

47. Walsh T, Casadei S, Coats KH, Swisher E, Stray SM, Higgins J, et al. Spectrum of mutations in BRCA1, BRCA2, CHEK2, and TP53 in families at high risk of breast cancer. JAMA. 2006;295(12):1379–88.

48. Arsenic R, Lehmann A, Budczies J, Koch I, Prinzler J, Kleine-Tebbe A, et al. Analysis of PIK3CA mutations in breast cancer subtypes. Appl Immunohistochem Mol Morphol. 2014;22(1):50–6.

49. Ikenoue T, Kanai F, Hikiba Y, Obata T, Tanaka Y, Imamura J, et al. Functional analysis of PIK3CA gene mutations in human colorectal cancer. Cancer Res. 2005;65(11):4562–7.

50. Gymnopoulos M, Elsliger MA, Vogt PK. Rare cancer-specific mutations in PIK3CA show gain of function. Proc Natl Acad Sci U S A. 2007;104(13):5569–74.

51. Boyault S, Drouet Y, Navarro C, Bachelot T, Lasset C, Treilleux I, et al. Mutational characterization of individual breast tumors: TP53 and PI3K pathway genes are frequently and distinctively mutated in different subtypes. Breast Cancer Res Treat. 2012;132(1):29–39.

52. Kalinsky K, Jacks LM, Heguy A, Patil S, Drobnjak M, Bhanot UK, et al. PIK3CA mutation associates with improved outcome in breast cancer. Clin Cancer Res. 2009;15(16):5049–59.

53. Dunlap J, Le C, Shukla A, Patterson J, Presnell A, Heinrich MC, et al. Phosphatidylinositol-3-kinase and AKT1 mutations occur early in breast carcinoma. Breast Cancer Res Treat. 2010;120(2):409–18.

54. Hutter RV. Pathological parameters useful in predicting prognosis for patients with breast cancer. Monogr Pathol. 1984;25:175–85.

55. McGuire WL, Clark, GM, Dressler LG and Owens, MA. Role of steroid hormone receptors as prognostic factors in primary breast cancer. NCI Monogr. 1986;1:19–23.

56. Huang YE, Iijima M, Parent CA, Funamoto S, Firtel RA,Devreotes P, et al. Receptor-mediated regulation of PI3Ks confines PI(3,4,5)P3 to the leading edge of chemotaxing cells. Mol Biol Cell. 2003;14(5):1913–22.

57. Cizkova M, Susini A, Vacher S, Cizeron-Clairac G, Andrieu C, Driouch K, et al. PIK3CA mutation impact on survival in breast cancer patients and in ER alpha, PR and ERBB2-based subgroups. Breast Cancer Res. 2012;14(1):R28.

58. Baselga J, Cortés J, Im SA, Clark E, Ross G, Kiermaier A, et al. Biomarker analyses in CLEOPATRA: a phase III, placebo-controlled study of pertuzumab in human epidermal growth factor receptor 2-positive, first-line metastatic breast cancer. J Clin Oncol. 2014;32(33):3753–61.

59. Joensuu H, Kellokumpu-Lehtinen PL, Bono P, Alanko T, Kataja V, Asola R, et al. Adjuvant docetaxel or vinorelbine with or without trastuzumab for breast cancer. N Engl J Med. 2006;354(8):809–20.

60. Loi S, Michiels S, Lambrechts D, Fumagalli D, Claes B, Kellokumpu-Lehtinen PL, et al. Somatic mutation profiling and associations with prognosis and trastuzumab benefit in early breast cancer. J Natl Cancer Inst. 2013;105(13): 960–7.

61. Fu X, Osborne CK, Schiff R. Biology and therapeutic potential of PI3K signaling in ER+/HER2-negative breast cancer. Breast. 2013;22 Suppl 2:S12–8.

62. Harle A, Lion M, Lozano N, Merlin JL. Clinical, diagnostic significance and theranostic interest of PIK3CA gene mutations in breast cancer. Bull Cancer. 2013;100(10):947–54.

8

Comparison of time-motion analysis of conventional stool culture and the BD MAX™ Enteric Bacterial Panel (EBP)

Joel E. Mortensen[1][*], Cindi Ventrola[1], Sarah Hanna[1] and Adam Walter[2]

Abstract

Background: Conventional bacterial stool culture is one of the more time-consuming tests in a routine clinical microbiology laboratory. In addition, less than 5 % of stool cultures yield positive results. A molecular platform, the BD MAX™ System (BD Diagnostics, Sparks, MD) offers the potential for significantly more rapid results and less hands-on time. Time-motion analysis of the BD MAX Enteric Bacterial Panel (EBP) (BD Diagnostics, Quebec, Canada) on the BD MAX System was compared to conventional stool culture in the microbiology laboratory of a tertiary care pediatric hospital.

Methods: The process impact analysis of time-motion studies of conventional cultures were compared to those of EBP with 86 stool specimens. Sample flow, hands-on time, processing steps, and overall turnaround time were determined and analyzed. Data were obtained and analyzed from both standard operating procedures and direct observation. A regression analysis was performed to ensure consistency of measurements. Time and process measurements started when the specimens were logged into the accessioning area of the microbiology laboratory and were completed when actionable results were generated.

Results: With conventional culture, negative culture results were available from 41:14:27 (hours:minutes:seconds) to 54:17:19; with EBP, positive and negative results were available from 2:28:40 to 3:33:39.

Conclusions: This study supports the suggestion that use of the EBP to detect commonly encountered stool pathogens can result in significant time savings and a shorter time-to-result for patients with acute bacterial diarrhea.

Keywords: Time-motion analysis, BD MAX™, Diarrhea, Bacterial stool pathogens

Background

The World Health Organization has reported that, worldwide, there are nearly 1.7 billion cases of diarrheal disease every year and that diarrheal disease is the second leading cause of death in children under five years old [1, 2]. Each year, diarrhea results in approximately 760,000 preventable deaths of children under the age of five years. Diarrhea in this age group is also a leading cause of malnutrition. Most cases of this disease are related to unsafe drinking-water, inadequate sanitation, and poor hygiene [1, 2].

Detection and identification of the etiological agents of acute bacterial diarrhea are important for both the treatment of individual patients and for the management of diarrheal diseases of public health importance. Conventional bacterial culture remains the gold standard for the aforementioned detection, even though stool culture has relatively low sensitivity and requires a significant amount of labor. The use of nucleic acid amplification methods to detect and identify the etiological agents of acute bacterial diarrhea could have a significant impact on the laboratory diagnostic process, clinical approach, and epidemiology of this disease [3–5].

The objective of this study was to examine the laboratory impact of a new molecular platform (use of the BD MAX Enteric Bacterial Panel on the BD MAX System) on turnaround time, associated laboratory processes, and the cost of providing results with this system compared to conventional culture methods. Results of both

* Correspondence: joel.mortensen@cchmc.org
[1]Department of Laboratory Medicine, Cincinnati Children's Hospital, MLC1010, 3333 Burnet Ave, 45229 Cincinnati, OH, USA
Full list of author information is available at the end of the article

conventional culture (including a commercial immunoassay for shiga-toxin) and the EBP, which include tests for the detection of *Salmonella* spp., *Shigella* spp./ Enteroinvasive *Escherichia coli* (EIEC), *Campylobacter* spp. (*jejuni* and *coli*), and Shiga toxin 1 and 2 genes in stool specimens were evaluated. Lean and Six Sigma processes were used to analyze the time from sample receipt to actionable result for conventional stool culture and the EBP. The following "events or decisions per specimen" were determined: any action or thought process that must occur to process and issue a result, the overall distance traveled per sample as a measure of efficiency, and the operating costs of the two systems [6].

(The results of this study were presented, in part, at the 24th European Congress of Clinical Microbiology and Infectious Diseases, Barcelona, Spain, May 10–13, 2014 and at the 114th General Meeting of the American Society for Microbiology, Boston MA, May 17–20, 2014.)

Methods

Lean and Six Sigma processing analysis were performed to evaluate time-to-results for both culture and EBP testing. By design, this study did not involve human subjects or any patient information. Observations were performed without patient identifiers and additional testing was carried out on discarded, anonymous samples. Any sample ordered for routine stool culture was eligible for inclusion in the study.

Culture

Clinical stool samples were immediately accessioned and plated upon arrival in the laboratory following standard laboratory practices. They were not stored prior to culture. Sample flow, hands-on time, processing steps, overall turnaround time, and specimen travel distance were measured by two independent observers over the course of three separate observation periods; each observation period was five days. To eliminate any potential of operator-to-operator bias during the study, 11 different laboratory technologists were observed performing all pre-analytical, analytical, and post-analytical culture procedures which occurred at five different laboratory stations: specimen receipt, specimen plating and incubation, culture reading, automated identification (Vitek 2 System, bioMérieux, Marcy l'Etoile, France) and shiga-toxin testing (Immunocard STAT! EHEC, Meridian Bioscience, Cincinnati, Ohio, USA).

In brief, for this study, stool samples that were submitted for routine culture were transported in Cary Blair Transport Medium (Meridian Bioscience, Inc.). Specimens were processed within 2 h of receipt. Initially, samples were inoculated onto the following agar media: 5 % sheep blood, MacConkey, Sorbitol MacConkey, Hektoen, Campy CVA (BD Diagnostics, Sparks, MD, USA).

Cultures were incubated under standard conditions. Suspected bacterial pathogens were identified using the Vitek 2 System (bioMerieux) and standard conventional methodologies as needed. Additional testing may have included the following: Salmonella serotyping and Shigella serotyping Becton, Dickinson and Company, Sparks, MD, USA) and Remel RIM E. coli O157:H7 Latex Test (Remel, Lenexa, KS, USA).

Additional data were obtained and analyzed from laboratory Standard Operating Procedures (SOP) used routinely in this particular laboratory. In order to ensure consistency during the study, a regression analysis of measurements, processing, and adherence to the SOP was performed. Correlation studies were performed on independent data sets to ensure no bias was falsely introduced by operator-to-operator performance [7]. The following elements were analyzed: elapsed time, distance traveled, processing steps performed, and clinical decisions, from the time the specimens were logged into the accessioning area until the time actionable results were generated. Processing was observed and data were collected during each of the following notable events: specimen arrival, specimen accessioning, specimen plating and preparation, specimen incubation, first-day plate reading and workup, subsequent day(s) reading, including *Campylobacter* spp. cultures reading, automated identification and additional workup, shiga-toxin broth inoculation, shiga-toxin rapid testing, and verification of results, and entering results into the laboratory/hospital information system.

EBP testing

Methods similar to those used to evaluate culture processes were measured and analyzed: elapsed time, distance traveled, processing steps, and clinical decisions (also from the time specimens were logged into the accessioning area to the time actionable results were generated). Processing was observed and data were collected during each of the following notable events: specimen arrival, specimen accessioning, control preparation, specimen preparation, instrument preparation, worklist preparation, instrument processing, and result verification. For BD MAX testing, the samples were batched and tested in different batch sizes. Batch sizes ranged from 4 to 24 samples in increments of 4 to mimic routine clinical testing.

Cost analysis

Standard institutional cost analysis was used to determine the costs for conventional culture and for EBP. The main cost components of the analysis were labor, direct materials and supplies, and general shared costs (Test Site Burden). Hands-on time (minutes) for each step of the cultures and the EBP was multiplied by the average hourly technologist salary/min of labor to determine labor costs. The quantity of each item and the cost of each item used in culture and EBP testing were derived from institutional inventory data. Institutional overhead or Test Site Burden is the cost for basic services such as lights and heat and the cost of common shared laboratory equipment such as incubators, repeat pipettes, etc.

Institutional review board

It was determined that this study did not meet regulatory criteria for research involving human subjects because the research did not obtain data through intervention or interaction with the individual or identifiable private information. All observations of process were made without any patient identifiers available to the observer. All specimens tested on the BD MAX were anonymous, discarded samples that were only used after clinical testing was completed and for which no patient identifiers were used.

Results

86 patient specimens were examined. No pathogens under consideration in this study (i.e., *Salmonella, Campylobacter, Shigella* and shiga toxin producing organisms) were detected by culture or BD MAX EBP.

To enable a comparison, simultaneously, 84 alternate specimens tested by EBP were processed across six batches of differing size (4 to 24 samples each) on the BD MAX platform. Processing and turnaround times of routine cultures were compared to the process and turnaround times of EBP testing. The mean time to reportable result for 86 routine cultures was 44:37:00 (hours:minutes:seconds) (+/– 8 h, 10 min) (Fig. 1). If potential pathogens

were detected that required additional testing, the time to final result ranged from 97:18:17 to 145:27:11.

Although the time to perform EBP testing is approximately two hours, EBP is designed and best used to batch specimen testing at reasonable intervals as determined by each laboratory. If a reasonable operational model is two EBP runs per day (one in the morning, one in the afternoon), the time to reportable EBP results would be, at most, 07:06:00 (no standard deviation; all variability dependent upon batch size and timing of run). Hands-on time per specimen was 0:01:30 (+/– 19 s). With an assumption of two EBP runs per day and 90 s hands-on time/specimen, there was an 85 % reduction of time to reportable results compared to culture.

Process Steps for Culture and EBP

Technologists made an average of 141 and 25 decisions per culture and EBP test, respectively. Thus, EBP testing required 82 % fewer decisions than did culture (Table 1). The number of steps and processes in each unique laboratory can be represented by a spaghetti diagram of process flow for culture and for EBP testing (Fig. 2).

Cost analysis

Detailed costs are listed in Table 2. The basic labor to process and handle a stool culture was 0:15:00 – 0:17:00. Approximately 20 % of the cultures required additional process steps to rule out potential pathogens; these additional steps resulted in additional labor (0:35:00 – 0:40:00) and supplies. The EBP required 0:01:28 hands on time.

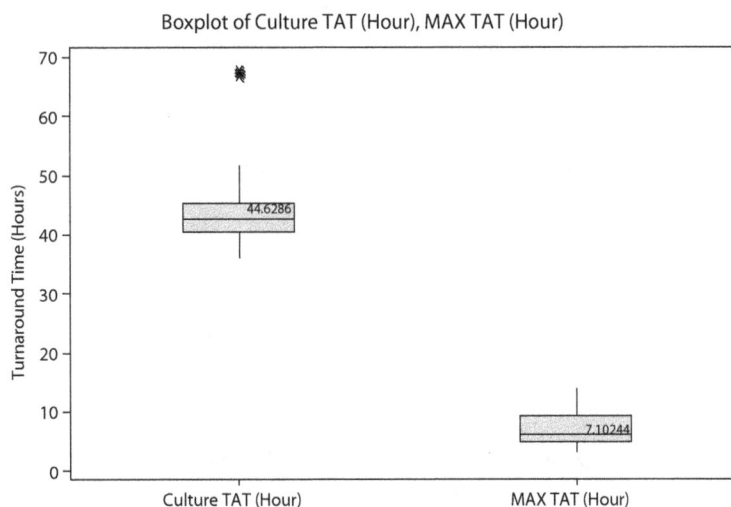

Fig. 1 The mean turnaround time (TAT) to reportable results for 86 routine stool cultures and 84 samples tested with BD MAX EBP. Legend. *Represents 4 outlying culture results that required additional testing for confirmation of the results. All final culture results were negative for pathogens

Table 1 Average Number of Process Steps (Decisions/Manipulations) Involved in Routine Culture and BD MAX EBP Testing

Process Steps	Routine Culture	EBP
Receipt	3	3
Accession	7	1
Routine culture		
Blood agar	43	-
MacConkey agar	26	-
Hektoen	26	-
Sorbitol MacConkey	14	-
Shiga toxin testing	4	-
Sample Preparation	-	8
System operation	-	13
Total activities	141	25

Discussion

A number of molecular platforms have been evaluated for specific specimen types, including stool, and potential pathogens in clinical laboratory settings and have been shown to be highly sensitive and specific when compared to conventional methods [3–5]. The BD MAX platform has been evaluated for the detection of MRSA and more recently stool pathogens [8, 9]. Recently, several investigators have recognized that beyond scientific validation, these platforms need to be evaluated for their impact on the operations and the time to reportable results in clinical laboratories [7, 10–12].

One of the more challenging parts of this study was accounting for all of the costs. The lack of positive samples with target stool pathogens did not allow a complete determination of the costs and labor associated with routine stool cultures. A community outbreak of acute bacterial diarrhea might significantly impact both labor and supplies for both of the methods in this study. In addition, it was difficult to account for the individual variability between technologists in the workup of stool cultures. Differences in individual technologists and their experience could have affected the extent of work and supplies needed for a culture. Nonetheless, including multiple technologists in the performance of this study more accurately represents real-world performance of the two methods than, for example, performing the study with specified research technologists. The use of a significant amount of shared equipment for routine cultures makes complete accounting for the portion of the cost of equipment such as water baths, incubators, storage rack, microscopes, etc. assigned to each culture difficult. At our institution, we use the somewhat arbitrary "Test Site Burden" as one mechanism of sharing these

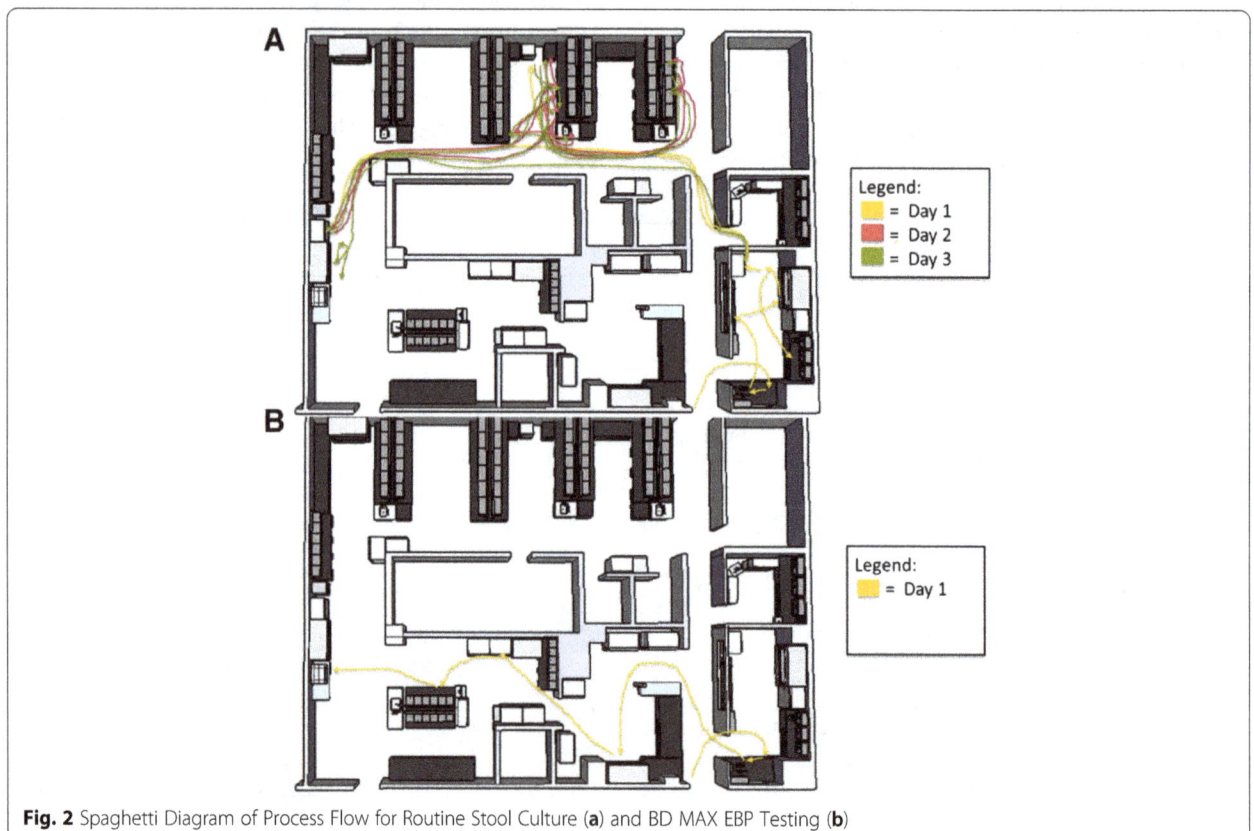

Fig. 2 Spaghetti Diagram of Process Flow for Routine Stool Culture (**a**) and BD MAX EBP Testing (**b**)

Table 2 Cost Analysis of Routine Stool Cultures and BD MAX EBP Testing

	Stool Culture			EBP		
	Cost/Unit	#Units	Cost	Cost/Unit	#Units	Cost
Basic test						
Labor -Technologist time (minutes)	0.45	15 - 17	6.75 – 7.65	0.45	1.48	0.67
Information System labels	0.05	3	0.15	0.05	2	0.1
5 % Sheep Blood agar plate	0.25	1	0.25			
MacConkey agar plate	0.25	1	0.25			
Campy agar plate and BioBag	2.39	1	2.39			
Hektoen Enteric agar plate	0.31	1	0.31			
MacConkey Sorbitol agar plate	0.44	1	0.44			
Shiga toxin test kit and MacConkey Broth	13.52	1	13.52			
Disposable 10 µl loop				0.02	1	0.02
Enteric Panel Kit				30 – 35.00	1	30 – 35.00
MAX test cartridge				0.40 – 0.65	1	0.40 – 0.65
Test site burden	1.00	2	2.00	1.00	1	1.00
Additional workup*						
Labor -Technologist time (minutes)	0.45	35-40	15.75 – 18.00			
5 % Sheep Blood agar plate	0.25	1-3	0.25 – 0.75			
Vitek-Gram negative ID card	6.00	1-3	6.00 – 18.00			
RIM EC O157:H7 test	0.59	1	0.59			
Total Cost (in $)			$26.06 – 64.30			$32.19–37.44

*20 % of cultures required additional labor and supplies to rule out potential pathogens

costs. An additional impact within the laboratory is the shift in supplies storage. A significant number of different media and tests are need for routine cultures and most of these require refrigerated storage. A move to the EBP assay would reduce the number of tests and the amount of media. In addition, adoption of the system would shift much of that storage to room temperature.

In contrast to culture, the cost of operating the BD MAX was more easily captured. However, there are several additional issues that affect the cost of operating the EBP assay that a clinical laboratory would need to consider. Because of how the disposables are constructed, samples can be run in various size batches. To optimize and reduce cost, the ideal batch size is 24. To optimize and reduce turnaround time, the ideal batch size is as small as possible. Use of fewer stools samples per batch would have a minor effect on the cost of the test. The cost of the EBP would not change with a positive result; however, a positive EBP would require a follow-up culture to allow serotyping, antimicrobial susceptibility testing as appropriate, and epidemiological studies, including time and supplies to send isolates to the State Public Health Laboratory. Depreciation of instruments is an important consideration if the instrumentation is purchased outright. Our analysis did not include the cost of the analyzer as that cost per assay is directly related to the volume of assays performed on the instrument. Finally, the cost of

service contracts is often not considered as part of the cost of a test, but can represent a significant cost to the operations of the laboratory.

As clinical microbiology laboratories move from traditional culture based methods to instrument based molecular methods, we need to look carefully at scientific merits of the various options, but we need also to look at the turnaround time of results, associated laboratory processes, and the cost of providing results with this system compared to conventional culture methods in our laboratories.

Conclusion

This study supports the suggestion that use of the BD MAX EBP can save significant time (over that required by culture) in the laboratory diagnosis of acute bacterial diarrhea caused by *Salmonella* spp., *Shigella* spp./(EIEC), *Campylobacter* spp. (*jejuni* and *coli*), and Shiga toxin producing *E. coli* which are responsible for 95 % of acute bacterial gastroenteritis. The use of a flexible and focused approach to identifying enteric pathogens (bacteria, viruses & parasites) based on patient history or risk, clinical presentation or clinician's preference is aligned with widely recommended clinical algorithms which not only potentially streamline laboratory testing and workflow in a cost effective manner, but also provide physicians with timely results which improve the standard of care for common causes of gastroenteritis. As additional nucleic amplification assays become available, the impact of the use of focused versus comprehensive panels will continue to be evaluated for their respective clinical relevance, cost and work flow implications.

Abbreviations
EBP: Enteric bacterial panel; EIEC: Enteroinvasive *Escherichia coli*; SOP: Standard operating procedures; MRSA: Methicillin resistant *Staphylococcus aureus*.

Competing interests
AW is an employee of BD Diagnostics. JEM has received honoraria from BD Diagnostics. Other authors have no competing interests.

Authors' contributions
JEM conceived the study, analyzed the data and authored the manuscript. CV performed data collection, participated in the process measurements and performed the cost analysis. SH performed the BD MAX testing and data collection, and participated in the process measurements. AW contributed to the study design and performed the process measurements. All authors have reviewed the manuscript and accept responsibility for its content.

Acknowledgements
BD Diagnostics (Sparks, MD) provided financial support and supplies for this project. BD Diagnostics did not design the study, interpret the data, write the manuscript or control submission of the manuscript for publication.

Author details
[1]Department of Laboratory Medicine, Cincinnati Children's Hospital, MLC1010, 3333 Burnet Ave, 45229 Cincinnati, OH, USA. [2]BD Diagnostics, Sparks, MD, USA.

References
1. WHO/UNICEF. Ending preventable child deaths from pneumonia and diarrhoea by 2025:The integrated Global Action Plan for Pneumonia and Diarrhoea (GAPPD). New York, N.Y: The United Nations CHildren's Fund(UNICEF)/World Health Organization (WHO); 2013.
2. Johansson EW, Wardlaw T, Binkin N, Brocklehurst C, Dooley T. Diarrhoea: why children are still dying and what can be done, (UNICEF). New York, N.Y: The United Nations CHildren's Fund(UNICEF)/World Health Organization (WHO); 2009.
3. Navidad JF, Griswold DJ, Gradus MS, Bhattacharyya S. Evaluation of Luminex xTAG gastrointestinal pathogen analyte-specific reagents for high-throughput, simultaneous detection of bacteria, viruses, and parasites of clinical and public health importance. J Clin Microbiol. 2013;51:3018–24.
4. Buchan BW, Olson WJ, Pezewski M, Marcon MJ, Novicki T, Uphoff TS, et al. Clinical evaluation of a real-time PCR assay for identification of Salmonella, Shigella, Campylobacter (Campylobacter jejuni and C. coli), and shiga toxin-producing Escherichia coli isolates in stool specimens. J Clin Microbiol. 2013;51(12):4001–7.
5. Patel A, Navidad J, Bhattacharyya S. Site-specific Clinical Evaluation of the Luminex xTAG Gastrointestinal Pathogen Panel for the Detection of Infectious Gastroenteritis in Fecal Specimens. J Clin Microbiol. 2013;52(8):3068–71.
6. Schweikhart SA, Dembe AE. The application of Lean and Six Sigma techniques to clinical and translational research. J Invest Med. 2009;57(7):748–55.
7. Felder RA, Foster ML, Lizzi MJ, Pohl BR, Diemert DM, Towns BG. Process evaluation of a fully automated molecular diagnostics system. J Assoc Lab Autom. 2009;14:262–8.
8. Widen R, Healer V, Silber S. Laboratory Evaluation of the BD MAX MRSA assay. J Clin Microbiol. 2014;52(7):2686–8.
9. Harrington SM, Buchan B, Doern C, Fader R, Ferraro MJ, Pillai D, et al. Multi-center evaluation of the BD MAX™ Enteric Bacterial Panel PCR assay for the rapid detection of Salmonella spp., Shigella spp., Campylobacter spp. (C. jejuni and C. coli), and Shiga toxin 1 and 2 genes. ASM General Meeting, 2014.
10. Hassell LA, Glass CF, Yip C, Eneff PA. The combined postive impact of Lean methology and Ventana Symphony autostainer on histology lab workflow. BMC Clin Path. 2010;10:2–10.
11. Felder RA, Jackson KD, Walter AM. Process Evaluation of an Open Architecture Real-Time Molecular Laboratory Platform. J Lab Autom. 2014;19(5):468–73.
12. Williams JA, Eddleman L, Pantone A, Martinez R, Young S, Van Der Pol B. Time-Motion Analysis of Four Automated Systems for the Detection of Chlamydia trachomatis and Neisseria gonorrhoeae by Nucleic Acid Amplification Testing. J Lab Autom. 2013;19(4):423–6.

9

Expression of a-Tocopherol-Associated protein (TAP) is associated with clinical outcome in breast cancer patients

Xi Wang[1][*][†], Brian Z. Ring[2][†], Robert S. Seitz[3], Douglas T. Ross[4], Kirsten Woolf[1], Rodney A. Beck[5], David G. Hicks[1] and Shuyuan Yeh[1]

Abstract

Background: The role of vitamin E in breast cancer prevention and treatment has been widely investigated, and the different tocopherols that comprise this nutrient have been shown to have divergent associations with cancer outcome. Our previous studies have shown that a-Tocopherol-associated protein (TAP), a vitamin E binding protein, may function as a tumor suppressor-like factor in breast carcinogenesis. The current study addresses the association of TAP expression with breast cancer clinical outcomes.

Methods: Immunohistochemical stain for TAP was applied to a tissue microarray from a breast cancer cohort consisting of 271 patients with a median follow-up time of 5.2 years. The expression of TAP in tumor cells was compared with patient's clinical outcome at 5 years after diagnosis. The potential role of TAP in predicting outcome was also assessed in clinically relevant subsets of the cohort. In addition, we compared TAP expression and Oncotype DX scores in an independent breast cancer cohort consisting of 71 cases.

Results: We demonstrate that the expression of TAP was differentially expressed within the breast cancer cohort, and that ER+/PR ± tumors were more likely to exhibit TAP expression. TAP expression was associated with an overall lower recurrence rate and a better 5-year survival rate. This association was primarily in patients with ER+ tumors; exploratory analysis showed that this association was strongest in patients with node-positive tumors and was independent of stage and treatment with chemotherapy. TAP expression in ER/PR negative or triple negative tumors had no association with clinical outcome. In addition, we did not observe an association between TAP expression and Oncotype DX recurrence score.

Conclusions: The significant positive association we found for a-Tocopherol-associated protein with outcome in breast cancer may help to better define and explain studies addressing a-tocopherol's association with cancer risk and outcome. Additionally, further studies to validate and extend these findings may allow TAP to serve as a breast-specific prognostic marker in breast cancer patients, especially in those patients with ER+ tumors.

Keywords: Breast cancer, a-Tocopherol-associated protein (TAP), Vitamin E

* Correspondence: xi_wang@urmc.rochester.edu
[†]Equal contributors
[1]Department of Pathology, University of Rochester Medical Center, Rochester, NY 14642, USA
Full list of author information is available at the end of the article

Table 1 Cohort characteristics. *P* value for difference between proportion of clinical characteristic within TAP positive and negative patients determined with a two-proportion z-test, except for age and tumor size for which a *t*-test was employed

	All cases		TAP negative		TAP positive		
	No. of patients	%	No. of patients	%	No. of patients	%	*P* value
Total	271		183		88		
Grade							
1	34	12.5	20	10.9	14	15.9	0.33
2	105	38.7	59	32.2	46	52.3	0.02
3	92	33.9	78	42.6	14	15.9	0.03
Unknown	40	14.8	26	14.2	14	15.9	nd
Stage							
I	97	35.8	60	32.8	37	42	0.18
II	137	50.6	94	51.4	43	48.9	0.39
III	31	11.4	23	12.6	8	9.1	0.4
Unknown	6	2.2	6	3.3		0	nd
Age (avg, range)							
	58.1 (26–89)		56.9 (26–87)		62.6 (35–89)		<0.001
T							
T1	138	50.9	82	44.8	56	63.6	0.01
T2	101	37.3	74	40.4	27	30.7	0.19
T3	14	5.2	12	6.6	2	2.3	0.41
T4	8	3	6	3.3	2	2.3	0.47
Unknown	10	3.7	9	4.9	1	1.1	nd
N							
N0	150	55.4	97	53	53	60.2	0.2
N1	108	39.9	74	40.4	34	38.6	0.43
N2	6	2.2	5	2.7	1	1.1	0.46
Unknown	7	2.6	7	3.8		0	nd
M							
M0	258	99.2	172	98.9	86	100	1
M1	2	0.8	2	1.1		0	nd
Unknown	11		9		2		nd
Tumor size (avg, cm)							
	2.09		2.39		1.83		<0.001
Received chemotherapy							
no	133	49.1	75	41	58	65.9	1
yes	130	48	101	55.2	29	33	1
Unknown	8	3	7	3.8	1	1.1	nd
ER							
ER-	65	24	58	31.7	7	8	0.1
ER+	197	72.7	120	65.6	77	87.5	0
Unknown	9	3.3	5	2.7	4	4.5	nd
HER2							
HER2-	116	42.8	85	46.4	31	35.2	1
HER2+	72	26.6	43	23.5	29	33	1
Unknown	83	30.6	55	30.1	28	31.8	nd

Table 1 Cohort characteristics. *P* value for difference between proportion of clinical characteristic within TAP positive and negative patients determined with a two-proportion z-test, except for age and tumor size for which a *t*-test was employed *(Continued)*

Hormone therapy								
No	77	26.7	57	28.8	20	22.2	0.28
yes	187	64.9	120	60.6	67	74.4	0.03
Unknown	24	8.3	21	10.6	3	3.3	nd

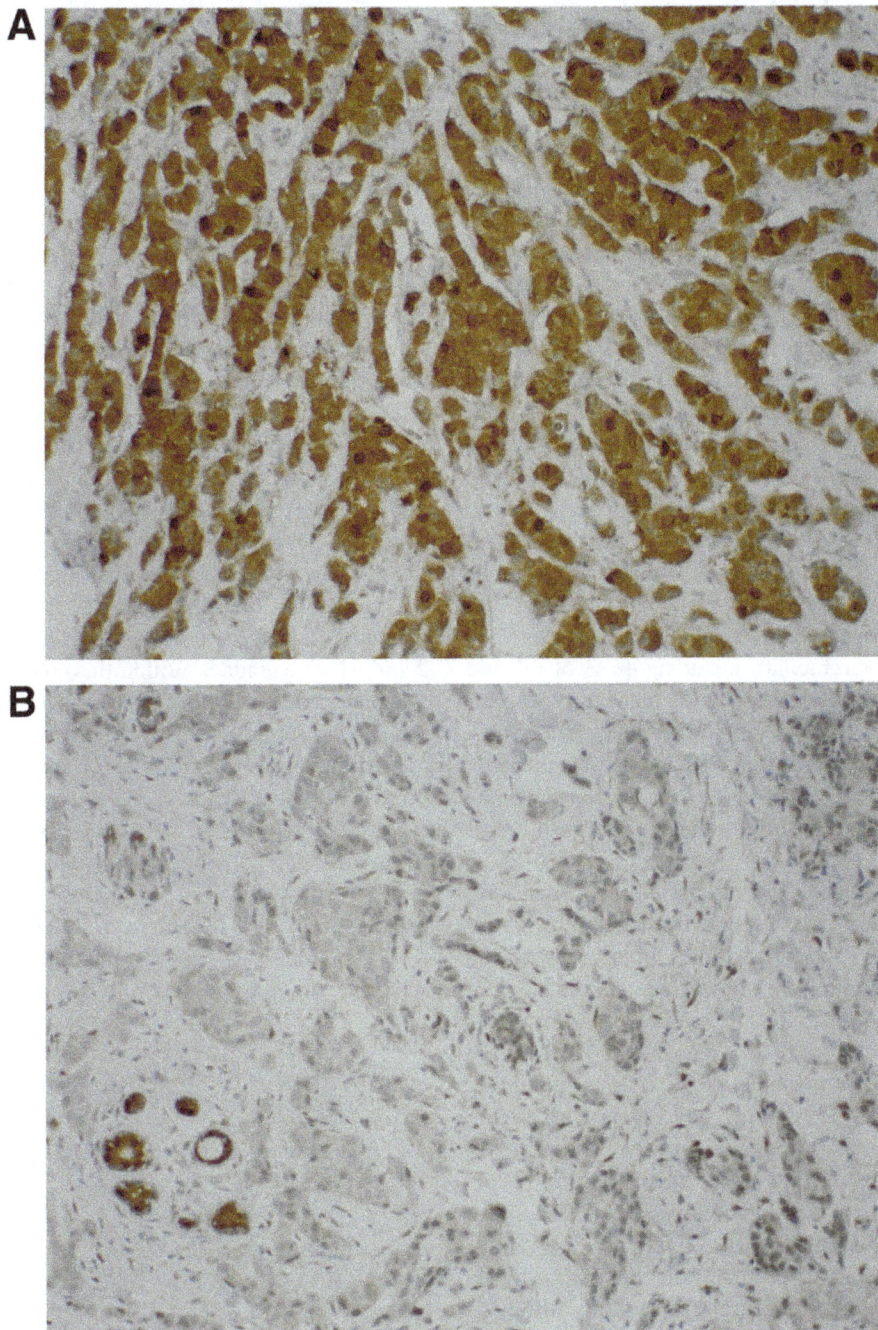

Fig. 1 Invasive ductal carcinoma showing TAP staining positive (**a**), and negative with the positive internal control of normal/benign TDLU (**b**)

Background

Breast cancer is the most common malignant tumor in women worldwide, comprising 16 % of all female cancers. Epidemiological studies have shown that vitamin E has a potential utility in the prevention and treatment of human malignancies, including breast cancer [1–3]. However clinical trials on the effectiveness of dietary supplementation with vitamin E or α-tocopherol, the principle and most active vitamin E isoform in human plasma, as an aid in the prevention of cancer have not produced evidence of a consistent association with decreased cancer occurrence [4, 5]. The inconstancies between epidemiological studies and intervention trials may be due to differing roles for the tocopherols that comprise vitamin E or unexplained genetic diversity in the study populations affecting how they utilized vitamin E.

Our previous studies have shown that α-Tocopherol-associated protein (TAP), a vitamin E binding protein [6], is selectively expressed in human breast, prostate, liver and brain tissue and its expression can be evaluated by immunohistochemical staining [7, 8]. We have shown that, while TAP can facilitate vitamin E retention in cancer cells and promote vitamin E-mediated anti-proliferation effects, it can also act as a tumor suppressor-like protein in a vitamin E-independent fashion. Overexpression of TAP in prostate cancer cells was shown to suppress cell growth; and a TAP siRNA knockdown in a prostate cell line led to increased cell growth [7]. In human breast, we identified that TAP is typically co-expressed with ER in sporadic normal/benign luminal cells in terminal ductal lobular units, and that TAP showed decreased expression in 57 % of invasive breast carcinomas, including 46 % of ER and PR positive carcinomas, and 80 % of high grade carcinomas [9]. Another study has shown that TAP mRNA level is negatively associated with tumor stage and lymph node status in breast cancer [10]. TAP expression therefore may be a candidate for a marker of less aggressive breast carcinoma.

Despite the advances in multidisciplinary treatment, breast cancer remains the second most common cause of death related to cancer in women. In addition to the routine pathologic characteristics of breast cancer, such as tumor size, grade, vascular invasion, lymph node metastasis, ER/PR/Her2 status etc., genes which may have an association with tumor biology and help in predicting recurrence, therapeutic response and survival have been studied widely. Currently there are at least nine gene expression signatures showing some correlation with certain clinical breast cancer outcomes [11–16]. The genes included in these panels are diverse but largely related to cell cycle regulation and proliferation, the ER pathway, and to a lesser degree, the immune system. Although these gene panels have similar outcomes performance, they exhibit a large degree of discordance in the assignment of a particular breast tumor to a specific prognostic group [11]. More accurate prognostic predictive gene signatures will depend on better understanding of the genes specifically involved in breast cancer carcinogenesis.

To further investigate if TAP expression is associated with clinical outcome in breast carcinomas, we studied TAP expression in a breast cancer cohort of 271 patients diagnosed with invasive breast carcinomas with median follow up time of 5.2 years. In addition, in an independent cohort of 71 breast cancer cases, we compared TAP expression with the Oncotype DX recurrence score to determine if there was a correlation between TAP expression and this clinically available multigene prognostic/predictive assay.

Methods

A tissue micro-array comprising 288 patient samples from a primary invasive breast cancer cohort from the Clearview Cancer Institute (CCI, AL, U.S.A.), consisting of all available patient samples collected from 1990 to 2001, was constructed. The patient average age was 58.9 (range 26–89), with an average tumor size 2.21 cm (range 0.2–8.0) and a median follow up time of 5.2 years. Ninety eight tumors were stage 1, 141 stage 2, and 33 stage 3. One hundred fifty four patients had negative lymph nodes, while 118 patients had positive lymph node(s). One hundred thirty two patients had received chemotherapy plus hormonal therapy, while 156 were untreated or treated with hormonal therapy only. No patients had been treated with Herceptin. Thirty six tumors were grade 1, 106 were grade 2 and 93 were grade 3. Within this cohort, 271 patients had complete follow-up and TAP expression data. The composition of this set of patients is as shown in Table 1.

An independent cohort of 71 invasive breast carcinomas for which Oncotype DX (Genomic Health, Inc.) recurrence scores had been determined were identified from the files of the Department of Pathology and Laboratory Medicine at Strong Memorial Hospital (Rochester, NY). All cases were hormone receptor positive, Her2 negative, and lymph node negative. A representative whole tissue section was cut from each tumor.

Table 2 TAP and hormone receptor status, patient counts. P value for difference between proportion of TAP positive and negative patients determined with a two-proportion z-test

	TAP-	TAP+	P value
Hormone Receptor Negative (ER & PR-)	48	6	<0.001
ER-	58	7	<0.001
Hormone Receptor Positive (ER or PR+)	127	78	<0.001
ER+	120	77	0.001
HR positive/ HER2-	56	29	0.003
HR positive/ HER2+	31	28	0.35

This study was approved by the Huntsville Hospital Institutional Review Committee. Archived tumor samples were provided by the Clearview Cancer Institute of Huntsville Alabama and corresponding anonymized patient data was provided via an institutional review board–approved database. An IRB exemption for the use of the tissue samples was granted by the Huntsville Hospital Institutional Review Committee as all patient data were a) anonymized, b) consent was unnecessary, and c) only excess tissue was used.

Tissue arrays were processed as previously described [17]. TAP antibody was generated in house as previously published. Immunohistochemical staining for TAP was performed on tissue micro-array and whole tissue sections with the method we described previously [8]. TAP expression was classified as positive or negative, with positive expression defined as any cytoplasmic and/or nuclear staining (Fig. 1). Commercial antibodies for ER, PR, and HER2 were stained by a commercial service (US Labs Inc). ER and PR were considered positive if at least

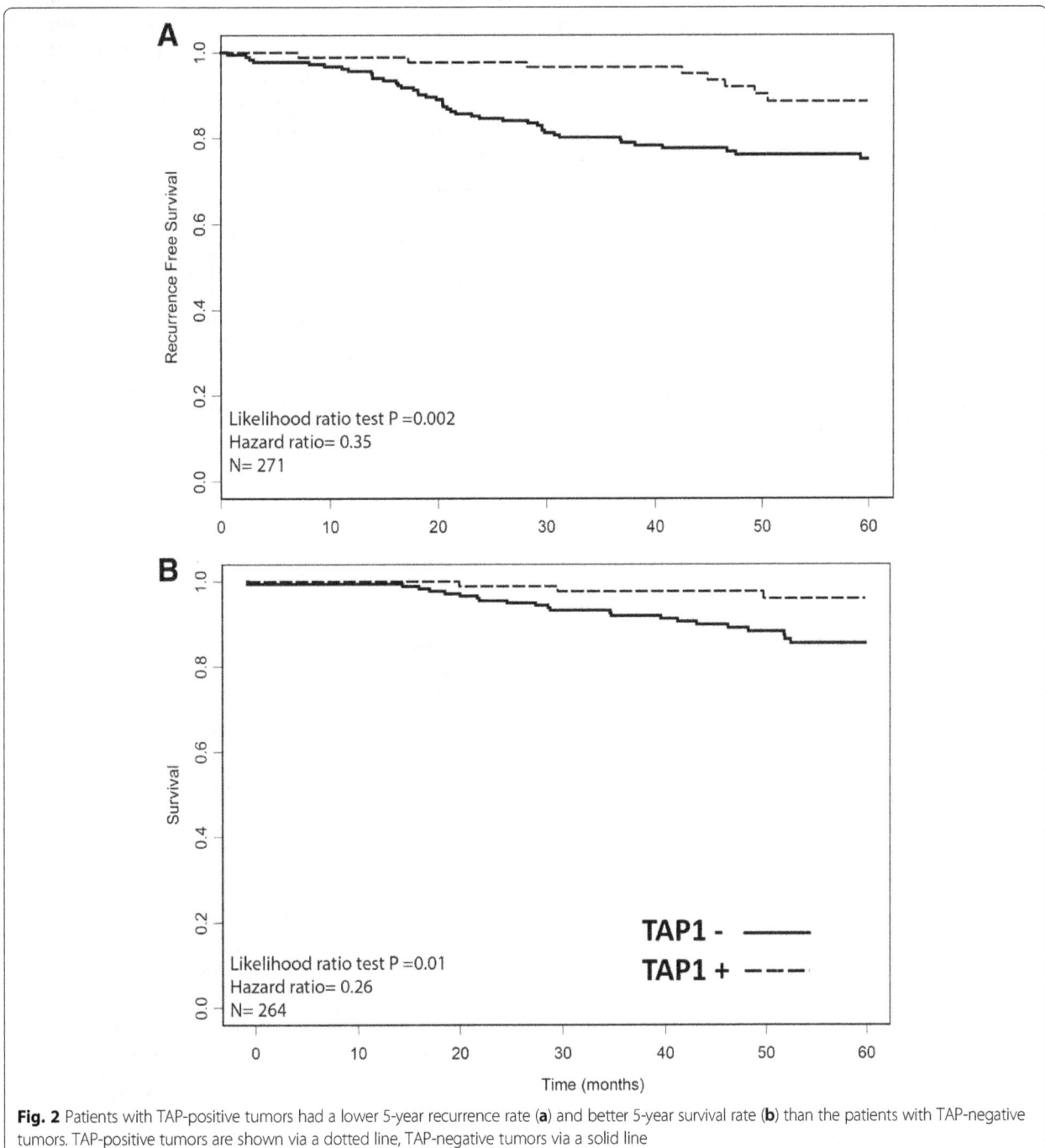

Fig. 2 Patients with TAP-positive tumors had a lower 5-year recurrence rate (**a**) and better 5-year survival rate (**b**) than the patients with TAP-negative tumors. TAP-positive tumors are shown via a dotted line, TAP-negative tumors via a solid line

1 % of the cells examined exhibited any nuclear staining, and HER2 was scored positive when intense membrane staining in more than 10 % of invasive tumor cells was observed.

In assessing association with outcome, the likelihood ratio test was used in univariate analyses, and the Wald test for multivariate models. All p values are presented as two sided, with a value of less than 0.05 being considered significant.

Results

In the CCI breast cohort of 271 breast carcinoma samples, we observed positive TAP staining in 88 (32 %) and negative staining in 183 (68 %) tumors. Consistent with our previous findings, we found that ER+/PR ± tumors are more likely to exhibit TAP expression than hormone negative tumors (Table 2). Overall, patients with TAP-positive tumors had a lower 5-year recurrence rate ($N = 271$, $p = 0.002$) and better 5-year survival rate ($N = 264$, $p = 0.010$) (Fig. 2a, b). This positive association with outcome was conserved in all ER-positive tumors, regardless of PR status (5 year recurrence, HR = 0.35, $p = 0.02$, 5 year survival, HR = 0.141, $p = 0.014$) (Fig. 3a, b). This association was

also significant at 10 years post diagnosis (10 year survival HR = 0.21, $p = 0.0024$; 10 year recurrence HR = 0.55, $p = 0.023$). Looking further at the clinically relevant ER+/PR±/Her2- patients, significant associations were also observed (5 year recurrence, HR = 0.17, $p = 0.035$, 5 year survival, HR = <0.001, $p = 0.007$, $N = 81$). TAP was not prognostic of 5 year recurrence in ER+/HER2+ cases (HR = 0.38 $p = 0.22$, $N = 57$), ER-/HER2-(HR < 0.01, $p = 0.23$, $N = 32$), or ER-/HER2+ cases (HR = 4.1 $p = 0.28$, $N = 15$). Tumors negative for ER and PR had a non-significant association with 5-year recurrence and survival (Fig. 3c, d). In triple negative patients the association remained non-significant, though low patient numbers ($N = 25$) makes it difficult to draw conclusions from this subset analysis. Exploratory analysis showed that the association with outcome was even stronger in node-positive patients (5-year recurrence: $N = 118$, $p = 0.0001$; 5-year survival: $N = 114$, $p = 0.0036$), but it was not significant in node-negative patients (5-year recurrence: $N = 151$ and $p = 0.98$; 5-year survival: $N = 150$ and $p = 0.72$) (Fig. 4a-d). Within PR subsets (ER+/PR- and ER+/PR+), TAP did not have a significant association with recurrence ($p = 0.102$ and 0.098, respectively), though the hazard ratio remained low.

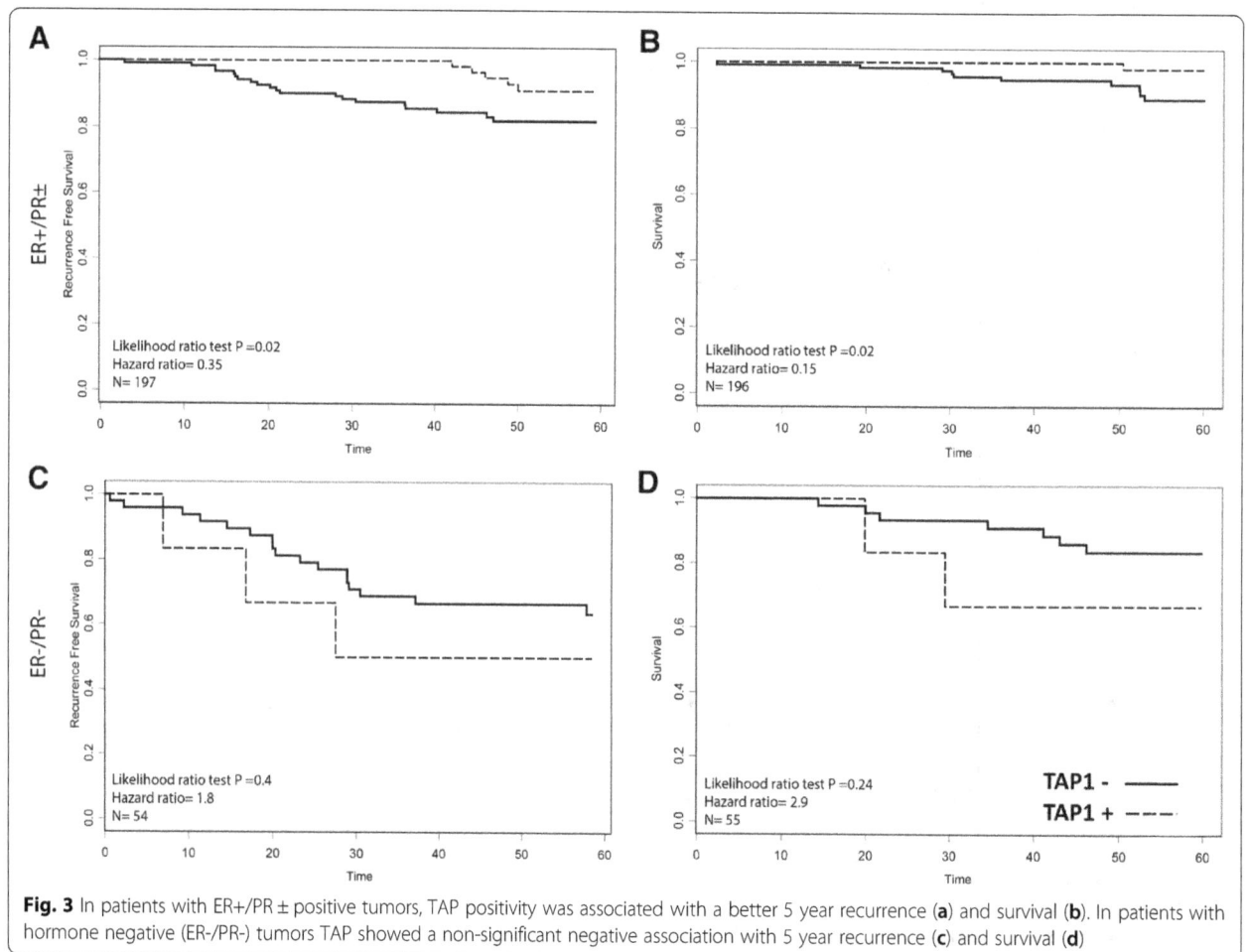

Fig. 3 In patients with ER+/PR ± positive tumors, TAP positivity was associated with a better 5 year recurrence (**a**) and survival (**b**). In patients with hormone negative (ER-/PR-) tumors TAP showed a non-significant negative association with 5 year recurrence (**c**) and survival (**d**)

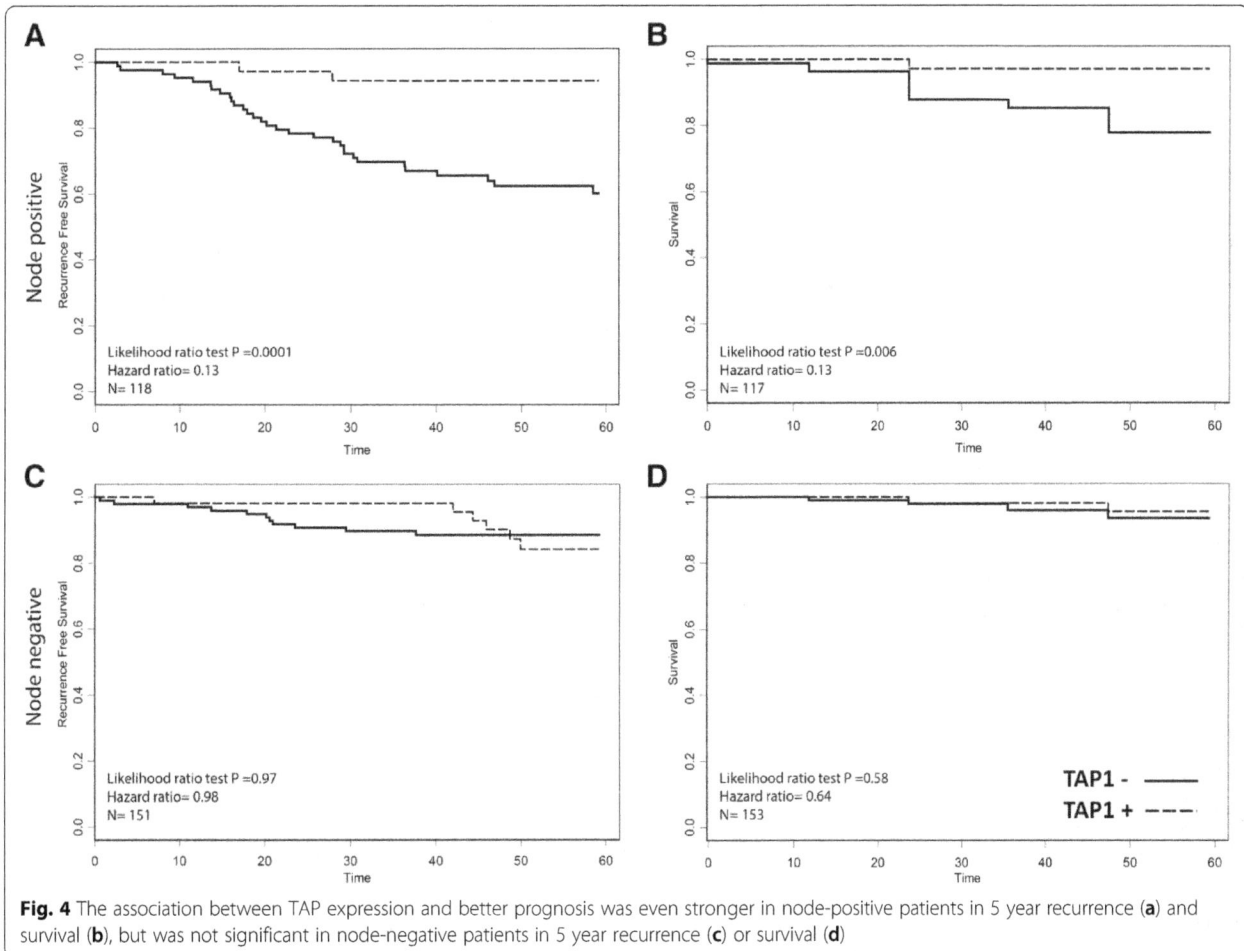

Fig. 4 The association between TAP expression and better prognosis was even stronger in node-positive patients in 5 year recurrence (**a**) and survival (**b**), but was not significant in node-negative patients in 5 year recurrence (**c**) or survival (**d**)

Furthermore, TAP was independent of PR when assessed as a multivariable model (data not shown).

In an exploratory multivariate analysis of TAP status and common clinical variables, TAP was independent of age, stage, hormonal therapy and chemotherapy status with 5 year recurrence as the outcome measurement in all patients (Table 3). TAP was not independent of grade, which suggests that grade and TAP were measuring a shared aspect of cell biology. Indeed, there was a significant negative association between grade and TAP (p < 0.0001 via chi-square). TAP positive tumors were more likely to represent low grade tumors compared to TAP negative tumors. In patients with ER+/PR ± tumors, TAP expression was independent of stage and age in predicting 5 year recurrence; while in patients with ER+/PR±/Her2- tumors, TAP was not independent of stage (5 year recurrence HR = 0.18, $p = 0.110$). However, only 81 patients were included in this subset. When looking at 5 year survival, TAP expression was independent of age and stage, but not chemotherapy status or tumor grade.

In the study of tumors with a known Oncotype DX recurrence score, TAP was positive in 47 of the 71 tumors (66.2 %), with 29 of 43 (67.4 %) in a low risk group, 16 of 24 (66.7 %) in an intermediate risk group, and 2 of 4 (50 %) in a high risk group (Table 4). There was no association observed between TAP expression and Oncotype DX recurrence risk using a Fisher's exact test ($P = 0.60$).

The limitation of the study includes relatively small sample size in the CCI breast cohort and Oncotype DX cohort. Ki67 labeling index data and the status of vascular invasion were not available for analysis.

Discussion

Genes involved in cell proliferation have been shown to comprise a major component of many of the available gene expression signatures used to predict clinical outcome in breast cancer patients [11–16]. TAP has also been implicated in the control of cellular proliferation and other aspects of tumor growth. Researchers demonstrated that vitamin E derivatives can inhibit cell proliferation and colony formation of breast cancer cell lines, and induce apoptosis of the tumor cells [18–21]. As a vitamin E binding protein, TAP can promote vitamin E retention and thus increase its concentration in cells. Our previous studies have demonstrated that TAP can promote vitamin E-induced inhibition of tumor cell

Table 3 Association of TAP and other clinical variables with outcome using Cox proportional hazard regression. TAP, chemotherapy, grade, stage and age are shown as individual and multivariable models. Variables with a significant association with survival or recurrence are shown in bold

	5 year survival			5 year recurrence			5 year recurrence, ER+/PR±		
	HR	p	N	HR	p	N	HR	p	N
TAP	0.26 (0.08, 0.87)	0.01	264	0.35 (0.16, 0.74)	0.002	271	0.35 (0.13, 0.92)	0.02	197
Hormone therapy	0.54 (0.25, 1.2)	0.12	262	0.68 (0.38, 1.2)	0.21	261	1.8 (0.55, 6.2)	0.28	192
Chemotherapy	4.34 (1.63, 11.6)	0.001	262	2.51 (1.37, 4.6)	0.002	263	2.2 (1, 4.84)	0.05	193
Grade	4.44 (1.74, 11.3)	<0.001	230	2.3 (1.34, 3.93)	0.001	231	2.5 (1.24, 5.05)	0.007	175
Stage	3.35 (1.82, 6.16)	<0.001	264	2.71 (1.76, 4.17)	<0.001	265	2.66 (1.47, 4.83)	0.001	195
Age	0.98 (0.95, 1.01)	0.193	264	0.98 (0.97, 1)	0.054	265	0.97 (0.94, 1)	0.058	195
TAP	0.28 (0.08, 0.95)	0.04	264	0.38 (0.18, 0.81)	0.012	265	0.37 (0.14, 0.98)	0.045	195
Stage	3.25 (1.76, 6)	<0.001		2.63 (1.71, 4.06)	<0.001		2.57 (1.41, 4.69)	0.002	
TAP	0.55 (0.16, 1.93)	0.35	230	0.54 (0.23, 1.24)	0.15	231	0.51 (0.19, 1.39)	0.19	174
Grade	3.93 (1.52, 10.18)	0.005		2.05 (1.19, 3.52)	0.01		2.3 (1.15, 4.59)	0.018	
TAP	0.28 (0.08, 0.94)	0.039	264	0.38 (0.18, 0.82)	0.014	265	0.37 (0.14, 0.98)	0.045	195
Age	0.99 (0.96, 1.02)	0.37		0.98 (0.96, 1.01)	0.16		0.97 (0.94, 1.01)	0.097	
TAP	0.27 (0.08, 0.90)	0.032	262	0.37 (0.17, 0.78)	0.0093	261	0.35 (0.13,0.93)	0.036	192
Hormone therapy	0.58 (0.27, 1.3)	0.17		0.73 (0.41, 1.3)	0.3		1.77 (0.53, 5.9)	0.35	
TAP	0.34 (0.1, 1.14)	0.081	262	0.42 (0.2, 0.91)	0.027	263	0.38 (0.14, 1.01)	0.052	193
Chemotherapy	3.69 (1.37, 9.92)	0.01		2.16 (1.17, 4.01)	0.014		1.94 (0.87, 4.3)	0.1	
TAP	0.33 (0.1, 1.13)	0.078	262	0.41 (0.19, 0.89)	0.023	263	0.38 (0.14, 1.03)	0.057	193
Stage	2.77 (1.42, 5.4)	0.003		2.44 (1.53, 3.9)	0		2.42 (1.27, 4.61)	0.007	
Chemotherapy	2.21 (0.79, 6.17)	0.13		1.35 (0.7, 2.59)	0.37		1.23 (0.53, 2.85)	0.63	
TAP	0.32 (0.1, 1.1)	0.07	262	0.41 (0.19, 0.89)	0.024	263	0.39 (0.15, 1.06)	0.065	193
Stage	2.8 (1.43, 5.47)	0.003		2.44 (1.53, 3.9)	0		2.53 (1.34, 4.76)	0.004	
Chemotherapy	2.98 (0.89, 10)	0.077		1.34 (0.61, 2.94)	0.47		0.85 (0.31, 2.32)	0.75	
Age	1.02 (0.98, 1.06)	0.35		1 (0.97, 1.03)	0.98		0.97 (0.94, 1.01)	0.19	

proliferation and also regulate tumor cell growth in a vitamin E-independent fashion [7]. We also showed that TAP is selectively expressed in normal/benign breast luminal epithelium, but not in many other organ systems [8]. TAP expression is down-regulated at the mRNA and protein levels in several human breast cancer cell lines and in human breast carcinomas compared to a nonmalignant cell line and to normal/benign breast tissue. We extended these observations in current study, which showed that TAP expression is associated with an overall more favorable outcome, both in terms of tumor recurrence and survival rate in breast cancer patients. These findings, taken together, suggest that TAP is a regulator of cell proliferation that can affect breast carcinogenesis and tumor prognosis.

Breast cancer is a heterogeneous group of diseases. The biological features and clinical behavior of individual tumors are frequently different, even within the morphologically low grade, ER+/PR+/Her2- subtype, which is generally considered to be a group with a better prognosis. It is important to identify novel markers which

can predict clinical outcomes in this group. We have reported that TAP is co-expressed with ER in the normal/benign breast luminal epithelium of terminal ductal lobular units, where breast carcinogenesis is most likely to be initiated, and that TAP is down regulated in 46 % of ER and PR positive breast carcinomas, indicating that the loss of TAP expression may be associated with the process of hormonal carcinogenesis [9]. Here we have demonstrated that TAP expression in ER+/PR±/Her2- tumors is associated with a significantly better 5-year recurrence free and survival rate. This finding could be clinically significant in terms of further predicting tumor

Table 4 Comparison of TAP positivity and OncoTypeDx Recurrence scores

Recurrence Score	TAP +	TAP -	Total
1	29	14	43
2	16	8	24
3	2	2	4
Total	47	24	71

behaviors of ER+/PR±/Her2- subtype breast carcinomas. Currently, there are few breast carcinogenesis-related oncogenes and tumor suppressor genes that are implicated in the clinical treatment and prognosis. Her2 and p53, the most widely evaluated cancer-related genes, are only altered in approximately 20-25 % of breast carcinomas, primarily in ER/PR negative tumors [22]. In contrast, TAP is altered in 57 % of breast carcinomas, including 46 % ER/PR+ tumors, thus may serve as a useful complement to existing biomarkers.

OncotypeDX has been used to guide clinical approaches for ER-positive, lymph node-negative breast cancer patients. Even though TAP expression is associated with better clinical outcome in ER-positive tumors, we did not identify any association between TAP expression and OncotypeDX recurrence scores in the additional cohort. This may suggest that TAP expression is associated with a different aspect(s) of tumor biology than is OncotypeDX and may be a useful complement in predicting patient outcome and tumor subclassification. Further study with a larger population of ER+ tumors is needed to help validate these findings.

Several studies have demonstrated a protective effect of vitamin E on the occurrence of several cancers (for review see [3]). However clinical trials have found little support for dietary supplementation [23]. The disparity of these results could be due to vitamin E not being cancer preventive at the supra-nutritional level, significant roles for other vitamin E isoforms, such as γ- and δ-tocopherols [24], or genetic diversity among dietary intervention trial participants contributing to unrecognized heterogeneity in how they utilized vitamin E. Our study found considerable heterogeneity among the tumors in expression of TAP, the vitamin E binding protein, and its significant association with cancer progression. This finding suggests a possible role for TAP in the interplay between vitamin E and cancer progression. Stratification of trial participation by TAP expression may be an interesting and important aspect for the elucidation of how dietary vitamin E supplementation may affect cancer risk and prognosis.

Conclusions

In summary, we demonstrated that TAP, as a proliferation-related gene in breast carcinogenesis, is associated with a better 5-year clinical outcome, particularly in node-positive and ER+ breast cancer patients. TAP may serve as a prognostic marker, especially in those patients with ER+ low grade breast cancers, and may also serve to stratify studies assessing the role and utility of vitamin E or α-tocopherol supplementation for the prevention of cancer.

Competing interests
All authors declare no conflict of interests.

Authors' contributions
XW, RS, DTR, DGH and SY conceived of the study, and participated in its design and coordination. BZR performed the statistical analysis and figure preparation. KW and RAB performed the immunohistochemical assays. XW and BZR wrote the manuscript. All authors read and approved the final manuscript.

Acknowledgements
The authors wish to thank Yanling Wang for her technical assistance.

Author details
[1]Department of Pathology, University of Rochester Medical Center, Rochester, NY 14642, USA. [2]Institute for Genomic and Personalized Medicine, School of Life Science and Technology, Huazhong University of Science and Technology, Wuhan, China. [3]Insight Genetics Inc., Nashville, TN, USA. [4]CardioDx, Inc., Redwood City, CA, USA. [5]Conversant Biologics, Huntsville, AL, USA.

References

1. Wada S. Cancer preventive effects of vitamin E, vol. 13, 2011/04/07 edn.
2. Kline K, Yu W, Sanders BG. Vitamin E and breast cancer. J Nutr. 2004;134(12 Suppl):3458S–62S.
3. Ju J, Picinich SC, Yang Z, Zhao Y, Suh N, Kong AN, et al. Cancer-preventive activities of tocopherols and tocotrienols. Carcinogenesis. 2010;31(4):533–42.
4. Klein EA, Thompson Jr IM, Tangen CM, Crowley JJ, Lucia MS, Goodman PJ, et al. Vitamin E and the risk of prostate cancer: the Selenium and Vitamin E Cancer Prevention Trial (SELECT). JAMA. 2011;306(14):1549–56.
5. Lee IM, Cook NR, Gaziano JM, Gordon D, Ridker PM, Manson JE, et al. Vitamin E in the primary prevention of cardiovascular disease and cancer: the Women's Health Study: a randomized controlled trial. JAMA. 2005;294(1):56–65.
6. Zimmer S, Stocker A, Sarbolouki MN, Spycher SE, Sassoon J, Azzi A. A novel human tocopherol-associated protein: cloning, in vitro expression, and characterization. J Biol Chem. 2000;275(33):25672–80.
7. Ni J, Wen X, Yao J, Chang HC, Yin Y, Zhang M, et al. Tocopherol-associated protein suppresses prostate cancer cell growth by inhibition of the phosphoinositide 3-kinase pathway. Cancer Res. 2005;65(21):9807–16.
8. Wang X, Ni J, Hsu CL, Johnykutty S, Tang P, Ho YS, et al. Reduced expression of tocopherol-associated protein (TAP/Sec14L2) in human breast cancer. Cancer Invest. 2009;27(10):971–7.
9. Johnykutty S, Tang P, Zhao H, Hicks DG, Yeh S, Wang X. Dual expression of alpha-tocopherol-associated protein and estrogen receptor in normal/benign human breast luminal cells and the downregulation of alpha-tocopherol-associated protein in estrogen-receptor-positive breast carcinomas. Mod Pathol. 2009;22(6):770–5.
10. Tam KW, Ho CT, Lee WJ, Tu SH, Huang CS, Chen CS, et al. Alteration of alpha-tocopherol-associated protein (TAP) expression in human breast epithelial cells during breast cancer development. Food Chem. 2013;138(2–3):1015–21.
11. Reyal F, van Vliet MH, Armstrong NJ, Horlings HM, de Visser KE, Kok M, et al. A comprehensive analysis of prognostic signatures reveals the high predictive capacity of the proliferation, immune response and RNA splicing modules in breast cancer. Breast Cancer Res. 2008;10(6):R93.
12. Paik S, Shak S, Tang G, Kim C, Baker J, Cronin M, et al. A multigene assay to predict recurrence of tamoxifen-treated, node-negative breast cancer. N Engl J Med. 2004;351(27):2817–26.
13. Paik S, Tang G, Shak S, Kim C, Baker J, Kim W, et al. Gene expression and benefit of chemotherapy in women with node-negative, estrogen receptor-positive breast cancer. J Clin Oncol. 2006;24(23):3726–34.
14. Teschendorff AE, Naderi A, Barbosa-Morais NL, Pinder SE, Ellis IO, Aparicio S, et al. A consensus prognostic gene expression classifier for ER positive breast cancer. Genome Biol. 2006;7(10):R101.
15. van de Vijver MJ, He YD, van't Veer LJ, Dai H, Hart AA, Voskuil DW, et al. A gene-expression signature as a predictor of survival in breast cancer. N Engl J Med. 2002;347(25):1999–2009.
16. Wang Y, Klijn JG, Zhang Y, Sieuwerts AM, Look MP, Yang F, et al. Gene-expression profiles to predict distant metastasis of lymph-node-negative primary breast cancer. Lancet. 2005;365(9460):671–9.

17. Ring BZ, Seitz RS, Beck R, Shasteen WJ, Tarr SM, Cheang MC, et al. Novel prognostic immunohistochemical biomarker panel for estrogen receptor-positive breast cancer. J Clin Oncol. 2006;24(19):3039–47.

18. Anderson K, Simmons-Menchaca M, Lawson KA, Atkinson J, Sanders BG, Kline K. Differential response of human ovarian cancer cells to induction of apoptosis by vitamin E Succinate and vitamin E analogue, alpha-TEA. Cancer Res. 2004;64(12):4263–9.

19. Malafa MP, Neitzel LT. Vitamin E succinate promotes breast cancer tumor dormancy. J Surg Res. 2000;93(1):163–70.

20. Neuzil J, Weber T, Gellert N, Weber C. Selective cancer cell killing by alpha-tocopheryl succinate. Br J Cancer. 2001;84(1):87–9.

21. Yu W, Simmons-Menchaca M, Gapor A, Sanders BG, Kline K. Induction of apoptosis in human breast cancer cells by tocopherols and tocotrienols. Nutr Cancer. 1999;33(1):26–32.

22. Hamilton A, Piccart M. The contribution of molecular markers to the prediction of response in the treatment of breast cancer: a review of the literature on HER-2, p53 and BCL-2. Ann Oncol. 2000;11(6):647–63.

23. Stratton J, Godwin M. The effect of supplemental vitamins and minerals on the development of prostate cancer: a systematic review and meta-analysis. Fam Pract. 2011;28(3):243–52.

24. Lu G, Xiao H, Li GX, Picinich SC, Chen YK, Liu A, et al. A gamma-tocopherol-rich mixture of tocopherols inhibits chemically induced lung tumorigenesis in A/J mice and xenograft tumor growth. Carcinogenesis. 2010;31(4):687–94.

10

High Molecular Weight (HMW): total adiponectin ratio is low in hiv-infected women receiving protease inhibitors

Fierdoz Omar[1*], Joel A Dave[2], Judy A King[1], Naomi S Levitt[2] and Tahir S Pillay[1,3]

Abstract

Background: At the time of the study, the HIV-treatment policy in South Africa included highly active antiretroviral therapy (HAART) regimens 1 (nucleotide reverse transcriptase inhibitors (NRTIs) only), and 2 (protease inhibitors (PI) and NRTIs). HAART is associated with the lipodystrophy syndrome, insulin resistance and reduced total adiponectin (TA) levels. The high molecular weight (HMW):TA ratio is a superior marker of insulin resistance. The aim of this study was to establish whether HMW:TA ratios are low in patients on PIs and whether they correlate with insulin resistance.

Methods: This was a cross-sectional study undertaken in an antiretroviral clinic at a tertiary hospital. The participants were 66 HIV-infected females: 22 were on regimen 2 (PI group), 22 on regimen 1 (non-PI) and 22 treatment naïve (TN), matched for BMI and age. Patients with a history of diabetes or impaired glucose tolerance were excluded. Serum adiponectin multimers were analysed using the AlpcoTM Adiponectin (Multimeric) enzyme immunoassay. Waist hip ratios (WHR), glucose and insulin levels were assessed, and HOMA-IR and QUICKI calculated. Data were analysed non-parametrically and multivariate analysis was performed.

Results: TA and HMW levels were lower in the treatment groups than in the TN group. HMW:TA was lower in the PI than in the non-PI and TN groups, and in the non-PI than in the TN groups. HMW:TA correlated negatively with waist, insulin and HOMA-IR, independently of BMI and duration of therapy. HOMA-IR and QUICKI did not differ among the groups.

Conclusion: HMW:TA is significantly decreased with HAART (particularly with PIs, but also with non-PIs) and may be a more sensitive marker of insulin resistance in these patients than conventional markers or HMW and total adiponectin individually.

Keywords: HMW adiponectin, Lipodystrophy syndrome, HMW: adiponectin ratio, Protease inhibitors, Insulin resistance

Background

Adiponectin is an insulin-sensitising hormone found in multimeric forms in the circulation with the high molecular weight (HMW) 16-18mer (>400 kDa) being the predominant and active form [1].

Although an adipokine, unlike other hormones secreted by adipocytes, adiponectin levels are reduced in people with increased central body fat [1], insulin resistance, type 2 diabetes mellitus and atherosclerosis, as well as in individuals with lipoatrophy and lipohypertrophy [1]. HMW adiponectin has been shown to correlate better with insulin sensitivity than total adiponectin (TA) [2] and the HMW:TA ratio to be a better predictor of coronary artery disease than TA [3]. The ratio has also been shown to be suppressed in type 2 diabetes mellitus patients with coronary artery disease even when HMW and TA levels were unchanged [4].

In HIV-associated lipodystrophy, a syndrome consisting of fat redistribution, dyslipidaemia and insulin resistance, adiponectin levels are significantly lower, demonstrating a

* Correspondence: fierdoz.omar@nhls.ac.za
[1]Division of Chemical Pathology, C17 NHLS, Groote Schuur Hospital, University of Cape Town, Anzio Road Observatory, Cape Town 7925, South Africa
Full list of author information is available at the end of the article

negative correlation with abdominal visceral fat mass and insulin resistance [5,6]. This syndrome is associated with antiretroviral (ARV) therapy, particularly protease inhibitors (PIs) (but also nucleotide- and nucleoside reverse transcriptase inhibitors such as stavudine (d4T), zidovudine (AZT)) and didanosine (ddI) [7,8]. In such patients, thiazolidinedione administration, via peroxisome proliferator-activated receptor γ activation, leads to improved insulin sensitivity [9] with upregulation of adiponectin levels, specifically the HMW form [10,11]. Adiponectin administration in mice markedly ameliorates protease-induced dyslipidaemia, suggesting that hypoadiponectinaemia may be partially responsible for the metabolic derangements associated with PIs [12].

In South Africa, the National Department of Health had two highly active antiretroviral therapy (HAART) regimens at the time of this study. The first regimen consisted of d4T, lamivudine (3TC) and either efavirenz (EFV) or nevirapine i.e. a combination of two nucleotide reverse transcriptase inhibitors (NRTIs) and one non-nucleotide reverse transcriptase inhibitor (NNRTIs); while the second regimen consisted of AZT and lopinavir/ritonavir (LPV/r). AZT and ddI are nucleotide- and nucleoside reverse transcriptase inhibitors, respectively, while LPV/r is a PI.

The purpose of this study was to establish whether PI therapy was associated with lower HMW:TA ratios in HIV-infected patients, and to examine associated biochemical evidence of insulin resistance in these patients.

Methods

This cross-sectional study was performed in accordance with the Helsinki Declaration. The protocol was approved by the University of Cape Town Faculty of Health Sciences Research Ethics Committee with reference number REC 450/2006. Sixty-six HIV-infected African females were enrolled into the study into three groups, viz. PI (Regimen 2 for at least six months), non-PI (Regimen 1 for at least six months) and treatment naïve (TN) groups, each consisting of 22 patients. Subjects were recruited from the ARV clinic at Groote Schuur Hospital, with the non-PI and TN groups matched to the PI group for body mass index (BMI) and age. Exclusion criteria included a history of impaired glucose tolerance or diabetes mellitus, active acute opportunistic infections, renal failure and pregnancy. Written informed consent was obtained. Waist and hip circumferences, weight and height were measured, and the BMI and waist: hip ratio (WHR) calculated. A 75 g OGTT was performed and blood samples drawn at 0 and 120 min. Glucose was measured at both time points and insulin and multimeric adiponectin in the 0 min sample only. Samples were centrifuged and stored at −70°C until analysis. The homeostatic model assessment for insulin resistance (HOMA-IR) and quantitative insulin-sensitivity check index (QUICKI) were calculated.

Adiponectin was analysed using the Alpco™ Adiponectin (Multimeric) enzyme immunoassay (sensitivity 0.04 ng/mL and coefficient of variation (CV) <15%), insulin by the Bayer ACS180 auto-analyser (CV 12%), and glucose by the Bayer Alera chemistry analyser.

Statistical analysis

Results were analysed non-parametrically, using the Mann–Whitney U, Kruskall-Wallis and Spearman correlation tests. Multivariate analyses and power calculations were performed. A p-value of 0.05 was considered significant.

Results
Patient characteristics

In the PI group, 21 patients received LPV/r and one Atazanavir for at least six months, with the median duration on PIs being 11.5 months. The median duration on regimen 1 drugs prior to progression to regimen 2 was 15 months. Four (18%) patients received d4T and 13 (59%) AZT, as part of their regimen. The median total duration on these drugs were 15.5 and nine months, respectively. In the non-PI group, 21 of the 22 patients received either AZT or d4T, with median durations of 12 and 10 months, respectively.

The median (interquartile range (IQR)) age and BMI among the groups were 36 (29; 42) years and 27 (24; 30), respectively. Waist measurement and WHR did not differ among the groups (Table 1).

Adiponectin levels in serum (Figure 1 and Table 1)

TA levels were within the reference interval (3.5 – 22 mg/L) [13] in all groups. However, total and HMW adiponectin levels were significantly lower in both treatment groups compared to the naïve group, with no significant difference between the PI and non-PI groups. In contrast, the HMW:TA ratio differed among all three groups and was significantly lower in the PI group than in both the non-PI and TN groups, and lower in the non-PI group than in the TN group. This difference was maintained when adjusting for BMI (data not shown) (Table 1 and Figure 1).

Traditional markers of insulin resistance

There were no significant differences among the groups for insulin, fasting and 2-h glucose, and the derived parameters HOMA-IR and QUICKI (Table 1). However, 15 (23%) of the entire study sample of HIV-infected patients had insulin resistance, defined as HOMA-IR >1.95 [14], and their HMW:TA ratios were lower (p = 0.0059) (median 0.31, IQR 0.22 and 0.47) compared to those without insulin resistance (median 0.50, IQR 0.40 and 0.57). Similarly, 40 (60%) of the entire sample of HIV-infected patients were overweight (BMI ≥25) and had

Table 1 Adiponectin and markers of insulin resistance among the treatment groups (A), duration of therapy among the groups (B)

	(A) Adiponectin and markers of insulin resistance among the treatment groups				
	PI *Median (IQR)*	Non-PI *Median (IQR)*	TN *Median (IQR)*	Units	p-value
Age	34.5 (29.8; 41.0)	34.5 (31.3; 41.0)	35.5 (29.0; 41.0)	Years	0.986
BMI	27.7 (24.9; 30.4)	25.0 (23.8; 29.5)	25.7 (22.9; 29.7)	-	0.586
Waist	89 (82; 95)	83 (80; 93)	82 (76; 88)	cm	0.194
WHR	0.87 (0.82; 0.93)	0.85 (0.79; 0.89)	0.84 (0.80; 0.90)	-	0.315
Fasting insulin	5.5 (2.7; 10.1)	3.1 (2.1; 5.7)	4.4 (2.0; 8.0)	mIU/L	0.365
Fasting glucose	86 (81; 90)	91 (83; 98)	91 (85; 97)	mg/dL	0.145
2 hour glucose	104 (80; 113)	94 (85; 109)	94 (81; 109)	mg/dL	0.877
HOMA-IR	1.18 (0.54; 2.09)	0.72 (0.50; 1.17)	1.05 (0.41; 1.73)	-	0.479
QUICKI	0.37 (0.34; 0.42)	0.41 (0.37; 0.43)	0.38 (0.35; 0.45)	-	0.234
Total adiponectin	5.6 (3.4; 9.4)	7.3 (4.0; 8.7)	9.0 (7.6; 12.1)	ng/mL	0.039*
HMW adiponectin	2.2 (1.0; 3.9)	3.5 (1.8; 5.1)	5.3 (3.8; 7.0)	ng/mL	0.002*
HMW:Total adiponectin	0.35 (0.29; 0.42)	0.48 (0.41; 0.56)	0.56 (0.52; 0.61)	-	<0.0001**
(B) Duration of therapy among the treatment groups					
Regimen 1	15 (8.5; 21.5)	12 (9.5; 20.0)	-	Months	
Regimen 2	11.5 (9.3; 14.0)	-	-	Months	
d4T	15.5 (9.8; 22.3)	10 (8; 17.5)	-	Months	
AZT	9 (5; 16.5)	12 (11; 15.0)	-	Months	

The Kruskall-Wallis and Mann–Whitney U tests were used to assess differences among the groups collectively and individually, respectively. PI, protease inhibitor group; Non-PI, non-protease inhibitor group; TN, treatment-negative group; IQR, interquartile range; HMW, high molecular weight. *p < 0.05; **p < 0.001. Multiply by the following conversion factor for SI units: glucose 0.0555 (mmol/L); insulin 6.945 (pmol/L).

significantly lower (p = 0.0475) HMW:TA ratios (median 0.44, IQR 0.31 and 0.54) than those who were not overweight (median 0.50, IQR 0.44 and 0.58).

HMW, TA, and their ratio correlated negatively (p <0.05) with waist, BMI, fasting insulin and HOMA-IR, even when adjusted for BMI (Table 2). While HMW, TA, and their ratio correlated positively (p < 0.05) with QUICKI, this significance was lost when adjusting for BMI. When adjusting for both BMI and total duration of therapy, only the HMW:TA ratio maintained a significant correlation with fasted insulin, HOMA-IR and QUICKI, while all three adiponectin parameters remained significantly associated with waist. TA, HMW and their ratio maintained their association with waist, fasting insulin and HOMA-IR when adjusting for duration of therapy alone. HMW and HMW:TA also remained significantly associated with QUICKI when adjusting for duration of therapy alone.

Discussion

Altered body composition and insulin resistance are components of the HIV–associated lipodystrophy syndrome [7]. This syndrome is primarily seen in HIV-infected patients on HAART, with a 17% risk of developing lipodystrophy after the first year of HAART and each additional 6 month period associated with a 45% risk [15]. These findings are particularly associated with PIs, but similar findings have been seen in some patients on nucleotide and nucleoside analogues such as d4T, AZT and ddI [8].

Adiponectin has been implicated in the pathogenesis of HIV– associated lipodystrophy [12], with PI administration in mice producing a dose-related reduction in adiponectin levels and administration of recombinant adiponectin ameliorating the associated dyslipidaemia.

It was therefore somewhat surprising that TA levels were well within the reference interval in all our study groups. However, they were significantly lower in the HIV-infected patients on HAART therapy (both PIs and non-PIs) than in those not receiving treatment.

The active HMW form of adiponectin has been shown to correlate better with insulin sensitivity than TA [16], and has been shown to be low in HIV-infected patients with insulin resistance [10]. In our study, HMW adiponectin levels were significantly lower in patients receiving both PIs and non-PIs, but also in those receiving only non-PIs. This finding in the latter group, may be attributed to the use of d4T (16 (66%) patients) or AZT (5 (23%) patients), drugs which have both been associated with lipodystrophy [17].

The HMW:TA ratio is a superior marker of insulin resistance compared to total and HMW adiponectin levels individually [18]. It is also an independent risk factor for coronary vascular disease (CVD) [19]. Previous studies have shown increased cardiovascular risk in HIV-infected

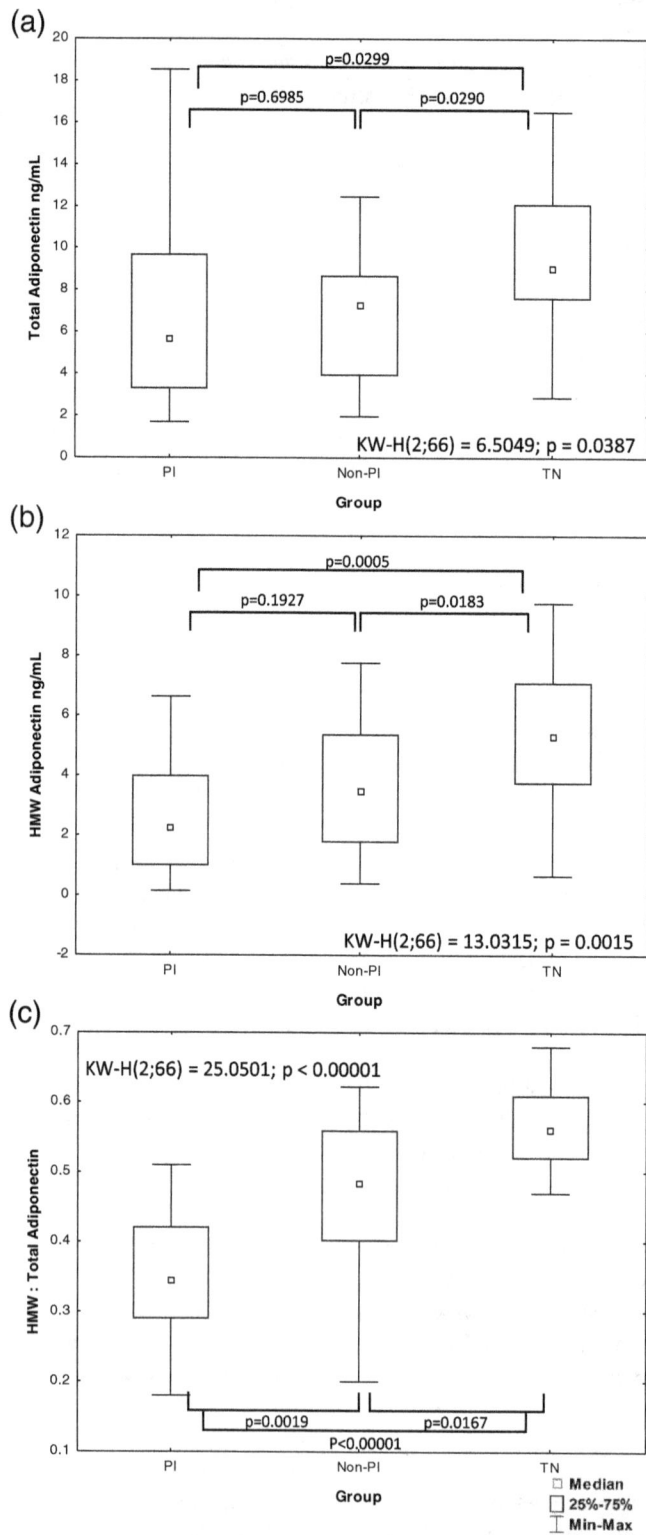

Figure 1 Distribution of (a) Total adiponectin, (b) HMW adiponectin, and (c) HMW: total adiponectin ratio among the three groups.
HMW, high molecular weight; PI, protease inhibitor group; Non-PI, non-protease inhibitor group; TN, treatment-negative group; KW, Kruskall-Wallis; p <0.05 considered significant.

Table 2 The relationship between adiponectin and various markers of insulin resistance before and after adjusting for BMI and duration of therapy, separately and together

Relationship between adiponectin and markers of insulin resistance

| | Univariable | | | Multivariable | | | | | | | | |
| | | | | Adjusted for BMI | | | Adjusted for duration of therapy | | | Adjusted for BMI and duration of therapy | | |
	b	95% CI	p-value	b	95% CI	p-value	b	95% CI	p-value	b	95% CI	p-value
Total Adiponectin												
Waist	−0.27	(−0.3895,−0.1420)	0.0001**	−0.28	(−0.5153,−0.0517)	0.019*	−0.29	(−0.4582,−0.1161)	0.002*	−0.35	(−0.6479,−0.0492)	0.028*
Fasted Insulin	−0.28	(−0.4683,−0.0906)	0.005*	−0.21	(−0.3945,−0.0164)	0.037*	−0.28	(−0.5408,−0.0266)	0.036*	−0.24	(−0.4935,0.0099)	0.067
HOMA-IR	−1.11	(−1.8677,−0.3428)	0.006*	−0.81	(−1.5741,−0.0551)	0.040*	−1.21	(−2.3196,−0.1036)	0.038*	−1.07	(−2.1435,0.0051)	0.058
QUICKI	14.20	(1.2607,27.1444)	0.035*	8.24	(−4.8207,21.3036)	0.221	15.25	(−0.2780,30.7806)	0.061	11.29	(−4.4271,26.9992)	0.167
HMW Adiponectin												
Waist	−0.17	(−0.2484,−0.0923)	0.0001**	−0.19	(−0.3350,−0.0429)	0.014*	−0.16	(−0.2637,−0.0627)	0.003*	−0.19	(−0.3674,−0.0109)	0.044*
Fasted Insulin	−0.17	(−0.2941,−0.0547)	0.006*	−0.13	(−0.2475,−0.0078)	0.041*	−0.17	(−0.3204,−0.0169)	0.035*	−0.14	(−0.2918,0.0048)	0.065
HOMA-IR	−0.69	(−1.1753,−0.2091)	0.007*	−0.51	(−0.9903,−0.0273)	0.042*	−0.72	(−1.3745,−0.0666)	0.037*	−0.64	(−1.2681,−0.0022)	0.056
QUICKI	9.38	(1.2388,17.5231)	0.027*	5.67	(−2.5563,13.9009)	0.182	9.97	(0.9112,19.0352)	0.037*	7.66	(−1.5098,16.8289)	0.110
HMW: TA												
Waist	−0.007	(−0.0102,−0.0042)	0.000**	−0.011	(−0.0165,−0.0054)	0.0003**	−0.16	(−0.2637,−0.0627)	0.003*	−0.007	(−0.0130,−0.0016)	0.016*
Fasted Insulin	−0.008	(−0.0123,−0.0030)	0.002*	−0.006	(−0.0109,−0.0014)	0.013*	−0.007	(−0.0119,−0.0025)	0.005*	−0.006	(−0.0111,−0.0018)	0.009*
HOMA-IR	−0.03	(−0.0497,−0.0123)	0.002*	−0.03	(−0.0442,−0.0063)	0.011*	−0.03	(−0.0509,−0.0103)	0.005*	−0.03	(−0.0479,−0.0084)	0.008*
QUICKI	0.42	(0.1036,0.7331)	0.011*	0.30	(−0.0230,0.6253)	0.073	0.44	(0.1586,0.7148)	0.004*	0.38	(0.0911,0.6598)	0.014*

HMW, high molecular weight; b, coefficient; CI, confidence interval. *p < 0.05; **p < 0.001.

patients, including those on HAART [20,21]. We found this ratio to be significantly lower in the PI and less so (but nevertheless still significantly so) in the non-PI groups. This may imply an increased risk for CVD in patients on HAART (consistent with the findings of others) [20,21], with the risk for CVD increased when both PIs and non-PIs are being used. This significantly lower HMW:TA ratio in patients receiving both PIs and NRTIs (with the majority, i.e. 17 of 22, of patients also receiving a thymidine analogue) confirms previous findings that protease inhibitors and thymidine analogues induce metabolic complications synergistically [7]. A limitation in this study is that the PI group also contained the nucleoside analogue ddI. Further studies are needed in the absence of so called d-drugs to confirm the contribution of PI drugs to the changes seen in this study.

Our patient groups were selected to exclude the presence of overt diabetes, and therefore it was not surprising that fasting glucose was not abnormal in any of the groups. On the other hand, we were surprised by the lack of difference in all measures of glucose tolerance and insulin sensitivity among the groups (Table 1), despite the difference seen among the groups in total and HMW adiponectin. However, a larger study sample may be required to verify this. The sample size was sufficiently powered (75.5%) to detect a difference in HMW: TA, but not to verify the lack of significant differences demonstrated for the insulin resistance markers. A further limitation is that visceral and subcutaneous adiposity were not quantitatively assessed. Notwithstanding, the relationship between insulin resistance markers and adiponectin, previously shown [5], was demonstrated here, with the HMW:TA ratio shown to be significantly lower in patients (in all groups) with established insulin resistance (HOMA-IR greater than 1.95 [21]) and also significantly lower in patients with BMI greater than or equal to 25 than in those with lower BMIs. Furthermore, adiponectin levels (high, total and their ratio) correlated negatively with HOMA-IR and positively with QUICKI. The HMW:TA ratio also correlated negatively with waist, waist hip ratio (data not shown), fasting insulin levels and BMI (data not shown) - all markers of insulin resistance. While BMI and duration of drug therapy collectively contribute to the association seen between the markers of insulin resistance and the TA and HMW adiponectin forms, they do not affect the associations seen with the HMW:TA ratio.

Conclusion

These data demonstrate that both PI- and non-PI-containing HAART regimens significantly lower the HMW:TA ratio in HIV patients, with the ratio more significantly decreased in the PI-containing regimen, implying that PIs and NRTIs have an additive effect on the HMW:TA ratio. Although the HMW:TA ratio correlated

negatively with indirect markers of insulin resistance, insulin resistance was not demonstrated to be associated with ARV drugs. We therefore propose that the HMW:TA ratio may be an earlier or more sensitive marker of insulin resistance in HIV-infected patients on HAART than conventional markers or HMW and total adiponectin individually.

Abbreviations
HMW: High molecular weight; HIV: Human immunodeficiency virus; PI: Protease inhibitor; d4T: Stavudine; AZT: Zidovudine; HAART: Highly active antiretroviral therapy; 3TC: Lamivudine; EFV: Efavirenz; ddI: Didanosine; NRTI: nucleotide reverse transcriptase inhibitors; NNRTI: non-nucleotide reverse transcriptase inhibitor; LPV/r: Liponavir/ritonavir; TA: Total adiponectin; ARV: Antiretroviral; non-PI: non-protease inhibitor; BMI: Body mass index; TN: Treatment naive; WHR: Waist: hip ratio; HOMA-IR: Homeostatic model assessment for insulin resistance; QUICKI: Quantitative insulin-sensitivity check index; CV: Coefficient of variation; IQR: interquartile range; CVD: coronary vascular disease; KW: Kruskall-Wallis.

Competing interests
The authors declare that they have no competing interests.

Authors' contributions
FO: carried out the analysis, produced the data, analysed the data and produced the draft of the manuscript. JD, DL: physicians, under whose care the patients fell; obtained the blood samples. JAK: assisted with obtaining the data and the laboratory analysis; TSP: conceptualised the study, designed the study, obtained the funding and supervised the research. All authors read and approved the final manuscript.

Authors' information
FO: Chemical Pathologist; JD, Consultant Endocrinologist ; NL, Professor of Diabetes and Endocrinology; TSP: Professor and Chair, Chemical Pathology and Clinical Pathology.

Acknowledgements
The authors wish to acknowledge Dr Andrew Boulle for assistance with statistical analysis. This project was funded by the National Health Laboratory Service, National Research Foundation of South Africa, World Diabetes Foundation and the Department of Health. This work was submitted as part fulfilment for the MMed degree in Chemical Pathology at the University of Cape Town.
This paper was supported by a grant from the National Health Laboratory Service Research Trust Fund, the National Research Foundation, the World Diabetes Foundation and the Department of Health.

Author details
[1]Division of Chemical Pathology, C17 NHLS, Groote Schuur Hospital, University of Cape Town, Anzio Road Observatory, Cape Town 7925, South Africa. [2]Division of Diabetic Medicine and Endocrinology, Groote Schuur Hospital and University of Cape Town, Cape Town, South Africa. [3]Department of Chemical Pathology, University of Pretoria and NHLS Tshwane Academic Division/Steve Biko Academic Hospital, Tshwane, South Africa.

References
1. Swarbrick MM, Havel PJ: **Physiological, pharmacological, and nutritional regulation of circulating adiponectin concentrations in humans.** *Metab Syndr Relat Disord* 2008, **6**(2):87–102.
2. Fisher FM, Trujillo ME, Hanif W, Barnett AH, McTernan PG, Scherer PE, Kumar S: **Serum high molecular weight complex of adiponectin correlates better with glucose tolerance than total serum adiponectin in indo-asian males.** *Diabetologia* 2005, **48**(6):1084–1087.
3. El-Menyar A, Rizk N, Al Nabti AD, Hassira SA, Singh R, Abdel Rahman MO, Suwaidi JA: **Total and high molecular weight adiponectin in patients with coronary artery disease.** *J Cardiovasc Med (Hagerstown)* 2009, **10**(4):310–315.

4. Aso Y, Yamamoto R, Wakabayashi S, Uchida T, Takayanagi K, Takebayashi K, Okuno T, Inoue T, Node K, Tobe T, Inukai T, Nakano Y: **Comparison of serum high-molecular weight (HMW) adiponectin with total adiponectin concentrations in type 2 diabetic patients with coronary artery disease using a novel enzyme-linked immunosorbent assay to detect HMW adiponectin.** *Diabetes* 2006, **55**(7):1954–1960.

5. Addy CL, Gavrila A, Tsiodras S, Brodovicz K, Karchmer AW, Mantzoros CS: **Hypoadiponectinemia is associated with insulin resistance, hypertriglyceridemia, and fat redistribution in human immunodeficiency virus-infected patients treated with highly active antiretroviral therapy.** *J Clin Endocrinol Metab* 2003, **88**(2):627–636.

6. Tong Q, Sankale JL, Hadigan CM, Tan G, Rosenberg ES, Kanki PJ, Grinspoon SK, Hotamisligil GS: **Regulation of adiponectin in human immunodeficiency virus-infected patients: Relationship to body composition and metabolic indices.** *J Clin Endocrinol Metab* 2003, **88**(4):1559–1564.

7. Carr A, Samaras K, Burton S, Law M, Freund J, Chisholm DJ, Cooper DA: **A syndrome of peripheral lipodystrophy, hyperlipidaemia and insulin resistance in patients receiving HIV protease inhibitors.** *AIDS* 1998, **12**(7):F51–8.

8. Haubrich RH, Riddler SA, DiRienzo AG, Komarow L, Powderly WG, Klingman K, Garren KW, Butcher DL, Rooney JF, Haas DW, Mellors JW, Havlir DV, AIDS Clinical Trials Group (ACTG) A5142 Study Team: **Metabolic outcomes in a randomized trial of nucleoside, nonnucleoside and protease inhibitor-sparing regimens for initial HIV treatment.** *AIDS* 2009, **23**(9):1109–1118.

9. Sutinen J, Kannisto K, Korsheninnikova E, Fisher RM, Ehrenborg E, Nyman T, Virkamaki A, Funahashi T, Matsuzawa Y, Vidal H, Hamsten A, Yki-Jarvinen H: **Effects of rosiglitazone on gene expression in subcutaneous adipose tissue in highly active antiretroviral therapy-associated lipodystrophy.** *Am J Physiol Endocrinol Metab* 2004, **286**(6):E941–9.

10. Qurashi S, Mynarcik DC, McNurlan MA, Ahn H, Ferris R, Gelato MC: **Importance of the high-molecular-mass isoform of adiponectin in improved insulin sensitivity with rosiglitazone treatment in HIV disease.** *Clin Sci (Lond)* 2008, **115**(6):197–202.

11. Blumer RM, van der Valk M, Ackermans M, Endert E, Serlie MJ, Reiss P, Sauerwein HP: **A rosiglitazone-induced increase in adiponectin does not improve glucose metabolism in HIV-infected patients with overt lipoatrophy.** *Am J Physiol Endocrinol Metab* 2009, **297**(5):E1097–104.

12. Xu A, Yin S, Wong L, Chan KW, Lam KS: **Adiponectin ameliorates dyslipidemia induced by the human immunodeficiency virus protease inhibitor ritonavir in mice.** *Endocrinology* 2004, **145**(2):487–494.

13. Nien JK, Mazaki-Tovi S, Romero R, Erez O, Kusanovic JP, Gotsch F, Pineles BL, Gomez R, Edwin S, Mazor M, Espinoza J, Yoon BH, Hassan SS: **Plasma adiponectin concentrations in non-pregnant, normal and overweight pregnant women.** *J Perinat Med* 2007, **35**(6):522–531.

14. Jennings CL, Lambert EV, Collins M, Joffe Y, Levitt NS, Goedecke JH: **Determinants of insulin-resistant phenotypes in normal-weight and obese black african women.** *Obesity (Silver Spring)* 2008, **16**(7):1602–1609.

15. Martinez E, Mocroft A, Garcia-Viejo MA, Perez-Cuevas JB, Blanco JL, Mallolas J, Bianchi L, Conget I, Blanch J, Phillips A, Gatell JM: **Risk of lipodystrophy in HIV-1-infected patients treated with protease inhibitors: A prospective cohort study.** *Lancet* 2001, **357**(9256):592–598.

16. Seino Y, Hirose H, Saito I, Itoh H: **High molecular weight multimer form of adiponectin as a useful marker to evaluate insulin resistance and metabolic syndrome in japanese men.** *Metabolism* 2007, **56**(11):1493–1499.

17. Bogner JR, Vielhauer V, Beckmann RA, Michl G, Wille L, Salzberger B, Goebel FD: **Stavudine versus zidovudine and the development of lipodystrophy.** *J Acquir Immune Defic Syndr* 2001, **27**(3):237–244.

18. Hara K, Horikoshi M, Yamauchi T, Yago H, Miyazaki O, Ebinuma H, Imai Y, Nagai R, Kadowaki T: **Measurement of the high-molecular weight form of adiponectin in plasma is useful for the prediction of insulin resistance and metabolic syndrome.** *Diabetes Care* 2006, **29**(6):1357–1362.

19. Wang W, Xing W, Zhang H, Ding M, Shang L, Lau WB, Wang X, Li R: **Reduced high molecular weight adiponectin is an independent risk factor of cardiovascular lesions in hypercholesterolemic patients.** *Clin Endocrinol (Oxf)* 2012.

20. Dolan SE, Hadigan C, Killilea KM, Sullivan MP, Hemphill L, Lees RS, Schoenfeld D, Grinspoon S: **Increased cardiovascular disease risk indices in HIV-infected women.** *J Acquir Immune Defic Syndr* 2005, **39**(1):44–54.

21. Friis-Moller N, Sabin CA, Weber R, d'Arminio Monforte A, El-Sadr WM, Reiss P, Thiebaut R, Morfeldt L, De Wit S, Pradier C, Calvo G, Law MG, Kirk O, Phillips AN, Lundgren JD, Data Collection on Adverse Events of Anti-HIV Drugs (DAD) Study Group: **Combination antiretroviral therapy and the risk of myocardial infarction.** *N Engl J Med* 2003, **349**(21):1993–2003.

11

Challenging dedifferentiated liposarcoma identified by *MDM2*-amplification, a report of two cases

Suvi Lokka[1†], Andreas H Scheel[1,2*†], Sebastian Dango[3,4], Katja Schmitz[2], Rudolf Hesterberg[3], Josef Rüschoff[1] and Hans-Ulrich Schildhaus[2]

Abstract

Background: Liposarcoma is the most frequent soft tissue sarcoma. Well differentiated liposarcoma may progress into dedifferentiated liposarcoma with pleomorphic histology. A minority additionally features myogenic, osteo- or chondrosarcomatous heterologous differentiation. Genomic amplification of the *Mouse double minute 2 homolog (MDM2)* locus is characteristic for well differentiated and dedifferentiated liposarcomas. Detection of *MDM2* amplification may supplement histopathology and aid to distinguish liposarcoma from other soft tissue neoplasia.

Case presentation: Here we present two cases of dedifferentiated liposarcoma with challenging presentation. Case 1 features a myogenic component. As the tumour infiltrated the abdominal muscles and showed immunohistochemical expression of myogenic proteins, rhabdomyosarcoma had to be ruled out. Case 2 has an osteosarcomatous component resembling extraosseous osteosarcoma. The *MDM2* status was determined in both cases and helped making the correct diagnosis. Overexpression of MDM2 and co-overexpression of Cyclin-dependent kinase 4 is demonstrated by immunohistochemistry. The underlying *MDM2* amplification is shown by fluorescence in situ hybridisation. Since low grade osteosarcoma may also harbour *MDM2* amplification it is emphasised that the amplification has to be present in the lipomatous parts of the tumour to distinguish liposarcoma from extraosseous osteosarcoma.

Conclusions: The two cases exemplify challenges in the diagnoses of dedifferentiated liposarcoma. Liposarcoma often has pleomorphic histology and additionally may feature heterologous components that mimic other soft tissue neoplasms. Amplification of *MDM2* is characteristic for well differentiated and dedifferentiated liposarcomas. Determination of the *MDM2* status by in situ hybridisation may assist histopathology and help to rule out differential diagnoses.

Keywords: Dedifferentiated Liposarcoma, Liposarcoma with osteoblastic component, *MDM2*, Fluorescence in situ hybridisation

Background

Liposarcoma (LS) is the most common soft tissue sarcoma with about 20% [1]. They are categorized into five subtypes according to WHO classification [2,3] (Table 1). The majority are well differentiated liposarcomas/atypical lipomatous tumours (ALT; 40%). About 10% progress to

* Correspondence: scheel@patho-nordhessen.de
†Equal contributors
[1]Institute of Pathology Nordhessen, Germaniastr. 7, 34119 Kassel, Germany
[2]Department of Pathology, University Medical Centre Göttingen, Robert-Koch-Str. 38, 37077 Göttingen, Germany
Full list of author information is available at the end of the article

dedifferentiated liposarcoma [3] (DDLPS). LS are usually located in the deep soft tissue. ALT are most frequently located in the limbs, particularly the thighs while DDLPS are most frequent in the retroperitoneum. LS affect adults, the incidence peaks around 60 years.

Histomorphology of DDLPS usually shows remains of ALT with an abrupt shift to dedifferentiated neoplastic tissue. The dedifferentiated tissue is most commonly non lipogenic and pleomorphic, reminiscent of undifferentiated pleomorphic sarcoma (formerly called malignant fibrous histiocytoma). Additionally, heterologous differentiation

Table 1 Benign and malignant lipomatous tumors as listed by the current WHO-definition and _MDM2_-status

Entity	Dignity	ICD-O	MDM2 amplified
Lipoma	Benign	8850/0	no
Lipoblastoma	Benign	8851/0	no
Angiolipoma	Benign	8861/0	no
Myolipoma	Benign	8890/0	no
Chondroid lipoma	Benign	8862/0	no
Spindle cell lipoma	Benign	8854/0	no
Pleomorphic lipoma	Benign	8854/0	no
Hibernoma	Benign	8880/0	no
Well differentiated liposarcoma/atypical lipomatous tumor	Intermediate, locally aggressive	8851/1	yes
Dedifferentiated liposarcoma	Malignant	8858/3	yes
Myxoid liposacroma	Malignant	8852/3	no
Pleomorphic liposarcoma	Malignant	8854/3	no

occurs in about 10% of DDLPS and may present as myogenic, osteo/chondrosarcomatous or angiosarcomatous [4]. Thus DDLPS may mimic a broad spectrum of soft tissue tumours. The clinical prognosis of DDLPS is better than for other high grade sarcoma and is not affected by the presence of heterologous differentiation.

A hallmark of ALT and DDLPS is the genomic amplification of the _MDM2_ gene [5]. This can be detected by fluorescence in situ hybridization (FISH) and may facilitate diagnosis [6].

In this report we present two cases of DDLPS with challenging presentations. Both tumours featured heterologous components imitating other soft tissue sarcoma. _MDM2_ amplification was detected by FISH and helped to rule out potential differential diagnosis.

Case presentation

Case #1, clinical presentation
An 84 year old male obese (BMI 35 kg/m^2) patient presented with chronic anaemia, localized right abdominal pain and loss of appetite. A CT-scan unmasked a 4.2 × 2.7 × 7 cm hypodense (50HU) solid mass in the painful abdominal region [Figure 1A]. Staging laparoscopy was performed and revealed a whitish tumour in the subcutaneous fatty tissue. The adjacent abdominal skeletal muscles were infiltrated while the peritoneum was not compromised and the abdominal cavity was inconspicuous. Biopsies were taken and routine histology showed a malignant mesenchymal neoplasm. After discussion in an interdisciplinary tumour board wide resection with the aim of complete tumour removal was performed. The tumour region including the path of the laparoscopy, adjacent skin and peritoneum, inguinal canal and ductus deferens were removed en-bloc. The abdominal wall was reconstructed using an intraperitoneal onlay mesh graft technique (IPOM). Histological finding revealed

disseminated tumour growth into the cranio-lateral margin (R1). Reoperation yielded a complete tumour removal (R0). The patient recovered and was discharged from hospital 13 days after initial surgery. Soon after the patient was readmitted with ileus due to abdominal adhesions. Laparoscopy was performed and a 35 cm long small intestine segment was removed. Histology did not show any further tumour infiltrates. The patient recovered well and was in good health one year later.

Histologic and molecular findings
On gross examination the 13 × 10.5 × 6 cm specimen contained a 7 × 3.5 × 3.1 cm tumour with whitish/pale yellow cut surfaces [Figure 1B]. The tumour was mostly well delimited with focal areas of diffuse transition into the surrounding tissue. Haematoxylin and eosin (HE) staining showed a neoplasm with high cellularity and mostly spindle-shaped cells arranged in storiform patterns (Figure 2B). Focal transition into more well differentiated atypical adipose tissue were present (2A). Parts of the tumour showed myofibroblastic morphology with parallel, slender cells (2C). Immunohistochemistry (IHC) revealed coexpression of Actin and Desmin (2D) while Caldesmon and Myogenin were negative.

Neoplastic giant cells with nuclear vacuoles were present (Figure 3) and IHC stainings for CDK4 and MDM2 were positive (3B, C). Fluorescence in situ hybridization with a _MDM2_-specific probe (ZytoLight SPEC MDM2/CEN12 dual colour probe; ZytoVision, Bremerhaven, Germany) was supplemented. Groups of highly amplified _MDM2_ clusters were detected in all parts of the tumour (3D). Given morphologic and molecular findings, the neoplasm was identified as dedifferentiated liposarcoma with myofibroblastic component (ICD-O: C49.4 M8858/3 G3 (FNCLCC)).

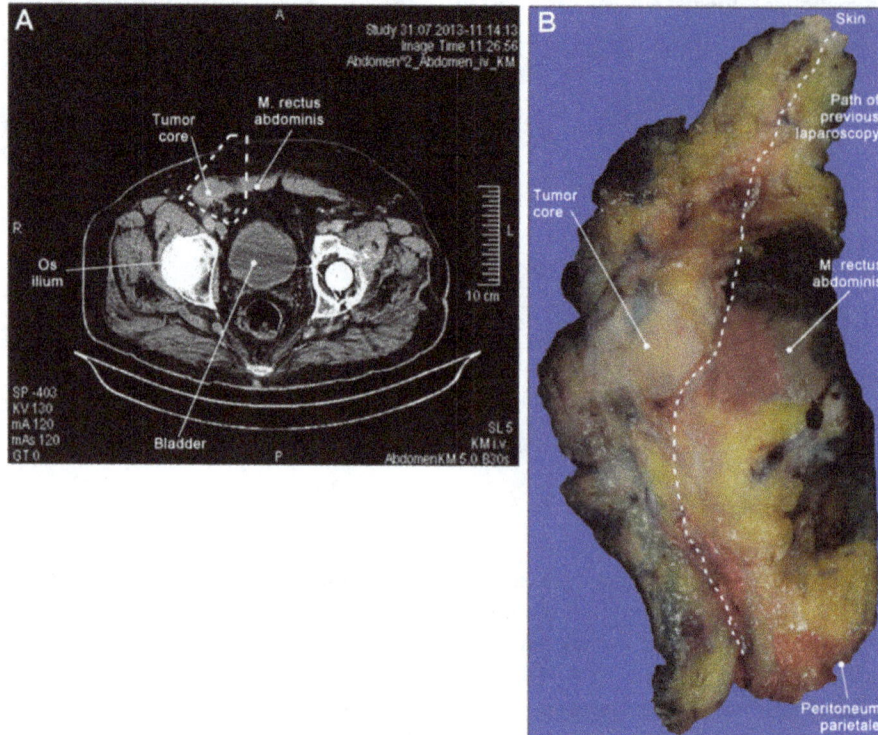

Figure 1 Clinical presentation of Case #1: Preoperative CT-scan (A) of the tumour in the lower left abdominal wall. Macroscopic presentation of the surgical specimen **(B)**; central parts of the tumour are well delimited ('core'); the path of the primary laparoscopy is visible. The tumour infiltrated the abdominal skeletal muscles but did not extra into the abdominal cavity.

Case #2, clinical presentation

A 66 year old male patient presented with acute abdomen. The pain was pronounced in the lower right abdomen. Emergency surgery was performed and revealed a ruptured cystic mass of the lower right abdominal wall with connection to the abdominal cavity. En bloc resection was performed. The mass was found to be contained in the soft tissue without connection to the pelvic bones. Given the emergency situation and rupture, excision in toto could not be guaranteed.

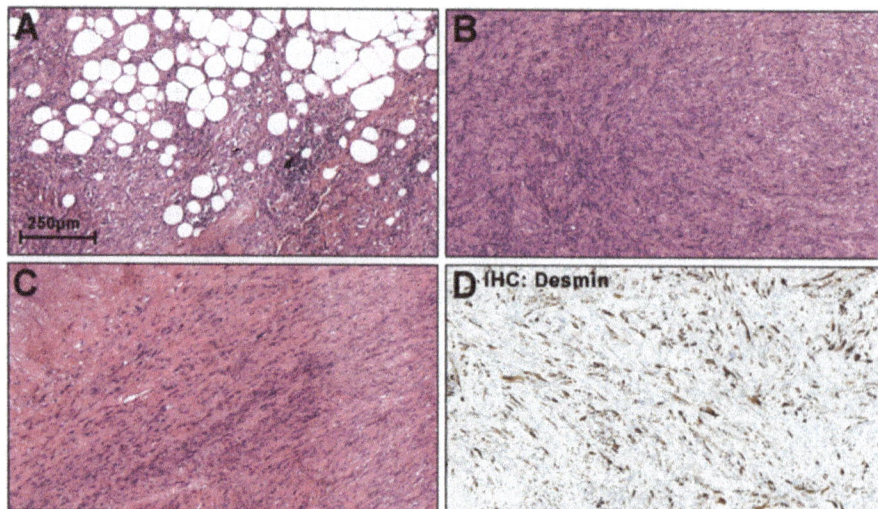

Figure 2 Histopathology of Case #1: The tumour shows patches of higher differentiated atypical lipomatous tissue (A) but mostly displays only poorly differentiated spindle-shaped cells (B). Prominent areas with myofibroblastic morphology were noticed **(C)** and immunohistochemistry was positive for Desmin **(D)** and Actin.

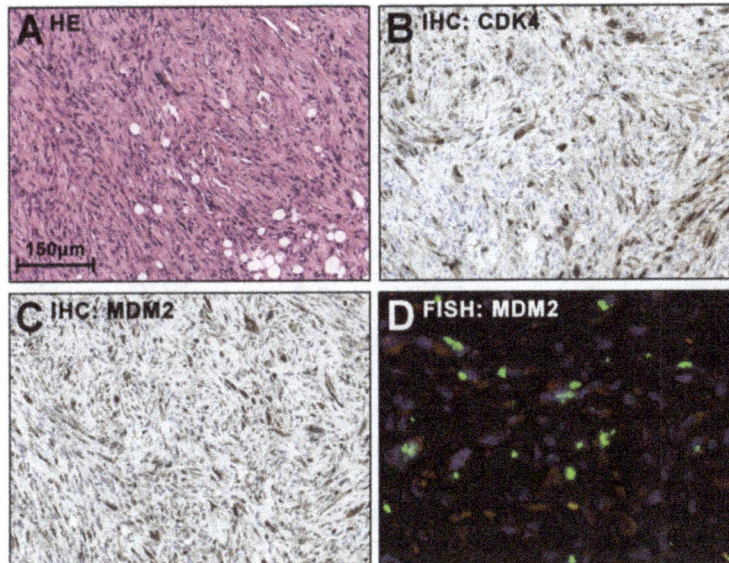

Figure 3 Molecular hallmarks of Case #1: Immunohistochemistry demonstrates co-overexpression of CDK4 (B) and MDM2 (C) in both the poorly and higher differentiated areas (A: HE-staining of corresponding region). Fluorescence in situ hybridisation shows strong amplification of the MDM2 locus as underlying genetic alteration (D; Green: MDM2 probe, Red: Chromosome 12 reference probe). The features are characteristic of dedifferentiated liposarcoma.

Histologic and molecular findings

Gross examination showed a 20 × 9 × 2.5 cm specimen with yellow-whitish, smooth surface. Cross sections showed soft and fatty tissue. The wall showed areas with solid, partially mineralized tissue with lamellar macroscopic appearance.

HE stainings showed a mesenchymal proliferation with high cellularity and mixed morphology (Figure 4): The cells were mostly of spindle-shaped appearance with high pleomorphy. Giant cells with segmented nuclei were present. Mitoses and few atypical mitoses were observed besides areas with no mitotic activity. Transitions into more differentiated fatty tissue were found (Figure 4A) as well as areas with osteoblastic/osteosarcomatous (4B) and fibrosarcomatous appearance (4C). FISH of the *MDM2* gene revealed highly amplified clusters in the

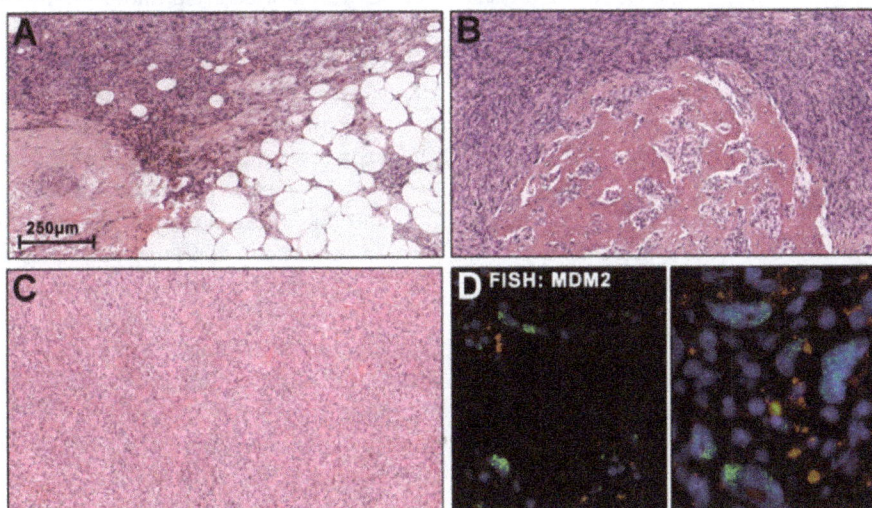

Figure 4 Histopathology and molecular hallmarks of Case #2: The tumour showed heterogeneous morphology. Most cells were spindle-shaped but giant cells with segmented nuclei were also present. Focally, transitions into higher differentiated lipomatous tissue were noticed (A). Other areas were of osteoblastic/osteosarcomatous (B) and fibrosarcomatous appearance (C). Fluorescence in situ hybridisation of the MDM2 gene revealed highly amplified clusters in the lipomatous (D, left), fibrosarcomatous and the osteosarcomatous regions (D, right).

lipomatous, fibrosarcomatous and the osteosarcomatous regions (4D, ZytoLight SPEC MDM2/CEN12 dual colour probe). The tumour was identified as dedifferentiated liposarcoma with heterologous differentiation (ICD-O: C49.4 M8858/3 G2 (FNCLCC)).

Course of disease

The patient was transferred to a medical centre specialized in abdominal and plastic surgery. Wide excision of the tumour area was performed about one month after initial surgery. Intraoperative two tumours on the small intestine were noticed and excised. Histology confirmed tumour implants of the liposarcoma both of which had been locally excised in sano. The patient recovered from the extended surgical procedures and no signs of recurrent disease were detectable during follow-up CT- and ultrasound-scans one year later.

Conclusions

Two cases of neoplasm of the lower abdominal wall were resolved as dedifferentiated liposarcomas. Each tumour featured mixed morphology, one with myofibroblastic and one with osteoblastic component. Histopathology was supplemented with detailed immunohistochemistry and in situ hybridization for MDM2. Both tumours showed high MDM2 amplification which is an almost pathognomonic finding given the localization and age of the patients.

ALT and DDLPS usually show a characteristic genomic amplification of 12q13-15 including the proto-oncogenes MDM2 (12q14.3-15) and CDK4 (12q14). Amplification may be detected by comparative genome hybridization or by FISH. CDK4 is often coamplified with MDM2 and the gene products may be detected by IHC. Ubiquitin ligase MDM2 accelerates protosomal degradation of master tumour suppressor protein p53 while cell cycle associated kinase CDK4 phosphorylates and activates the retinoblastoma gene product (Rb) [7,8]. Physiologically CDK4 is itself activated by D cyclines during G1 progression and inhibited by p16 (INK4a). Conversely p53 point mutations are rarely found in ALT and DDLPS.

The most widely used technique to determine the MDM2 status is currently dual colour FISH. Two probes specific for 12q14 and for the centromeric region of chromosome 12 are employed to detect amplification or polysomy. Cases are dichotomously classified by the ratio of MDM2 to centrosome; ≥2.0 are regarded as amplified and <2.0 as non-amplified. At least 50 non overlapping neoplastic cells should be counted [6]. In our own hands application of the threshold is usually not required since ALT and DDLPS invariably show high amplifications with clusters of >10 copies [Figures 2D, 3D].

Sensitivity of the FISH analysis has been reported to be 93.5%-100% in a case-dependent manner [6,9]. It also has a high specificity in distinguishing lipoma from ALT.

Benign lipomatous lesions do not harbour MDM2 amplifications [6,10]. Spindle cell lipoma are reported to frequently have chromosome 12 polysomy [6] while ALT and DDLPS close to always show MDM2 amplifications. On the other hand, myxoid liposarcomas and most pleomorphic liposarcomas do not harbour MDM2 amplifications. An exception from the rule of thumb that pleomorphic liposarcomas are MDM2 negative are cutaneous and subcutaneous pleomorphic liposarcoma which may be MDM2 amplified in very rare cases [11]. A recent study could demonstrate that peripheral undifferentiated sarcomas with MDM2 amplification correspond to DDLPS, even if a well-differentiated component was not present [12].

Overall, few non-liposarcomatous tumours are known to have increased MDM2 gene copy numbers. Most notably low grade osteosarcoma arising on the surface of bone may feature 12q14 amplifications [13] while extraosseous osteosarcoma are complex genomic sarcoma without recurrent MDM2 amplifications.

The two cases exemplify challenges in the diagnosis of DDLPS. Case #1 showed little remaining well differentiated liposarcomatous tissue and featured a myogenic component. Therefore, most important differential diagnosis was rhabdomyosarcoma. Localisation, epidemiology and molecular findings render this possibility unlikely: IHC for Myogenin was negative and the MDM2 amplification is not observed in tumours of myogenic origin.

Case #2 featured a striking osteosarcomatous component which could also reflect presence of an extraosseous osteosarcoma. Given the localisation close to a fascia ossifying myositis would be benign second differential diagnoses. Transitions into atypical lipomatous tissue were noticed and under the hypotheses of DDLPS hybridisation for MDM2 was performed. Low grade Osteosarcoma (OS) may also harbour amplified MDM2. Thus, the detection of MDM2-amplification in the osteosarcomatous parts is not suited to distinguish between low grade OS and DDLPS. However, the amplification in our case was present in all parts of the tumour, including the atypical adipocytes. Thus the malignant character of the atypical adipose tissue, i.e. the liposarcomatous tissue was confirmed. Also, the tumour did not have contact to bone and extraosseous OS do not harbour MDM2 amplifications. Thus, the combination of patient age, localisation, morphology and MDM2 status strongly argues for the osteosarcomatous tissue to be heterologous component of a DDLPS.

The current standard therapy of DDLPS is wide excision. No consensus exists about the minimal length of the resection margins and the widest resection possible should be archived [14]. This is particularly challenging in the retroperitoneum which may explain the high rates of local recurrences of DDLPS (20-100% depending on the respective study [3]). DDLPS may spread to distant sites in 15-20% of cases while ALT do not metastasise [2]. Case #2 exemplifies that scattered DDLPS tissue may easily spawn tumour implants. Both patients were in good health one year after treatment and showed no signs of recurrent disease. However, given the slow-growing behaviour of DDLPS careful follow-up investigations are necessary.

The recurrent *MDM2* amplification might be a key to targeted therapy of DDLPS: Experimental MDM2-inhibitors have been successfully employed in vitro to reactivate p53 and mediate apoptosis [15]. While the first generation of MDM2 inhibitors proved to be clinically intolerable several newly developed substances are currently undergoing phase I trials. Should they translate into approved drugs the *MDM2* status might become a predictive biomarker.

Keypoints

Liposarcoma is the most frequent soft tissue neoplasm. About 40% are well differentiated liposarcoma which may progress into dedifferentiated liposarcoma. The clinical prognosis is better compared to other high grade soft tissue sarcoma.

Dedifferentiated liposarcoma has pleomorphic histomorphology. The diagnosis is facilitated by the demonstration of remaining well differentiated liposarcomatous tissue.

A minority of cases may present a heterologous differentiation of myogenic, osteo-/chondrosarcomatous or angiosarcomatous appearance. These have to be distinguished from sarcoma of other origin.

Detection of MDM2 and CDK4 amplification and coexpression by FISH and IHC has a high specificity and may support classification of challenging cases.

Consent

Written informed consent was obtained from the patients for publication of this case report and any accompanying images. A copy of the written consent is available for review by the Editor of this journal.

Abbreviations
CDK4: Cyclin dependent kinase 4; FISH: Fluorescence in situ hybridization; FNCLCC: French Fédération Nationale des Centres de Lutte Contre le Cancer grading system; HE: Haematoxylin and eosin; IHC: Immunohistochemistry; MDM2: Murine double-minute 2; OS: Osteosarcoma.

Competing interests
The authors declare no conflicts of interest. The authors received no funding or financial compensation for the preparation of the manuscript.

Authors' contributions
The patient of case #1 was treated by RH and SD. The surgical specimens of both cases were examined by SL and AS. Histopathology was performed by SL and AS under guidance of JR. HUS was contacted for second opinion and for *MDM2*-FISH. FISH was performed by KS and HUS. The manuscript was drafted by SL, AS and SD under guidance of HUS and with contribution of all co-authors. The final manuscript was read and agreed upon by all authors.

Acknowledgements
The authors would like to thank Sara Hugo for excellent technical assistance.

Author details
[1]Institute of Pathology Nordhessen, Germaniastr. 7, 34119 Kassel, Germany. [2]Department of Pathology, University Medical Centre Göttingen, Robert-Koch-Str. 38, 37077 Göttingen, Germany. [3]Rotes Kreuz Krankenhaus, Department of Surgery, Hansteinstrasse 29, 34121 Kassel, Germany. [4]Department of General, Visceral, and Paediatric Surgery, University Medical Centre Göttingen, Robert-Koch-Str. 38, 37077 Göttingen, Germany.

References
1. Dei Tos AP: **Liposarcoma: New entities and evolving concepts.** *Ann Diagn Pathol* 2000, **4**:252–266.
2. WHO: In *Classification of Tumours of Soft Tissue and Bone.* 4th edition. Edited by Fletcher CDM, Bridge JA, Hogendoorn PCW, Mertens F, World Health Orgn. Geneva, Switzerland: WHO PRESS; 2013.
3. Mentzel T, Schneider-Stock R: **Lipogen differenzierte Tumoren.** In *Pathologie (Kopf-Hals-Region, Weichgewebstumoren, Haut).* 3rd edition. Edited by Klöppel G, Kreipe HH, Remmele W. Berlin - Heidelberg: Springer; 2008:401–403.
4. Nascimento AG: **Dedifferentiated liposarcoma.** *Semin Diagn Pathol* 2001, **18**:263–266.
5. Crago AM, Singer S: **Clinical and molecular approaches to well-differentiated and dedifferentiated liposarcoma.** *Curr Opin Oncol* 2011, **23**:373–378.
6. Weaver J, Downs-Kelly E, Goldblum JR, Turner S, Kulkarni S, Tubbs RR, Rubin BP, Skacel M: **Fluorescence in situ hybridization for MDM2 gene amplification as a diagnostic tool in lipomatous neoplasms.** *Mod Pathol* 2008, **21**:943–949.
7. Subhasree N, Jiangjiang Q, Kalkunte SS, Minghai W, Ruiwen Z: **The MDM2-p53 pathway revisited.** *J Biomed Res* 2013, **27**:254–271.
8. Brown VD, Phillips RA, Gallie BL: **Cumulative effect of phosphorylation of pRB on regulation of E2F activity.** *Mol Cell Biol* 1999, **19**:3246–3256.
9. Kashima T, Halai D, Ye H, Hing SN, Delaney D, Pollock R, O'Donnell P, Tirabosco R, Flanagan AM: **Sensitivity of MDM2 amplification and unexpected multiple faint alphoid 12 (alpha 12 satellite sequences) signals in atypical lipomatous tumour.** *Mod Pathol* 2012, **25**:1384–1396.
10. Kimura H, Dobashi Y, Nojima T, Nakamura H, Yamamoto N, Tsuchiya H, Ikeda H, Sawada-Kitamura S, Oyama T, Ooi A: **Utility of fluorescence in situ hybridization to detect MDM2 amplification in liposarcomas and their morphological mimics.** *Int J Clin Exp Pathol* 2013, **6**:1306–16.
11. Gardner JM, Dandekar M, Thomas D, Goldblum JR, Weiss SW, Billings SD, Lucas DR, McHugh JB, Patel RM: **Cutaneous and subcutaneous pleomorphic liposarcoma: a clinicopathologic study of 29 cases with evaluation of MDM2 gene amplification in 26.** *Am J Surg Pathol* 2012, **36**:1047–51.
12. Le Guellec S, Chibon F, Ouali M, Perot G, Decouvelaere AV, Robin YM, Larousserie F, Terrier P, Coindre JM, Neuville A: **Are peripheral purely undifferentiated pleomorphic sarcomas with MDM2 amplification dedifferentiated liposarcomas?** *Am J Surg Pathol* 2014, **38**:293–304.
13. Yoshida A, Ushiku T, Motoi T, Shibata T, Beppu Y, Fukayama M, Tsuda H: **Immunohistochemical analysis of MDM2 and CDK4 distinguishes low-grade osteosarcoma from benign mimics.** *Mod Pathol* 2010, **23**:1279–1288.
14. Thomas DM, O'Sullivan B, Gronchi A: **Current concepts and future perspectives in retroperitoneal soft-tissue sarcoma management.** *Expert Rev Anticancer Ther* 2009, **9**:1145–57.
15. Vassilev LT, Vu BT, Graves B, Carvajal D, Podlaski F, Filipovic Z, Kong N, Kammlott U, Lukacs C, Klein C, Fotouhi N, Liu EA: **In vivo activation of the p53 pathway by small-molecule antagonists of MDM2.** *Science* 2004, **303**:844–848.

Quantitative assessment of placental morphology may identify specific causes of stillbirth

Imogen Ptacek[1,2], Anna Smith[3], Ainslie Garrod[1,2], Sian Bullough[1,2], Nicola Bradley[1,2], Gauri Batra[3], Colin P. Sibley[1,2], Rebecca L. Jones[1,2], Paul Brownbill[1,2] and Alexander E. P. Heazell[1,2*]

Abstract

Background: Stillbirth is frequently the result of pathological processes involving the placenta. Understanding the significance of specific lesions is hindered by qualitative subjective evaluation. We hypothesised that quantitative assessment of placental morphology would identify alterations between different causes of stillbirth and that placental phenotype would be independent of post-mortem effects and differ between live births and stillbirths with the same condition.

Methods: Placental tissue was obtained from stillbirths with an established cause of death, those of unknown cause and live births. Image analysis was used to quantify different facets of placental structure including: syncytial nuclear aggregates (SNAs), proliferative cells, blood vessels, leukocytes and trophoblast area. These analyses were then applied to placental tissue from live births and stillbirths associated with fetal growth restriction (FGR), and to placental lobules before and after perfusion of the maternal side of the placental circulation to model post-mortem effects.

Results: Different causes of stillbirth, particularly FGR, cord accident and hypertension had altered placental morphology compared to healthy live births. FGR stillbirths had increased SNAs and trophoblast area and reduced proliferation and villous vascularity; 2 out of 10 stillbirths of unknown cause had similar placental morphology to FGR. Stillbirths with FGR had reduced vascularity, proliferation and trophoblast area compared to FGR live births. Ex vivo perfusion did not reproduce the morphological findings of stillbirth.

Conclusion: These preliminary data suggest that addition of quantitative assessment of placental morphology may distinguish between different causes of stillbirth; these changes do not appear to be due to post-mortem effects. Applying quantitative assessment in addition to qualitative assessment might reduce the proportion of unexplained stillbirths.

Keywords: Stillbirth, Unexplained Stillbirth, Placental Morphometry, Fetal Growth Restriction, Villous vascularity, Avascular villi

* Correspondence: alexander.heazell@manchester.ac.uk
[1]Institute of Human Development, Faculty of Medical and Human Sciences, University of Manchester, Oxford Rd, Manchester M13 9PL, UK
[2]Maternal and Fetal Health Research Centre, 5th floor (Research), St Mary's Hospital, Oxford Road, Manchester M13 9WL, UK
Full list of author information is available at the end of the article

Background

Histological examination of the placenta is one of the most frequently performed investigations to identify the cause of death in cases of stillbirth [1]; its application in this context is recommended by international guidelines [2–4]. A recent systematic review found large variations in the methodological quality of studies of placental examination after stillbirth, with few studies of high quality [5]. Interpretation of the results of such studies is further complicated by the use of different classification systems and a lack of consensus in terminology used to describe placental lesions which results in a large variation in the proportion of stillbirths attributed to a placental "cause" from 11–65 % [5]. Such qualitative placental assessment, combined with varied terminology, has some deficiencies. Firstly, qualitative assessment of placental lesions may introduce bias, particularly if assessors are not blinded to outcome. Furthermore, qualitative assessment may lead to inter-observer variation in diagnoses, which ranged from 25–91 % in one study [6]. The significance of specific abnormalities to stillbirth has also been questioned by Pathak et al. who describe placental abnormalities in a significant proportion of apparently healthy live-born infants [7]. Finally, identification of a specific lesion does not imply a single cause. For example, appearances of fetal thrombotic vasculopathy have been associated with various pathologies including: cytomegalovirus infection [8], umbilical cord accidents [9] or specific patterns of umbilical cord coiling [10]. Similarly, changes of maternal underperfusion may be related to hypertensive disorders [11] and antiphospholipid syndrome [12].

Recently, significant advances have been made in the development of modern classification systems [13–15] that reduce the proportion of unexplained stillbirths [16]. These classification systems have given greater recognition to the role of placental pathology in the aetiology of stillbirth [13–15] and progress has been made in reducing the variation of placental histological findings [6]. However, these clinically-orientated descriptions of placental phenotype have not yet been adopted into widespread practice, in part due to continued debate about terminology which varies between clinical and research studies [17]. Research studies have employed quantitative descriptions of placental morphology by stereology and morphometry to describe differences in placental structure in clinical conditions related to stillbirth such as fetal growth restriction (FGR) [18] and reduced fetal movements [19]. We aimed to use these quantitative methods to objectively evaluate placental appearances of different causes of stillbirth. Firstly, we hypothesised that specific causes of stillbirth would be associated with a morphometric phenotype. Secondly, we

hypothesised that morphological abnormalities associated with stillbirth would differ from live births with the same condition. To be of diagnostic value, any observed changes should not represent artefacts of storage or cessation of fetal blood flow after death. Since we have already described the effects of placental storage on placental structure [20], here we address a third hypothesis that there is an acute effect of post-stillbirth fetoplacental haemostasis on placental morphology.

Methods
Placental tissue samples

To address the first hypothesis we obtained placental tissue from cases of stillbirth, defined as the birth of an infant with no signs of life after 24 weeks gestation. Parents gave permission for the use of samples for research at the time of consent for post-mortem examination. A favourable ethical opinion was given by the Greater Manchester South Research Ethics Committee (09/H1012/11) and approval given from the Research and Innovation Division of Central Manchester University Hospitals NHS Foundation Trust to conduct the study. Cases of stillbirth were classified using the ReCoDe system [15] by a multidisciplinary meeting following a full panel of investigations including: post-mortem, histopathological examination of the placenta, chromosomal analysis and maternal biochemical, haematological, immunological and serological tests. We obtained samples from the following classifications of stillbirth: cord accident ($n = 8$), diabetes ($n = 5$), FGR ($n = 10$), hypertension ($n = 8$), infection ($n = 8$) and from stillbirths of an unknown cause ($n = 10$). For comparison, matched placental samples were used from appropriately-grown live born infants and preterm births (26–36 weeks) (demographics shown in Table 1). Samples from live births were collected following written informed consent as part of the Maternal and Fetal Research Centre (MFHRC) Biobank (08/H1010/55). To address the second hypothesis, placental samples were taken from a further cohort of stillbirths attributed to FGR ($n = 13$) and from live births with FGR ($n = 13$) with the same ethical approvals as described above. FGR was defined as a customised birthweight <5th centile (demographics shown in Table 2). To address the final hypothesis, placental tissue was obtained from appropriately grown ($n = 7$) and FGR ($n = 5$) live births following written informed consent as part of the MFHRC biobank previously described. For all cases, maternal and infant demographic information was recorded from medical case notes and post-mortem reports (for stillbirths). An estimate of the duration of in utero retention was made according to

Table 1 Demographic characteristics of samples from live births and stillbirths from known and unknown causes. Birthweight was significantly lower in stillbirths from FGR and hypertension than live births (P < 0.01); all other variables did not significantly differ between groups. Data are presented as median with range in parentheses except for estimated time of retention in utero where number of cases are presented

		Live births	Preterm birth	Cord	Diabetes	Hypertension	Infection	FGR	Unknown
Number of Samples		10	7	8	5	8	9	10	10
Maternal Age (years)		32 (28–37)	27 (18–41)	28 (21–36)	34 (31–40)	33 (27–37)	30 (25–32)	30 (22–32)	28 (21–31)
Gravidity		1 (1–5)	3 (1–6)	1 (1–1)	4 (2–7)	1 (1–2)	1 (1–3)	1 (1–4)	1 (1–2)
Parity		0 (0–4)	0 (0–4)	0 (0–0)	1 (1–2)	0 (0–0)	0 (0–2)	0 (0–2)	0 (0–0)
Gestation at delivery (weeks)		37 (37–38)	31 (26–36)	30 (27–38)	28 (28–40)	31 (26–35)	38 (24–41)	34 (26–38)	31 (27–39)
Birthweight (g)		3090 (2805–3430)	1821 (786–2760)	1300 (702–2750)	3120 (1473–3590)	1110 (399–1730)	2680 (494–2985)	1065 (564–2230)	2170 (892–3150)
Estimated in utero retention time	0 h - <24 h	N/A	N/A	0	1	4	4	2	2
	≥24 h - <48 h			1	0	2	2	4	3
	≥48 h - <96 h			2	1	0	2	2	1
	≥96 h - <1 week			3	1	1	0	0	2
	≥1 week			2	2	1	1	2	2

Table 2 Demographic details of samples used for experimental comparisons. The left hand columns relate to samples obtained from cases of FGR that were live or stillborn; all these samples had a birthweight <5th centile. The right hand columns relate to samples used for perfusion experiments. Data are presented as median with range in parentheses

	FGR live birth	FGR still birth	Appropriate for gestational age - placental perfusion	FGR - placental perfusion
Number of Samples	13	13	7	5
Maternal Age (years)	32 (20–40)	23 (19–42)	33 (27–36	31 (23–39))
Gravidity	2 (1–9)	2 (1–3)	2 (2–4)	1 (1–5)
Parity	1 (0–8)	0 (0–2)	2 (1–2)	1 (0–5)
Gestation at delivery (weeks)	37 (30–41)	35 (28–38)	39 (39–39)	38 (35–39)
Birthweight (g)	1389 (536–3060)	1010 (385–2000)	3740 (2910–3940)	2262 (1900–2440)
Mode of delivery (% Caesarean)	69	0	71	89
Infant gender (% Female)	54	62	57	78

Genests' descriptions of findings at post-mortem and from histopathological examination of the placenta [21–23].

Tissue from live births was obtained within 30 min of delivery. For assessment of placental morphology biopsies of villous tissue were dissected from the centre, middle and edge of the placenta. Tissue was fixed in 4 % neutral buffered formalin for 24 h before being wax embedded. For stillbirth samples three blocks of placental tissue not obtained from specific lesions were obtained for each placenta.

Placental perfusion
Unless otherwise stated, all reagents were supplied by Sigma-Aldrich Chemical Company (Poole, UK). To examine the acute impact of continued maternal blood flow in the absence of fetal blood flow single-sided (maternal) ex vivo human placental lobule perfusion was adapted from the dual-sided perfusion model [24]. Perfusion was performed on placentas from normal pregnancy ($n = 7$) and placentas from pregnancies complicated by FGR ($n = 5$). An intact peripheral lobule was selected, devoid of post-partum tears, deep decidual damage and marginal membrane separations. Prior to perfusion two villous biopsies were sampled from neighbouring lobules taken 5 cm apart, and fixed immediately in 4 % neutral buffered formalin forming "pre-perfusion samples". The fetal artery and vein on the chorionic surface, serving the villous trees within the lobule designated for perfusion, were each ligated using sutures (Mersilk 3/0, Ethicon, supplied by NuCare, UK) to confine a static fetal blood pool within the fetal vasculature of the associated cotyledons. The maternal surface was cannulated using five 10 cm lengths of polythene tubing (Smiths Medical, UK) arising from a perfusion manifold (Harvard Apparatus, UK). The distal ends of the cannulae were cut into apices and inserted through the decidual surface of the lobule with an even spatial distribution. The perfusate was modified Earle's bicarbonate buffer (EBB 117 mM NaCl, 10.7 mM KCl, 5.6 mM D-glucose, 3.6 mM CaCl, 1.8 mM NaH_2PO_4, 13.6 mM $NaHCO_3$, 0.04 mM L-arginine, 0.8 mM $MgSO_4$, 3.5 % (w/v) dextran, 0.1 % (w/v) bovine serum albumin, 5000 IU/L Heparin sodium) equilibrated with 95 % O_2 / 5 % CO_2 to pH 7.4 and warmed to 37 °C, delivered by a roller pump (Watson Marlow, UK) at 14 ml/min. Lobule preparations were only considered acceptable for experimentation when maternal-side perfusion was established within 30 min of delivery. Open-circuit perfusion was for 6 h, and then the physiological buffer was switched to a 4 % neutral buffered formalin at $T = 6$ h for a 10 min maternal-side perfusion fixation period. Following this, the lobule was excised and two further full thickness (vertical and horizontal) biopsies slices were taken as the "post-perfusion samples". These wide tissue sections where then immersion fixed in 4 % neutral buffered formalin for 24 h before being wax embedded. Placental structure in these biopsies was examined as described above.

Immunohistochemistry
Placental cell turnover, structure and vascularity were assessed using antibodies specific for Ki67 (Dako, Ely, Cambridgeshire, UK; 0.16 µg/ml), cytokeratin 7 (Dako; 0.9 µg/ml) and CD31 (Dako; 0.16 µg/ml). The number of leukocytes was assessed by an antibody specific for CD45 (Dako; 0.4 µg/ml). Negative controls were performed using non-immune mouse IgG (Dako) at matching concentrations to the primary antibody. Immunohistochemistry was performed as previously described with antigen retrieval performed by microwaving the sections for 10 min in 0.01 M sodium citrate buffer [19, 20].

Quantification of syncytial nuclear aggregates (SNAs, also known as syncytial knots) was conducted on sections stained with haematoxylin and eosin as previously described [19, 20]. Dewaxed and rehydrated sections were stained with Harris's haematoxylin for 10 min before differentiation in acid-alcohol. Slides were stained with eosin for 2 min, rinsed in cold tap water, and dehydrated and mounted as described above.

For all analyses images were captured using an Olympus BX41 light microscope (Southend-on-Sea, UK) and QIcam Fast 1394 (QImaging, BC, Canada) and Image Pro Plus 6.0 and 7.0 (Media Cybernetics Inc., MD, USA). During image acquisition and analysis the presumed cause of stillbirth was concealed

from the observer. Between images the microscope was taken out of focus to prevent selection bias, if the randomly selected image was not mostly of terminal villi another area was identified. Five random images of terminal villi were taken of each section, giving a total of 15 images per placenta for each component evaluated.

Assessment of placental structure

The number of SNAs were counted and total villous area measured using image analysis software, expressed

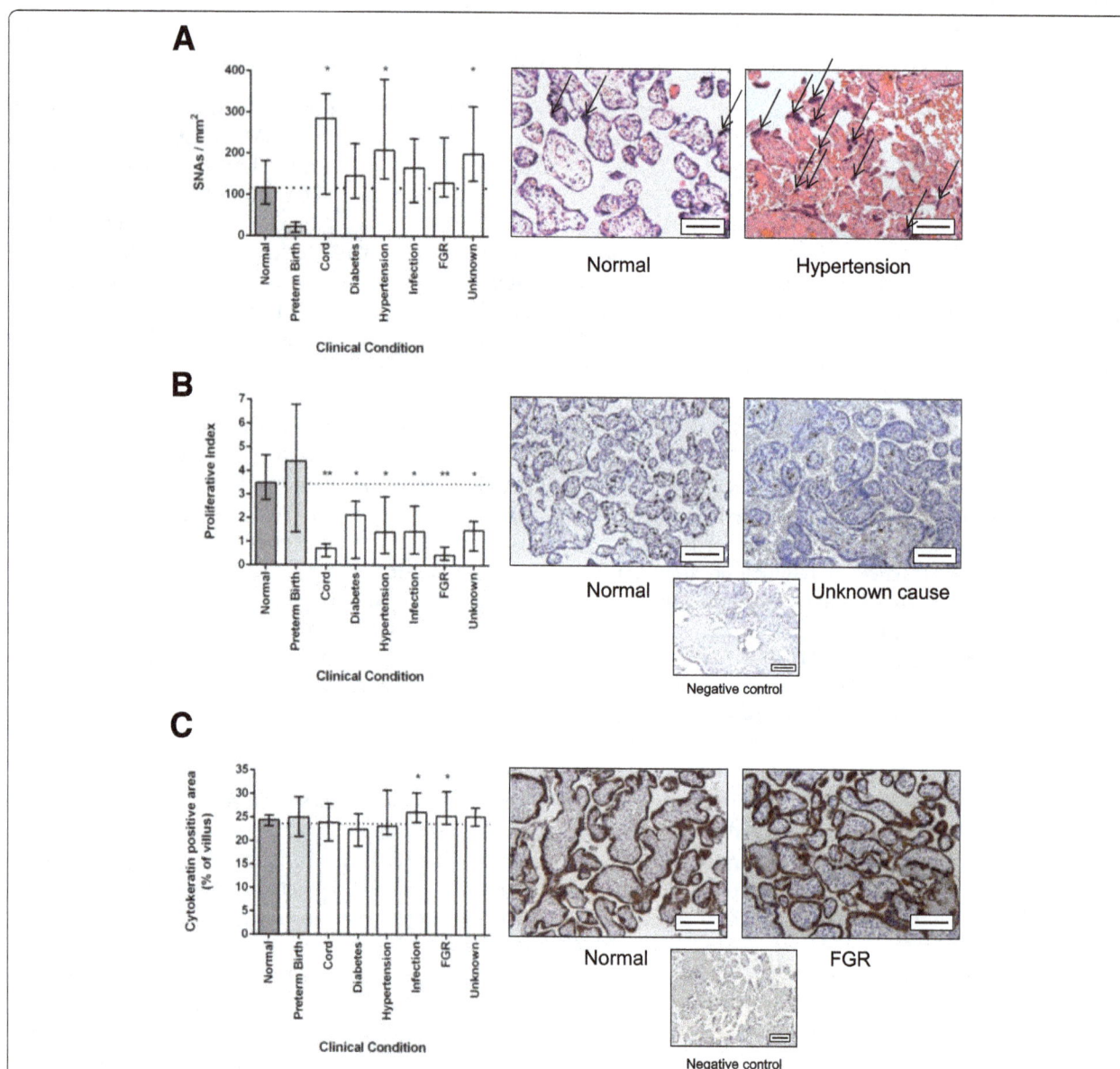

Fig. 1 a Assessment of syncytial nuclear aggregates (SNAs) in different causes of stillbirth compared to healthy live births. SNAs are shown by open arrows in representative images from normal pregnancy and stillbirth associated with hypertension. **b** Assessment of proliferation in different causes of stillbirth compared to healthy live births. **c** Assessment of trophoblast area in different causes of stillbirth compared to healthy live births. Negative control images shown in small panel beneath representative images of normal pregnancy and FGR. Scale bar = 50 μm in all images. Graphs show median and range, * $p < 0.05$, ** $p < 0.01$, *** $p < 0.001$. Dotted line indicates median level of healthy control

as the number of SNAs per mm^2 of villous tissue as previously described [25]. Proliferative index was the number of Ki67 positive nuclei as a proportion of total nuclei as previously described [19, 20]. Vascularity was expressed as the number of capillaries per terminal villus and the percentage of avascular villi (defined as a villus with no evidence of CD-31 immunostaining or morphological evidence of vessels) [19, 20]. Trophoblast area was expressed as the proportion of villous area positive for CK-7 immunostaining. The number of leukocytes was assessed by the number of CD45 positive cells per 1,000 nuclei.

Statistical analysis

For comparison of different causes of stillbirth data from each variable was compared to the median level in healthy controls using Wilcoxon signed rank test. Cases of FGR that were live-born were compared to those who were stillborn using Mann-Whitney U test. Data from pre- and post-perfusion samples were compared using Wilcoxon matched-pairs test. Demographic variables were compared using Kruskal-Wallis test with Dunn's post-hoc test for multiple comparisons and Mann-Whitney U test for single comparisons. For all statistical tests a p-value of 0.05 was considered to be statistically

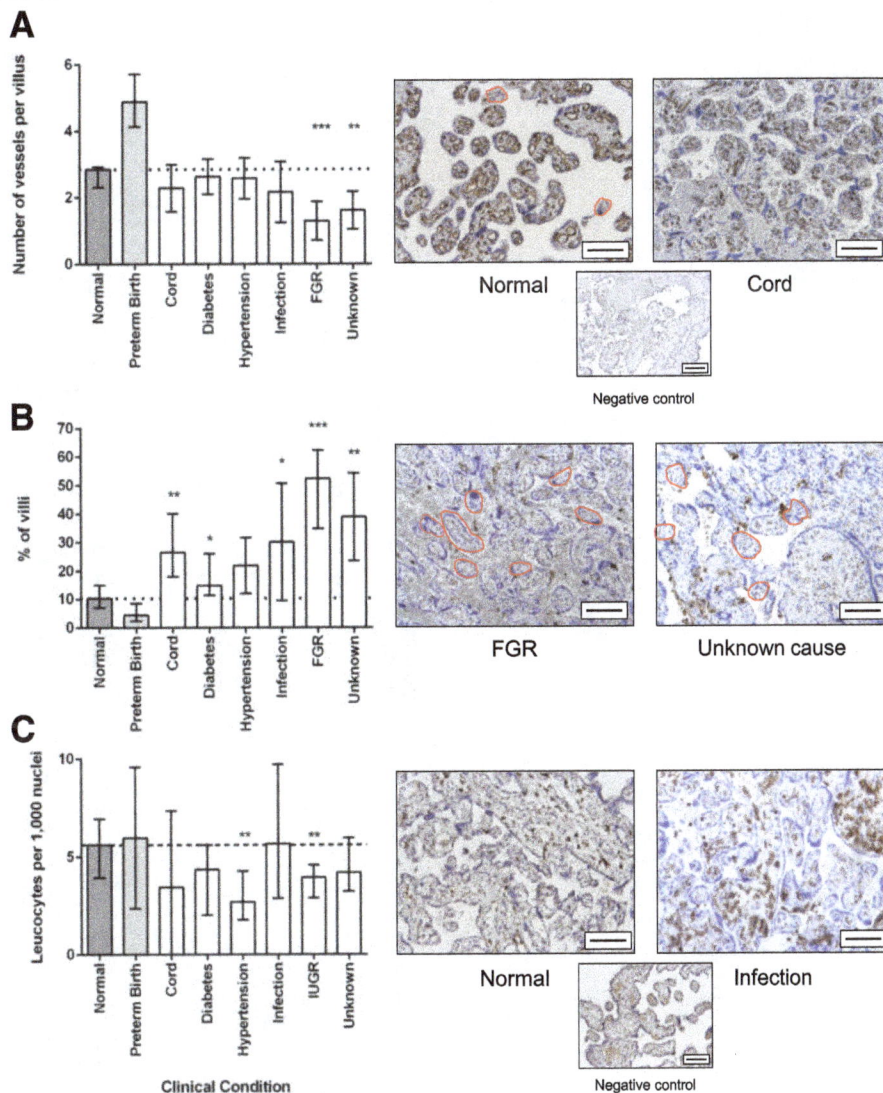

Fig. 2 a Assessment of villous vascularity in different causes of stillbirth compared to healthy live births. **b** Proportion of avascular villi in different causes of stillbirth compared to healthy live births. Avascular villi are highlighted in red. **c** Assessment of the number of leukocytes in different causes of stillbirth compared to healthy live births. Negative control images shown in small panel beneath representative images of normal pregnancy and FGR. Scale bar = 50 μm in all images. Graphs show median and range, * $p < 0.05$, ** $p < 0.01$, *** $p < 0.001$. Dotted line indicates median level of healthy control

Table 3 Pattern of placental morphology in placental samples from stillbirths of unknown cause ($n = 10$) demonstrating two samples with a very similar pattern to samples from FGR (highlighted in grey)

Sample	SNAs	Proliferation	Vascularity	Avascular villi	Trophoblast	Leukocytes	Profile
Unknown 1	Low	High	Unchanged	High	Low	Low	Not similar
Unknown 2	High	Unchanged	Low	High	Unchanged	Unchanged	Not similar
Unknown 3	High	Low	Low	High	High	Unchanged	Similar to FGR
Unknown 4	High	Unchanged	High	Unchanged	Unchanged	Unchanged	Not similar
Unknown 5	High	Low	Low	High	High	Unchanged	Similar to FGR
Unknown 6	High	Unchanged	Low	High	Unchanged	Unchanged	Not similar
Unknown 7	Unchanged	Unchanged	Low	High	Unchanged	Unchanged	Not similar
Unknown 8	Unchanged	High	Low	High	Increased	Low	Not similar
Unknown 9	High	Unchanged	Low	High	Increased	High	Not similar
Unknown 10	Unchanged	Unchanged	Low	High	Increased	Unchanged	Not similar

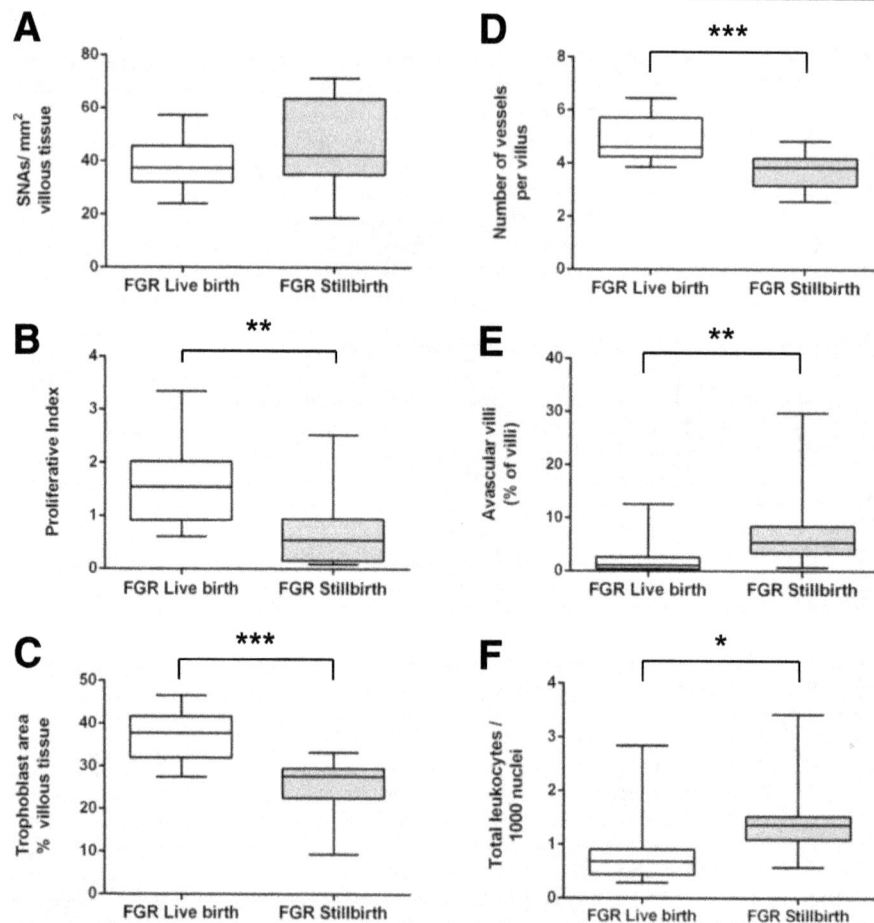

Fig. 3 Assessment of placental morphometry in live births associated with FGR compared to stillbirths associated with FGR. Graphs present data for **a**) Syncytial nuclear aggregates (SNAs) **b**) Proliferation, **c**) Trophoblast area, **d**) Villous vascularity, **e**) Proportion of avascular villi and **f**) Number of Leukocytes. Graphs show median and range, * $p < 0.05$, ** $p < 0.01$, *** $p < 0.001$

significant. All statistical analyses were carried out using GraphPad PRISM (Version 6, La Jolla, CA).

Results

Placental morphology in different causes of stillbirth

In comparison to normal pregnancy, SNAs were increased in stillbirths attributed to cord accident, hypertension, FGR and in stillbirths with an unknown aetiology (Fig. 1a). This was in contrast to fewer SNAs

seen in preterm live births. Proliferation was reduced in all cases of stillbirth, but was particularly reduced in those cases attributed to cord accident or FGR (Fig. 1b). The median trophoblast area (measured as cytokeratin-7 positive area) was increased in stillbirths attributed to infection and FGR (Fig. 1c). The median number of blood vessels identified by CD31 immunostaining was significantly reduced in stillbirths attributed to FGR and those with an unknown cause (Fig. 2a). The number of

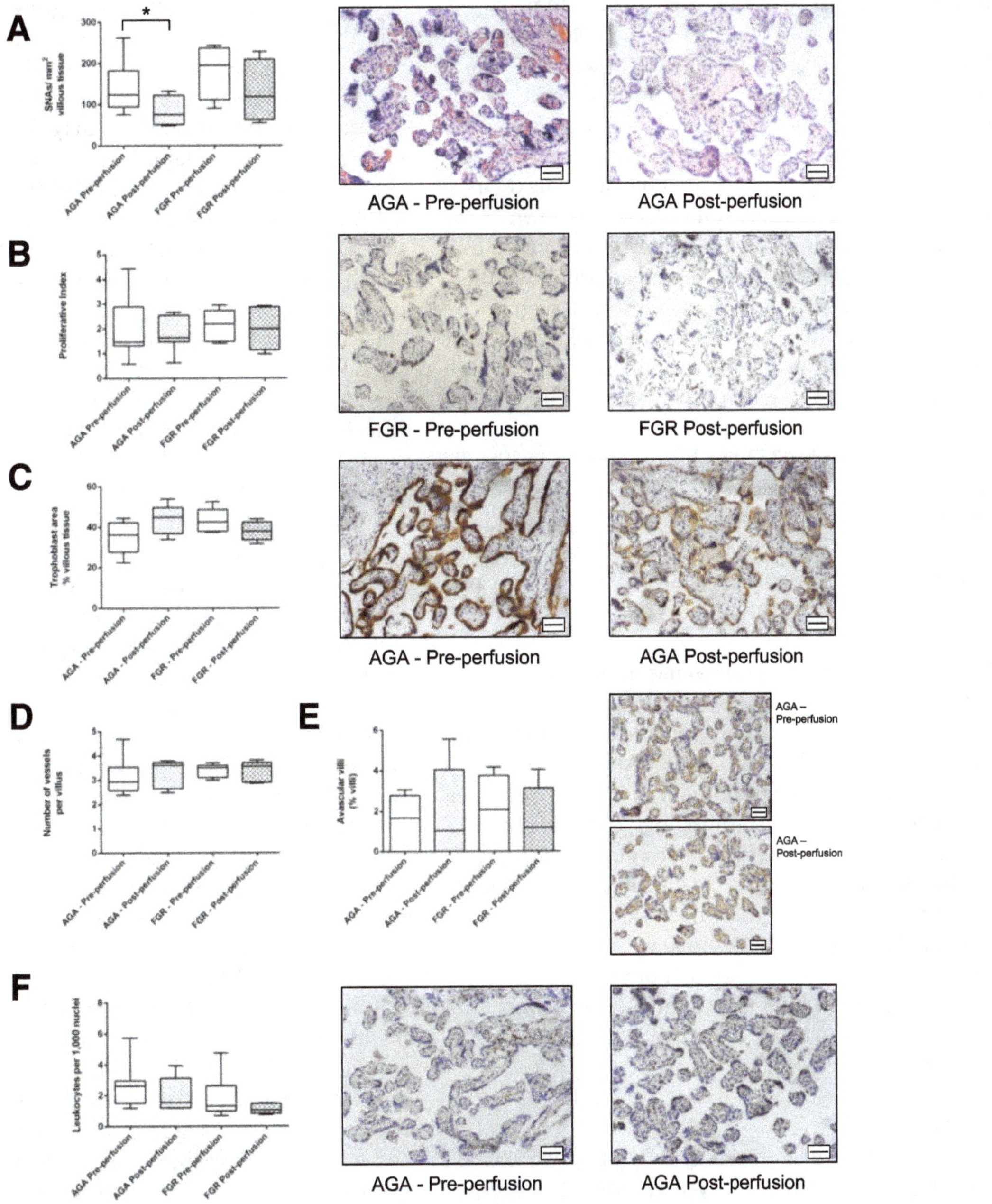

Fig. 4 Assessment of placental morphometry before and after maternal-side only placental perfusion in normal and FGR placentas. Graphs present data for a reduction in **a**) syncytial nuclear aggregates (SNAs), but no change in **b**) Proliferation, **c**) Trophoblast area, **d**) Villous vascularity, **e**) Proportion of avascular villi and **f**) Number of Leukocytes. Graphs show median and range, * $p < 0.05$. Representative images of each feature are shown. Scale bar = 50 μm in all images

avascular villi was significantly increased in these conditions, although an increase in avascular villi was also seen in stillbirths attributed to cord compression and hypertension (Fig. 2b). These changes were in contrast to an increase in vascularity and reduction in avascular villi observed in preterm live births. The median number of leukocytes was reduced in stillbirths attributed to maternal hypertension and FGR compared to healthy controls (Fig. 2c). It is important to note that in some variables, notably the number of leukocytes in cases of infection, there was a wide range in measurements obtained. The cause of stillbirth with the most placental differences from healthy pregnancies was FGR, which has increased numbers of SNAs, reduced proliferation, increased trophoblast area, fewer blood vessels per villus, more avascular villi and decreased numbers of leukocytes. Interestingly, the condition with next most frequent abnormalities was stillbirths of unknown cause. When the individual profiles of stillbirths from unknown cause are examined, two had a similar profile to those with FGR and others had similar features such as increased density of SNAs and reduced vascularity (Table 3). None of the features examined altered according to the estimated duration of in utero retention (Additional file 1: Figure S1).

When compared to FGR live births, FGR stillbirths did not have increased numbers of SNAs but had reduced proliferation and trophoblast area, fewer blood vessels per villus and a greater proportion of avascular villi. Leukocytes were increased in FGR stillbirths compared to FGR live births (Fig. 3).

Effect of short-term fetoplacental haemostasis on placental morphology

To assess changes that may happen in utero after cessation of fetal blood flow, placental tissue was examined before and after maternal-side only placental perfusion in placental tissue from healthy and FGR pregnancies. Perfusion in this manner for 6 h was not associated with any changes in proliferation, trophoblast area, villous vascularity or the proportion of avascular villi (Fig. 4). Maternal-side only perfusion was associated with a reduction in the number of SNAs in normal tissue (Fig. 4a). There was a consistent trend towards lower numbers of leukocytes in perfused tissue from both appropriately-grown and FGR pregnancies ($p = 0.08$).

Discussion

This pilot study demonstrates that objective assessment of placental morphology may provide additional information on placental villous structure in cases of stillbirth and in some cases, such as in FGR, can differentiate between specific causes of stillbirth and healthy live-born infants. In other cases, such as

stillbirths attributed to maternal diabetes, there were no morphological differences from live-born infants, which is consistent with few histopathological abnormalities in stillbirths related to diabetes [26]. When the morphometric profile was applied to ten stillbirths of unknown cause, two had a very similar placental profile to FGR, which suggests that some stillbirths that currently have no identified cause (despite intensive investigation) may actually result from FGR in a fetus that was not small, i.e. infants who have a birthweight >10th centile but whose growth rate was slowing down. These preliminary findings suggest that addition of objective assessment of placental morphology to histological examination with the use of a modern classification system may further decrease the proportion of unexplained stillbirths. However, further research is needed to understand the role that abnormalities of placental structure and function have in the aetiology of stillbirth both in the presence of a small fetus and when the birthweight is within an accepted normal range [27].

The findings in FGR stillbirths are consistent with other stereological and morphometric assessment of FGR placentas including: increased SNAs [25], reduced villous vascularity [28], reduced proliferation [29] and number of cytotrophoblasts [28]. The pattern seen in FGR stillbirths was also consistent with the placental morphology in women with reduced fetal movements [19], who are at increased risk of stillbirth [30]. However, some results differ from other studies, one of which describes a positive relationship between trophoblast area and birthweight [31]. The reduced trophoblast area in stillbirth FGR compared to healthy live births contrasts with an increased area relative to live born FGR infants. This observation may result from thicker syncytiotrophoblast covering hypoplastic villi; application of stereological techniques is required to explore this observation in greater depth.

The findings of this study are consistent with the Stillbirth Collaborative Research Network (SCRN) case-control study which found increased presence of placental lesions in stillbirths, including: diffuse terminal villous immaturity, inflammation, vascular degeneration in the chorionic plate, intra-placental thrombi, avascular villi and parenchymal infarction [32]. The SCRN study found differences in lesions depending on gestation. Avascular villi and fetal vascular thrombi were more frequently seen in term stillbirths than those occurring at earlier gestations. Whereas, chorioamnionitis was seen less frequently in stillbirths than live births at 24 weeks' gestation, but more frequently in term stillbirths compared to matched live births [32]. The SCRN study provides evidence that different causes of stillbirth have a different placental phenotype and addition evidence that gestation may affect the cause of stillbirth. Our study demonstrated that some features (SNAs and villous vascularity) were altered in preterm compared to term live births. Critically, these changes were in the opposite direction to that seen in stillbirth, so the morphology changes seen in cases of stillbirth cannot be attributed to their preterm gestation.

The finding that the placental phenotype of FGR stillbirths had reduced villous vascularity, increased avascular villi and increased leukocyte infiltration compared to live-born FGR may imply that FGR stillbirths result from a more severe placental phenotype. However, these differences must be interpreted cautiously, as differences between live and stillbirth may also result from artefacts from cessation of fetoplacental blood flow after fetal death, differences in mode of delivery or from storage prior to fixation. Our previous experimental data suggest that storage prior to fixation for ≤48 h does not alter any of the indices measured here [20]. Studying the effects of in utero retention is more challenging. We attempted to model this by maternal-side only placental perfusion for 6 h, finding that this did not reproduce any of the differences between FGR stillbirths and live births. However, the duration of perfusion was limited by the experimental technique and it cannot reproduce the in utero environment (e.g. presence of the maternal immune system). Placental changes may be altered by the duration of in utero retention, as evident by changes in histopathological appearances of the placenta in fetal maceration [33]. Thus, further study is needed to determine the effects of potential confounders, particularly in utero retention, on the quantitative measures used in this study. This could be explored by evaluating the morphology of stillbirths with known in utero retention time (e.g. intrapartum events, feticide for structural anomaly). The possibility that morphological changes might arise from differences in mode of delivery should also be considered, as Caesarean section is rarely used in cases of stillbirth, but is frequently employed in live born FGR infants; this can be resolved by detailed study of placental morphology after vaginal delivery and Caesarean section.

The study reported here is strengthened by a detailed assessment of multiple aspects of placental morphology with blinding of assessor to study group or pregnancy outcome. We also have compared cases of stillbirth to appropriately-grown healthy controls and preterm births primarily recruited for research rather than clinical cases with indication(s) for perinatal histology. The use of objective techniques that also have been used to evaluate related conditions allows comparison between different clinical situations. However, this study does have limitations: although 50 samples from well-characterised stillbirths have been analysed, this only amounts to ≤10 samples per group and these were obtained from a single

Paediatric and Perinatal Pathology department. Unfortunately, at the time of collection the collection protocols between the clinical histopathological service and research laboratories were slightly different resulting in different numbers of samples obtained per placenta potentially introducing a bias between samples from stillbirths and live births. However, we believe the chance of selection bias to be low as placental tissue was randomly sampled and blocks of specific lesions were not used in either protocol. Samples were divided into groups based upon the classification of stillbirth determined by multidisciplinary review (involving obstetricians, midwives, sonographers and pathologists) and, although this was made as robust as possible, it is possible that the cause of death was different from that attributed in the perinatal review process.

Conclusion

Due to the critical role played by the placenta in determining the outcome of pregnancy and the role of placenta failure in the aetiology of stillbirth [34], placental histology is a frequently employed investigation that can provide important information for clinicians and parents regarding the reasons for their child's death [35]. When combined with a modern classification system, histological examination of the placenta reduces the proportion of unexplained stillbirths [36, 37]. Our preliminary findings suggest that addition of objective measurement of placental structure may add to understanding of the cause of stillbirth. These quantitative observations need to be related to established qualitative descriptions; in some cases such as avascular villi and fetal thrombotic vasculopathy this may be straightforward, in others, such as placental maturation disorders, this may be more complex. Prior to clinical application further studies are needed to develop normal ranges for these morphological characteristics at different gestational ages and to determine the effects of in utero retention on these indices. Then blinded studies of randomly sampled cases of stillbirth from multiple populations are needed to ensure the findings presented here are sufficiently sensitive and specific for diagnostic use.

Additional file

Additional file 1: Figure S1. Assessment of placental morphometry in stillbirths (irrespective of cause) grouped by estimated time of in utero retention according to Genest's criteria [21–23]. Graphs present data for A) Syncytial nuclear aggregates (SNAs) B) Proliferation, C) Trophoblast area, D) Villous vascularity, E) Proportion of avascular villi and F) Number of Leukocytes per 1,000 nuclei. Graphs present the median and interquartile range for each group. There is no statistically significant difference of the frequency of the morphological feature and the groups divided by in utero retention.

Abbreviations

EBB: Earles' Bicarbonate Buffer; FGR: Fetal growth restriction; MFHRC: Maternal and Fetal Health Research Centre; ReCoDe: Relevant Condition at Death (Classification System); SCRN: Stillbirth Collaborative Research Network; SNA: Syncytial nuclear aggregate.

Competing interests

The authors confirm that they have no conflicts of interest to report in relation to this manuscript.

Authors' contributions

AEPH, GB, CPS, RLJ and PB conceived the study and designed the experiments. IP, SA, AG, SB, NB and AEPH conducted the experiments and completed the analysis. All authors contributed to the development and writing of the manuscript.

Acknowledgements

This work was funded by Tommy's - The Baby Charity, Holly Martin Stillbirth Research Fund and Tunbridge Wells Sands. The Maternal and Fetal Health Research Centre is supported by funding from Tommy's the Baby Charity, an Action Research Endowment Fund, the Manchester Biomedical Research Centre and the Greater Manchester Comprehensive Local Research Network. The funders did not have any role in the data acquisition, analysis, writing of the manuscript or decision to publish the findings. The authors wish to acknowledge all those who donated placental tissue, particularly bereaved parents who wished to contribute to research efforts to understand stillbirth. The authors wish to thank Mr James Horn for assistance with immunoperoxidase staining.

Author details

[1]Institute of Human Development, Faculty of Medical and Human Sciences, University of Manchester, Oxford Rd, Manchester M13 9PL, UK. [2]Maternal and Fetal Health Research Centre, 5th floor (Research), St Mary's Hospital, Oxford Road, Manchester M13 9WL, UK. [3]Department of Histopathology, Royal Manchester Children's Hospital, Central Manchester University Hospitals NHS Foundation Trust, Manchester Academic Health Science Centre, Manchester M13 9WL, UK.

References

1. Turner K, Sebire NJ, Evans M, on behalf of MBRRACE-UK. Pathological and Histological Investigations. In: Draper ES, Kurinczuk JJ, Kenyon S, on behalf of MBRRACE-UK, editors. MBRRACE-UK Perinatal Confidential Enquiry: Term, singleton, normally formed antepartum stillbirth. Leicester: Department of Health Sciences, University of Leicester; 2015. p. 61–4.
2. American College of Obstetricians and Gynecologists. ACOG Practice Bulletin No. 102: management of stillbirth. Obstet Gynecol. 2009;113(3): 748–61.
3. Royal College of Obstetricians and Gynaecologists. Green-Top Guideline 55 - Late Intrauterine Fetal Death and Stillbirth. London: Royal College of Obstetricians and Gynaecologists; 2010.
4. Flenady V, King J, Charles A, Gardener G, Ellwood D, Day K, McCowan L, Kent A, Tudehope D, Richardson R et al. PSANZ Clinical Practice Guideline for Perinatal Mortality. Version 2.2. 2009. http://www.psanzpnmsig.org
5. Ptacek I, Sebire NJ, Man JA, Brownbill P, Heazell AE. Systematic review of placental pathology reported in association with stillbirth. Placenta. 2014; 35(8):552–62.
6. Turowski G, Berge LN, Helgadottir LB, Jacobsen EM, Roald B. A new, clinically oriented, unifying and simple placental classification system. Placenta. 2012;33(12):1026–35.
7. Pathak S, Lees CC, Hackett G, Jessop F, Sebire NJ. Frequency and clinical significance of placental histological lesions in an unselected population at or near term. Virchows Arch. 2011;459(6):565–72.
8. Iwasenko JM, Howard J, Arbuckle S, Graf N, Hall B, Craig ME, et al. Human cytomegalovirus infection is detected frequently in stillbirths and is associated with fetal thrombotic vasculopathy. J Infect Dis. 2011;203(11): 1526–33.
9. Ryan WD, Trivedi N, Benirschke K, Lacoursiere DY, Parast MM. Placental histologic criteria for diagnosis of cord accident: sensitivity and specificity. Pediatr Dev Pathol. 2012;15(4):275–80.
10. Ernst LM, Minturn L, Huang MH, Curry E, Su EJ. Gross patterns of umbilical cord coiling: correlations with placental histology and stillbirth. Placenta. 2013;34(7):583–8.
11. Veerbeek JH, Nikkels PG, Torrance HL, Gravesteijn J, Post Uiterweer ED, Derks JB, et al. Placental pathology in early intrauterine growth restriction associated with maternal hypertension. Placenta. 2014;35(9): 696–701.
12. Viall CA, Chamley LW. Histopathology in the placentae of women with antiphospholipid antibodies: A systematic review of the literature. Autoimmun Rev. 2015;14(5):446–71.
13. Korteweg FJ, Gordijn SJ, Timmer A, Erwich JJ, Bergman KA, Bouman K, et al. The Tulip classification of perinatal mortality: introduction and multidisciplinary inter-rater agreement. BJOG. 2006;113(4):393–401.
14. Flenady V, Froen JF, Pinar H, Torabi R, Saastad E, Guyon G, et al. An evaluation of classification systems for stillbirth. BMC Pregnancy Childbirth. 2009;9:24.
15. Gardosi J, Kady SM, McGeown P, Francis A, Tonks A. Classification of stillbirth by relevant condition at death (ReCoDe): population based cohort study. Br Med J. 2005;331(7525):1113–7.
16. Vergani P, Cozzolino S, Pozzi E, Cuttin MS, Greco M, Ornaghi S, et al. Identifying the causes of stillbirth: a comparison of four classification systems. Am J Obstet Gynecol. 2008;199(3):319 e311–314.
17. Barbaux S, Erwich JJ, Favaron PO, Gil S, Gallot D, Golos TG, et al. IFPA meeting 2014 workshop report: Animal models to study pregnancy pathologies; new approaches to study human placental exposure to xenobiotics; biomarkers of pregnancy pathologies; placental genetics and epigenetics; the placenta and stillbirth and fetal growth restriction. Placenta. 2015;36 Suppl 1:S5–10.
18. Mayhew TM, Manwani R, Ohadike C, Wijesekara J, Baker PN. The placenta in pre-eclampsia and intrauterine growth restriction: studies on exchange surface areas, diffusion distances and villous membrane diffusive conductances. Placenta. 2007;28(2-3):233–8.
19. Warrander LK, Batra G, Bernatavicius G, Greenwood SL, Dutton P, Jones RL, et al. Maternal perception of reduced fetal movements is associated with altered placental structure and function. PLoS One. 2012;7(4):e34851.
20. Garrod A, Batra G, Ptacek I, Heazell AE. Duration and method of tissue storage alters placental morphology - implications for clinical and research practice. Placenta. 2013;34(11):1116–9.
21. Genest DR. Estimating the time of death in stillborn fetuses: II. Histologic evaluation of the placenta; a study of 71 stillborns. Obstet Gynecol. 1992; 80(4):585–92.
22. Genest DR, Singer DB. Estimating the time of death in stillborn fetuses: III. External fetal examination; a study of 86 stillborns. Obstet Gynecol. 1992; 80(4):593–600.
23. Genest DR, Williams MA, Greene MF. Estimating the time of death in stillborn fetuses: I. Histologic evaluation of fetal organs; an autopsy study of 150 stillborns. Obstet Gynecol. 1992;80(4):575–84.
24. Brownbill P, McKeeman GC, Brockelsby JC, Crocker IP, Sibley CP. Vasoactive and permeability effects of vascular endothelial growth factor-165 in the term in vitro dually perfused human placental lobule. Endocrinology. 2007; 148(10):4734–44.
25. Heazell AE, Moll SJ, Jones CJ, Baker PN, Crocker IP. Formation of syncytial knots is increased by hyperoxia, hypoxia and reactive oxygen species. Placenta. 2007;28(Supplement 1):S33–40.
26. Edwards A, Springett A, Padfield J, Dorling J, Bugg G, Mansell P. Differences in post-mortem findings after stillbirth in women with and without diabetes. Diabet Med. 2013;30(10):1219–24.
27. Heazell AE, Whitworth MK, Whitcombe J, Glover SW, Bevan C, Brewin J, et al. Research priorities for stillbirth: process overview and results from UK Stillbirth Priority Setting Partnership. Ultrasound Obstet Gynecol. 2015;46(6): 641–7.
28. Chen C-P, Bajoria R, Aplin JD. Decreased vascularization and cell proliferation in placentas of intrauterine growth-restricted fetuses with abnormal umbilical artery flow velocity waveforms. Am J Obstet Gynecol. 2002;187(3):764–9.
29. Heazell AE, Sharp AN, Baker PN, Crocker IP. Intra-uterine growth restriction is associated with increased apoptosis and altered expression of proteins in the p53 pathway in villous trophoblast. Apoptosis. 2011;16:135–44.

30. Heazell AE, Froen JF. Methods of fetal movement counting and the detection of fetal compromise. J Obstet Gynaecol. 2008;28(2):147–54.

31. Daayana S, Baker P, Crocker I. An image analysis technique for the investigation of variations in placental morphology in pregnancies complicated by preeclampsia with and without intrauterine growth restriction. J Soc Gynecol Investig. 2004;11(8):545–52.

32. Pinar H, Goldenberg RL, Koch MA, Heim-Hall J, Hawkins HK, Shehata B, et al. Placental findings in singleton stillbirths. Obstet Gynecol. 2014;123(2 Pt 1): 325–36.

33. Stanek J, Biesiada J. Relation of placental diagnosis in stillbirth to fetal maceration and gestational age at delivery. J Perinat Med. 2014; 42(4):457–71.

34. Heazell AE, Worton SA, Higgins LE, Ingram E, Johnstone ED, Jones RL, et al. IFPA Gabor Than Award Lecture: Recognition of placental failure is key to saving babies' lives. Placenta. 2015;36 Suppl 1:S20–8.

35. Korteweg FJ, Erwich JJ, Holm JP, Ravise JM, van der Meer J, Veeger NJ, et al. Diverse placental pathologies as the main causes of fetal death. Obstet Gynecol. 2009;114(4):809–17.

36. Heazell AE, Martindale EA. Can post-mortem examination of the placenta help determine the cause of stillbirth? J Obstet Gynaecol. 2009;29(3):225–8.

37. Korteweg FJ, Erwich JJ, Timmer A, van der Meer J, Ravise JM, Veeger NJ, et al. Evaluation of 1025 fetal deaths: proposed diagnostic workup. Am J Obstet Gynecol. 2012;206(1):53 e51–12.

13

SOD2 immunoexpression predicts lymph node metastasis in penile cancer

Lara Termini[1*], José H Fregnani[2], Enrique Boccardo[3], Walter H da Costa[4], Adhemar Longatto-Filho[5,6,7], Maria A Andreoli[1], Maria C Costa[1], Ademar Lopes[4], Isabela W da Cunha[8], Fernando A Soares[8], Luisa L Villa[1,9] and Gustavo C Guimarães[4]

Abstract

Background: Superoxide dismutase-2 (SOD2) is considered one of the most important antioxidant enzymes that regulate cellular redox state in normal and tumorigenic cells. Overexpression of this enzyme in lung, gastric, colorectal, breast cancer and cervical cancer malignant tumors has been observed. Its relationship with inguinal lymph node metastasis in penile cancer is unknown.

Methods: SOD2 protein expression levels were determined by immunohistochemistry in 125 usual type squamous cell carcinomas of the penis from a Brazilian cancer center. The casuistic has been characterized by means of descriptive statistics. An exploratory logistic regression has been proposed to evaluate the independent predictive factors of lymph node metastasis.

Results: SOD2 expression in more than 50% of cells was observed in 44.8% of primary penile carcinomas of the usual type. This expression pattern was associated with lymph node metastasis both in the uni and multivariate analysis.

Conclusions: Our results indicate that SOD2 expression predicts regional lymph node metastasis. The potential clinical implication of this observation warrants further studies.

Keywords: Penile cancer, Superoxide Dismutase-2, Lymph node metastasis

Background

Malignant penile tumors are rare in developed countries but exhibit relatively high prevalence in some developing countries. Regional lymph node metastasis is one of the most important prognostic factors in patients with penile carcinoma due to its correlation with the advanced pathological stage of the tumor and tumor-related death [1]. Other factors affecting prognosis are histological grade, tumor thickness, perineural invasion, lymphovascular invasion and pattern of invasion [2,3].

About 50% of the cases in which palpable suspicious lymph node were present, subsequent pathologic analysis failed to find any evidence of metastatic disease in the lymph nodes [4,5]. Conversely, 20% of lymph nodes with no clinical signal of disease display micro metastases [6]. Therefore there is a need to identify other markers that may predict the occurrence of inguinal metastasis, perineural and vascular invasion. The use of these markers could be valuable to better define the subset of patients that will benefit from different therapeutic approaches [2-7].

Several studies have shown that superoxide dismutase 2 (SOD2 or manganese superoxide dismutase) protein expression is up-regulated in colorectal, lung, gastric/esophageal, and cervical cancer cells when compared to normal tissues [8-11]. However, the relationship between SOD2 expression and penile cancer has not been addressed, mainly in terms of regional lymph node metastasis. This study aimed to evaluate the association of SOD2 immunoexpression with inguinal lymph node metastasis and its clinical implication.

Methods

Tissue samples

Penile samples from 125 patients were obtained from the Department of Anatomic Pathology, Medical and

* Correspondence: terminilara@gmail.com
[1]Santa Casa de São Paulo, INCT-HPV at Santa Casa Research Institute, School of Medicine, Rua Marquês de Itú, 381, 01223-001 São Paulo, Brazil
Full list of author information is available at the end of the article

Research Center, A. C. Camargo Cancer Center, São Paulo, Brazil. No patient had distant metastasis at the diagnosis and all of them underwent tumor resection between 1953 and 2000. Lymphadenectomy has been performed in 50.4% of the cases and no patient received postoperative radiotherapy. Pathologic T stage was classified according to the TNM system of the International Union Against Cancer, 7th edition [12]. Ethical approval for this study was granted by the Hospital A.C. Camargo Institutional Research Ethics Committee (Project Number 1369/10).

Lymph node status has been defined using the pathologic information from the lymphadenectomy performed in 63 men (pN status). Patients who had not undergone lymph node resection had their lymph node status based on a retrospective longitudinal analysis of regional recurrence. Since no patient received inguinal or pelvic radiation as part of the treatment, those cases with no lymphadenectomy and no regional recurrence in a 3-year follow-up period had their lymph node status classified as "negative" (n = 46). Nevertheless, nine men without lymphadenectomy developed lymphonodal metastatic recurrence during follow-up after penectomy (median time to recurrence: 7.1 months; range: 1.4 – 22.1 months) and consequently they were considered as having "positive nodes" (tumor progression not previously detected). It was not possible to clearly define the regional lymph node status in seven cases with no previous lymphadenectomy. Although they did not have regional recurrence, the follow-up period was less than three years (median follow-up: 24.1 months; range: 8.7 – 35.8 months). These samples were not included in the uni and multivariate analyses.

Immunohistochemical SOD2 detection

After deparaffinization in xylene and rehydration, antigen retrieval was performed by incubation in boiling citrate buffer pH 6.0 for 20 minutes. Endogenous peroxidase activity was inactivated with 3% hydrogen peroxide. Nonspecific avidin-binding was also blocked (DAKO, X0590, Carpinteria, CA, USA). Samples were incubated with an anti-SOD2 polyclonal antibody (Santa Cruz Biotechnology, sc-18504, Santa Cruz, CA, USA), 1:100 in 1% bovine serum albumin-phosphate buffered solution for 30 minutes at 37°C and for 18 hours at 4°C. Slides were then incubated for 30 minutes at 37°C with biotinylated rabbit anti-goat IgG, (Vector, BA5000, Burlingame, CA, USA) diluted 1:500, followed by incubation for 30 minutes at 37°C with the complex streptavidin and peroxidase (StreptABComplex/HRP Duet Mouse/Rabbit, DakoCytomation, K0492, Glostrup, Denmark), diluted 1:200 and developed using 100 mg of 3,3'-diaminobenzidine tetrahydrochloride (Sigma, D-5637, St Louis, MO, USA), 6% H_2O_2 in dimethyl sulphoxide

and counterstained with Harris' hematoxylin. Sections derived from an ovarian papillary serous adenocarcinoma were used as a positive control for SOD2 expression.

In order to verify the specimen quality for immuno-histochemistry, all samples were also checked using a cytokeratin panel, which was positive in all cases. In addition, positivity rate of SOD2 expression was analyzed according to the year of patient's admission (1950–1959; 1960–1969; 1970–1979; 1980–1989; 1990–2000) and no statistically significant difference was found. Thus, specimen quality was considered adequate for analysis.

Evaluation of tissue staining

Positive immunohistochemical reactions were evaluated considering the percentage of stained tumoral cells. Only tissue cores with more than 25% of tumor cells were analyzed. The evaluation was performed by examining the tumor core under X200 magnification. For the statistical analysis, reactions were scored as exhibiting less than 50% stained cells or more than 50% stained cells, as previously reported by our group [11]. Immunohistochemical evaluation was performed independently and blindly by two observers (ALF and FAS). The very few discordant results were discussed by both observers and a final score was established.

Statistical analysis

The casuistic has been characterized by means of descriptive statistics. Fisher's exact test was employed to compare categorical variables in the univariate analysis. Exploratory logistic regression has been proposed to evaluate the independent predictive factors of inguinal lymph node metastasis. Variables with p value less than 0.10 were included in the multivariate model, which was conducted using a stepwise forward technique. The significance level was set at 5% for all tests.

DNA extraction

For DNA extraction, several 5 μm sections of the paraffin-embedded samples were collected in 1.5-ml microtubes. Samples were treated with xylene and digested with proteinase-K according to standard protocols described previously [13]. The microtome blade was changed after each block was cut and all the surrounding area and apparatus were cleaned with xylene and ethanol after processing each sample to avoid contamination between the samples. DNA quality was checked by amplification of the human β-globin gene using PCO3+/PCO4+ primers [14].

HPV typing

HPV detection and genotyping using generic primers (GP5+/GP6+) and type specific probes (6, 11, 16, 18, 31,

Table 1 Characterization of the population study (n = 125)

Variable	Category	N	%
Age	<50 yo	43	34.4
	50 – 59 yo	41	32.8
	≥60 yo	41	32.8
pT (TNM)	pT1a	7	5.6
	pT1b	4	3.2
	pT2	52	41.6
	pT3	57	45.6
	pT4	5	4.0
Palpable suspicious regional lymph node	No	64	51.2
	Yes	59	47.2
	Unknown	2	1.6
Regional lymph node status	No metastasis	74	59.2
	Metastasis	44	35.2
	Unknown	7	5.6
Pattern of invasion	Pushing	14	11.2
	Infiltrating	101	80.8
	Unknown	10	8.0
Histological grade	Grade 1	15	12.0
	Grade 2	45	36.0
	Grade 3	65	52.0
Perineural invasion	No	83	66.4
	Yes	35	28.0
	Unknown	7	5.6
Vascular invasion	No	85	68.0
	Yes	33	26.4
	Unknown	7	5.6
Invasion of corpora cavernous	No	22	17.6
	Yes	60	48.0
	Missing data	43	34.4
Invasion of corpora spongiosum	No	4	3.2
	Yes	88	70.4
	Unknown	33	26.4
Invasion of urethra	No	42	33.6
	Yes	28	22.4
	Unknown	55	44.0
Tumor depth	≤5 mm	21	16.8
	>5 mm	92	73.6
	Unknown	12	9.6
HPV detection	No	99	79.2
	Yes	26	20.8
SOD2 expression	<50%	69	55.2
	>50%	56	44.8

33, 35, 39, 42, 45, 51, 52, 53, 54, 55, 56 and 58), respectively, was performed as previously described [15].

Results

In the present study we have analyzed by immunohistochemistry the association of SOD2 expression pattern with different tumor aggressiveness and progression variables in 125 primary SCC samples of the usual histological type. Characterization of the population studied is depicted in Table 1. A representative immunostaining for SOD2 in different penile tumor samples exhibiting <50% or >50% stained cells is presented in Additional file 1. Most of the cases was classified as pT2 or pT3 (87.2%) and 44 cases had regional lymph node metastasis at diagnosis. No cases with distant metastasis were observed. Fifty six tumors (44.8%) had SOD2 expression greater than 50%. In about 20% of the cases HPV infection was detected [see Additional file 2]. No relationship was observed between presence of HPV DNA and SOD2 expression (Table 2).

Table 3 shows the regional lymph node status according to the clinical and pathological variables. In the bivariate analysis, metastatic node was associated with palpable suspicious lymph node in the clinical exam (P < 0.001), tumor size (P = 0.045), histological grade (P = 0.013), perineural invasion (P < 0.001), vascular invasion (P = 0.010), tumor depth (P = 0.002) and SOD2 expression (P = 0.002). All these variables were included in the exploratory logistic regression (Table 4), which identified the following independent predictive factors of lymph node metastasis: palpable suspicious nodes (OR = 8.9; 95% CI: 2.7 – 29.2), tumor depth greater than 5 mm (OR = 11.6; 95% CI: 1.4 – 97.1), perineural invasion (OR = 9.6; 95% CI: 2.7 – 33.6) and SOD2 expression greater than 50% (OR = 3.4; 95% CI: 1.1 – 10.1).

Table 2 Number and percentage of cases according to HPV genotype and SOD2 expression

HPV genotype (*)	Category	SOD2 < 50% N	(%)	SOD2 > 50% N	(%)	P value
HPV-16	No	59	(54.6)	49	(45.4)	0.799
	Yes	10	(58.8)	7	(41.2)	
HPV-18	No	64	(54.2)	54	(45.8)	0.458
	Yes	5	(71.4)	2	(28.6)	
HPV non-16/non-18	No	67	(55.8)	53	(44.2)	0.656
	Yes	2	(40.0)	3	(60.0)	
High risk HPV	No	54	(53.5)	47	(46.5)	0.497
	Yes	15	(62.5)	9	(37.5)	

(*) HPV-16 (n = 17), HPV-18 (n = 7); HPV-11 (n = 3); HPV-6 (n = 3); HPV-35 (n = 1); HPV-39 (n = 1). HPV co-infection has been registered in four cases: HPV-6, 11 (n = 2); HPV 6, 11 and 16 (n = 1); HPV-16, 18 and 39 (n = 1).

Table 3 Number and percentage of cases with and without regional lymph node metastasis according to clinical and pathological variables

Variable	Category	No lymph node metastasis		Lymph node metastasis		P value
		N	(%)	N	(%)	
Age	< 50 yo	26	(65.0)	14	(35.0)	0.682
	50 – 59 yo	27	(65.9)	14	(34.1)	
	≥60 yo	21	(56.8)	16	(43.2)	
Palpable suspicious regional	No	48	(84.2)	9	(15.8)	<0.001
Lymph node	Yes	24	(40.7)	35	(59.3)	
pT (TNM)	pT1a	7	(100.0)	0	(0.0)	0.045
	> pT1a	67	(60.4)	44	(39.6)	
Pattern of invasion	Pushing	6	(46.2)	7	(53.8)	0.368
	Infiltrating	60	(61.9)	37	(38.1)	
Histological grade	Grade 1	13	(86.7)	2	(13.3)	0.013
	Grade 2	30	(71.4)	12	(28.6)	
	Grade 3	31	(50.8)	30	(49.2)	
Perineural invasion	No	59	(75.6)	19	(24.4)	<0.001
	Yes	9	(26.5)	25	(73.5)	
Vascular invasion	No	55	(68.8)	25	(31.2)	0.010
	Yes	13	(40.6)	19	(59.4)	
Invasion of *corpora cavernous*	No	14	(66.7)	7	(33.3)	0.303
	Yes	28	(50.9)	27	(49.1)	
Invasion of *corpora spongiosum*	No	3	(75.0)	1	(25.0)	1.000
	Yes	50	(60.2)	33	(39.8)	
Invasion of urethra	No	26	(66.7)	13	(33.3)	0.436
	Yes	14	(56.0)	11	(44.0)	
Tumor depth	≤5 mm	18	(90.0)	2	(10.0)	0.002
	>5 mm	44	(51.2)	42	(48.8)	
HPV-16	No	64	(62.1)	39	(37.9)	1.000
	Yes	10	(66.7)	5	(33.3)	
HPV-18	No	68	(61.3)	43	(38.7)	0.255
	Yes	6	(85.7)	1	(14.3)	
SOD2 expression	<50%	49	(75.4)	16	(24.6)	0.002
	>50%	25	(47.2)	28	(52.8)	

Table 5 summarizes the patient's distribution according to the four predictive factors of inguinal lymph node metastasis found in the multivariate model.

Discussion

To the best of our knowledge, this is the first study analyzing the expression of SOD2 in a large series of penile carcinoma samples. SOD2 is one of three distinct superoxide dismutases isoforms found in mammals. This protein is found generally in the mitochondrial matrix and is an evolutionary conserved enzyme in a variety of organisms. Superoxide dismutases act as part of the cellular antioxidant system protecting the redox sensitive

cellular machinery from damage induced by reactive oxygen species (ROS). This enzyme's activity affects important cellular processes including cell growth, proliferation and differentiation. As a consequence the role of SOD2 in cancer is complex and multifactorial. In fact, the exact role of SOD2 and redox state in cancer onset and progression remains poorly understood. Interestingly, accumulating evidence suggest that reducing oxidative stress levels by increasing SOD2 expression may represent a double-edged sword in tumor development. Reducing oxidative stress may have anti-tumoral effect by preventing DNA damage. This is supported by the observation that SOD2 expression can reduce the

Table 4 Predictive factors for regional lymph node metastasis according to the exploratory logistic regression

Variable	Category	N	Adjusted OR (*)	95% CI	P value
Palpable suspicious regional lymph node	No	49	1.0	Reference	
	Yes	55	8.9	2.7 – 29.2	<0.001
Tumor depth	≤5 mm	20	1.0	Reference	
	>5 mm	84	11.6	1.4 – 97.1	0.023
Perineural invasion	No	71	1.0	Reference	
	Yes	33	9.6	2.7 – 33.6	<0.001
SOD2 expression	<50%	57	1.0	Reference	
	>50%	47	3.4	1.1 – 10.1	0.029

(*) Number of outcomes included in the analysis: 44 (regional lymph node metastasis).
OR: Odds ratio 95% CI: 95% confidence interval.

Table 5 Distribution of patients according to the combination of the predictive factors of inguinal lymph node metastasis found in the multivariate model

Palpable suspicious lymph node	Tumor depth	Perineural invasion	SOD2 expression (>50%)	Patients at risk	Patients with inguinal lymph node metastasis	
				n	n	(%)
No (*1)	≤5 mm	Absent	-	9	0	(0.0)
		Absent	+	4	0	(0.0)
		Present	-	2	0	(0.0)
		Present	+	0	NA	NA
	>5 mm	Absent	-	15	2	(13.3)
		Absent	+	10	2	(20.0)
		Present	-	2	0	(0.0)
		Present	+	7	5	(71.4)
Yes (*2)	≤5 mm	Absent	-	2	0	(0.0)
		Absent	+	0	NA	NA
		Present	-	1	0	(0.0)
		Present	+	2	2	(100.0)
	>5 mm	Absent	-	19	7	(36.8)
		Absent	+	12	8	(66.7)
		Present	-	7	7	(100.0)
		Present	+	12	11	(91.7)
All cases (*3)	≤5 mm	Absent	-	11	0	(0.0)
		Absent	+	4	0	(0.0)
		Present	-	3	0	(0.0)
		Present	+	2	2	(100.0)
	>5 mm	Absent	-	34	9	(26.5)
		Absent	+	24	10	(41.7)
		Present	-	9	7	(77.8)
		Present	+	19	16	(84.2)

NA: Data not available since any case was observed in this situation.
(*1) Eight cases were not included in this group because they did have either tumor depth or perineural information. SOD2 expression was positive in three of them. All those cases had no lymph node metastasis.
(*2) Four cases were not included in this group because they did have either tumor depth or perineural information. SOD2 expression was positive in one of them. All those cases had no lymph node metastasis.
(*3) Two cases with unknown clinical status of inguinal nodes were included in this group. Both cases had tumor depth > 5 mm, no perineural invasion, positive SOD2 expression and no lymph node metastasis.

malignant potential of several transformed cell lines [10,16]. Conversely, it can be anticipated that SOD2 upregulation may reduce the level of ROS in tumor cells. This may prevent the accumulation of life incompatible levels of DNA and other macromolecules damage, protecting neoplastic cells from intrinsic cell death mechanisms and favoring their survival and spread [8,9].

Analysis of SOD2 expression conducted in solid tumor samples including colorectal [17,18], gastric and esophageal [19,20], oral [21], lung [22-24], brain [25], cervical [11] and skin [26] carcinomas have often associated its up-regulation with metastasis and poor disease outcome. The molecular mechanisms underlying increased SOD2 and metastasis include the alteration of several cellular pathways. It has been observed that SOD2 overexpression increases matrix metalloproteinases (MMPs)-1, −2, −3, −7, −10, −9 and −11 mRNA levels. In the case of MMP-1 this has been attributed to the activation of the Ras/MAP/extracellular signal-regulated kinase signaling cascade. In the same study SOD2 upregulation was associated with enhanced metastatic potential of fibrosarcoma cells in an animal model [27]. Since MMPs play a critical role in the metastatic process it can be argued that the association between increased SOD2 and poor prognosis observed in certain tumors may be attributed to elevated MMP production/activity. A recent study showed that SOD2 expression was sufficient to overcome ROS mediated growth arrest in prostate carcinoma cells [28]. Besides it was observed that elevated SOD2 levels confer resistance to ROS mediated anoikis in mammary epithelial cells in a process dependent on NFκB activation [29]. Since anoikis resistance is essential for tumor metastasis the anti-anoikis activity of SOD2 implicates this enzyme in the metastatic process. We can, therefore, speculate that increased SOD2 levels may confer an adaptive advantage to tumor cells favoring disease establishment and progression.

We have previously reported that SOD2 is differentially expressed between normal and HPV immortalized keratinocytes [30]. Furthermore, we have recently shown that SOD2 protein expression level is a potential biomarker for the characterization of different stages of cervical neoplasia, which is etiologically linked with infection with high-risk HPV types [11]. A proportion of penile cancers are also associated with HPV, mostly HPV16. In fact, recent evidence suggests that these viruses, particularly HPV16, may be associated with up to 48% of all penile tumors [31].

In the present study no association between SOD2 expression and HPV infection was observed. HPV DNA was detected in 20.8% of the samples analyzed which is below the HPV positivity data reported by others [31,32]. This result is not due to quality of the DNA recovered from the paraffinized specimens since >98% of them tested positive for globin. The low proportion of HPV-positive specimens detected probably reflects the fact that in our study most of the samples analyzed are of SCC of the usual histological type, which is less frequently associated with HPV infection. Using exploratory logistic regression we observed that SOD2 expression in more than 50% of the cells was an independent predictive factor of lymph node metastasis as were other well documented clinical-pathologic variables such as palpable suspicious nodes, tumor depth >5 mm and perineural invasion [33-36].

Although SOD2 expression was clearly an independent predictive factor of inguinal lymph node metastasis in the multivariate model, its real contribution in clinical practice remains to be determined. Table 5 demonstrates that tumor depth information is able to determine itself the presence of node metastasis, regardless the status of inguinal node in the clinical exam and perineural invasion status. Our results show that SOD2 expression has some value by increasing the risk of metastasis when the tumor depth was greater than 5 mm. All cases of inguinal metastasis, but two, occurred when the tumor depth was greater than 5 mm. Interestingly, the two cases in which lymph node metastasis was observed when tumor depth was less than 5 mm had positive SOD2 immunoexpression. Coincidently, those cases had palpable suspicious lymph nodes in inguinal clinical exam. The implication of SOD2 expression in thin penile tumors is uncertain and should be interpreted with caution because a limited number of cases in this particular setting were observed. However, the potential clinical implications of this observation as well as the contribution of SOD2 assessment in clinical practice warrants further studies.

Conclusions

SOD2 expression predicts regional lymph node metastasis in usual type squamous cell carcinomas of the penis. Further studies are needed to determine the clinical implication of this factor.

Abbreviations

HPV: Human papillomavirus; ROS: Reactive oxygen species; SOD2: Superoxide dismutase 2 or manganese superoxide dismutase.

Competing interests

The authors declare that they have no competing interests.

Authors' contributions

LT conceived the study, participated in its design, was involved in immunohistochemical reactions, manuscript preparation and results discussion. JHF carried out statistical analysis, manuscript drafting and results discussion. EB was involved in co-ordination of the study, in manuscript drafting and results discussion. WHC was involved with statistical analysis and manuscript drafting. AL-F, IWC and FAS performed the revision and classification of all histopathological samples, and gave critical assistance in the Discussion section. MAA and MCC were involved HPV genotyping and immunohistochemical reactions. AL and GCG carried out data bank administration, including patients' clinical follow up data/samples collection. LLV participated in the study design and co-ordination. All authors have read and approved the final version of the manuscript.

Acknowledgements

We are grateful to Carlos Ferreira do Nascimento, Severino Ferreira, Romulo Akira, Luciane Tsukamoto Kagohara and Suely Nonogaki from the A. C. Camargo Cancer Center, São Paulo, Brazil for technical assistance. Financial support: Dr. Lara Termini (FAPESP 2005/57274-9); Dr. Luisa Lina Villa (FAPESP 2008/57889-1 and CNPq 573799/2008-3).

Author details

[1]Santa Casa de São Paulo, INCT-HPV at Santa Casa Research Institute, School of Medicine, Rua Marquês de Itú, 381, 01223-001 São Paulo, Brazil. [2]Teaching and Research Institute, Barretos Cancer Hospital, Rua Antenor Duarte Vilela, 1331, 14784-006 Barretos, Brazil. [3]Department of Microbiology, Institute of Biomedical Sciences, University of São Paulo, Av. Prof. Lineu Prestes, 1374 - Ed. Biomédicas II, Cidade Universitária, 05508-900 São Paulo, Brazil. [4]Pelvic Surgery Department, A. C. Camargo Cancer Center, Rua Prof. Antônio Prudente 211, 01509-010 São Paulo, Brazil. [5]Laboratory of Medical Investigation (LIM) 14, Department of Pathology, School of Medicine, University of São Paulo, Av. Dr. Arnaldo 455, 01246-903 São Paulo, Brazil. [6]Life and Health Sciences Research Institute, School of Health Sciences, ICVS/3B's - PT Government Associate Laboratory, University of Minho, Braga, Guimarães, Portugal. [7]Molecular Oncology Research Center, Barretos Cancer Hospital, Pio XII Foundation, Barretos, Rua Antenor Duarte Villela, 1331, 14784-400 Barretos, Brazil. [8]Department of Anatomic Pathology, A. C. Camargo Cancer Center, Rua Prof. Antônio Prudente 109, 01509-900 São Paulo, Brazil. [9]Department of Radiology and Oncology, School of Medicine, University of São Paulo and Cancer Institute of the State of São Paulo, ICESP, Av Dr Arnaldo 250, 01246-000 São Paulo, Brazil.

References

1. Guimarães GC, Rocha RM, Zequi SC, Cunha IW, Soares FA. Penile cancer: epidemiology and treatment. Curr Oncol Rep. 2011;13(3):231–9.
2. Guimarães GC, Lopes A, Campos RS, Zequi S d C, Leal ML, Carvalho AL, et al. Front pattern of invasion in squamous cell carcinoma of the penis: new prognostic factor for predicting risk of lymph node metastases. Urology. 2006;68(1):148–53.
3. Chaux A, Caballero C, Soares F, Guimarães GC, Cunha IW, Reuter V, et al. The prognostic index: a useful pathologic guide for prediction of nodal metastases and survival in penile squamous cell carcinoma. Am J Surg Pathol. 2009;33(7):1049–57.
4. Guimarães GC, Cunha IW, Soares FA, Lopes A, Torres J, Chaux A, et al. Penile squamous cell carcinoma clinicopathological features, nodal metastasis and outcome in 333 cases. J Urol. 2009;182(2):528–34.
5. Zhu Y, Zhang HL, Yao XD, Zhang SL, Dai B, Shen YJ, et al. Development and evaluation of a nomogram to predict inguinal lymph node metastasis in patients with penile cancer and clinically negative lymph nodes. J Urol. 2010;184(2):539–45.
6. Pompeo AC. Extended lymphadenectomy in penile cancer. Can J Urol. 2005;1:30–6. discussion 97–8.
7. Velazquez EF, Ayala G, Liu H, Chaux A, Zanotti M, Torres J, et al. Histologic grade and perineural invasion are more important than tumor thickness as predictor of nodal metastasis in penile squamous cell carcinoma invading 5 to 10 mm. Am J Surg Pathol. 2008;32(7):974–9.
8. Holley AK, Dhar SK, Xu Y, St Clair DK. Manganese superoxide dismutase: beyond life and death. Amino Acids. 2012;42(1):139–58.
9. Johnson F, Giulivi C. Superoxide dismutases and their impact upon human health. Mol Aspects Med. 2005;26(4–5):340–52.
10. Kinnula VL, Crapo JD. Superoxide dismutases in malignant cells and human tumors. Free Radic Biol Med. 2004;36(6):718–44.
11. Termini L, Filho AL, Maciag PC, Etlinger D, Alves VA, Nonogaki S, et al. Deregulated expression of superoxide dismutase-2 correlates with different stages of cervical neoplasia. Dis Markers. 2011;30(6):275–81.
12. American Joint Committee on Cancer. Penis, in AJCC Cancer Staging Handbook. 7th ed. New York: Springer; 2010. p. 447.
13. Shi SR, Cote RJ, Wu L, Liu C, Datar R, Shi Y, et al. DNA extraction from archival formalin-fixed, paraffin-embedded tissue sections based on the antigen retrieval principle: heating under the influence of pH. J Histochem Cytochem. 2002;50(8):1005–11.
14. Saiki RK, Scharf S, Faloona F, Mullis KB, Horn GT, Erlich HA, et al. Enzymatic amplification of beta-globin genomic sequences and restriction site analysis for diagnosis of sickle cell anemia. Science. 1985;230(4732):1350–4.
15. de Roda Husman AM, Walboomers JM, van den Brule AJ, Meijer CJ, Snijders PJ. The use of general primers GP5 and GP6 elongated at their 3' ends with adjacent highly conserved sequences improves human papillomavirus detection by PCR. J Gen Virol. 1995;76(Pt4):1057–62.
16. Ough M, Lewis A, Zhang Y, Hinkhouse MM, Ritchie JM, Oberley LW, et al. Inhibition of cell growth by overexpression of manganese superoxide dismutase (MnSOD) in human pancreatic carcinoma. Free Radic Res. 2004;38(11):1223–33.
17. Toh Y, Kuninaka S, Oshiro T, Ikeda Y, Nakashima H, Baba H, et al. Overexpression of manganese superoxide dismutase mRNA may correlate with aggressiveness in gastric and colorectal adenocarcinomas. Int J Oncol. 2000;17(1):107–12.
18. Janssen AM, Bosman CB, Kruidenier L, Griffioen G, Lamers CB, van Krieken JH, et al. Superoxide dismutases in the human colorectal cancer sequence. J Cancer Res Clin Oncol. 1999;125(6):327–35.
19. Janssen AM, Bosman CB, van Duijn W, Oostendorp-van de Ruit MM, Kubben FJ, Griffioen G, et al. Superoxide dismutases in gastric and esophageal cancer and the prognostic impact in gastric cancer. Clin Cancer Res. 2000;6(8):3183–92.
20. Hwang TS, Choi HK, Han HS. Differential expression of manganese superoxide dismutase, copper/zinc superoxide dismutase, and catalase in gastric adenocarcinomas and normal gastric mucosa. Eur J Surg Oncol. 2007;33(4):474–9.
21. Liu X, Wang A, Lo Muzio L, Kolokythas A, Sheng S, Rubini C, et al. Deregulation of manganese superoxide dismutase (SOD2) expression and lymph node metastasis in tongue squamous cell carcinoma. BMC Cancer. 2010;10:365.
22. Ho JC-m, Zheng S, Comhair SA, Farver C, Erzurum SC. Differential expression of manganese superoxide dismutase and catalase in lung cancer. Cancer Res. 2001;61(23):8578–85.
23. Kinnula VL, Crapo JD. Superoxide dismutases in the lung and human lung diseases. Am J Respir Crit Care Med. 2003;167(12):1600–19.
24. Svensk AM, Soini Y, Pääkkö P, Hiravikoski P, Kinnula VL. Differential expression of superoxide dismutases in lung cancer. Am J Clin Pathol. 2004;122(3):395–404.
25. Haapasalo H, Kyläniemi M, Paunul N, Kinnula VL, Soini Y. Expression of antioxidant enzymes in astrocytic brain tumors. Brain Pathol. 2003;13(2):155–64.
26. St Clair D, Zhao Y, Chaiswing L, Oberley T. Modulation of skin tumorigenesis by SOD. Biomed Pharmacother. 2005;59(4):209–14.
27. Nelson KK, Ranganathan AC, Mansouri J, Rodriguez AM, Providence KM, Rutter JL, et al. Elevated SOD2 activity augments matrix metalloproteinase expression: evidence for the involvement of endogenous hydrogen peroxide in regulating metastasis. Clin Cancer Res. 2003;9(1):424–32.
28. Das TP, Suman S, Damodaran C. Reactive oxygen species generation inhibits epithelial-mesenchymal transition and promotes growth arrest in prostate cancer cells. Mol Carcinog. 2014;53(7):537–47.
29. Kamarajugadda S, Cai Q, Chen H, Nayak S, Zhu J, He M, et al. Manganese superoxide dismutase promotes anoikis resistance and tumor metastasis. Cell Death Dis. 2013;4:e504.
30. Termini L, Boccardo E, Esteves GH, Hirata Jr R, Martins WK, Colo AE, et al. Characterization of global transcription profile of normal and HPV-immortalized keratinocytes and their response to TNF treatment. BMC Med Genomics. 2008;1:29.

31. Chaux A, Cubilla AL. The role of human papillomavirus infection in the pathogenesis of penile squamous cell carcinomas. Semin Diagn Pathol. 2012;29(2):67–71.

32. Anic GM, Giuliano AR. Genital HPV infection and related lesions in men. Prev Med. 2011;53:36–41.

33. Pizzocaro G, Algaba F, Horenblas S, Solsona E, Tana S, Van Der Poel H, et al. EAU penile cancer guidelines 2009. Eur Urol. 2010;57(6):1002–12.

34. Lopes A, Hidalgo GS, Kowalski LP, Torloni H, Rossi BM, Fonseca FP. Prognostic factors in carcinoma of the penis: multivariate analysis of 145 patients treated with amputation and lymphadenectomy. J Urol. 1996;156(5):1637–42.

35. Ornellas AA, Nóbrega BL, Wei Kin Chin E, Wisnescky A, da Silva PC, de Santos Schwindt AB. Prognostic factors in invasive squamous cell carcinoma of the penis: analysis of 196 patients treated at the Brazilian National Cancer Institute. J Urol. 2008;180(4):1354–9.

36. Cubilla AL. The role of pathologic prognostic factors in squamous cell carcinoma of the penis. World J Urol. 2009;27(2):169–77.

14

Ultrastructural characterization of primary cilia in pathologically characterized human glioblastoma multiforme (GBM) tumors

Joanna J Moser, Marvin J Fritzler and Jerome B Rattner[*]

Abstract

Background: Primary cilia are non-motile sensory cytoplasmic organelles that are involved in cell cycle progression. Ultrastructurally, the primary cilium region is complex, with normal ciliogenesis progressing through five distinct morphological stages in human astrocytes. Defects in early stages of ciliogenesis are key features of astrocytoma/glioblastoma cell lines and provided the impetus for the current study which describes the morphology of primary cilia in molecularly characterized human glioblastoma multiforme (GBM) tumors.

Methods: Seven surgically resected human GBM tissue samples were molecularly characterized according to IDH1/2 mutation status, EGFR amplification status and MGMT promoter methylation status and were examined for primary cilia expression and structure using indirect immunofluorescence and electron microscopy.

Results: We report for the first time that primary cilia are disrupted in the early stages of ciliogenesis in human GBM tumors. We confirm that immature primary cilia and basal bodies/centrioles have aberrant ciliogenesis characteristics including absent paired vesicles, misshaped/swollen vesicular hats, abnormal configuration of distal appendages, and discontinuity of centriole microtubular blades. Additionally, the transition zone plate is able to form in the absence of paired vesicles on the distal end of the basal body and when a cilium progresses beyond the early stages of ciliogenesis, it has electron dense material clumped along the transition zone and a darkening of the microtubules at the proximal end of the cilium.

Conclusions: Primary cilia play a role in a variety of human cancers. Previously primary cilia structure was perturbed in cultured cell lines derived from astrocytomas/glioblastomas; however there was always some question as to whether these findings were a cell culture phenomena. In this study we confirm that disruptions in ciliogenesis at early stages do occur in GBM tumors and that these ultrastructural findings bear resemblance to those previously observed in cell cultures. This is the first study to demonstrate that defects in cilia expression and function are a true hallmark of GBM tumors and correlate with their unrestrained growth. A review of the current ultrastructural profiles in the literature provides suggestions as to the best possible candidate protein that underlies defects in the early stages of ciliogenesis within GBM tumors.

Keywords: Primary cilia, Ciliogenesis, Cilium-pit, Centriole, Basal body, Distal appendages, Glioblastoma multiforme, EGFR amplification, IDH1/2 mutation, MGMT promoter methylation

* Correspondence: rattner@ucalgary.ca
Department of Biochemistry and Molecular Biology, Faculty of Medicine,
University of Calgary, Calgary, AB, Canada

Ultrastructural characterization of primary cilia in pathologically characterized human glioblastoma...

117

Background

Primary cilia are non-motile sensory cytoplasmic organelles that have been implicated in signal transduction, cell to cell communication, left and right pattern embryonic development, sensation of fluid flow, regulation of calcium levels, mechanosensation, growth factor signaling and cell cycle progression [1,2]. They are present in the central nervous system and depletion of primary cilia in pro-opiomelanocortin hypothalamic neurons have induced hyperphagia [3,4]. Central nervous system primary cilia are key organelles required for Sonic hedgehog signalling (Shh) [5-8] where components Patched, Smoothened, Suppressor of fused and Gli transcription factors concentrate in the primary cilium [9-11]. It is currently thought that an intact primary cilium is required to enable proper Shh pathway function [12]. Subventricular zone astrocytes extend their primary cilium into the cerebral spinal fluid (CSF) suggesting they play a role in sensing ion concentration, pH, osmolarity, and changes in protein or glucose levels [13]. It is possible that astrocyte primary cilia can sense concentrations of neurotransmitters, growth factors, hormones, osmolarity, ions, pH and fluid flow in the extracellular space and relay homeostatic information (or lack thereof) to the centrosome.

Defects in the formation and/or function of primary cilia underlie a variety of human diseases that impact neurological development and are broadly referred to as ciliopathies and include diseases such as Alström, Bardet-Biedl, Joubert, Meckel-Gruber and oral-facial-digital type 1 syndromes. Common neurological phenotypes include obesity, ataxia and mental retardation [14]. The expression and function of primary cilia has become a focus of attention in a number of normal and malignant cells and tissues but have not been characterized in human glioblastoma tissue samples. Given that primary cilia are linked to cell cycle regulation and progression, several studies have suggested that primary cilia may play a role in tumor formation [15,16].

Previously our group undertook a comparative investigation of primary cilia in cultured primary human astrocytes and compared them to those found in five human astrocytoma/glioblastoma cell lines [17]. We demonstrated that the primary cilium region in cultured astrocyte cells is structurally complex, with ciliogenesis progressing through five distinct stages (Figure 1), and included foci for endocytosis-based signalling [17].

Further, we documented that in each of the five astrocytoma/glioblastoma cell lines studied (U-87 MG, T98G, U-251 MG, U-373 MG, U-138 MG), fully formed primary cilia are either expressed at a very low level, are completely absent or do not proceed through all the stages of ciliogenesis [17]. In addition, we noted several defects in the structure of astrocytoma/glioblastoma centrioles, including abnormal length and appendage architecture, that were not observed in primary human astrocytes [17]. We concluded that aberrant ciliogenesis is common in cells derived from astrocytomas/glioblastomas and that this deficiency likely contributes to the phenotype of these malignant cells. These initial studies in astrocytoma/glioblastoma cell lines indicate that defects in primary cilium ciliogenesis do occur in glioblastoma cells and provided the impetus for this current study which characterizes the morphology of primary cilia and documents ciliogenesis defects in molecularly characterized human glioblastoma multiforme (GBM) tumors. Glioblastomas, although relatively uncommon with an annual incidence rate of 3–4 cases per 100,000 people, have disproportionately high morbidity and mortality rates with median survival pegged at 12–15 months [18,19]. Primary glioblastomas typically occur in patients older than 50 years of age and are characterized by epidermal growth factor receptor (EGFR) amplification and mutations, loss of heterozygosity of chromosome 10q and other abnormalities as reviewed in Wen and Kesari (2008) [20]. One of the most common defects in growth factor signalling involves EGFR [21] and amplification occurs almost exclusively in glioblastomas with 40-50% of patients containing EGFR amplification [20]. Isocitrate dehydrogenase (IDH) mutations are a strong predictor of a more favourable prognosis and a highly selective molecular marker for secondary glioblastomas [22]. Mutations of genes encoding *IDH1* and *IDH2*, as compared to no mutations, are associated with younger age and a better prognosis in adults with gliomas [23]. O^6-methylguanine-DNA methyltransferase (MGMT) promoter methylation silences the *MGMT* gene, decreasing DNA repair activity and increases the susceptibility of tumor cells to chemotherapeutic agents [20]. Recently it was shown that MGMT promoter methylation was associated with better overall survival in patients with GBM regardless of therapeutic intervention [24]. Given this burden of disease, it is important to determine the degree to which ciliogenesis is compromised in glioblastoma tumors as this information will inform the identity of altered mechanisms which may become targets for the development of future treatments.

Our hypothesis was that primary cilia in human GBM cells would be completely absent or show defects in the early stages of ciliogenesis. Our primary objective was to examine primary cilia expression and structure in human GBM tissue samples at both the light and ultrastructural level.

Methods

Ethics statement

Anonymized human brain tumor (GBM) tissue samples and basic clinico-pathologic data were obtained through the Clark Smith Brain Tumour and Tissue Bank at the

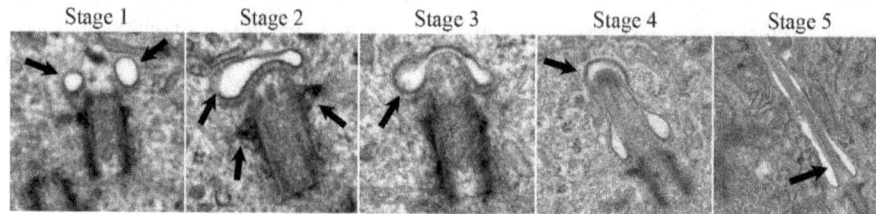

Figure 1 Primary ciliogenesis progresses through five morphologically distinct stages in human astrocytes. Key characteristics of each stage are indicated with arrows. Paired lateral vesicles are prominent at the distal end of the basal body in Stage 1. Distal appendages are triangular in appearance and reside at the distal end of the basal body (Stage 2). The paired lateral vesicles fuse to become a vesicular hat and become stretched by the outgrowth of the primary cilium and can be seen progressing through stages 2 through 4. Stage 5 shows a mature primary cilium with a surrounding cilium-pit. *Used with permission from Moser et al. BMC Cancer 2009, 9:448, Figure 2A © BioMed Central.*

University of Calgary and Calgary Laboratory Services, Calgary, AB (ethics approved for biobanking and previous patient consent granted at time of banking). Tissue was used according to the policies of the institutional review boards of Calgary Laboratory Services and the Calgary Health Region Ethics Board. Further ethics review and approval for this study (ID# E-23011) was provided by the Conjoint Health Research Ethics Board (University of Calgary, Calgary, AB).

GBM tissue samples

All samples were part of routine clinical care for diagnostic and treatment purposes and were designated as excess material by the consulting and consenting neuropathologist. Hematoxylin and eosin stained formalin-fixed paraffin-embedded sections were reviewed by a neuropathologist for confirmation of a diagnosis of high-grade glioma (glioblastoma WHO grade IV) as per World Health Organization criteria [18].

Molecular characterization of GBM tumors

Molecular characterization of IDH and EGFR was performed by the clinical Molecular Diagnostics Laboratory at Calgary Laboratory Services on formalin-fixed paraffin-embedded (FFPE) sections. Briefly, IDH1 and IDH2 mutational analyses were performed using a multiplexed SNaPshot® reaction and detection by capillary electrophoresis [25]. Analysis of EGFR amplification was performed by EGFR colorimetric *in situ* hybridization using standard methods with the EGFR probe #84-1300 (Zymed Laboratories), and scored by a neuropathologist as follows: 'amplified EGFR' indicates >10 signals/nucleus in >80% of tumor cells and 'not amplified' indicates 2 signals/nucleus in tumor cells.

Antigen retrieval method (ARM)

Slides containing the FFPE tissue sections were deparaffinised in xylene and passed through a graded ethanol series, rinsed with cold tap water and transferred to a Coplin jar on a hot plate containing a 100°C Tris-EDTA-Tween (w/v)

solution (0.121% Tris HCl, 0.0379% EDTA, 0.05% Tween-20, pH adjusted to 9.0). The sections were boiled for 60 minutes and then allowed to reach room temperature while remaining in the same solution. The slides were washed in phosphate buffered saline (PBS) for 10 minutes and processed for IIF.

Indirect immunofluorescence (IIF)

Formalin-fixed paraffin embedded tissue sections were treated with the above ARM (section 3.4.). Cells were blocked in 10% normal goat serum (NGS; Antibodies Incorporated, Davis, CA) and 2% bovine serum albumin (BSA; Sigma-Aldrich) for 30 minutes at room temperature (RT) and incubated with primary antibodies at appropriate working dilutions overnight at 4°C. Primary cilia were marked by mouse anti-acetylated tubulin at 1:100 dilution (Sigma, St. Louis, MO). After washing with PBS, cells were incubated for 2 hours in a dark chamber with Alexa Fluor (AF) 488 (green) secondary goat fluorochrome-conjugated antibodies at 1:100 dilution (Invitrogen). Slides were washed in several changes of PBS, cell nuclei counterstained with 4',6-diamidino-2-phenylindole (DAPI), mounted in Vectashield (Vector Laboratories, Burlingame, CA) and examined for IIF using a 100x objective on a Leica DMRE microscope equipped with epifluorescence and an Optronics camera. Appropriate IIF controls with no primary antibody revealed no detectable bleed-through between microscope filter sets.

Electron microscopy (EM)

Fresh GBM samples were immersed in a fixative containing 3% glutaraldehyde in Millonig's phosphate buffer and stored at 4°C for 48 hours. Samples were immersed post-fixation in 2% OsO_4 for 20 minutes and then dehydrated in ethanol and infiltrated with Polybed 812 resin (Polysciences Inc., Warrington, PA). Polymerization was performed at 37°C for 24 hours. Silver-gray sections were cut with an ultramicrotome (Leica) equipped with a diamond knife, stained with uranyl acetate and lead citrate and then examined in a H-700 Hitachi electron microscope. For each sample, 10 grids were examined on standard sections. Approximately 500 cells were examined in each tissue sample.

Results

We examined both formalin-fixed paraffin embedded (FFPE) and fresh-fixed tissue from seven cases of surgically resected brain tumors diagnosed by neuropathologists as grade IV glioblastoma/GBM using indirect immunofluorescence (IIF) and electron microscopy (EM), respectively.

The GBM tumors were molecularly characterized according to IDH 1/2 mutation status, EGFR amplification status and MGMT promoter status (Table 1). Our results showed that 71% of GBM patients had amplified levels of EGFR, 86% had no IDH1/2 mutations and 50% had methylated MGMT promoters (Table 1).

We examined the biopsy tissue from each of the 7 patients by light and electron microscopy. IIF examination of tissue from patient #1 showed typical primary cilia (Figure 2, top inset). Similarly, ultrastructural examination revealed a normal basal body with a fully formed mature primary cilium, consistent with normal morphology (Figure 2 compared to Figure 1). The cilium-pit was well defined (Figure 2) and the cilium contained well-formed microtubules with normal spacing between doublets (Figure 2, bottom inset). In addition, small vesicles were seen along the cilium microtubules and interfacing with the cilium-pit (Figure 2), which is consistent with previous findings that showed this is a site for endocytosis based signalling [17].

The GBM tissue from patient #2 failed to show abundant primary cilia by IIF. Ultrastructural examination revealed cells with basal bodies reminiscent of stage 1 ciliogenesis, however there were no paired vesicles present along the lateral sides of the distal end of the basal body/transition zone as observed in longitudinal and cross-sections (Figure 3A and inset compared to Figure 1). In addition to missing paired vesicles, patient #2 had basal bodies that presented with abnormal, vertically outstretched distal appendages (Figure 3B). Figure 3C shows another example of an abnormal basal body with

absent paired vesicles along the lateral sides of the distal end of the basal body/transition zone. Interestingly, the transition zone plate is present without the presence of the vesicles which suggests that the vesicles do not need to be present to allow the transition zone to form, but need to be present to allow ciliogenesis to progress beyond stage 1. In one rare example, a primary cilium which had progressed to stage 5 of ciliogenesis was found (Figure 3D). On close examination, this cilium displayed a disrupted ciliary membrane which was also the site of cytoplasmic extrusions into the surrounding environment (Figure 3D). These abnormal primary cilia also have a dark pericentriolar material (PCM)-like collection of material clumped along the transition zone of the primary cilium with darkening of the cilia microtubules at the proximal end of the cilium shaft (Figure 3D).

The tissue from patient #3 revealed an absence of mature primary cilia by IIF and ultrastructural examination showed that 70% of centrosome/basal body profiles were at stage 1 while the remaining 30% of profiles examined displayed stage 2/3 of ciliogenesis (Figure 4). Many of the immature cilia contained electron dense material along the cilium shaft (Figure 4 compared to Figure 1). The stretched vesicular hat that is so prominent in normal cells at stage 2/3 was irregular, thin and misshapen in patient #3 GBM cells (Figure 4). The microtubules of the cilium appear irregular, lack organization and do not display the normal architectural characteristics of the transition zone (Figure 4). There were no cilia in stages 4–5 observed for patient #3.

GBM tissue from patient #4 failed to display mature primary cilium by IIF. Ultrastructurally, patient #4 expressed basal bodies that were similar to stage 1 with a transition zone plate formed along the distal end (Figure 5A compared to Figure 1). It is important to note that in many of these electron microscope centrosome/basal body profiles there was only 1 vesicle present (as opposed to the normal 2 vesicles) at the distal end and the vesicle was positioned directly above the transition zone plate (as opposed to the normal lateral orientation beside the transition zone plate) (Figure 5A). The architecture of

Table 1 Molecularly characterized grade IV glioblastoma GBM tumors

Patient no.	IDH 1/2	EGFR amplification	MGMT promoter
1	No mutations detected	Amplified	Not assessed
2	No mutations detected	Amplified	Un-methylated
3	No mutations detected	Amplified	Un-methylated
4	IDH1 exon 4 R132H mutation detected; no mutation in exon 4 of IDH2	Amplified	Methylated
5	No mutations detected	Not amplified	Methylated
6	No mutations detected	Amplified	Methylated
7	No mutations detected	Not amplified	Un-methylated

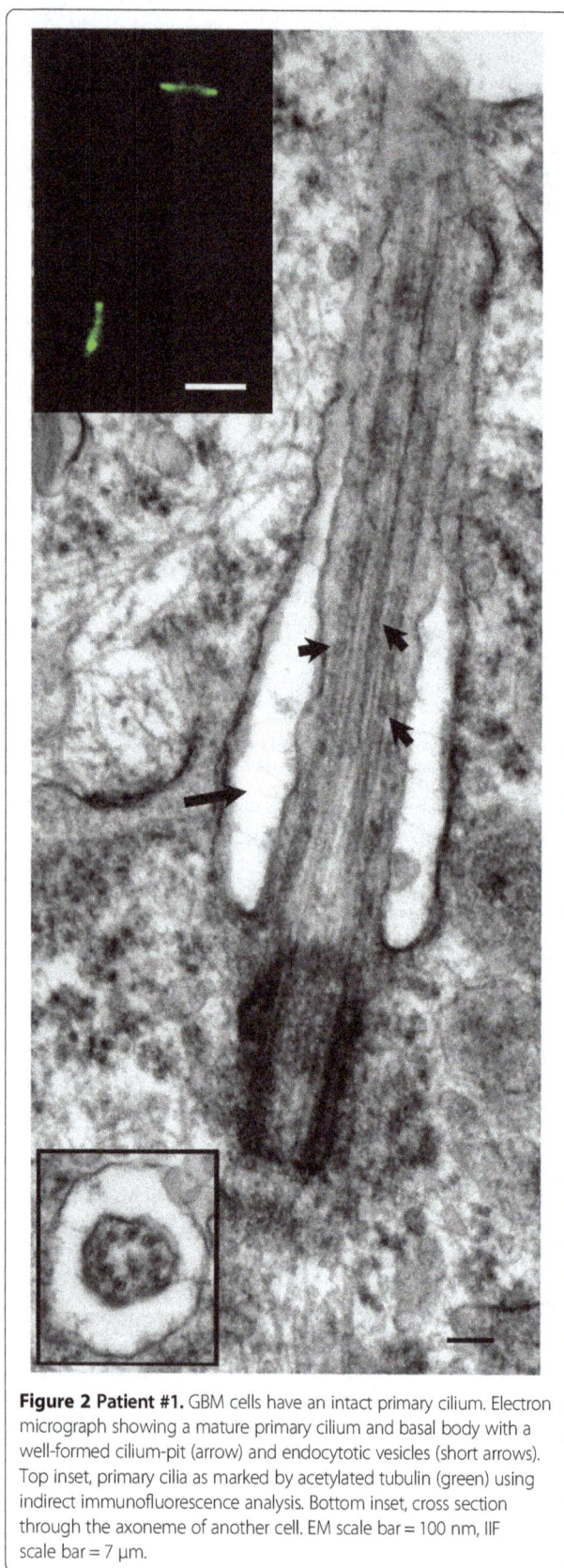

Figure 2 Patient #1. GBM cells have an intact primary cilium. Electron micrograph showing a mature primary cilium and basal body with a well-formed cilium-pit (arrow) and endocytotic vesicles (short arrows). Top inset, primary cilia as marked by acetylated tubulin (green) using indirect immunofluorescence analysis. Bottom inset, cross section through the axoneme of another cell. EM scale bar = 100 nm, IIF scale bar = 7 μm.

the distal appendages along the basal body was also abnormal given their outstretched vertical appearance (Figure 5A) as opposed to the normal horizontal appearance displayed in Figure 1. Figure 5B, illustrates a discontinuity present in one of the centriole microtubule blades, although this centriole was 357 nm in length (Figure 5B) which falls within normal parameters [17].

Samples from patient #5 did not show mature primary cilia by IIF. Ultrastructural examination revealed either basal bodies with an immature transition zone or profiles similar to stage 1 (Figure 6 compared to Figure 1). The transition zone was not visible in the electron micrograph centrosome/basal body profiles from this patient and we did not observe any paired vesicles similar to that seen in patient #2 (Figure 6). There also appears to be minimal PCM distributed in the cytoplasmic area surrounding the basal body and centriole (Figure 6).

There were no observable primary cilia staining by IIF in the GBM tissue from patient #6, although ultrastructural examination showed cilia at multiple stages (Figure 7). We observed profiles at stage 1 with a well-defined plate within the transition zone lacking paired laterally placed vesicles (Figure 7A). We observed many cilia at stage 1 with either multiple irregular abnormally shaped vesicles formed at the distal end of the basal body or 4 distinct vesicles above the plate within the transition zone (Figure 7B). In the latter case, distal appendages were absent. In rare cases, a cilium with a short axoneme was detected (Figure 7C). These cilia appeared to have a truncated cilium-pit so that the distal end of the cilium is continuous with the cytoplasm, a configuration reminiscent of a regressing cilium [26].

GBM tissue from patient #7 also did not show any primary cilia by IIF staining. Ultrastructurally, primary ciliogenesis occurred in profiles to a maximum of stage 2 (Figure 8 compared to Figure 1). These cells had vesicular hats that were misshaped and swollen (Figure 8A and B) and had outstretched, vertical distal basal body appendages (Figure 8B). These characteristics were similar to those observed in other astrocytoma/glioblastoma cell lines, particularly in U-373 MG and U-138 MG cells (Figure 2B in [17]).

Discussion

The expression of a primary cilium relies on two main events: 1) activation of ciliogenesis and 2) orderly progression through a series of developmental stages so that a structurally and functionally competent mature cilium is formed [27-29]. Our study illustrates that ciliogenesis was activated in all the GBM samples examined but cilium morphogenesis beyond stage 1 was rare in the majority of tumors. These findings support our previous examination of several astrocytoma/glioblastoma cell lines [17]. Thus,

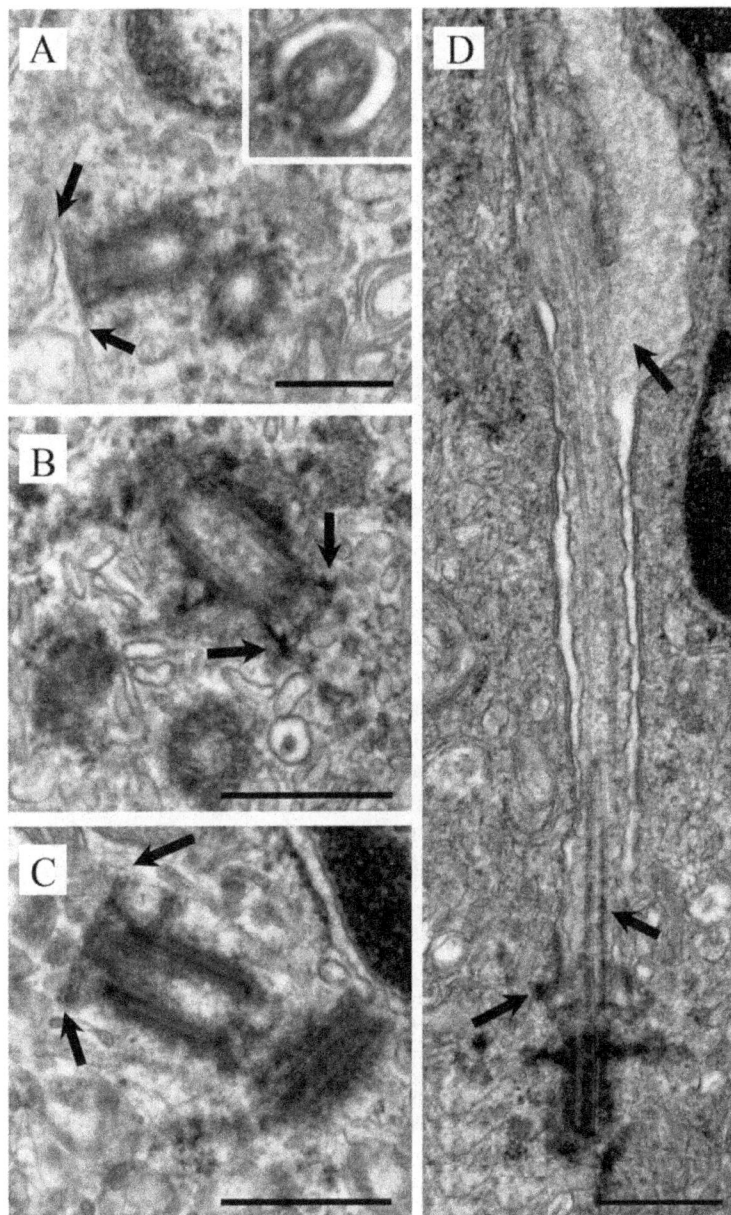

Figure 3 Patient #2. GBM cells are halted at stage 1 of ciliogenesis with rare cells progressing to stage 5. **(A)** Basal body and abnormal stage 1 cilium with absent paired lateral vesicles. Inset cross section through the transition zone from another cell. **(B)** Basal body and abnormal stage 1 cilium with vertically outstretched distal appendages and no vesicles. **(C)** Basal body with clear transition zone and abnormal stage 1 cilium with absent vesicles. **(D)** Rare occurrence of a primary cilium at stage 5 with abnormal destruction of the cilium-pit with cytoplasmic extrusion, darkened microtubules at proximal end of cilium and electron dense collection of material at the transition zone. EM scale bars = 500 nm.

cells from each of these sources (cell line or tumor tissue) express a similar defect or set of defects that targets the earliest stages of ciliogenesis and does not inhibit the cells ability to proliferate.

These findings are compatible with previous studies of melanoma, renal cell carcinoma and pancreatic cancer, which found that primary cilia loss was independent of Ki67 staining (cell proliferation marker) suggesting that cilia loss is not the result of altered cellular proliferation rates but rather may be due to aberrations in another mechanism that is inherent to ciliogenesis [30-32]. Yang and colleagues (2013) recently showed that cell cycle-related kinase (CCRK) and its substrate intestinal cell kinase inhibited ciliogenesis in a glioblastoma cell line [33]. Specifically, they showed that dysregulated high levels of CCRK are present in U-251 MG glioblastoma cells whereby knockdown of CCRK led to the formation of primary cilia indicating that CCRK depletion restored

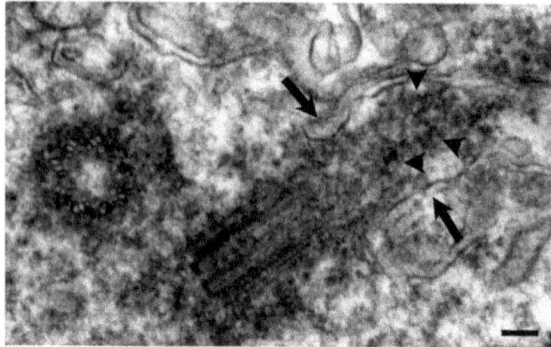

Figure 4 Patient #3. GBM cells are halted at stage 3 of ciliogenesis and display electron dense material clustered along the cilium shaft (arrow heads) and an irregular vesicular hat (arrows). EM scale bar = 100 nm.

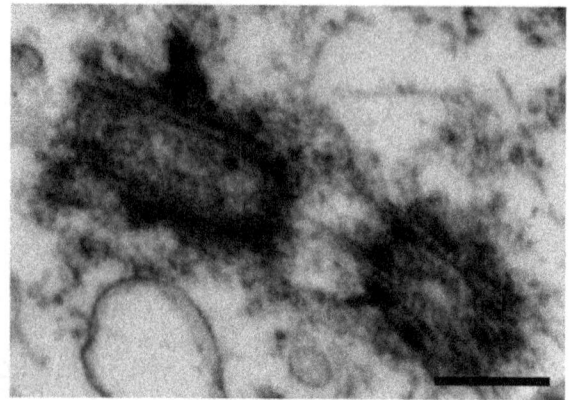

Figure 6 Patient #5. GBM cells were characterized by abnormal primary cilia that were halted at or before stage 1 of ciliogenesis with no evidence of paired vesicles or a transition zone plate. EM scale bar = 250 nm.

primary ciliogenesis [33]. Furthermore, it was demonstrated that the inhibition of ciliogenesis by over-expression of CCRK in U-251 MG glioblastoma cells promoted cell proliferation capacity [33].

From our ultrastructural studies in astrocytoma/glioblastoma cell lines and GBM tumor tissues it is interesting to note that profiles occasionally displayed centriole/ basal bodies with structural abnormalities (i.e. altered length or microtubule integrity). This suggests that it is possible for such structural alterations to be tolerated by the cycling cell, perhaps by being repaired, or that these defects underlie further aberrant cancer cell behaviour.

It is important to note that in the majority of previously published studies, IIF alone was used to evaluate ciliogenesis status. This technique alone does not allow for the precise identification or characterization of the earliest stages of ciliogenesis. Thus, truncated cilia such as that seen in a few patients within our study may be more common that previously indicated. Our ultrastructural data not only reveals a defect in early ciliogenesis but also shows that this defect specifically

affects the initial elaboration of the distal surface of the basal body and its ability to associate with Golgi derived vesicles. There have been a number of proteins shown to act at the distal end of the basal body, particularly at the distal appendage region, and they include; Cep170 [34], ninein [8,35], ε-tubulin [36], cenexin/ODF2 [37] (likely cenexin1 [38]) and by association Rab8a [39], centriolin/ Cep110 [8,40], Cep164 [41] and Cep123 [42] reviewed in [1]. For example, in neuronal primary cilia, B9-C2 containing proteins have been shown to collect at the base of the primary cilium in the transition zone [43-47] and physically interact and with ciliary protein localization [48] (and reviewed in [49]). One B9-C2 family gene in particular named Stumpy (or *B9d2*) is required for mammalian ciliogenesis where knockout mutants displayed nearcomplete loss of neuronal primary cilia with remaining cilia displaying dysmorphic stump-like ultrastructures [43].

Of particular interest, a distal appendage protein, Cep 123, has recently been shown to be required for initiation

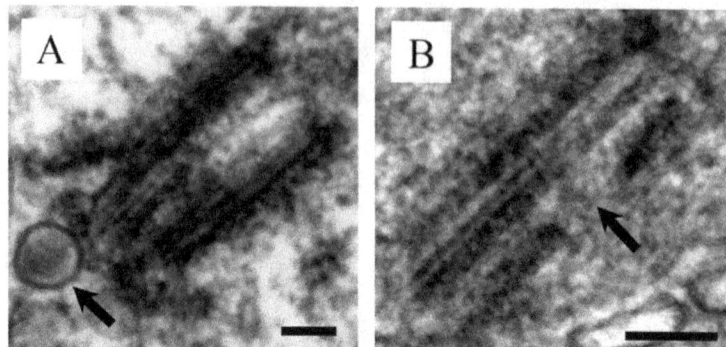

Figure 5 Patient #4. GBM cells were characterized by **(A)** primary cilia that were halted at stage 1 of ciliogenesis with a single vesicle present above the transition plate and abnormal distal appendages and **(B)** breakages in the basal body/centriole microtubules. EM scale bars = 100 nm.

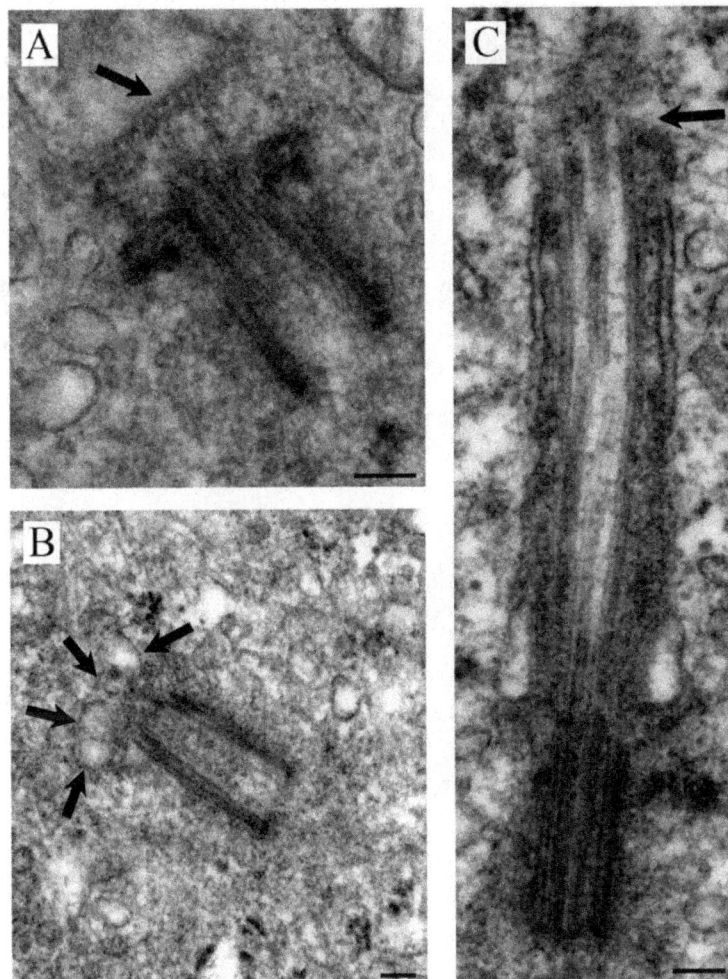

Figure 7 Patient #6. GBM cells were characterized by abnormal primary cilia at **(A, B)** stage 1/2 and **(C)** 4/5 of ciliogenesis with either absent lateral vesicles, aberrant supernumerary vesicles along the length of the transition zone plate or abrupt cessation of the cilium shaft. EM scale bars = 100 nm.

of ciliogenesis by modulation of capping the distal end of the mother centriole with a ciliary vesicle [42]. Sillibourne and colleagues (2013) showed that Cep123 is required for assembly of a primary cilium but not the maintenance of the axoneme in human retinal pigment epithelial (RPE1) cells [42]. Depletion of Cep123 using Cep 123 siRNA perturbed ciliary vesicle formation at the distal end of the basal body which suggests that distal appendage proteins are critical for progression of cilia beyond the early stages of ciliogenesis [42]. These knockdown studies are captured in Figure 6B by Sillibourne *et al.* (2013) [42] and are very similar in appearance to the abnormal early stages of ciliogenesis seen in our GBM tumors. Given this high degree of ultrastructural similarity, Cep123 may be the best candidate to explain the defects we observed in GBM tumors. Although a review of the glioblastoma literature does not highlight Cep123 as being defective in patients with GBM tumors, our study

suggests that it is a reasonable target for future expression studies and ultrastructural analysis in GBM tumors.

Limitations of the current study are small sample size and lack of normal brain tissue for comparison. Given the small incidence of malignant gliomas per year, we collected samples over a 5 year period and eliminated those samples that were not grade IV glioblastomas/ GBM. To respect the ethics of collection of normal human brain tissue from our patients, we compared the GBM patient results to those previously established in normal human astrocyte cells that were used between passages 3–5 in culture [17]. Although 10 grids were examined for each patient sample, there were noticeable differences between tumor samples in terms of cellularity and patient heterogeneity. It is important to emphasize that this is a complex mixture of cells and extracellular matrixof GBM brain tissue and that some cell types are ciliated whereas others are not ciliated. Because of the

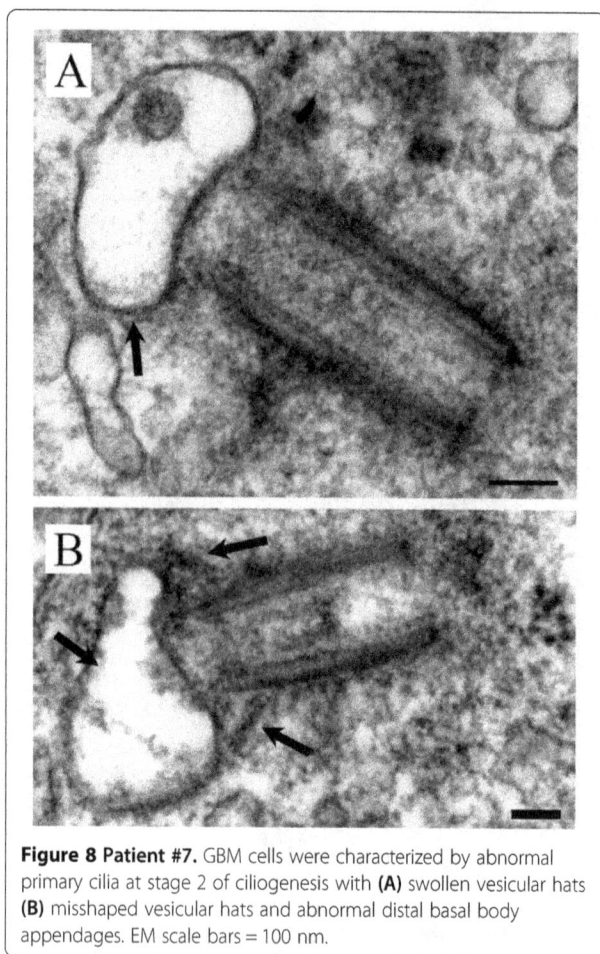

Figure 8 Patient #7. GBM cells were characterized by abnormal primary cilia at stage 2 of ciliogenesis with **(A)** swollen vesicular hats **(B)** misshaped vesicular hats and abnormal distal basal body appendages. EM scale bars = 100 nm.

tissue complexity and heterogeneity, it is impossible to identify all the cells which have the potential to undergo ciliogenesis. When we do see profiles, we can quantitate the number of cells undergoing abnormal ciliogenesis (including profiles at stages 3/4/5) which is summarized as follows. Patient #1: 20 cells with profiles, 2 cells with normal cilia, 0 cells with abnormal cilia. Patient #2: 9 cells with profiles, 0 cells with normal cilia, 2 cells with abnormal cilia. Patient #3: 20 cells with profiles, 0 cells with normal cilia, 2 cells with abnormal cilia. Patient #4: 22 cells with profiles, 0 cells with normal cilia, 0 cells with abnormal cilia. Patient #5: 20 cells with profiles, 0 cells with normal cilia, 0 cells with abnormal cilia. Patient #6: 30 cells with profiles, 0 cells with normal cilia, 3 cells with abnormal cilia. Patient #7: 15 cells with profiles, 0 cells with normal cilia, 0 cells with abnormal cilia. Taken together, only one patient expressed morphologically normal cilia. As a whole, we did see the same types of abnormalities in the early stages of ciliogenesis amongst tumor samples which suggests that early ciliogenesis defects are a generalized problem in GBM tumors. In summary, we can say that the large majority of grade 4 glioblastoma/ astrocytomas (i.e. GBM tumors) are likely to express

abnormal immature primary cilia suggesting that this defect may be a hallmark of GBMs. We have not detected a clear correlation between abnormal ciliogenesis and the 3 main molecular characterizations examined in these patient samples. It must be kept in mind that our patient sample size may not be sufficient to reveal correlations with molecular markers and this might require a larger study.

In summary, we found that ciliogenesis is activated in GBM tumors but the normal development of a mature cilium is perturbed at early stages of ciliogenesis. The aberrant ultrastructural profiles observed in our survey of GBM tumors and a review of the current ultrastructural profiles present in the literature suggest the possibility that at present the best possible candidate protein underlying defects in the early stages of ciliogenesis within GBM tumors might involve Cep123.

Conclusions

The major finding of this report is that primary ciliogenesis is disrupted at an early stage in the majority of human GBM tumors. This finding is important for several reasons. First, these results confirm astrocytoma/ glioblastoma cell culture data. Second, it indicates that defects in ciliogenesis are a hallmark of GBM tumor pathology and provides impetus for further study of the relationship between primary cilium defects and other brain tumors such as astrocytoma, oligodendroglioma and medulloblastoma. Third, it provides further evidence that the early stages of ciliogenesis are a critical time in the process of ciliogenesis, thus narrowing the number of target proteins that may underlie these defects. Fourth, it catalogues and describes the key basal body/cilium-related ultrastructural abnormalities that are common between GBM tumors. The ultrastructural description of this study informs which proteins are involved in early ciliogenesis defects and identifies candidates that are currently in the literature. In future, it will be important to elucidate which specific proteins are involved in this critical time period and whether alterations in their expression can restore ciliogenesis and thus restore cell cycle control.

Abbreviations

ARM: Antigen retrieval method; CCRK: Cell cycle-related kinase; CSF: Cerebral spinal fluid; DAPI: 4',6-diamidino-2-phenylindole; EM: Electron microscopy; EGFR: Epidermal growth factor receptor; FFPE: Formalin-fixed paraffin embedded; GBM: Glioblastoma multiforme; IIF: Indirect immunofluorescence; IDH: Isocitrate dehydrogenase; MGMT: O^6-methylguanine-DNA methyltransferase; PBS: Phosphate buffered saline; PCM: Pericentriolar material; RPE1: Retinal pigment epithelial; Shh: Sonic hedgehog signalling; WHO: World Health Organization.

Competing interests

The authors declare that they have no competing interests.

Authors' contributions

JJM and JBR obtained the molecular characterization data, carried out the electron microscopy studies, performed indirect immunofluorescence experiments and wrote the first draft of the manuscript. JJM, MJF and JBR conceived of the study design, participated in obtaining ethics approval, interpretation of the data, read, edited and approved the final manuscript. All authors read and approved the final manuscript.

Acknowledgements

We thank neuropathologists, Drs. Jennifer Chan and Leslie Hamilton, University of Calgary for providing the samples, diagnoses and clinico-pathological information on the tissues obtained from Calgary Laboratory Services. This work was supported in part by the Canadian Institutes for Health Research Grant MOP-57674 (MJF) and the Natural Sciences and Engineering Research Council of Canada Grant 690481 (JBR).

References

1. Moser JJ, Fritzler MJ, Ou Y, Rattner JB: The PCMbasal body/primary cilium coalition. *Semin Cell Dev Biol* 2010, 21:148–155.
2. Hassounah NB, Bunch TA, McDermott KM: Molecular pathways: the role of primary cilia in cancer progression and therapeutics with a focus on hedgehog signaling. *Clin Cancer Res* 2012, 18:2429–2435.
3. Davenport JR, Watts AJ, Roper VC, Croyle MJ, van Groen T, Wyss JM, Nagy TR, Kesterson RA, Yoder BK: Disruption of intraflagellar transport in adult mice leads to obesity and slow-onset cystic kidney disease. *Curr Biol* 2007, 17:1586–1594.
4. Satir P: Cilia biology: stop overeating now! *Curr Biol* 2007, 17:R963–R965.
5. Ingham PW: Transducing hedgehog: the story so far. *EMBO J* 1998, 17:3505–3511.
6. Dahmane N, Altaba A: Sonic hedgehog regulates the growth and patterning of the cerebellum. *Development* 1999, 126:3089–3100.
7. Wallace VA: Purkinje-cell-derived Sonic hedgehog regulates granule neuron precursor cell proliferation in the developing mouse cerebellum. *Curr Biol* 1999, 9:445–448.
8. Ou YY, Mack GJ, Zhang M, Rattner JB: CEP110 and ninein are located in a specific domain of the centrosome associated with centrosome maturation. *J Cell Sci* 2002, 115:1825–1835.
9. Corbit KC, Aanstad P, Singla V, Norman AR, Stainier DYR, Reiter JF: Vertebrate Smoothened functions at the primary cilium. *Nature* 2005, 437:1018–1021.
10. Haycraft C, Banizs B, Aydin-Son Y, Zhang Q, Michaud EJ, Yoder BK: Gli2 and Gli3 localize to cilia and require the intraflagellar transport protein polaris for processing and function. *PLoS Genet* 2005, 1:e53.
11. Rohatgi R, Milenkovic L, Scott MP: Patched1 regulates hedgehog signaling at the primary cilium. *Science* 2007, 317:372–376.
12. Breunig JJ, Sarkisian MR, Arellano JI, Morozov YM, Ayoub AE, Sojitra S, Wang B, Flavell RA, Rakic P, Town T: Primary cilia regulate hippocampal neurogenesis by mediating sonic hedgehog signaling. *Proc Natl Acad Sci* 2008, 105:13127–13132.
13. Danilov AI, Gomes-Leal W, Ahlenius H, Kokaia Z, Carlemalm E, Lindvall O: Ultrastructural and antigenic properties of neural stem cells and their progeny in adult rat subventricular zone. *Glia* 2009, 57:136–152.
14. Badano JL, Mitsuma N, Beales PL, Katsanis N: The ciliopathies: an emerging class of human genetic disorders. *Annu Rev Genomics Hum Genet* 2006, 7:125–148.
15. Wong SY, Seol AD, So PL, Ermilov AN, Bichakjian CK, Epstein EH, Dlugosz AA, Reiter JF: Primary cilia can both mediate and suppress Hedgehog pathway-dependent tumorigenesis. *Nat Med* 2009, 15:1055–1061.
16. Han YG, Kim HJ, Dlugosz AA, Ellison DW, Gilbertson RJ, Alvarez-Buylla A: Dual and opposing roles of primary cilia in medulloblastoma development. *Nat Med* 2009, 15:1062–1065.
17. Moser JJ, Fritzler MJ, Rattner JB: Primary ciliogenesis defects are associated with human astrocytoma/glioblastoma cells. *BMC Cancer* 2009, 9:448.
18. Louis D, Ohgaki H, Wiestler O, Cavenee W, Burger P, Jouvet A, Scheithauer B, Kleihues P: The 2007 WHO classification of tumours of the central nervous system. *Acta Neuropathol* 2007, 114:547.
19. Ostrom QT, Gittleman H, Farah P, Ondracek A, Chen Y, Wolinsky Y, Stroup NE, Kruchko C, Barnholtz-Sloan JS: CBTRUS Statistical Report: Primary Brain and Central Nervous System Tumors Diagnosed in the United States in 2006-2010. *Neuro Oncol* 2013, 15(suppl 2):ii1–ii56.
20. Wen PY, Kesari S: Malignant gliomas in adults. *N Engl J Med* 2008, 359:492–507.
21. Furnari FB, Fenton T, Bachoo RM, Mukasa A, Stommel JM, Stegh A, Hahn WC, Ligon KL, Louis DN, Brennan C, Chin L, DePinho RA, Cavanee WK: Malignant astrocytic glioma: genetics, biology, and paths to treatment. *Genes Dev* 2007, 21:2683–2710.
22. Nobusawa S, Watanabe T, Kleihues P, Ohgaki H: IDH1 mutations as molecular signature and predictive factor of secondary glioblastomas. *Clin Cancer Res* 2009, 15:6002–6007.
23. Yan H, Parsons DW, Jin G, McLendon R, Rasheed BA, Yuan W, Kos I, Batinic-Haberle I, Jones S, Riggins GJ, Friedman H, Friedman A, Reardon D, Herndon J, Kinzler KW, Velculescu VE, Vogelstein B, Bigner DD: IDH1 and IDH2 mutations in gliomas. *N Engl J Med* 2009, 360:765–773.
24. Zhang K, Wang XQ, Zhou B, Zhang L: The prognostic value of MGMT promoter methylation in Glioblastoma multiforme: a meta-analysis. *Fam Cancer* 2013, 12:449–458.
25. Perizzolo M, Winkfein B, Hui S, Krulicki W, Chan JA, Demetrick DJ: IDH mutation detection in formalin-fixed paraffin-embedded gliomas using multiplex PCR and single-base extension. *Brain Pathol* 2012, 22:619–624.
26. Williams NE, Frankel J: Regulation of microtubules in tetrahymena : I. electron microscopy of oral replacement. *J Cell Biol* 1973, 56:441–457.
27. Sorokin S: Centrioles and the formation of rudimentary cilia by fibroblasts and smooth muscle cells. *J Cell Biol* 1962, 15:363–377.
28. Hagiwara H, Ohwada N, Aoki T, Takata K: Ciliogenesis and ciliary abnormalities. *Med Electron Microsc* 2000, 33:109–114.
29. Hagiwara H, Ohwada N, Takata K: Cell Biology of normal and abnormal ciliogenesis in the ciliated epithelium. In *International Review of Cytology*, Volume 234. Academic Press: Kwang WJ; 2004:101–141. ISBN ISBN 9780123646385.
30. Tukachinsky H, Lopez LV, Salic A: A mechanism for vertebrate Hedgehog signaling: recruitment to cilia and dissociation of SuFuGli protein complexes. *J Cell Biol* 2010, 191:415–428.
31. Schraml P, Frew IJ, Thoma CR, Boysen G, Struckmann K, Krek W, Moch H: Sporadic clear cell renal cell carcinoma but not the papillary type is characterized by severely reduced frequency of primary cilia. *Mod Pathol* 2008, 22:31–36.
32. Seeley ES, Carrière C, Goetze T, Longnecker DS, Korc M: Pancreatic cancer and precursor pancreatic intraepithelial neoplasia lesions are devoid of primary cilia. *Cancer Res* 2009, 69:422–430.
33. Yang Y, Roine N, Makela TP: CCRK depletion inhibits glioblastoma cell proliferation in a cilium-dependent manner. *EMBO Rep* 2013, 14:741–747.
34. Guarguaglini G, Duncan PI, Stierhof YD, Holmstrom T, Duensing S, Nigg EA: The Forkhead-associated domain protein Cep170 Interacts with Polo-like Kinase 1 and serves as a marker for mature centrioles. *Mol Biol Cell* 2005, 16:1095–1107.
35. Mogensen MM, Malik A, Piel M, Bouckson-Castaing V, Bornens M: Microtubule minus-end anchorage at centrosomal and non-centrosomal sites: the role of ninein. *J Cell Sci* 2000, 113:3013–3023.
36. Chang P, Giddings TH, Winey M, Stearns T: epsilon-Tubulin is required for centriole duplication and microtubule organization. *Nat Cell Biol* 2003, 5:71–76.
37. Ishikawa H, Kubo A, Tsukita S, Tsukita S: Odf2-deficient mother centrioles lack distal/subdistal appendages and the ability to generate primary cilia. *Nat Cell Biol* 2005, 7:517–524.
38. Soung NK, Park JE, Yu LR, Lee KH, Lee JM, Bang JK, Veenstra TD, Rhee K, Lee KS: Plk1-dependent and -independent roles of an ODF2 splice variant, hCenexin1, at the centrosome of somatic cells. *Dev Cell* 2009, 16:539–550.
39. Si Y, Egerer J, Fuchs E, Haas AK, Barr FA: Functional dissection of Rab GTPases involved in primary cilium formation. *J Cell Biol* 2007, 178:363–369.
40. Gromley A, Jurczyk A, Sillibourne J, Halilovic E, Mogensen M, Groisman I, Blomberg M, Doxsey S: A novel human protein of the maternal centriole is required for the final stages of cytokinesis and entry into S phase. *J Cell Biol* 2003, 161:535–545.
41. Graser S, Stierhof YD, Lavoie SB, Gassner OS, Lamla S, Le Clech M, Nigg EA: Cep164, a novel centriole appendage protein required for primary cilium formation. *J Cell Biol* 2007, 179:321–330.
42. Sillibourne JE, Hurbain I, Grand-Perret T, Goud B, Tran P, Bornens M: Primary ciliogenesis requires the distal appendage component Cep123. *Biol Open* 2013.
43. Town T, Breunig JJ, Sarkisian MR, Spilianakis C, Ayoub AE, Liu X, Ferrandino AF, Gallagher AR, Li MO, Rakic P, Flavell RA: The stumpy gene is required for mammalian ciliogenesis. *Proc Natl Acad Sci* 2008, 105:2853–2858.

44. Garcia-Gonzalo FR, Corbit KC, Sirerol-Piquer MS, Ramaswami G, Otto EA, Noriega TR, Seol AD, Robinson JF, Bennett CL, Josifova DJ, García-Verdugo JM, Katsanis N, Hildebrandt F, Reiter JF: **A transition zone complex regulates mammalian ciliogenesis and ciliary membrane composition.** *Nat Genet* 2011, **43**:776–784.
45. Williams CL, Li C, Kida K, Inglis PN, Mohan S, Semenec L, Bialas NJ, Stupay RM, Chen N, Blacque OE, Yoder BK, Leroux MR: **MKS and NPHP modules cooperate to establish basal body/transition zone membrane associations and ciliary gate function during ciliogenesis.** *J Cell Biol* 2011, **192**:1023–1041.
46. Chih B, Liu P, Chinn Y, Chalouni C, Komuves LG, Hass PE, Sandoval W, Peterson AS: **A ciliopathy complex at the transition zone protects the cilia as a privileged membrane domain.** *Nat Cell Biol* 2012, **14**:61–72.
47. Zhang D, Aravind L: **Identification of novel families and classification of the C2 domain superfamily elucidate the origin and evolution of membrane targeting activities in eukaryotes.** *Gene* 2010, **469**:18–30.
48. Dowdle W, Robinson J, Kneist A, Sirerol-Piquer M, Frints S, Corbit K, Zaghloul N, van Lijnschoten G, Mulders L, Verver D, *et al*: **Disruption of a Ciliary B9 protein complex causes Meckel syndrome.** *Am J Hum Genet* 2011, **89**:94–110.
49. Gate D, Danielpour M, Levy R, Breunig J, Town T: **Basic biology and mechanisms of neural ciliogenesis and the B9 family.** *Mol Neurobiol* 2012, **45**:564–570.

15

Prevalence and predictors of Pap smear cervical epithelial cell abnormality among HIV-positive and negative women attending gynecological examination in cervical cancer screening center at Debre Markos referral hospital, East Gojjam, Northwest Ethiopia

Melkamu Getinet[1], Baye Gelaw[2], Abinet Sisay[1], Eiman A. Mahmoud[3] and Abate Assefa[2*]

Abstract

Background: Cervical cancer is the leading cause of cancer related death among women in developing countries. Cervical cancer is preceded by cervical surface epithelial cell abnormalities (ECA) which can be detected by Pap smear test. Simultaneous human papillomavirus and human immunodeficiency virus (HIV) infection increases cervical cancer. Data on the prevalence and predictors of ECA among women in Ethiopia is limited. Hence, we aimed to determine the prevalence and associated factors of ECA among women.

Methods: A comparative cross-sectional study was conducted among HIV+ and HIV- women attending gynecological examination in cervical cancer screening center at the Debre Markos referral hospital. The study subjects were stratified by HIV status and systematic random sampling method was used to recruit study participants. Cervical smears were collected for Pap smear examination. Logistic regression analysis was employed to examine the possible risk factors of cervical ECA.

Results: A total of 197 HIV+ and 194 HIV- women were enrolled in the study. The overall prevalence of cervical ECA was 14.1 % of which the prevalence of atypical squamous cells undetermined significance (ASCUS), low grade squamous intraepithelial lesion (SIL), high grade SIL, squamous cell carcinoma and ASC, cannot exclude high grade SIL (ASCH) were 5.1, 3.8, 4.1 and 1.0 %, 0.0 % respectively. Significantly higher prevalence of ECA (17.8 %) was observed among HIV+ women (COR 1.9, 95 % CI: 1.1 – 3.4, $p = 0.036$) as compared to HIV-women (10.3 %). Multiple sexual partnership (AOR 3.2, 95 % CI: 1.1 – 10.0, $p = 0.04$), early ages of first sexual contact (<15 years) (AOR 5.2, 95 % CI: 1.5 – 17.9, $p = 0.009$), parity greater than three (AOR 10.9, 95 % CI: 4.2 – 16.8, $p < 0.001$) and long term oral contraceptive pills (OCP) use (AOR 11.9, 95 % CI: 2.1 – 16.7, $p = 0.02$) were significant predictors of prevalence of ECA.

Conclusions: Cervical ECA is a major problem among HIV-infected women. Lower CD4+ T-cell counts of below 350 cells/μl, HIV infection, multiple sexual partnership, early age at first sexual contact, parity greater than three and long term OCP use were significant predictors of prevalence of ECA. Strengthening screening program in HIV+ women should be considered.

* Correspondence: abezew@gmail.com
[2]Department of Medical Microbiology, School of Biomedical and Laboratory Sciences, College of Medicine and Health Sciences, University of Gondar, Gondar, Ethiopia
Full list of author information is available at the end of the article

Background

Squamous intraepithelial lesions (SIL) are an abnormal growth of squamous epithelial cells of the ecto-cervix. Cervical epithelial cell abnormalities (ECA) represent a spectrum of SIL that lie along the pathway, from mild-to-severe dysplasia to invasive cancer [1]. Cervical carcinoma develops gradually through well characterized precursor lesions [2]. Greater than 99.7 % cervical cancer is attributed by *human papillomavirus* (HPV) infection. HPV usually causes a variety of benign papillo-matous lesions of the skin and mucosal basal epithelium [3, 4]. There are more than100 different HPV genotypes [5]. Based on oncogenic potential, HPV is classified as high-risk (HR) and low-risk (LR) oncogenic types. HR-HPV types, HPV 16, 18, 31, 33, 35, 39, 45, 51, 52, 56, 58, 59, 68 and 82, cause anogenital cancer [6], while infec-tion with LR-HPV types, HPV 6 and 11, is associated with benign genital warts. HR-HPV types are detected in 99 % of cervical cancer, and about 70 % of cervical cancer is due to HPV 16 and 18 [7].

More than half of sexually active people become in-fected with HPV during their lifetime [8]. It is estimated that in Ethiopia about 33.6 % of women in the general population has HPV infection [9]. Persistent infection with HR-HPV types over time leads to the development and progression of cervical intraepithelial neoplasia (CIN). Not all women who acquire HPV infection do de-velop CIN. Rather approximately 90 % of HPV infections clear within 2 years [10]. The peak of HPV infection in women occurs in the late teens and early twenties following sexual exposure [11, 12]. Cervical cancer asso-ciated with HPV infection also leads to infertility. There is higher incidence of ECA among women complaining of infertility [13].

Cervical ECA can be detected and classified by cyto-logical screening methods. Well organized programmes of regular gynecological screening and treatment of precancerous lesions have been very effective in prevent-ing cervical cancer [14, 15]. Cytological examination of cervical scrapping from clinically suspicious cases by Papanicolaou (Pap) cytological screening test can detect cervical ECA. The Pap smear identifies any changes in cells of the transformation zone of the cervix [16]. The Bethesda System 2001 classifies ECA into atypical squa-mous cell (ASC), low-grade squamous intraepithelial lesion (LSIL), high-grade squamous intraepithelial lesion (HSIL) and squamous cell carcinoma (SCC). ASC com-prises: ASC of undetermined significance (ASCUS) and ASC, cannot exclude HSIL (ASCH); LSIL encompasses: HPV, mild dysplasia, and CIN1; while HSIL includes: moderate and severe dysplasia, carcinoma in situ, CIN 2, and CIN 3. These categories promote specificity in the mode of treatment [17]. For patients with invasive le-sions the stage of a cervical cancer is the most important

factor in the selection of treatment modality. For women diagnosed with ASCUS and LSIL follow up with HPV-DNA testing, Pap smear or colposcopy within certain time interval is some of the management options. In general, noninvasive SIL identified using Pap smear only, are treated with superficial ablative procedures such as cryotherapy or laser therapy [18].

On a global level, 75 % of women has abnormal cervical cytology at least once in their life time which may progress to cervical cancer. Cervical cancer is the second most common women cancer worldwide of which 80 % occurs in developing countries. The higher prevalence of cervical ECA due to HPV was reported in African countries [19–21]. Current estimates indicates that in Ethiopia 4648 women are diagnosed annually with cervical cancer and 3235 die from the disease [9]. Several factors such as number of sexual partners and age of first sexual activity, smoking, immune-suppression, and presence of other sexually transmitted infection (STI) can increase the risk of developing cervical cancer [22]. Several studies revealed that human immunodeficiency virus (HIV) infection is associated with an increased risk of HPV related cervical ECA [23–25]. Mortality and morbidity due to cervical cancer is higher among HIV patients [26–28]. HIV infection and cervical cancer among women in Ethiopia are major public health prob-lems. More than 534,000 adult women are estimated to be infected with HIV and at risk of developing cervical cancer. However, Ethiopia has invested little in the infra-structure, training, and laboratory capacity required for successful cytological screening [29]. Though studies have shown that the prevalence of ECA is more common among HIV-infected than non HIV-infected women, such data in Ethiopia is limited. For the development of a ra-tional approach to the screening and the subsequent man-agement of precancerous cervical lesion in HIV-infected women, understanding of the specific risk factors associ-ated with ECA occurrence among HIV- positive women is very much important. The aim of this comparative study was to determine the prevalence of ECA and risk factors associated with its occurrence among HIV+ and HIV-women attending the Debre Markos referral hospital.

Methods

Study setting and design

A comparative cross-sectional study was conducted among HIV- and HIV + women attending at the Debre Markos referral hospital cervical cancer screening center from the 1st of March to the 30th of May, 2014. Debre Markos referral hospital is located in Debre Markos town in East Gojjam Zone 300 km North of Addis Ababa. According to July 2014 zonal statistical agency report, the town has an estimated population of 100,000. The hospital has cervical cancer screening and treatment center. The screening service is provided for all HIV+ women. All women attending the Debre Markos referral hospital during the study period for any gynecological problem were eligible for the study. Pregnant women, lactating women and women on menstrual cycle were excluded from the study. The sample size was determined using two population proportion formula with the assumption of 95 % confidence interval (CI), 5 % marginal error and 33.6 % prevalence of ECA among HIV-infected women (15) and 10 % nonresponse rate. Since there is no previous study done in Ethiopia among HIV-women, the prevalence of ECA was assumed to be 50 %. Using this assumptions the final sample size becomes 400 (200 HIV+ and 200 HIV- women). During the study period there were a total of 1600 HIV- and 2000 HIV+ women attending gynecological examination in cervical cancer screening center. The study subjects from both groups were selected by systematic random sampling method.

Socio-demographic and clinical information

Data was collected after obtaining written informed consent from each participant. A pre-tested structured questionnaire was used to collect socio-demographic and clinical information needed for the study. Socio-demographic and clinical information included in this study were age, marital status, age at first sexual intercourse, number of sexual partners, duration of oral contraceptive pills (OCP) use, condom use, alcohol use, smoking, prostitution, history of STI, CD4 + T-cell count and parity.

Cytopathological examination

The cervical smear specimens were collected by gynecologist. Cervical smears were taken with a wooden applicator stick, smeared on a microscopic slide, fixed immediately with 95 % ethanol and allowed to air dry. The smears were stained with Pap stain, examined and graded according to the criteria of Bethesda classification system [17]. To ensure the quality of Pap smear results, 20 randomly selected patients were evaluated by gynecologist with colposcopic examination and visual inspection. Moreover, representative smears were reexamined by pathologists at the University of Gondar hospital blinded from the first results. In this regard 30 randomly selected positive and negative slides were blindly rechecked by a pathologist.

HIV test and CD4+ T cell count

HIV counseling and testing based the national guideline was offered to participants unaware of their HIV status. Whole blood sample of 8 ml was collected from each study subject for HIV testing and CD4+ T-cell counts. HIV testing was done based on current national rapid HIV testing algorithms. For all HIV+ women, CD4+ T-cell counts were determined by Fluorescent Activated Cell Sorter (FACS) count (Becton Dickinson) at Debre Markos referral hospital.

Statistical analysis

Data was initially registered in a registration book and transferred to excel Microsoft spread sheet. Data was cleaned and checked for completeness before analysis using SPSS version 20 computer software. Descriptive statistical analysis was used to determine the socio – demographic and clinical characteristics of study participants and prevalence of cervical ECA. The prevalence of ECA was stratified by study subjects' HIV status. Associations of patient characteristics with ECA were assessed using a series of bivariate logistic regression analysis. Then, to control simultaneously for the possible confounding effects of the different variables; a multivariable model was fitted with stepwise variable selection among variables having p-value ≤ 0.2 at bivariate analysis. In both bivariate and multivariate analyses, the associations were expressed in odds ratios (OR) and 95 % CI. For all cases p-value <0.05 were considered statistically significant.

Ethical approval

The study was reviewed and approved by ethical review committee of School of Biomedical and Laboratory Sciences, College of Medicine and Health sciences, University of Gondar and official permission was obtained from Debre Markos referral hospital higher management. A written informed consent was obtained from each study participant. All Pap smear positive results were referred to the department of obstetrics and gynecology for immediate treatment. The patients record were made anonymous and any identifying information were removed prior to analysis. Individual records were coded and accessed only by research staff members.

Results

Consistency of microscopy and colposcopic examinations

Pap smear microscopic examination was undertaken initially by trained laboratory technologist. Results obtained were compared with results obtained by a pathologist and gynecologist for consistency. In this regard, ten positive Pap smeared slides were given to three of the readers and examined blindly. There was no discrepancy between the results of the laboratory technologist and the pathologist or the gynecologist results except for one sample that was diagnosed as LSIL by the laboratory technologist but as ASCUS by the pathologist (Table 1).

Table 1 Consistency of the results of the 3 readers

Sample No	Reader A			Reader B			Reader C		
	Method	Result	Grade	Method	Result	Grade	Method	Result	Grade
20	Msy	ECA	1	Msy	ECA	1	Cpy	ECA	-
55	Msy	ECA	2	Msy	ECA	2	Cpy	ECA	-
90	Msy	ECA	3	Msy	ECA	3	Cpy	ECA	-
111	Msy	ECA	1	Msy	ECA	1	Cpy	ECA	-
146	Msy	ECA	2	Msy	ECA	2	Cpy	ECA	-
244	Msy	ECA	2	Msy	ECA	1	Cpy	ECA	-
281	Msy	ECA	1	Msy	ECA	1	Cpy	ECA	-
307	Msy	ECA	1	Msy	ECA	1	Cpy	ECA	-
331	Msy	ECA	3	Msy	ECA	3	Cpy	ECA	-
343	Msy	ECA	1	Msy	ECA	1	Cpy	ECA	-

Reader A trained data collector, *Reader B* pathologist, *Reader C* Gynecologist, *Msy* Microscopy, *Cpy* Colposcopy, *ECA* Epithelial cell abnormality, *Grade 1* atypical squamous cell undetermined significance, *Grade 2* Low grade squamous intraepithelial lesion, *Grade 3* High grade squamous intraepithelial lesion, *Grade 4* squamous cell carcinoma

Socio-demographic data and clinical characteristics of the patients

A total of 400 women (200 HIV+ and 200 HIV- women) were enrolled in the study, but 9 patients (3 HIV+ and 6 HIV-) were excluded because the smears were not adequate for evaluation. Therefore, further analyses were restricted to 391 study subjects. The mean age of the study subjects was 35.02 years with standard deviation of ±8.41 years. Two hundred and thirty (58.8 %) of the women were married, and only 65 (16.6 %) were employed. Majority of the study participants (59.1 %) were urban dwellers. Hundred and seventy six (45.0 %) of the women had no formal education (Table 2).

The number of life time sexual partners, greater than two, was higher in HIV+ women (66.6 %) as compared to HIV- ones (33.6 %). First sexual contact at early age (<18 years) was also higher among HIV+ women (56.0 %) than HIV- women (44.0 %). About 26.1 % of the study subjects had a history of STI. Two hundred and sixty seven participants (68 %) were accustomed to alcohol intake and 0.8 % was currently smoking. About 5.4 % of women used OCP for greater than 5 years and only 14.8 % of the women used condom. The number of parity greater than two was lower in HIV+ women compared to that of HIV- women (Table 3).

Clinical examination and Pap smear results

Clinical investigation was also conducted for all study subjects and 16.4 % (64/391) were found to have abnormal clinical findings. Among patients who had abnormal clinical results, 60.9 %(39/64) were positive for HIV. Abnormal vaginal discharge and contact bleeding were the most common clinical findings. In 56 (14.3 %) of the women abnormal vaginal discharge was observed, whereas 8 (2.0 %) of the women had contact bleeding. Pap smear examination revealed that

55 (14.1 %) patients were positive for cervical ECA. Higher prevalence of ECA (17.8 %) was observed in HIV+ women, of which the prevalence of ASCUS was 5.6 % (n = 11), 0.0 % ASCH, 6.1 % LSIL (n = 12), 5.1 % HSIL (n = 10) and 1.0 % SCC (n = 2). On the other hand, a 10.3 % cervical ECA prevalence was found among HIV- women with a prevalence of 4.6 % (n = 9), 0(0.0 %), 1.5 % (n = 3), 3.1 % (n = 6) and 1.0 % (n = 2) for ASCUS, ASCH, LSIL, HSIL and SCC respectively (Table 4).

The prevalence of cervical ECA was high (51.9 %) among HIV+ women with CD4 + T-cell count <200 cells/μl. The prevalence of ECA among women with CD4 + T-cell counts of 200–349 cells/μl and 350–500 cells/μl were 18.5 % (n = 10) and 12.7 % (n = 7), respectively. On the other hand, relatively low prevalence (6.6 %) of ECA was found among women with CD4 + T-cell count greater than 500/ μl (Fig. 1).

Risk factor analysis for cervical epithelial cell abnormality

Both bivariate and multivariate logistic regression analyses were employed to determine factors associated with ECA. All variables tested in the bivariate logistic regression analysis were entered into multivariate analyses if they have p-value of ≤0.2. The highest prevalence of cervical ECA (25.0 %) was observed in older age women (>45 years of old). Moreover, bivariate analysis showed that the prevalence of ECA was significantly higher among patients within the age groups of 30–45 years old and above (crude odds ratio (COR) 2.5, 95 % CI: 1.2 – 5.1, $p = 0.012$; COR 4.2, 95 % CI: 1.7 – 10.5, $p = 0.002$ respectively) as compared to younger women. Residence, educational status, condom use, smoking and alcohol consumption were not associated with the development of ECA.

Table 2 Socio-demographic characteristics of women attending cervical cancer screening center at Debre Markos referral hospital

Characteristics	HIV status		Total n %	
	Positive n (%)	Negative n (%)		
Age(in year)				
<30	73(49.0)	76(51)	149	38.1
30-45	102(51.5)	96(48.5)	198	50.6
>45	22(50.0)	22(50.0)	44	11.3
Marital status				
Married	92(40.0)	138(60.0)	230	58.8
Single	10(32.3)	21(67.7)	31	7.9
Divorced	49(69.0)	22(31.0)	71	18.2
Widowed	46(78.0)	13(22.0)	59	15.1
Marital status				
Orthodox	185(52.4)	168(47.6)	353	90.3
Muslim	5(31.2)	11(68.8)	16	4.1
Protestant	7(31.8)	15(68.2)	22	5.6
Residence				
Rural	70(43.8)	90(56.2)	160	40.9
Urban	127(55.0)	104(45.0)	231	59.1
Educational status				
Illiterate	96(54.5)	81(45.5)	176	45.0
Primary school	59(58.4)	41(40.6)	101	25.8
Secondary& above	42(37.2)	71(62.8)	113	28.9
Occupation				
Employed	24(36.9)	41(63.1)	65	16.6
House wife/Farmer	81(41.9)	112(58.1)	193	49.4
No work	32(68.1)	15(31.9)	47	12.0
Daily laborer	20(90.9)	2(9.1)	22	5.6
Commercial sex worker	8(50.0)	8(50.0)	16	4.1
Others	32(66.7)	16(33.3)	48	12.3

HIV Human immunodeficiency virus

The higher proportion of cervical ECA (63.6 %) was accounted by HIV+ women. Even though HIV infection was not found as an independent risk factor for ECA in multivariate analysis, in the bivariate analysis it was significantly associated with developing ECA (COR 1.9, 95 % CI:1.1 – 3.4, $P = 0.036$). A downward trend of the prevalence of ECA along the increment of CD4+ T-cell counts was observed among HIV+ women. Significantly higher prevalence of ECA were observed in HIV+ women with CD4+ T-cell counts <200 cells/µl (adjusted OR (AOR) 14.1, 95 % CI: 6.7 – 16.4, $p < 0.001$) and between 200 and 349 cells/µl all (AOR 9.6, 95 % CI: 1.8 – 11.5, $p = 0.008$) as compared to patients with CD4+ T-cell counts of above 500 cells/µl.

Women with a previous history of multiple lifetime sexual partners (more than two), were at high risk for developing ECA when compared to their counterparts with one or two sexual partner (AOR 3.2, 95 % CI: 1.0 – 10, $p = 0.048$). Early age at first sexual contact (<15 years) was also identified as a significant risk factor for the development of ECA (AOR 5.2, 95 % CI: 1.5– 17.9, $p = 0.009$). Association of marital status for the development of ECA was analyzed. Widowed (AOR3.2, 95 % CI: 1.2 – 8.8, $p = 0.021$) and divorced (AOR 3.0; 95 % CI: 1.1 – 8.1; $p = 0.029$) women were at higher risk than women who are married. Women with high parity (parity greater than four) were ten folds more likely to develop ECA (AOR10.9, 95 % CI; 4.2 – 16.8, $p < 0.001$) than women with parity lower than three. OCP users for more than five years were found to be at higher risk of developing ECA (AOR11.9, 95 % CI: 2.1 – 16.7, $p = 0.02$) (Table 5).

Discussion

The study showed that microscopic examination of Pap smear results by a trained laboratory technologist are comparable with the microscopic examination results of the same preparation observed by a pathologist. The current accepted practice is for the Pap smear to be examined by pathologist, while nurse responsibility is collection of the sample of cervical cells, and the technician responsibility is to prepare the slides with the pathologist responsible for slide readings and final reporting of findings. The comparable accuracy of the trained technologist reports of the Pap smear to the pathologist reports may indicate the possible utilization of trained technicians in the interpretations of Pap smears at the peripheral health facility where there is no pathologist.

In this study, 16.4 % of the women had abnormal clinical findings. The most prevalent clinical finding (13.4 %) was abnormal vaginal discharge but only 2.0 % of the women had contact bleeding. Vaginal discharge is often a normal and regular occurrence. There are, however, types of discharge that may suggest underlying infectious etiology. Such abnormal discharge was considered when the vaginal discharge was yellow or green in color, chunky in consistency, and have a foul odor. Most abnormal discharges in the study were caused by yeast or bacterial infection. The prevalence of abnormal gynecological findings such as abnormal vaginal discharge and contact bleeding of the current study was relatively lower than abnormal clinical findings reported from India which was 20 % and 6.7 % respectively [30].

In this study, the overall prevalence of cervical ECA based on Pap smear test was 14.1 % in which the prevalence of ASCUS, ASCH, LSIL, HSIL and SCC were 5.1, 0.0, 3.8, 4.1 and 1.0 % respectively. The prevalence of ECA among HIV+ women was 17.8 % which is quite

Table 3 Behavioral and clinical characteristics of women attending cervical cancer screening unit at Debre Markos referral hospital

Variable		HIV status		Total	
		Positive n (%)	Negative n (%)	N	%
No. of life time sexual partner	1-2	106(41.7)	148(58.3)	254	65.0
	>2	91(66.4)	46(33.6)	137	35.0
Age of 1st sexual contact	<18	160(56.0)	126(44.0)	286	73.1
	18-20	25(32.0)	53(68.0)	78	19.9
	>20	12(44.4)	15(55.6)	27	6.9
Alcohol use	Yes	142(53.2)	125(46.8)	267	68.3
	No	55(44.4)	69(55.6)	124	31.7
Smoking	Yes	2(66.7)	1(33.3)	3	0.8
	No	195(50.3)	193(49.7)	388	99.2
History of STI	Yes	66(64.7)	36(35.3)	102	26.1
	No	131(45.3)	158(54.7)	289	73.9
Duration of OCP usage	<5 years	43(55.8)	34(44.2)	77	19.7
	>5 years	13(61.9)	8(38.1)	21	5.4
Condom use	Always	40(69.0)	18(31.0)	58	14.8
	Some times	52(46.8)	59(53.2)	111	28.4
	Never	105(47.3)	117(52.7)	222	56.8
Parity	≤2	122(52.6))	110(47.4)	232	59.3
	3-4	39(49.4)	40(50.6)	79	20.2
	>4	36(45.0)	44(55.0)	80	20.5

HIV Human immunodeficiency virus, *OCP* Oral contraceptive pills, *STI* Sexually transmitted infection

higher than from that of ECA among HIV- women. Relatively concordant results on the prevalence of ECA among HIV-infected women were reported from Tanzania (17 %) [31] and Thailand (15.4 %) consisting of ASCUS 2.8 %, LSIL 8.5 %, and HSIL 3.5 % [32]. On the other hand, lower prevalence of ECA (2.8 %) was reported among Turkish women of which 2.2 % was ASCUS, 0.5 % LSIL, 0.1 % HSIL and 0.0 % SCC [33]. In different regions of Nigeria, Pap smear screening have shown a lower prevalence of HPV induced cervical ECA (7.6 – 13.2 %) [34, 35]. Similarly, based on Bethesda

Table 4 The prevalence of epithelial cell abnormality among women attending cervical cancer screening unit at Debre Markos referral hospital

Cervical cytology result		HIV status		Total tested	
		Positive	Negative	n	%
NIL		162(82.2 %)	174(89.7 %)	336	85.9
ECA		35(17.8 %)	20(10.3 %)	55	14.1
Types of ECA	ASCUS	11(5.6 %)	9(4.6 %)	20	5.1
	LSIL	12(6.1 %)	3(1.5 %)	15	3.8
	HSIL	10(5.1 %)	6(3.1 %)	16	4.1
	SCC	2(1.0 %)	2(1.0 %)	4	1.1

NIL Negative for intraepithelial lesion, *ECA* Cervical epithelial cell abnormality, *ASCUS* atypical squamous cell undetermined significance, *LSIL* Low grade squamous intraepithelial lesion, *HSIL* High grade squamous intraepithelial lesion, *SCC* squamous cell carcinoma, *HIV* Human immunodeficiency virus

System ECA classification, the study conducted in Nigeria among young females indicated that the prevalence of ASCUS was 7 %, LSIL 12.2 %, HSIL 7.7 % and SCC 0.7 % [35]. Another study among Italian women also reported 2.8 % ASCUS, 6.2 % LSIL and 1.7 % HSIL cervical cytological abnormalities [36]. In contrast, higher prevalence of HPV induced cervical ECA was observed in South Africa in which 41.7, 70.2 and 83 % were ASCUS, LSILS and HSIL, respectively [21]. In

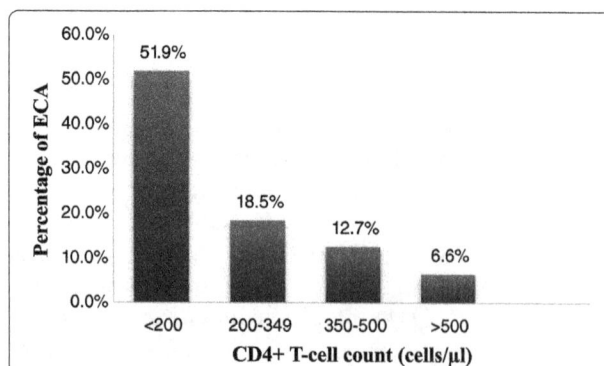

Fig. 1 Proportion of cervical epithelial cell abnormality (ECA) compared with the CD4 + T-cell count level of HIV+ women. Increasing prevalence of cervical ECA was observed along with the concomitant decreasing of CD4 + T-cell count which indicates a direct relationship between the occurrence of cervical ECA and CD4 + T-cell count level

Table 5 Bivariate and multivariate analysis of risk factors for cervical ECA among women attending cervical cancer screening unit at Debre Markos referral hospital

Variables		Cervical ECA		COR (95 % CI)	P	AOR (95 % CI)	P
		Yes	No				
		No (%)	No (%)				
Age (in year)	<30	11(7.4)	138(92.6)	1		1	
	30-45	33(16.7)	165(83.3)	2.5(1.22, 5.11)	0.012	0.8(0.30, 2.09)	0.648
	>45	11(25.0)	33(75.0)	4.2(1.67, 10.47)	0.002	0.6(0.18, 2.25)	0.493
Marital status	Married	21(9.1)	209(90.9)	1		1	
	Single	1(3.2)	30(96.8)	0.3(0.04, 2.55)	0.290	1.2(0.11,12.43)	0.869
	Divorced	15(21.1)	56(78.9)	2.7(1.29, 5.50)	0.008	3.2(1.19, 8.77)	0.021
	Widowed	18(30.5)	41(69.5)	4.4(2.14, 8.91)	0.000	3.0(1.12, 8.09)	0.029
Education	NFE	35(19.8)	142(80.2)	2.6(0.87, 7.69)	0.087	2.2(0.69, 6.67)	0.181
	Primary	16(9.5)	152(90.5)	1		1	
Occupation	Employed	6(9.2)	59(90.8)	1		1	
	HW	28(18.3)	165(81.7)	1.8(0.29, 10.76)	0.275	0.4(0.10, 1.88)	0.536
	DL	10(16.7)	50(83.3)	2.9(0.64, 12.86)	0.167	0.3(0.05, 1.86)	0.205
	CSW	4(18.2)	18(81.8)	1.6(0.27,9.93)	0.004	0.1(0.01, 0.95)	0.046
	Others	7(14.6)	41(85.4)	2.6(0.80, 8.25)	0.081	0.8(0.17, 1.16)	0.112
Age of 1st sex (in year)	<15	42(23.5)	137(76.5)	7.7(2.68, 22.28)	<0.001	5.2(1.49, 17.95)	0.009
	15-18	9(8.4)	98(91.6)	2.3(069, 7.77)	0.173	2.4(0.61, 9.49)	0.208
	>18	4(3.8)	101(96.2)	1		1	
No. of sexual partner	1-2	21(8.3)	233(91.7)	1		1	
	3-4	34(24.8)	103(75.2)	3.6(1.84, 6.96)	<0.001	3.2(1.00, 10.03)	0.048
History of STI	Yes	21(20.6)	81(79.4)	1.9(1.06, 3.53)	0.029	1.5(0.67, 3.42)	0.314
	No	34(11.8)	255(88.2)	1		1	
OCP user (in year)	<5	7(9.1)	70(90.9)	1		1	
	≥5	16(76.2)	5(23.8)	30.0(7.6, 118.37)	<0.001	11.9(2.11, 16.69)	0.020
	No	14(11.3)	110(88.7)	1		1	
Parity	≤2	13(5.6)	219(94.4)	1		1	
	3-4	6(10.7)	50(89.3)	3.2(1.36, 7.30)	0.007	1.7(0.53, 5.44)	0.362
	>4	36(35.0)	67(65.0)	7.9(3.67, 16.92)	<0.001	10.9(4.16, 16.75)	<0.001
HIV status	Negative	20(10.3)	174(89.7)	1		1	
	Positive	35(17.8)	162(82.2)	1.9(1.04, 3.38)	0.036	1.4(0.62, 3.16)	0.410
CD4 + T-cell count (cells/ μl)	<200	14(51.9)	13(48.1)	15.3(4.33, 54.31)	<0.001	14.1(6.69, 16.4)	<0.001
	200-349	10(18.5)	44(81.5)	3.2(0.95, 11.01)	0.060	9.6(1.79, 11.54)	0.008
	350-500	7(12.7)	48(87.3)	2.1(0.57, 7.52)	0.265	5.8(0.98,31.62)	0.052
	>500	4(6.6)	57(93.4)	1		1	

HIV Human immunodeficiency virus, *COR* crude odds ratio, *AOR* adjusted odds ratio, *CI* confidence interval, *P* p- value, *OCP* Oral contraceptive pills, *STI* Sexually transmitted infection, *NFE* No formal education, *CSW* Commercial sex worker, *HW* House wife, *DL* Daily laborer

another study carried among Turkish women, higher prevalence of ECA (54.8 %) was observed. The prevalence of ASCUS was 36.7 %, LSIL 16.8 %, HSIL 1.3 % [37]. The discrepancy in the prevalence of ECA between these studies may be due to differences in the study population. Higher prevalence of ECA observed from our finding and the report from South Africa may be due to the inclusion of high number of

HIV-infected women. HIV is reported as one of the independent risk factor for development of cervical ECA and cervical cancer.

Women in the age groups of 30 years and older were at greater risk of developing ECA in the present study. There are also some other study findings which indicate that older age women had greater risk for the development of ECA. Cervical cancer mortality, usually occurring among unscreened women, increases with age, with the maximum mortality rate reported for white women between age 45 years and 70 years, and for black women in their 70s [38, 39]. Mortality among women with negative Pap smear screening is low at all ages. The prevalence of SCC and ASCUS were 36.4 and 81.8 % respectively among women <30 years of age. ASCUS was found to be highest in the youngest age group women in this study.

The study participants were stratified by their HIV status and data of 197 (50.4 %) HIV+ and 194 (49.6 %) HIV- women were analyzed. We found higher prevalence of cervical ECA (17.8 %) among HIV+ women as compared to HIV- women (10.3 %). This finding was very similar to the study finding reported from Brazil where ECA was more common in the HIV+ group (12.1 %) compared to the HIV- group (5.4 %) [40]. In a study finding reported from India, all cervical ECA (26.35 %) were found among HIV+ women [41]. HIV infection is one of the major risk factor that contributes for the growth of cervical ECA. HIV leads to an increased risk of CIN and cervical cancer [40]. Up to 20 % of HIV co-infected patients develop HPV-induced premalignant lesions of the uterine cervix within three years of HIV diagnosis [42]. Progression of an untreated HPV-induced dysplastic lesion can lead to invasive cervical cancer, an AIDS defining illness [43].

Moreover, the prevalence of ECA in this study was significantly higher among HIV+ women with lower CD4 + T-cell counts of < 350 cells/μl. Statistically significant downward trends of the prevalence of ECA along the increment of CD4+ T-cell counts in HIV+ women was observed in the present study. Similarly, higher prevalence of ECA among HIV+ women with lower CD + T-cell counts of <200 cells/μl was reported [40, 44]. There are study reports that documented the higher risk of cervical ECA when CD4+ T-cell counts fall below < 200 cells/μl [25, 28]. Decreased CD4+ T-cells count and increased HIV-RNA levels are risk factors for CIN. In addition, it has also been shown that with decreasing numbers of CD4+ T-cells, there is an increase in both frequency and severity of cervical dysplasia in HIV-infected women [36, 45]. Significant correlation was reported between low levels of CD4+ T-cells, high HIV-viral load and risk of CIN [46]. A Brazilian study demonstrated that immunosuppressed women had a higher risk of lesion recurrence as compared to women with a CD4+ T-cells count > 200 cells/μl [47].

In our study widowed (30.5 %) and divorced (21.1 %) women were significantly at higher risk for the development of ECA when compared to married (9.1 %) women. This difference might be due to divorced and widowed women may have multiple

sexual partners when compared to married women. This finding is supported by the report from Ghana in which higher prevalence of ECA (21.3 %) was observed in polygamous women when compared to monogamous women (13.9 %) [48]. In this study, women with a history of STI were 1.5 times more likely to develop cervical ECA than women with no history of STI. Previous reports also demonstrated that genital infections were risk factors for the acquisition of HPV infection and the progression of cervical cancer [35, 43, 44].

We identified earlier initiation of first sexual contact (<15 years) as a significant risk factor for the development of ECA. Women with previous history of multiple life time sexual partners (more than two) were also at high risk for developing ECA which is supported by the study reported from Tanzania (44). Another most important finding of this study was that women with higher parity (greater than four) were 10.9 times more likely to develop ECA as compared to women with parity less than three. OCP users for more than 5 years had higher risk for the presence of ECA than their counterparts. Similar study supported that the prevalence of cervical cancer associated death in Ghana [48] among OCP users was higher.

Limitation

The limitation of this study is that the number of study participants is relatively small for an epidemiological study; the results may only be applied to Northwest Ethiopia. Most of the study subjects were patients with gynecological problems which may not represent the general population. The result of this study also may not represent the hospital catchment population for most of women attending the cervical screening center are HIV+. The short duration of the study did not allow the adequate follow up of the disease progression. Moreover, the study didn't further assess the etiology of the ECA.

Conclusions

Women infected with HIV had a greater risk of developing cervical ECA than HIV- women. There was a downward trend of the prevalence of ECA along the increment of CD4+ T-cell counts among HIV-infected women. Lower CD4+ T-cell counts of below 350 cells/μl, earlier initiation of first sexual contact (at the age of <15 years), parity greater than four, being widowed and divorced, multiple sexual partnership (more than three partners) and long term OCP use were significant predictors of increased risk of cervical ECA. Hence, cytological screening program should be targeting specifically HIV+ women. Awareness creation on risk factors as multiple sexual partnership and sexual initiation at earlier age should be provided.

Abbreviations
ASCUS: Atypical squamous cell undetermined significance; CIN: Cervical intraepithelial neoplasia; ECA: Cervical epithelial cell abnormality; HIV: Human immunodeficiency virus; HR: High risk; HPV: *Human papillomavirus*; HSIL: High grade squamous intraepithelial lesion; LR: Low risk; LSIL: Low grade squamous intraepithelial lesion; NIL: Negative for intraepithelial lesion; OCP: Oral contraceptive pills; SCC: Squamous cell carcinoma; SIL: Squamous intraepithelial lesion; STI: Sexually transmitted infection.

Competing interests
The authors declare that they have no competing interests.

Authors' contributions
MG proposed the initial idea for the study. MG, BG and AA contributed to the study design. MG and AS collected all the data. All authors analyzed and interpreted the data. MG drafted the manuscript. All authors contributed to the writing of the manuscript. AA prepared the manuscript for publication. All authors read and approved the final manuscript.

Authors' information
MG: MSc in medical microbiology; BG: PhD, associate professor of medical microbiology; AA: MSc, lecturer in clinical microbiology; AS: MD, gynecologist, EM: Professor, MD, MPH, Pathology, Director of Global Health Program.

Acknowledgements
We would like to thank Debre Markos hospital for all the help and support provided during data collection, cytopathological examination and other laboratory investigation. We also thank the Amhara Regional Health Bureau for financial support. We gratefully acknowledge all study participants for their participation in the study. Lastly we would like to acknowledge University of Gondar department of pathology for examination of Pap smear slides.

Author details
[1]Debre Markos Referral Hospital, Debre Markos, Ethiopia. [2]Department of Medical Microbiology, School of Biomedical and Laboratory Sciences, College of Medicine and Health Sciences, University of Gondar, Gondar, Ethiopia. [3]Department of Basic Sciences, College of Osteopathic Medicine, Touro University, Vallejo, CA, USA.

References
1. Tornesello ML, Buonaguro L, Giorgi-Rossi P, Buonaguro FM. Viral and cellular biomarkers in the diagnosis of cervical intraepithelial neoplasia and cancer. Biomed Res Int. 2013;2013:519619.
2. Saslow D, Castle PE, Cox JT, Davey DD, Einstein MH, Ferris DG, et al. American Cancer Society Guideline for human papillomavirus (HPV) vaccine use to prevent cervical cancer and its precursors. CA Cancer J Clin. 2007;57:7–28.
3. Trottier H, Franco EL. The epidemiology of genital human papillomavirus infection. Vaccine. 2006;24 Suppl 1:S1–15.
4. Pande S, Jain N, Prusty BK, Bhambhani S, Gupta S, Sharma R, et al. Human papillomavirus type 16 variant analysis of E6, E7, and L1 genes and long control region in biopsy samples from cervical cancer patients in north India. J Clin Microbiol. 2008;46:1060–6.
5. Gagnon S, Hankins C, Tremblay C, Forest P, Pourreaux K, Coutlée F, et al. Viral polymorphism in human papillomavirus types 33and 35 and persistent and transient infection in the genital tract of women. J Infect Dis. 2004;190:1575–85.
6. Ault KA. Epidemiology and natural history of human papillomavirus infections in the female genital tract [Review]. Infect Dis Obstet Gynecol. 2006;Suppl:40470.
7. Bosch F, Sanjose S. Chapter 1: human papillomavirus and cervical cancer–burden and assessment of causality. J Natl Cancer Inst Monogr. 2003;3–13.
8. Gillison ML, Broutian T, Pickard RK, Tong ZY, Xiao W, Kahle L, et al. Prevalence of oral HPV infection in the United States, 2009–2010. JAMA. 2012;307:693–703.
9. World Health Organization (WHO). Human Papillomavirus and Related Cancers. Summary Report Update. 2010. Available at: http://screening.iarc.fr/doc/Human%20Papillomavirus%20and%20Related%20Cancers.pdf.. Accessed on Dec 23, 2013.
10. Franco EL, Villa LL, Sobrinho JP, Prado JM, Rousseau MC, Désy M, et al. Epidemiology of acquisition and clearance of cervical human papillomavirus infection in women from a high-risk area for cervical cancer. J Infect Dis. 1999;180:1415–23.
11. Kerr DJ, Fiander AN. Towards Prevention of Cervical Cancer in Africa. 2009. Available at: www.afrox.org. Accessed on Dec 15, 2013.
12. Hariri S, Unger ER, Sternberg M, Dunne EF, Swan D, Patel S, et al. Prevalence of genital human papillomavirus among females in the United States, the National Health and Nutrition Examination Survey, 2003–2006. J Infect Dis. 2011;204:566–73.
13. Abdull Gaffar B, Kamal MO, Hasoub A. The prevalence of abnormal cervical cytology in women with infertility. Diagn Cytopathol. 2010;38:791–4.
14. Hailu A, Mariam DH. Patient side cost and its predictors for cervical cancer in Ethiopia: a cross sectional hospital based study. BMC Cancer. 2013;13:69.
15. Cutts FT, Franceschi S, Goldie S, Castellsague X, de Sanjose S, Garnett G, et al. Human papillomavirus and HPV vaccines: a review. Bull. 2007; 85(9):719–26.
16. Luyten A, Buttmann-Schweiger N, Luyten K, Mauritz C, Reinecke-Lüthge A, Pietralla M, et al. Early detection of CIN3 and cervical cancer during long-term follow-up using HPV/Pap smear co-testing and risk-adapted follow-up in locally organized screening programs. Int J Cancer. 2014;135:1408–16.
17. Solomon D, Davey D, Kurman R, Moriarty A, O'Connor D, Prey M, et al. Bethesda 2001 Workshop: The 2001 Bethesda System: terminology for reporting results of cervical cytology. JAMA. 2002;287:2114–9.
18. Mayrand MH, Duarte-Franco E, Rodrigues I, Walter SD, Hanley J, Ferenczy A, et al. Human papillomavirus DNA versus Papanicolaou screening tests for cervical cancer. N Engl J Med. 2007;357:1579–88.
19. Richter K, Becker P, Horton A, Dreyer G. Age-specific prevalence of cervical human papillomavirus infection and cytological abnormalities in women in Gauteng Province, South Africa. S Afr Med J. 2013;103:313–7.
20. Allan B, Marais DJ, Hoffman M, Shapiro S, Williamson AL. Cervical human papillomavirus (HPV) infection in South African women: implications for HPV screening and vaccine strategies. J Clin Microbiol. 2008;46:740–2.
21. Firnhaber C, Van Le H, Pettifor A, Schulze D, Michelow P, Sanne IM, et al. Association between cervical dysplasia and human papillomavirus in HIV seropositive women from Johannesburg South Africa. Cancer Causes Control. 2010;21:433–43.
22. Daniel T, Juana S. Human Papillomavirus infection and cervical cancer: pathogenesis and epidemiology. 2007. Available at: http://www.formatex.org/microbio/pdf/pages680-688.pdf. Accessed on Dec 8, 2013.
23. Kravchenko J, Akushevich I, Sudenga SL, Wilson CM, Levitan EB. ShresthaS: Transitional probability-based model for HPV clearance in HIV-1-positiveadolescent females. PLoS One. 2012;7:e30736.
24. Abraham AG, D'Souza G, Jing Y, Gange SJ, Sterling TR, Silverberg MJ, et al. Invasive cervical cancer risk among HIV-infected women: a North American multi-cohort collaboration prospective study. J Acquir Immune Defic Syndr. 2013;62:405–13.
25. Terry R. Management of patients with atypical squamous cells of undetermined significance (ASCUS) on Papanicolaou smears. J Am Osteopath Assoc. 1996;96(8):465–8.
26. Elfström KM, Herweijer E, Sundström K, Arnheim-Dahlström L. Current cervical cancer prevention strategies including cervical screening and prophylactic human papillomavirus vaccination: a review. Curr Opin Onco. 2014;26:120–9.
27. Palefsky J. HPV infection and HPV-associated neoplasia in immunocompromised women. Int J Gynaecol Obstet. 2006;94:S56–64.
28. Anastos K, Hoover DR, Burk RD, Cajigas A, Shi Q, Singh DK, et al. Risk factors for cervical precancer and cancer in HIV-infected, HPV-positive Rwandan women. PLoS One. 2010;5:e13525.
29. Combating-Cervical-Cancer-in-Ethiopia.pdf. 2010. http://www.pathfinder.org/publications-tools/pdfs/Combating-Cervical-Cancer-in-Ethiopia.pdf. Accessed on Feb 15, 2015.
30. Srivastava S, Gupta S, Roy JK. High prevalence of oncogenic HPV-16 in cervical smears of asymptomatic women of eastern Uttar Pradesh, India: a population-based study. J Biosci. 2012;37:63–72.

31. Obure J, Olola O, Swai B, Mlay P, Masenga G, Walmer D. Prevalence and
     severity of cervical squamous intraepithelial lesion in a tertiary hospital in
     northern Tanzania. Tanzan J Health Res. 2009;11:163–9.
32. Chalermchockcharoenkit A, Chayachinda C, Thamkhantho M, Komoltri C.
     Prevalence and cumulative incidence of abnormal cervical cytology among
     HIV-infected Thai women: a 5.5-year retrospective cohort study. BMC Infect
     Dis. 2011;11:8.
33. Açikgöz A, Ergör G. Cervical cancer risk levels in Turkey and compliance to
     the national cervical cancer screening standard. Asian Pac J Cancer Prev.
     2011;12:923–7.
34. Patricia A, Marco T, Suelene B. Cervical Cytopathology in a Population of
     HIV-Positive and HIV-Negative Women. J Trop Med. 2012;869758.
35. Durowade KA, Osagbemi GK, Salaudeen AG, Musa OI, Akande TM,
     Babatunde OA, et al. Prevalence and risk factors of cervical cancer among
     women in an urban community of Kwara State, north central Nigeria. J Prev
     Med Hyg. 2012;53:213–9.
36. Meloni A, Pilia R, Campagna M, Usai A, Masia G, Caredda V, et al. Prevalence
     and molecular epidemiology of human papillomavirus infection in Italian
     women with cervical cytological abnormalities. J Public Health Res.
     2014;3:157.
37. Atilgan R, Celik A, Boztosun A, Ilter E, Yalta T, Ozercan R. Evaluation of
     cervical cytological abnormalities in Turkish population. Indian J Pathol
     Microbiol. 2012;55:52–5.
38. Saslow D, Runowicz CD, Solomon D, Moscicki AB, Smith RA, Eyre HJ, et al.
     American Cancer Society guideline for the early detection of cervical
     neoplasia and cancer. CA Cancer J Clin. 2002;52:342–62.
39. National Institutes of Health Consensus Development Conference
     Statement: cervical cancer, April 1–3. National Institutes of Health Consensus
     Development Panel. J Natl Cancer Inst Monogr. 1996;1996:vii–xix.
40. Heard I, Tassie JM, Schmitz V, Mandelbrot L, Kazatchkine MD, Orth G.
     Increased risk of cervical disease among human immunodeficiency
     virus-infected women with severe immunosuppression and high human
     papillomavirus load(1). Obstet Gynecol. 2000;96:403–9.
41. Lima MA, Tafuri A, Araújo AC, Lima LM, Melo VH. Cervical intraepithelial
     neoplasia recurrence after colonization in HIV-positive and HIV-negative
     women. IntJ Gynecol Obstet. 2009;104:100–04.
42. Jamieson DJ, Duerr A, Burk R, Klein RS, Paramsothy P, Schuman P, et al.
     Characterization of genital human papillomavirus infection in women who
     have or who are at risk of having HIV infection. Am J Obstet Gynecol.
     2002;186:21–7.
43. Hatuvedi AK, Madeleine MM, Biggar RJ, Engels EA. Risk of human
     papillomavirus -associated cancers among persons with AIDS. J Natl Cancer
     Inst. 2009;101:1120–30.
44. Kafuruki L, Rambau PF, Massinde A, Masalu N. Prevalence and predictors of
     cervical intraepithelial neoplasia among HIV infected women at Bugando
     Medical Centre, Mwanza-Tanzania. Infect Agent Cancer. 2013;8(1):45.
45. Harris TG, Burk RD, Palefsky JM, Massad LS, Bang JY, Anastos K, et al.
     Incidence of cervical squamous intraepithelial lesions associated with HIV
     sero-status, CD4 cell counts, and human papillomavirus test results. JAMA.
     2005;293:1471–6.
46. Hawes SE, Critchlow CW, Sow PS, Touré P, N'Doye I, Diop A, et al. Incident
     high-grade squamous intraepithelial lesions in Senegales women with and
     without human immunodeficiency virus type 1 (HIV-1) and HIV-2. J Natl
     Cancer Inst. 2006;98:100–9.
47. Russomano F, Paz BR, Camargo MJ, Grinstejn BG, Friedman RK, Tristao MA,
     et al. Recurrence of cervical intraepithelial neoplasia in human
     immunodeficiency virus-infected women treated by means of
     electrosurgical excision of the transformation zone (LLETZ) in Rio de Janeiro,
     Brazil. Sao Paulo Med J. 2013;131(6):405–10.
48. Domfeh A, Wiredu E, Adjei A, Ayeh-Kumi P, Adiku T, Tettey Y, et al. Cervical
     human papillomavirus infection in Accra, Ghana. Ghana Med J. 2008;42:71–8.

16

A putative role for homocysteine in the pathophysiology of acute bacterial meningitis in children

Roney Santos Coimbra[1*], Bruno Frederico Aguilar Calegare[2], Talitah Michel Sanchez Candiani[3] and Vânia D'Almeida[2]

Abstract

Background: Acute bacterial meningitis frequently causes cortical and hippocampal neuron loss leading to permanent neurological sequelae. Neuron death in acute bacterial meningitis involves the excessive activation of NMDA receptors and p53-mediated apoptosis, and the latter is triggered by the depletion of NAD + and ATP cellular stores by the DNA repair enzyme poly(ADP-ribose) polymerase. This enzyme is activated during acute bacterial meningitis in response to DNA damage induced, on its turn, by reactive oxygen and nitrogen species. An excess of homocysteine can also induce this cascade of events in hippocampal neurons.
The present work aimed at investigating the possible involvement of homocysteine in the pathophysiology of meningitis by comparing its concentrations in cerebrospinal fluid (CSF) samples from children with viral or acute bacterial meningitis, and control individuals.

Methods: Homocysteine and cysteine concentrations were assessed by high-performance liquid chromatography in CSF samples from nine patients with acute bacterial meningitis, 13 patients with viral meningitis and 18 controls (median age: 4 years-old; range: <1 to 13) collected by lumbar puncture at admission at the Children's Hospital Joao Paulo II - FHEMIG, from January 2010 to November 2011.

Results: We found that homocysteine accumulates up to neurotoxic levels within the central nervous system of patients with acute bacterial meningitis, but not in those with viral meningitis or control individuals. No correlation was found between homocysteine and cysteine concentrations and the cerebrospinal fluid standard cytochemical parameters.

Conclusions: Our results suggest that HCY is produced intrathecally in response to acute bacterial meningitis and accumulates within the central nervous system reaching potentially neurotoxic levels. This is the first work to propose a role for HCY in the pathophysiology of brain damage associated with acute bacterial meningitis.

Keywords: Acute bacterial meningitis, Homocysteine, Neurotoxicity

Background

Meningitis is the inflammation of the meninges, the protective membranes covering the brain and the spinal cord. According to the etiology, meningitis is classified as viral (VM), also called aseptic meningitis, or bacterial (BM). VM is mainly caused by enteroviruses and is considered to be typically benign, with an auto-limited course being rarely associated to bad prognostic. As opposite, acute BM is ranked among the ten leading causes of death by infectious diseases worldwide [1]. The main etiological agents of BM are *Streptococcus pneumoniae*, *Neisseria meningitidis*, and *Haemophilus influenzae* type b. Despite significant advances in antimicrobial and intensive care therapies in the last decades, mortality rates associated with BM remain as high as 30%, and among the patients who survive the infection, 30 to 50% have permanent neurological sequelae which include deafness, sensory-motor deficits, seizure disorders, cerebral palsy, mental retardation, and learning impairment associated to neuronal injury [2].

* Correspondence: roney.s.coimbra@cpqrr.fiocruz.br
[1]Biosystems Informatics, Research Center Rene Rachou, FIOCRUZ, Av. Augusto de Lima 1715, Belo Horizonte, MG Zip Code: 30190-002, Brazil
Full list of author information is available at the end of the article

The neurological sequelae associated to meningitis are mainly due to neuron loss by necrosis in the cerebral cortex, and by apoptosis in the hippocampal dentate granule cells [3-5]. The cascade of events that triggers neuronal apoptosis during BM involves the excessive activation of the DNA repair enzyme poly(ADP-ribose) polymerase (PARP) which synthesizes ADP-ribose polymers in response to DNA damage [6]. This process comes at a very high-energy cost depleting NAD + and ATP and thereby causing cell death. PARP may provide a linkage between oxidative DNA damage and apoptosis or necrosis during BM depending upon the severity of the ATP and NAD + withdrawal. Homocysteine (HCY) is a sulfur amino acid produced from methionine by a methylation cycle [7]. HCY induces neuronal apoptotic death by over stimulating N-methyl-D-aspartate (NMDA) receptors [8,9] and by enhancing the production of free radicals [10,11], two hallmarks of the pathophysiology of acute BM [12-14]. Furthermore, elevated HCY levels in the nucleus of cells may induce DNA strand breaks by disturbing the DNA methylation cycle [15]. Consistent with this hypothesis, Kruman et al. [16] have shown a major role for PARP activation in HCY-induced neuronal apoptosis and increased neuronal vulnerability to excitotoxicity.

Thus, this study aims to investigate the possible involvement of HCY in the pathophysiology of meningitis by comparing its levels and those of cysteine (CYS), another sulfur amino acid two steps downstream to HCY in the same pathway, in cerebrospinal fluid (CSF) samples from infant patients with acute BM, VM, and control children.

Methods

HCY and CYS levels were assessed by high-performance liquid chromatography (HPLC) in CSF samples collected by lumbar puncture from 40 children (median age: 4 years-old; range: <1 to 13 years) at admission at the Children's Hospital João Paulo II – FHEMIG, Belo Horizonte, Brazil, with suspected meningitis from January 2010 to November 2011. The cohort comprised: a) nine patients with acute BM confirmed by CSF culture and/or latex agglutination test, being six infected with pneumococci and three with meningococci; b) 13 patients with VM, who had clinical signs of meningitis but presented normal or slightly altered cytochemical parameters in CSF, and negative CSF and blood latex and culture for bacterial pathogens [1]; c) 18 controls subjects attending the hospital because of a suspect of meningitis, but who had no infection of the central nervous system (CNS) or neurodegenerative diseases at the definitive diagnostic. The standard CSF cytochemical parameters assessed for diagnostic purpose immediately after puncture were protein and glucose concentrations,

white blood cell count and percentage of polymorphonuclear neutrophils [17]. Patients previously treated with antibiotics, or whose CSF samples contained more than 50 erythrocytes per mm^3, indicating blood contamination due to puncture accident, were excluded. All patients included in this study survived meningitis, but one children who had pneumococcal meningitis developed total hearing loss in one ear. An aliquot of the CSF sample was centrifuged at 5.000 rpm for 10 minutes, at 4°C, and the supernatant was stored at -80°C.

HCY and CYS concentrations in CSF samples were measured by high-performance liquid chromatography (HPLC) with fluorimetric detection after derivatization of sulfur amino acids with fluorescent 7-fluorobenzofurazan-4-sulfonic acid as previously published [18]. Calibration curves were linear up to 200 μM and 800 μM for homocysteine and cysteine, respectively. The limit of detection for homocysteine was 0.16 μM. For statistical analysis, HCY and CYS concentrations below the detection limit of the method were arbitrarily assigned to zero.

The variances of medians of all groups were compared using the Kruskal-Wallis test and, subsequently, pairs of groups were compared using the Dunn's test. Correlations were tested using the Spearman's test. The threshold for statistical significance was p <0.05. These statistical analyses were performed with the package GraphPad Prism 5.01 (GraphPad Software, Inc., La Jolla, CA, USA).

This study was approved by the Brazilian Committee for Ethical Research (process number: 25000.199054/2008-18). The guardians of all patients were informed about the study and signed a consent form.

Results and discussion

The HCY and CYS medians of the three groups varied significantly (p <0.005). HCY and CYS concentrations were increased in the CSF of patients with BM, regardless of the pathogen when compared to controls or patients with VM (Table 1). The median concentration of HCY in the CSF of patients with BM (0.69 μM) was higher than the lowest concentration reported to induce apoptosis in cultured hippocampal neurons (0.5 μM) [16]. In addition, for one patient with BM, the HCY and CYS levels were measured in CSF samples collected at admission during the acute infection and after cure (HCY: 0.690 vs. 0 μM; CYS: 51.231 vs. 0 μM). These results indicate that the HCY and CYS levels were increased during acute BM, dropping to normal levels after cure. No correlations were found between HCY or CYS levels and the standard CSF cytochemical parameters.

This is the first work reporting the association between increased HCY levels within the CNS and the pathophysiology of acute BM. The specific increase in HCY concentrations in the CSF of children with acute

Table 1 Cytochemical parameters in the CSF of patients with meningitis and controls

	BM (n =9) Mean ± SD (range)	Median	VM (n =13) Mean ± SD (range)	Median	Ctrl (n =18) Mean ± SD (range)	Median
HCY (µM)	1.08 ± 1.43 (0.0 – 4.37)	0.69*†	0 (-)	0*	0.05 ± 0.16 (0.0 – 0.52)	0†
CYS (µM)	30.77 ± 18.46 (13.37 – 67.64)	29.34*†	8.41 ± 5.49 (0.0 – 19.92)	8.19*	7.72 ± 4.70 (0.0 – 16.48)	8.33†
% PMN	77.89 ± 27.86 (5 – 95)	86*	35.92 ± 37.38 (0 – 95)	19	16.22 ± 26.43	3.5*
WBC /µL	1383 ± 2131 (18 – 5600)	120*	75.38 ± 92.96 (8 – 348)	50†	4.05 ± 4.10 (1 – 9)	2.5*†
Protein (mg/dL)	157.83 ± 136.1 (35 – 441)	117*†	32.67 ± 12.49 (20 – 56.6)	26*	33.34 ± 18.98 (20 – 85)	26.15†
Glucose (mg/dL)	48 ± 15.67 (20 – 71)	48	53 ± 19.62 (40 – 72)	57.5	60.94 ± 9.59 (50 – 84)	60

BM = bacterial meningitis; VM = viral meningitis; Ctrl = controls; HCY = homocysteine; CYS = cysteine; WBC = white blood cell; PMN = polymorphonuclear neutrophils; SD = standard deviation; * or † = p <0.05.

BM, and the absence of correlation between HCY and CYS or the standard CSF cytochemical parameters indicate that the local production of HCY in the intrathecal space is part of the host response to the pneumococci or meningococci invasion of the CNS. The intrathecal accumulation of HCY at potentially neurotoxic levels [16] strongly support the hypothesis that this sulphur amino acid may play a pivotal role in the pathophysiological processes that lead to neuron death and brain damage associated with acute BM. In agreement with these conclusions, Qureshi et al. [19] have previously reported increased HCY levels in CSF samples of adults with tuberculous meningitis compared to those with aseptic meningitis or controls. However, these authors did not investigate HCY levels in children with acute BM. The HCY concentrations in adult patients with aseptic meningitis and control adults reported by Qureshi et al. were higher than those reported herein for children. This may be explained by the differences in the average age of the patients enrolled in these two studies. Indeed, previously reported reference values for HCY in the CSF from healthy adults ranged from 1.28 to 0.66 µM [20], while for healthy children these reference values were lower than 0,10 µM [21].

Conclusions

The results presented herein, in the light of the current biomedical literature, suggest that the excess of homocysteine within the central nervous system may play a pivotal role in the pathophysiology of acute bacterial meningitis. Further investigations with larger cohorts and additional studies using animal models are still needed in order to assess the association between increased HCY levels within the CNS and the development of brain damage and permanent neurological sequelae after acute BM. If this association can be definitely established, new adjuvant therapies to prevent brain damage in BM will be conceivable targeting key enzymes of the homocysteine pathway.

Abbreviations
BM: Bacterial meningitis; CNS: Central nervous system; CSF: Cerebrospinal fluid; CYS: Cysteine; HCY: Homocysteine; HPLC: High-performance liquid chromatography; NMDA: N-methyl-D-aspartate; PARP: Poly(ADP-ribose) polymerase; VM: Viral meningitis.

Competing interests
The authors declare that they have no competing interests.

Authors' contributions
RSC – conceived, designed and coordinated this study, did the biochemical and statistical analysis, and wrote the manuscript. BFAC – contributed significantly to the biochemical analysis and critically reviewed the manuscript. TMSC – recruited the patients, collected the samples and clinical data, and critically reviewed the manuscript. VD'A – contributed significantly to the experimental design, data analysis, and critically reviewed the manuscript. All authors read and approved the final manuscript.

Acknowledgements
This work received financial support from FAPEMIG, CNPq, FAPESP and AFIP.

Author details
[1]Biosystems Informatics, Research Center Rene Rachou, FIOCRUZ, Av. Augusto de Lima 1715, Belo Horizonte, MG Zip Code: 30190-002, Brazil. [2]Department of Psychobiology, Universidade Federal de São Paulo (UNIFESP/EPM), São Paulo, SP, Brazil. [3]Children's Hospital João Paulo II – FHEMIG, Belo Horizonte, MG, Brazil.

References

1. Somand D, Meurer W: **Central nervous system infections.** *Emerg Med Clin North Am* 2009, **27**(1):89–100. ix.
2. Bedford H, de Louvois J, Halket S, Peckham C, Hurley R, Harvey D: **Meningitis in infancy in England and Wales: follow up at age 5 years.** *BMJ* 2001, **323**(7312):533–536.
3. Gerber J, Brück W, Stadelmann C, Bunkowski S, Lassmann H, Nau R: **Expression of death-related proteins in dentate granule cells in human bacterial meningitis.** *Brain Pathol* 2001, **11**(4):422–431.
4. Nau R, Soto A, Brück W: **Apoptosis of neurons in the dentate gyrus in humans suffering from bacterial meningitis.** *J Neuropathol Exp Neurol* 1999, **58**(3):265–274.
5. Gianinazzi C, Grandgirard D, Imboden H, Egger L, Meli D, Bifrare Y, Joss P, Tauber M, Borner C, Leib S: **Caspase-3 mediates hippocampal apoptosis in pneumococcal meningitis.** *Acta Neuropathol* 2003, **105**(5):499–507.
6. Koedel U, Winkler F, Angele B, Fontana A, Pfister H: **Meningitis-associated central nervous system complications are mediated by the activation of poly(ADP-ribose) polymerase.** *J Cereb Blood Flow Metab* 2002, **22**(1):39–49.
7. Finkelstein J: **The metabolism of homocysteine: pathways and regulation.** *Eur J Pediatr* 1998, **157**(Suppl 2):S40–S44.
8. Lipton S, Kim W, Choi Y, Kumar S, D'Emilia D, Rayudu P, Arnelle D, Stamler J: **Neurotoxicity associated with dual actions of homocysteine at the N-methyl-D-aspartate receptor.** *Proc Natl Acad Sci U S A* 1997, **94**(11):5923–5928.
9. Pullan L, Olney J, Price M, Compton R, Hood W, Michel J, Monahan J: **Excitatory amino acid receptor potency and subclass specificity of sulfur-containing amino acids.** *J Neurochem* 1987, **49**(4):1301–1307.
10. Outinen P, Sood S, Liaw P, Sarge K, Maeda N, Hirsh J, Ribau J, Podor T, Weitz J, Austin R: **Characterization of the stress-inducing effects of homocysteine.** *Biochem J* 1998, **332**(Pt 1):213–221.
11. Huang R, Huang S, Lin B, Wei J, Liu T: **Homocysteine thiolactone induces apoptotic DNA damage mediated by increased intracellular hydrogen peroxide and caspase 3 activation in HL-60 cells.** *Life Sci* 2001, **68**(25):2799–2811.
12. Leib S, Kim Y, Ferriero D, Tauber M: **Neuroprotective effect of excitatory amino acid antagonist kynurenic acid in experimental bacterial meningitis.** *J Infect Dis* 1996, **173**(1):166–171.
13. Kolarova A, Ringer R, Tauber M, Leib S: **Blockade of NMDA receptor subtype NR2B prevents seizures but not apoptosis of dentate gyrus neurons in bacterial meningitis in infant rats.** *BMC Neurosci* 2003, **4**:21.
14. Gerber J, Nau R: **Mechanisms of injury in bacterial meningitis.** *Curr Opin Neurol* 2010, **23**(3):312–318.
15. Blount B, Mack M, Wehr C, MacGregor J, Hiatt R, Wang G, Wickramasinghe S, Everson R, Ames B: **Folate deficiency causes uracil misincorporation into human DNA and chromosome breakage: implications for cancer and neuronal damage.** *Proc Natl Acad Sci U S A* 1997, **94**(7):3290–3295.
16. Kruman I, Culmsee C, Chan S, Kruman Y, Guo Z, Penix L, Mattson M: **Homocysteine elicits a DNA damage response in neurons that promotes apoptosis and hypersensitivity to excitotoxicity.** *J Neurosci* 2000, **20**(18):6920–6926.
17. Negrini B, Kelleher K, Wald E: **Cerebrospinal fluid findings in aseptic versus bacterial meningitis.** *Pediatrics* 2000, **105**(2):316–319.
18. Pfeiffer C, Huff D, Gunter E: **Rapid and accurate HPLC assay for plasma total homocysteine and cysteine in a clinical laboratory setting.** *Clin Chem* 1999, **45**(2):290–292.
19. Qureshi G, Baig S, Bednar I, Halawa A, Parvez S: **The neurochemical markers in cerebrospinal fluid to differentiate between aseptic and tuberculous meningitis.** *Neurochem Int* 1998, **32**(2):197–203.
20. Hyland K, Bottiglieri T: **Measurement of total plasma and cerebrospinal fluid homocysteine by fluorescence following high-performance liquid chromatography and precolumn derivatization with o-phthaldialdehyde.** *J Chromatogr* 1992, **579**(1):55–62.
21. Surtees R, Bowron A, Leonard J: **Cerebrospinal fluid and plasma total homocysteine and related metabolites in children with cystathionine beta-synthase deficiency: the effect of treatment.** *Pediatr Res* 1997, **42**(5):577–582.

17

Parotid gland, an exceptional localization of sebaceous carcinoma

Mouna Khmou[1,2]*, Karima Laadam[1,2] and Nadia Cherradi[1,2]

Abstract

Background: Sebaceous carcinoma (SC) is a rare malignancy, occurring predominantly in eyelids. Till date, only 25 cases of sebaceous carcinoma (SC) of the parotid gland have been reported in world literature.

Case presentation: A 33 year-old male presented with left sided laterocervical mass. Clinical examination showed enlargement of the left parotid gland, with cervical lymphadenopathy. No skin lesions were found. A resection of the gland was performed. Pathological findings were consistent with primary sebaceous carcinoma of the parotid gland.

Conclusion: Sebaceous carcinoma of the parotid gland is extremely uncommon. Clinical and radiological features are not specific. The aim of this report, is to describe histopathological, and immunohistochemical findings of this rare entity, and discuss differential diagnosis.

Keywords: Parotid, Gland, Sebaceous, Carcinoma, Rare

Background

Sebaceous glands are holocrine adnexal components of the skin, usually found in close association with hair follicles [1]. Sebaceous tumors are uncommon, and their classification is controversial [2] Predominantly occurs in eyelids [3], other sites may exceptionally be involved. In the English literature, only 25 cases of sebaceous carcinoma (SC) of the parotid gland have been reported [4]. Sebaceous carcinoma is defined by the WHO as "a malignant tumor composed of sebaceous cells of varying maturity that are arranged in sheets and/or nests with different degrees of pleomorphism, nuclear atypia, and invasiveness" [5]. Diagnosis may be difficult, given the low incidence and inconsistencies in histopathologic classification. Regardless of the location, sebaceous carcinomas must be considered as an aggressive neoplasm with a potential for regional and distant metastasis [2].

We report an additional case, discuss the clinical and pathologic features ; and briefly review of the literature,

Case presentation

A 33 year-old Moroccan male presented with left sided laterocervical mass, which had persisted for four months. No personal or family history was noted. He had no previous history of smoking, alcohol use, or irradiation. The mass had slowly grown with occasional pain. He had no fever, chills, or weight loss. Upon physical examination, the left parotid gland was enlarged, firm, with cervical lymphadenopathy, no skin lesions were found. Ultrasonography and computed tomography revealed a solid mass involving the parotid gland. A biopsy revealed a poorly differentiated carcinoma.

The patient underwent tumor excision. The excised mass measuring 21,5 × 9 × 6 cm, with skin tag measuring 11 × 10 cm. The cut surface of the tumor was firm tan-gray, lobulated, measuring 6 × 5,5 × 5 cm, with, apparently normal looking, salivary gland tissue at the peripheral margin (Fig. 1). Meticulous and extensive sampling of the tumor was done.

Histopathological examination revealed a lobulated tumor with expansive growth within parotid parenchyma (Fig. 2). It was composed of nests of two cell populations : large foamy cells with centrally located nuclei and vacuolated clear cytoplasm, surrounded by closely packed smaller basaloid cells with scanty cytoplasm (Fig. 3). Large tumor cells showed sebaceous differentiation (Fig. 4), with cellular pleomorphism, high mitotic

* Correspondence: mouna.khmou@yahoo.fr
[1]Department of Pathology, Hospital of Specialities, Rabat, Morocco
[2]Faculty of Medicine and Pharmacy Rabat, University Mohammed V Rabat, Rabat, Morocco

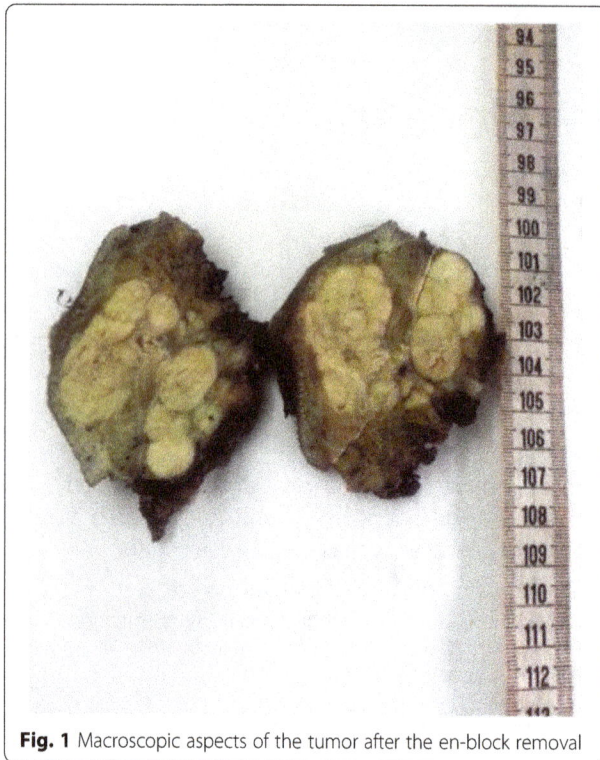

Fig. 1 Macroscopic aspects of the tumor after the en-block removal

activity (Fig. 5) and necrosis. Some areas showed squamous islands with keratin pearl formation. Periodic acid–Schiff (PAS) was negative in the foamy, large cells.

Immunohistochemical staining of the tumor showed expression of epithelial membrane antigen (EMA) (Fig. 6), pancytokeratin, and p63 in all neoplastic cells, and focaly B-Catenin. They lacked expression of CK5/6, CEA, S100, CD10, Vimentin, melan A, and CD45. The diagnosis of Sebaceous carcinoma of the parotid gland was made.

Since a recent literature review report a relation between sebaceous carcinoma and MSH2 mutation, we evaluated by immunohistochemistry MLH1 and MSH2 protein expression. Strong nuclear expression of both proteins was found (Figs. 7 and 8). All surgical margins were microscopically negative. A staging computerised tomography (CT), gastrointestinal endoscopy and colonoscopy were preformed and no tumor was found. Thus, the Muir-Torre syndrome was excluded. Adjuvant radiotherapy was decided. The patient is alive without signs of tumor recurrence after 1 year of follow-up.

Discussion

Sebaceous carcinoma was first described in the salivary glands by Rauch and Masshoff in [6]. It is a rare and aggressive malignant neoplasm usually occurring in the head and neck region [3], involving in 75 % the periocular region, particularly the upper eyelid in elderly women [2]. Only handful cases of primary salivary sebaceous carcinoma had been described, most of them involving the parotid gland, rarely the submandibular and minor salivary glands [7].

The histogenesis of sebaceous carcinoma in the parotid gland remain unclear. Sebaceous differentiation of salivary ducts is seen in both normal and chronic sialadenitis [3]. The parotid gland in the present case had mild chronic inflammation. The current hypothesis is that sebaceous carcinoma arises from pluripotent stem cells, which can differentiate into sebaceous cells [7]. It

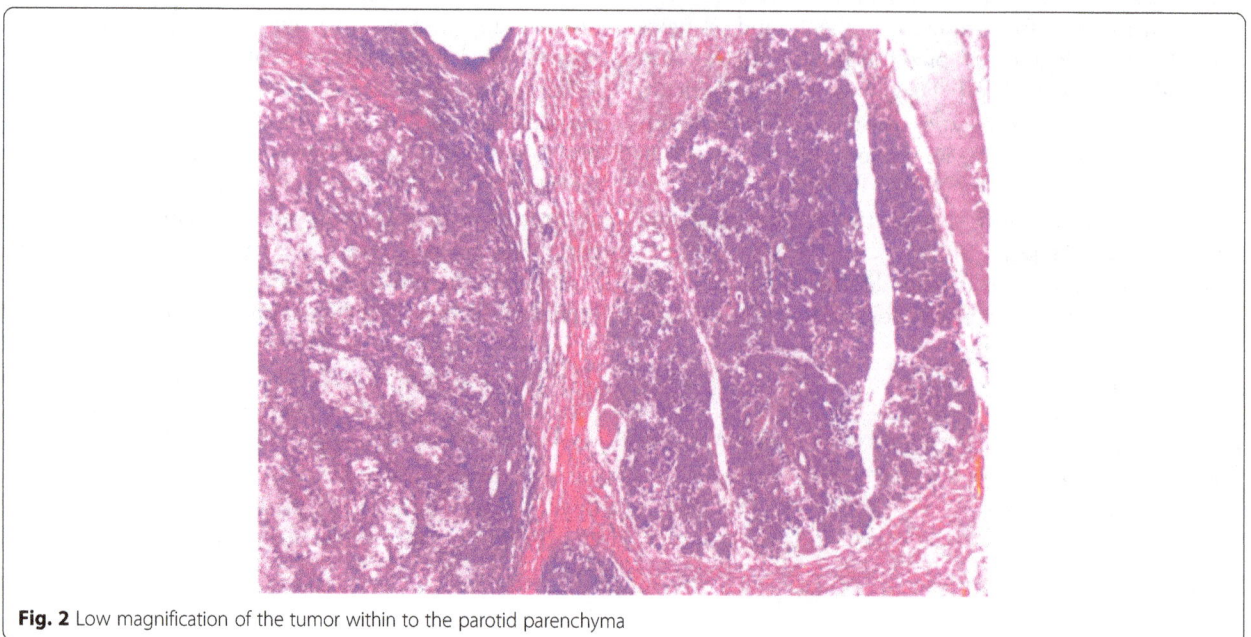

Fig. 2 Low magnification of the tumor within to the parotid parenchyma

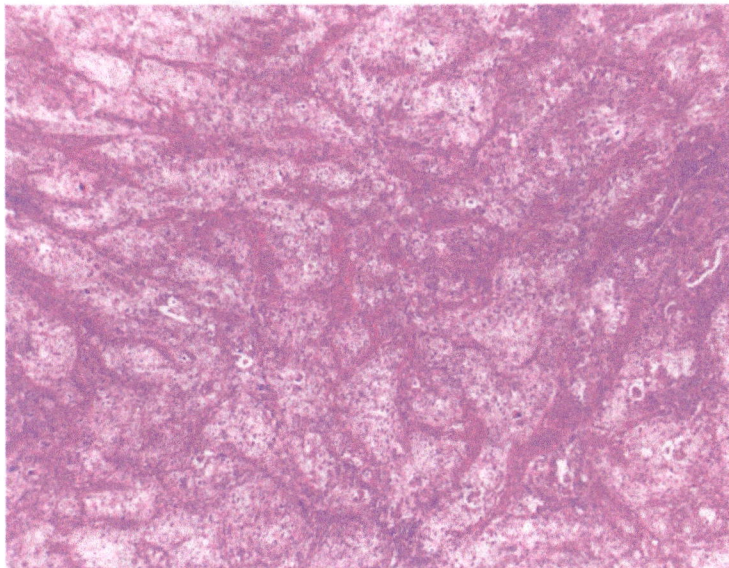

Fig. 3 The tumor lobules composed of large foamy cells surrounded by basaloid cells

is accepted that sebaceous lymphadenocarcinoma arises from sebaceous lymphadenoma, but SC of the salivary glands seems to be a de-novo lesion [2]. SC can be part of Muir-Torre syndrome (MTS), and it was suggested that expression of retinoid X receptor beta and gamma could be related to the development of SC [8]. Muir-Torre syndrome is a phenotypic variant of hereditary non-polyposis colorectal cancer (HNPCC) or Lynch syndrome. Germline mutation in hMSH2 and hMLH1 genes are often associated with this disorder [9]. The result for DNA mismatch repair genes in sporadic sebaceous carcinoma is inconclusive [3]. The most common site for sebaceous neoplasms in Muir Torre Syndrome is the eyelids and nose, and after extensive review of the literature, the association between parotid sebaceous carcinoma in Muir Torre Syndrome has been reported only once. In this present case, no association with Muir-Torre syndrome was established, and immunohisto-chemical staining showed normal nuclear expression of MLH1 and MSH2 in tumor cells.

SC in the parotid gland is reported to occur in both genders with the same incidence, and may have an increased frequency in the asian population [2]. This tumor has a bimodal age distribution, with a peak in the second decade and another one in the seventh decade of life (with a range of 6–92 years) [4].

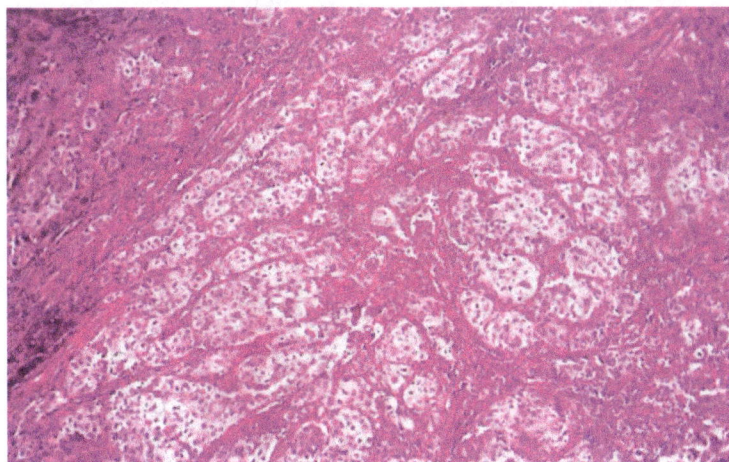

Fig. 4 numerous cells with sebaceous differentiation

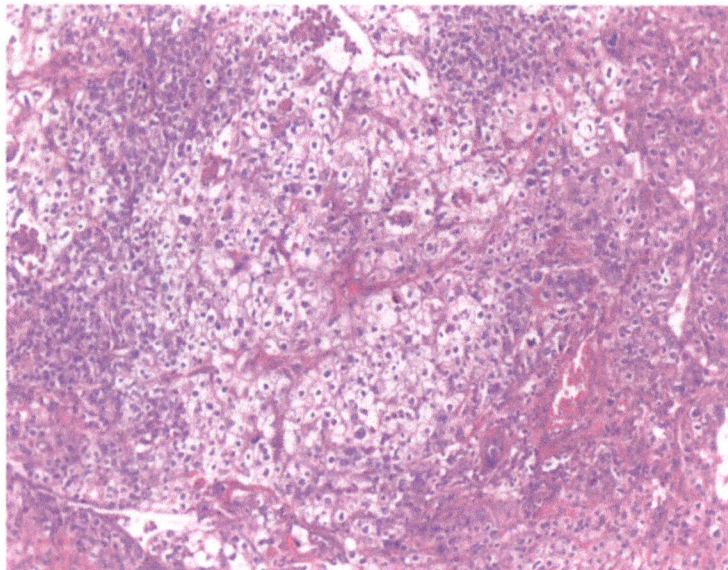

Fig. 5 Tumor cells showing nuclear atypia and mitosis

Clinically, the duration of symptoms is highly variable and ranges from few months to 20 years. SC typically present as slowgrowing swellings with variable pain, facial nerve involvement, and fixation to the overlying skin. Rare cases have arisen from a preexisting pleomorphic adenoma [10]. Our patient has no history of an untreated or recurrent pleomorphic adenoma ; also an extensive sampling of the tumor was done, and no area of residual benign mixed tumour, was found.

Grossly, tumors range in size from 0.6 to 8.5 cm, frequently appear to be well circumscribed or partially encapsulated [5], gray to tan on the cut surface [11]. Microscopically, the tumor consists of sheets, nests, or cords with expansive growth. Duct-like structures may be numerous and cystic spaces of varying sizes are occasionally present. The tumor may exhibit, pleomorphic cells with variable degrees of cytologic atypia [11]. In well-differentiated tumors, the cells have hyperchromatic nuclei and abundant, cytoplasmic foamy vacuolization,

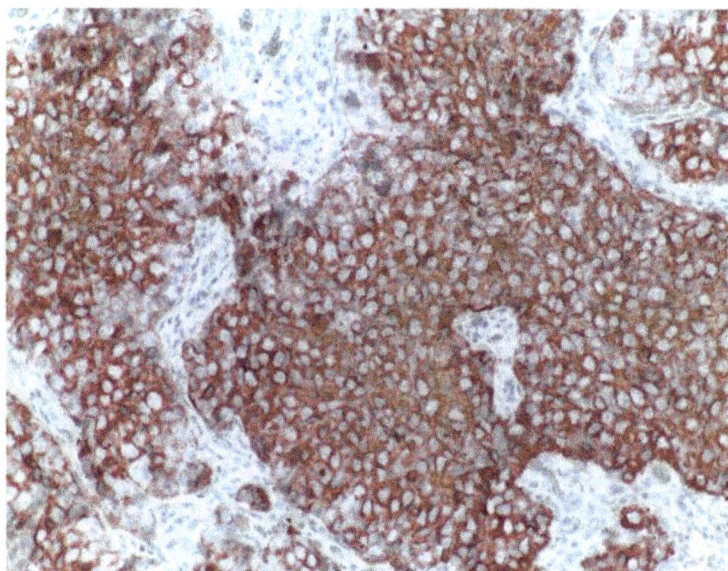

Fig. 6 Immunohistochemistry shows positive staining for EMA

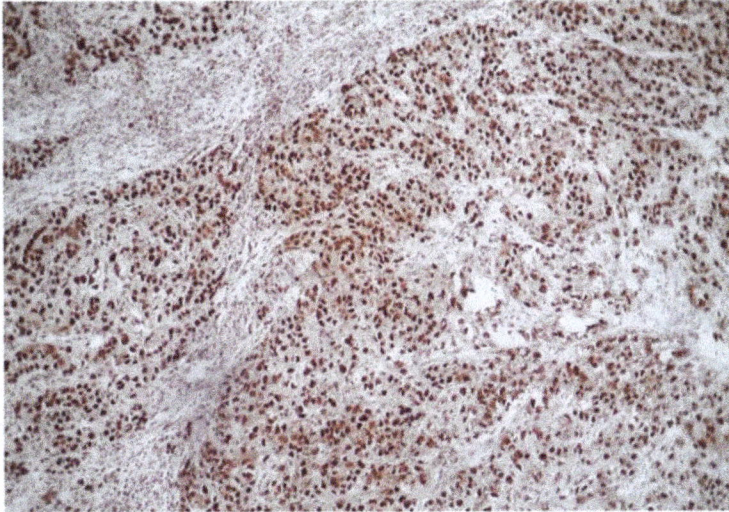

Fig. 7 Immunohistochemistry shows positive staining for MSH2 in tumor cells and lymphocytes

giving a typical sebaceous appearance [5]. Typically, sebaceous neoplasic cells are located in the central parts of the nests, which peripherally show more undifferentiated cells with scarcer cytoplasm. A transition is observed between sebaceous and undifferentiated cells [12]. Squamous differentiation in sebaceous neoplasms is common [3]. Scattered mucous cells, xanthogranulomatous reaction and oncocytic metaplasia are occasional findings [11]. A positive lipid stain, such as oil-red-O or Sudan IV, is helpful for establishing the diagnosis [1], but in most cases not possible because frozen sections are not always available [3].

Immunohistochemically, Androgen receptor (AR) is useful in the diagnosis of poorly differentiated sebaceous carcinomas [3], but there are no studies of AR in SC of the salivary glands [2]. On the contrary, SC of the breast is known to be positive for AR, indicating that expression of this receptor may be related to the site of tumor origin [2]. EMA and HMFG1 (human milk fat globule1) are expressed mainly by the sebaceous cells both in the cytoplasm and membrane, but are negative in most of the basaloid peripheral cells [2]. Several case reports and case series have confirmed the usefulness of immunohistochemistry in diagnosing SC [4]. But since most reported cases have no extensive information on this issue, further studies are needed to determine the most useful immunohistochemistry panel in the diagnosis of SC.

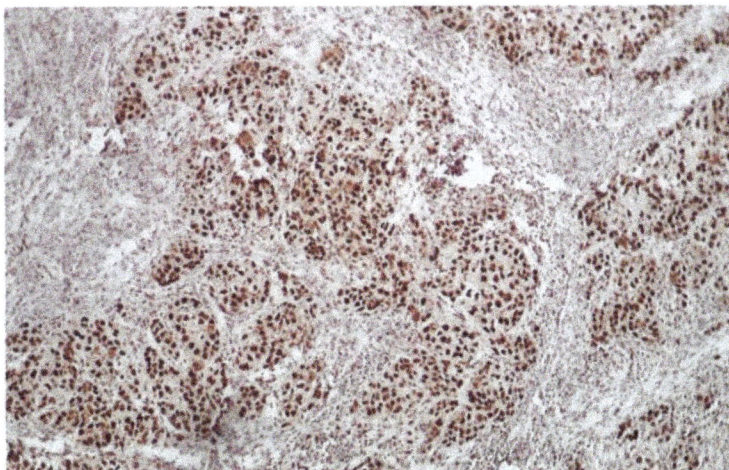

Fig. 8 Immunohistochemistry shows positive staining for MLH1 in tumor cells

Sebaceous carcinoma must be distinguished from mucoepidemoid carcinoma, poorly differentiated squamous carcinoma, basal cell carcinoma, and metastatic clear cell renal carcinoma [4].

Unlike mucoepidemoid carcinoma, PAS and D-PAS in SC stains negative. Malignant squamous cells may accumulate glycogen and demonstrate clear cytoplasm. Which can be confirmed by PAS staining, and positivity of CK5/6 on immunohistochemistry.

The lack of lymphoid tissue did not support a diagnosis of sebaceous lymphadenocarcinoma [9].

Sebaceous Epithelial-Myoepithelial Carcinoma (EMC) must be considered as a differential diagnosis. This tumor is composed by bilayered ductal structures composed of inner epithelial-type cells and outer myoepithelial cells with clear cytoplasmic. The key feature to distinguish sebaceous EMC from sebaceous carcinoma is to reveal the myoepithelial nature of the tumor cells. Mostly by using myoepithelial markers, such as calponin, a-SMA, MSA, p63, CK 14, S-100 protein, and vimentin, on immunohistochemistry [13].

The treatment of choice is wide surgical excision. Parotidectomy, extended parotidectomy, and/or neck dissection maybe required to achieve complete resection [4]. Postoperative radiotherapy and chemotherapy, in tumors with a high microscopic grade or clinical stage, has occasionally been proposed [5, 9]. Out of reported cases, 9 were treated with radiotherapy. Although most reported cases have no information on the tumor progression only 1 case treated with radiotherapy recurred [4]. This indicates the beneficial role of radiotherapy as treatment option in SC of the parotid. Our patient has no signs of tumor recurrence after 1 year after adjuvant radiotherapy. Metastasis may occur in the lung, brain, and regional lymph nodes [4].

There are too few reported cases to make accurate prognostic statements. Although extraocular cases were considered less aggressive, this is no longer accepted [2]. At least 6 cases of SC of the salivary glands have been described with recurrence and metastasis [12].

Conclusion

In summary, primary sebaceous carcinoma of the salivary glands is extremely rare and aggressive tumor, and because of its rarity, clinicopathological characteristics and histogenesis are not fully understood.

Abbreviations

SC, Sebaceous carcinoma; PAS, periodic acid–Schiff; EMA, epithelial membrane antigen; MTS, Muir-Torre syndrome; HMFG1, human milk fat globule1; EMC, Epithelial-Myoepithelial Carcinoma

Acknowledgements
We would like to thank Professor Mohamed Oukabli, Head-Department of Pathology, Mohamed V Teaching Military Hospital, Rabat.

Funding
None.

Authors' contributions
MK analyzed and interpreted the patient data, drafted the manuscript and made the figures. NC performed the histological examination, proposed the study, supervised MK and revised the manuscript. KL had made substantial contributions to analysis and interpretation of patient data. All authors read and approved the final manuscript.

Competing interest
The authors declare that they have no competing interests.

References
1. Bailet JW, Zimmerman MC, Arnstein DP, Wollman JS, Mickel RA. Sebaceous Carcinoma of the Head and Neck Case Report and Literature Review. Arch Otolaryngol Head Neck Surg. 1992;118:1245–9.
2. Altemani A, Vargas PA, Cardinali I, Aguiar SS, Lopes M, Soares AB, Speight PM, Almeida OP. Sebaceous carcinoma of the parotid gland in children: An immunohistochemical and ploidy study. Int J Oral Maxillofac Surg. 2008;37:433–40.
3. Wang H, Yao J, Solomon M, Axiotis CA. Sebaceous carcinoma of the oral cavity: a case report and review of the literature Hangjun Wang. Oral Surg Oral Med Oral Pathol Oral Radiol Endod. 2010;110:e37–40.
4. Takada Y, Kawamoto K, Baba S, Takada T, Inoue T, Tomoda K. Sebaceous Carcinoma of the Parotid Gland: A Case Report. Case Rep Oncol. 2015;8:106–12.
5. Barnes L, Eveson JW, Reichart P, et al. WHO classification of tumours, pathology and genetics, head and neck tumours. Lyon: IARC Press; 2005. p. 231.
6. Rauch S, Masshoff W. Sialoma resembling sebaceous gland. Frankf Z Pathol. 1959;69:513–25.
7. Das K, Karmakar A. Sebaceous carcinoma of parotid gland. Gomal J Med Sci. 2014;12:122-3.
8. Chakravarti N, El-Naggar AK, Lotan R, Anderson J, Diwan AH, Saadati HG, Diba R, Prieto VG, Esmaeli B. Expression of retinoid receptors in sebaceous cell carcinoma. J Cutan Pathol. 2006;33:10–7.
9. Neelakantan IV, Di Palma S, Smith CE, McCoombe A. Parotid Sebaceous Carcinoma in Patient with Muir Torre Syndrome, Caused by MSH2 Mutation. Head Neck Pathol. 2015 Nov 17. doi:10.1007/s12105-015-0670-9. [Epub ahead of print].
10. Cohn ML, Callender DL, El-Naggar AK. Sebaceous carcinoma ex-pleomorphic adenoma: a rare phenotypic occurrence. Ann Diagn Pathol. 2004;8:224–6.
11. Barnes L. Informa Healthcare; USA. Diseases of the Salivary Glands, Surgical Pathology of the Head and Neck. 2009;1:567–8. Third Edition.
12. Ohara N, Taguchi K, Yamamoto M, Nagano T, Akagi T. Sebaceous carcinoma of the submandibular gland with high-grade malignancy: Report of a case. Pathol Int. 1998;48:287–91.
13. Shinozaki A, Nagao T, Endo H, Kato N, Hirokawa M, Mizobuchi K, Komatsu M, Igarashi T, Yokoyama M, Masuda S, Sano K, Izumi M, Fukayama M, Mukai K. Sebaceous Epithelial-Myoepithelial Carcinoma of the Salivary Gland: Clinicopathologic and Immunohistochemical Analysis of 6 Cases of a New Histologic Variant. Am J Surg Pathol. 2008;32:913–23.

18

Monocarboxylate Transporter 1 (MCT1) is an independent prognostic biomarker in endometrial cancer

Ayşe Latif[1], Amy L. Chadwick[1,2], Sarah J. Kitson[2], Hannah J. Gregson[2], Vanitha N. Sivalingam[2], James Bolton[3], Rhona J. McVey[3], Stephen A. Roberts[4], Kay M. Marshall[1], Kaye J. Williams[1], Ian J. Stratford[1] and Emma J. Crosbie[2,5]* (iD)

Abstract

Background: Endometrial cancer (EC) is a major health concern due to its rising incidence. Whilst early stage disease is generally cured by surgery, advanced EC has a poor prognosis with limited treatment options. Altered energy metabolism is a hallmark of malignancy. Cancer cells drive tumour growth through aerobic glycolysis and must export lactate to maintain intracellular pH. The aim of this study was to evaluate the expression of the lactate/proton monocarboxylate transporters MCT1 and MCT4 and their chaperone CD147 in EC, with the ultimate aim of directing future drug development.

Methods: MCT1, MCT4 and CD147 expression was examined using immunohistochemical analysis in 90 endometrial tumours and correlated with clinico-pathological characteristics and survival outcomes.

Results: MCT1 and MCT4 expression was observed in the cytoplasm, the plasma membrane or both locations. CD147 was detected in the plasma membrane and associated with MCT1 ($p = 0.003$) but not with MCT4 ($p = 0.207$) expression. High MCT1 expression was associated with reduced overall survival ($p = 0.029$) and remained statistically significant after adjustment for survival covariates ($p = 0.017$).

Conclusion: Our data suggest that MCT1 expression is an important marker of poor prognosis in EC. MCT1 inhibition may have potential as a treatment for advanced or recurrent EC.

Keywords: Endometrial cancer, Monocarboxylate transporters, Hypoxia, Glycolysis

Background

In 2012, it is estimated that more than 30,000 new diagnoses of endometrial cancer (EC) were made worldwide. In the UK, EC is the fourth most common cancer in women, with more than 9000 new cases diagnosed in 2013 [1]. EC usually presents at an early stage following the onset of postmenopausal bleeding and is generally cured by hysterectomy and bilateral salpingo-oophorectomy. However, surgery can be dangerous for obese and elderly women, with significant risk of anaesthetic and surgical complications. Mainstay treatment for advanced EC includes cytotoxic chemotherapy and/or hormonal therapy. However, women with advanced, recurrent or metastatic disease have a poor prognosis with only 7-12 months median survival [2–4]. There is therefore a clear unmet clinical need for new therapies to modify disease outcome.

The rising incidence of EC over the last three decades has paralleled the obesity epidemic [1]. Clinical and epidemiological studies have shown that women with obesity and type II diabetes have an increased risk of EC [5–7]. In obese and diabetic women, tissues involved in insulin-mediated glucose uptake (such as the liver) become insulin resistant, leading to hyperglycaemia and hyperinsulinaemia [8]. The increased risk of EC is further

* Correspondence: Emma.crosbie@manchester.ac.uk
[2]Gynaecological Oncology Research Group, Division of Cancer Sciences, Faculty of Biology, Medicine and Health, University of Manchester, Level 5 – Research, St Mary's Hospital, Oxford Road, Manchester M13 9WL, UK
[5]Department of Obstetrics and Gynaecology, St Mary's Hospital, Central Manchester University Hospitals NHS Foundation Trust, Manchester Academic Health Science Centre, Manchester, UK
Full list of author information is available at the end of the article

influenced by high levels of circulating glucose acting as an energy source and contributing to metabolic adaptations in rapidly proliferating tumour cells. Most malignancies have been shown to utilise aerobic glycolysis as the predominant energy pathway (known as "the Warburg effect") [9]. As a consequence, large amounts of lactic acid are produced, which must be exported out of cells by monocarboxylate transporters (MCTs), to avoid acid-induced apoptosis.

MCTs are transmembrane proteins encoded by the SLC16A family of genes. Among all 14 MCT family members, four MCTs (MCT1-MCT4) are characterized as lactate/proton symporters. In particular, MCT4 (efflux of lactate) and MCT1 (both influx and efflux of lactate) are among the most important regulators of intracellular pH homeostasis in tumours and other high glycolytic tissues [10, 11]. Upregulation of MCTs has been shown in many malignancies including colorectal [12, 13], cervix [14], breast [15, 16], prostate [17], central nervous system [18, 19], soft tissue [20], gastrointestinal [21, 22], oral cavity [23], urothelial [24] and lung carcinomas [25] and high expression is associated with poor prognosis. Both MCT1 and 4 require association with the ancillary protein CD147 (also known as EMMPRIN or Basigin) for plasma membrane expression and activity [26–28]. CD147 is a pleiotropic plasma membrane glycoprotein that stimulates the synthesis of several matrix metalloproteinases, thus promoting tumour invasion [29–31]. Maturation and cell surface expression of CD147 is also dependent on MCT1 or MCT4 expression [32]. CD147 is upregulated [31] and linked to poor prognosis in malignancies of various origins, including endometrium [33].

The potential role of MCTs in tumour metabolism has promoted their emergence as new targets for cancer therapy. Despite evidence that MCT1, MCT4 and CD147 are poor prognostic factors in several cancer types, their significance in EC is not known. The aim of this study was to analyse the expression of MCT1, MCT4 and CD147 in EC and relate these findings to clinico-pathological features and survival outcomes.

Methods
Case selection
Ethical approval for this study was obtained from NRES Committee London - Fulham (reference 12/LO/0364). It was conducted in accordance with the conditions and principles outlined in the EU Directive 2001/20/EC and Good Clinical Practice, including the Data Protection Act 1998. Tumour tissues were obtained from 90 sequential EC patients who underwent hysterectomy (between 2011 and 2013) and donated their tumours for future research at St Mary's Hospital, Manchester, UK. All participants provided written, informed consent for their clinical data and tumour samples to be stored

anonymously and used for future research. Their paraffin-embedded tumour specimens were retrieved from the pathology archives and cut into 4-µm serial sections for immunohistochemical analysis. The median age of the cohort was 67 years (IQR range 57.7-74 years) and there were 47 endometrioid (EEC) and 43 non-endometrioid (Non-EEC) tumours. The non-EEC group comprised tumours of carcinosarcoma ($n = 11$), clear-cell ($n = 9$), serous ($n = 6$), mixed ($n = 16$) and undifferentiated (n = 1) histology. Mixed tumours were clear cell/high grade endometrioid ($n = 13$), clear cell/ high grade serous ($n = 2$) or high grade serous/ endometrioid (n = 1). Clinico-pathological data were obtained from patients' hospital medical records, original pathology results and death certificates, where appropriate, including age at diagnosis, Body Mass Index (BMI), tumour histological type, grade, Federation of Gynecology and Obstetrics (FIGO) 2009 stage, tumour size, lymphovascular space involvement (LVSI), depth of myometrial invasion, last follow-up date, date of recurrence, type of recurrence, death and cause of death (Table 1). The average follow up time was 32.4 months and there were 28 recurrences and 22 deaths, of which 12 were EC-specific.

Immunohistochemistry (IHC)
All IHC was performed using a fully automated IHC platform Leica BOND-MAX together with Bond™ Polymer Refine Detection kit (DS9800) and on-board retrieval system. The detection kit is based on a biotin-free, polymeric horseradish peroxidase (HRP)-linker antibody conjugate system for the detection of tissue-bound mouse and rabbit IgG and some mouse IgM primary antibodies. It is intended for staining sections of formalin-fixed, paraffin-embedded tissue on the Bond™ automated system. The sections were quenched using hydrogen peroxide and subjected to MCT1 (Santa Cruz, sc-365,501, 1:100 dilution), MCT4 (Santa Cruz, sc-376,140, 1:100 dilution) and CD147 (Fitzgerald Industries International, Clone UM-8D6, 1:100 dilution) primary antibody according to standard validated Protocol F written by Leica. Negative (isotype) controls were used for quality assurance. Following addition of post primary reagents the primary antibody was refined and visualized using the substrate chromogen, 3,3'-Diaminobenzidine tetrahydrochloride hydrate (DAB) via a brown precipitate. Tissue sections were counterstained with haematoxylin to visualize cell nuclei and were permanently mounted.

Immunohistochemical evaluation
Immunoreaction in sections was evaluated for whole cell staining in whole tumour sections. A semi-quantitative scoring system was devised to take into account

Table 1 Expression of MCT1, MCT4 and CD147 in EC tumours and their correlation with clinico–pathological characteristics

	N = 90 (%)	MCT1 (N = 89)			MCT4 (N = 87)			CD147 (N = 87)		
		Low (<200) N = 48 (53.9%)	High (≥200) N = 41 (46.1%)	p	Low (<200) N = 59 (67.8%)	High (≥200) N = 28 (32.2%)	p	Low (<200) N = 31 (35.6%)	High (≥200) N = 56 (64.4%)	p
Age of Onset (Median, IQR years)	67 (57.7–74)	69 (58.2–74.7)	67 (56–73)	0.917	67 (56–74)	69.5 (61.5–75.2)	0.760	67 (61–73)	68 (56–75)	0.836
BMI (Median)	29.4 (26–37.8)	29 (26.1–35.1)	39 (26–39.5)	0.764	30.7 (26–39.4)	28 (26.2–34.9)	0.596	28.2 (23.2–34.9)	30.2 (26.3–39.5)	0.557
Diabetic, N (%)				0.094			0.949			0.678
Yes (0)	71 (78.9%)	41 (58.6%)	29 (41.4%)		46 (67.6%)	22 (32.4%)		25 (36.8%)	43 (63.2%)	
No (1)	19 (21.1%)	7 (36.8%)	12 (63.2%)		13 (68.4%)	6 (31.6%)		6 (31.6%)	13 (68.4%)	
Grade, N (%)				0.218			0.313			0.737
I/II	42 (46.7%)	25 (60.9%)	16 (39.1%)		30 (73.1%)	11 (26.9%)		15 (37.5%)	25 (62.5%)	
III	48 (53.3%)	23 (47.9%)	25 (52.1%)		29 (63.1%)	17 (36.9%)		16 (34.1%)	31 (65.9%)	
Histological Type, N (%)				0.614			0.409			0.988
Endometrioid (1)	47 (52.2%)	26 (56.5%)	20 (43.5%)		26 (56.5%)	20 (43.5%)		16 (35.6%)	29 (64.4%)	
a Non-endometrioid (2)	43 (47.8%)	22 (51.2%)	21 (48.8%)		22 (51.2%)	21 (48.8%)		15 (35.7%)	27 (64.3%)	
FIGO 2009 Stage, N (%)				0.752			0.988			0.026
I	58 (64.4%)	31 (54.4%)	26 (45.6%)		37 (66.1%)	19 (33.9%)		25 (44.6%)	31 (55.4%)	
II	11 (12.2%)	5 (45.5%)	6 (54.5%)		9 (81.8%)	2 (18.2%)		2 (18.2%)	9 (81.8%)	
III	19 (21.1%)	10 (52.6%)	9 (47.4%)		12 (66.7%)	6 (33.3%)		4 (22.2%)	14 (77.8%)	
IV	2 (2.2%)	2 (100%)	0 (0%)		1 (50.0%)	1 (50.0%)		0 (0%)	2 (100%)	
Tumour Size, N (%)				0.234			0.866			0.117
Less than 2 cm (1)	9 (10.0%)	5 (55.6%)	4 (44.4%)		7 (77.8%)	2 (22.2%)		4 (50.0%)	4 (50.0%)	
2–5 cm (2)	46 (51.1%)	28 (62.2%)	17 (37.8%)		32 (71.1%)	13 (28.9%)		19 (43.2%)	25 (56.8%)	
Bigger than 5 cm (3)	11 (26.7%)	10 (41.7%)	14 (58.3%)		16 (72.7%)	6 (27.3%)		6 (25.0%)	18 (75.0%)	
Missing	24 (26.7%)									
LVSI, N (%)				0.928			0.692			0.948
No (0)	50 (55.6%)	26 (53.1%)	23 (46.6%)		33 (67.3%)	16 (32.7%)		17 (35.4%)	31 (64.6%)	
Yes (1)	37 (41.1%)	20 (54.1%)	17 (45.9%)		25 (71.4%)	10 (28.6%)		13 (36.1%)	23 (63.9%)	
Missing	3 (3.3%)									
Depth of Myometrial Invasion, N (%)				0.680			0.203			0.512
Less than (<) 50%	50 (55.6%)	26 (52.0%)	24 (48.0%)		36 (73.5%)	13 (26.5%)		16 (32.7%)	33 (67.3%)	
More than or equal to (≥) 50%	40 (44.4%)	22 (56.4%)	17 (43.6%)		23 (60.5%)	15 (39.5%)		15 (39.5%)	23 (60.5%)	

a Non-EEC tumours are composed of tumours with carcinosarcoma, mixed, clear cell, serous and undifferentiated histology

differences in staining intensity and distribution in different tumours. The observed staining intensities were given a score 0–3, from zero intensity staining (0) to high intensity staining (3), each staining intensity was multiplied by the percentage of tumour cells staining positively at each intensity. This gave a score range of 0-300. The tumours were separated into two groups as 'low expression <200' and 'high expression ≥200'. Immunohistochemical evaluation was performed by two blinded independent observers and discrepancies were settled by consensus to determine the final score.

Statistical analysis

All data was stored and analysed using SPSS statistical software (version 22). Comparisons between staining positivity and clinico-pathological characteristics were made using Chi- square (χ^2), Fishers exact test (as appropriate) or Mann Whitney U test (for continuous variables). Pearson correlation coefficients were calculated to assess the association between metabolic markers and/ or clinico-pathological characteristics. Overall survival (OS), cancer specific survival (CSS) and recurrence-free survival (RFS) were analysed using Kaplan-Meier curves and compared using the Log-rank (Mantel-Cox) tests. Analyses adjusted for previously identified prognostic factors were performed using Cox proportional hazards models using a large covariate set (grade, FIGO 2009 stage, tumour size, LVSI and depth of myometrial invasion). Further, given the low event number a simpler model adjusted for grade and stage was also fitted. As CSS and RFS endpoints had fewer events a model which just

adjusted for grade as a stratification variable was used for these endpoints. In all statistical analyses threshold for significance was $p < 0.05$.

Results

MCT1, MCT4 and CD147 expression, distribution and subcellular localization in EC

In this study, immunohistochemical evaluation of MCT1, MCT4 and CD147 was performed in 90 EC (47 endometrioid [EEC] and 43 non-endometrioid [non-EEC]) tumours. All aforementioned markers were expressed at varying levels. Representative images of tumour sections stained for MCT1, MCT4 and CD147 are shown in Fig. 1. MCT1 was expressed in the cytoplasm, the plasma membrane or in both locations. MCT4 and CD147 were always expressed in the plasma membrane accompanied by some degree of cytoplasmic staining (Fig. 1).

MCT1 and MCT4 staining patterns were highly variable both within and between tumours. MCT1 was generally observed in peripheral zones (Fig. 2a) whereas MCT4 was expressed in central zones of the same tumour (Fig. 2b). Strong CD147 expression was mainly observed in those areas that were heavily stained with MCT1 (Fig. 2c). In contrast, in areas with strong MCT4 expression CD147 expression was weaker (Fig. 2c). Stromal and myometrial expression of MCT1 and MCT4 was also seen (Fig. 2d-i). In some, stromal and glandular staining displayed high contrast; malignant glands showed strong MCT1 expression whilst stromal staining was negative (or mild) or vice versa. In others, MCT1 and MCT4 expression was similar across stromal and glandular tumour compartments. Although the nucleus

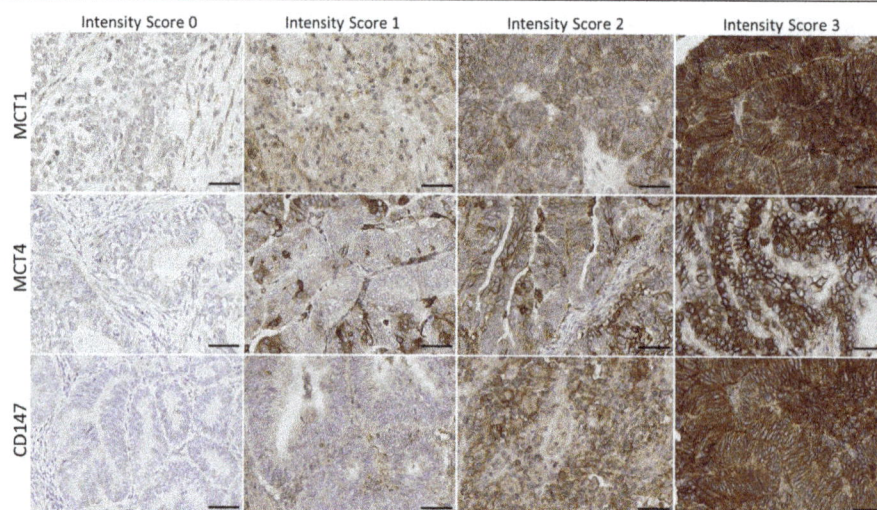

Fig. 1 Representative immunohistochemical reactions for intensity score 0, 1, 2 and 3 for MCT1, MCT4 and CD147 expression in non-EEC tumours. The expression of MCT1 was localized to the cytoplasm, the plasma membrane or both locations. MCT4 and CD147 expression was always observed in the plasma membrane with some level of cytoplasmic staining. Scale bars represent 50 μm

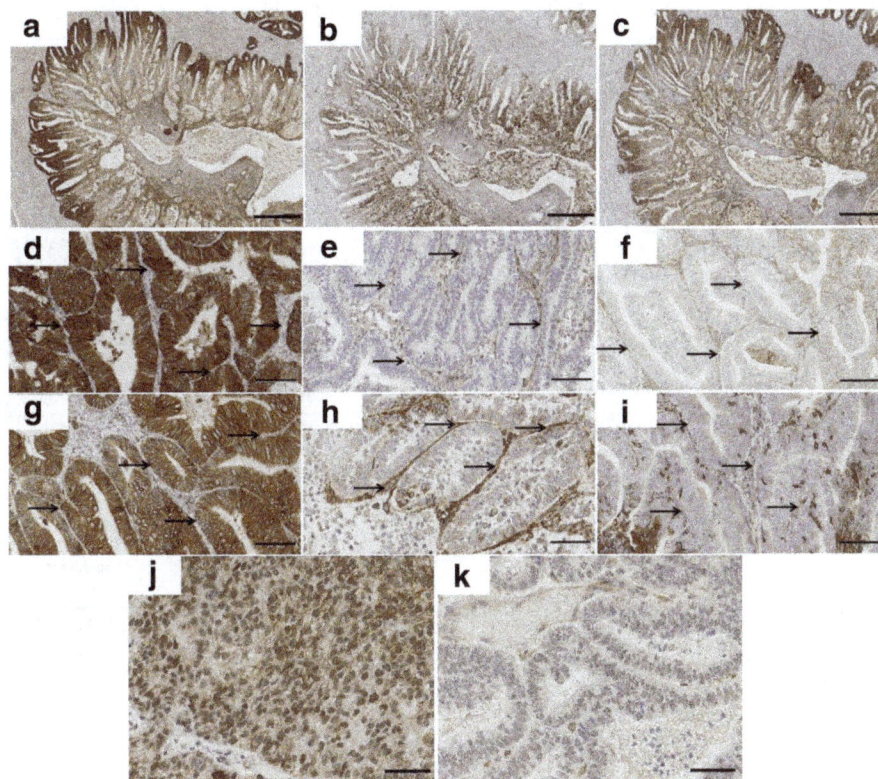

Fig. 2 Representative examples of MCT1, MCT4 and CD147 distribution and subcellular localization in EC tumours. **a** MCT1 and **b** MCT4 were found to dominate different zones of the same tumour, peripheral and central zones, respectively. **c** CD147 expression was observed in the same zone with MCT1. In some, strong glandular staining for **d** MCT1 and **g** MCT4 was observed with no stromal staining. In others, stromal expression of **e** MCT1 and **h** MCT4 were higher than glandular staining. Some tumours showed similar levels of **f** MCT1 and **i** MCT4 expression in both glandular and stromal tumour compartments. In more than half of the tumours, nuclear MCT1 staining (**j** and **k**) was observed. Arrows indicate stromal compartment between malignant glands. Scale bars represent 500 μm, 100 μm and 50 μm in (**a-c**), (**d-i**) and (**j-k**), respectively

is not a usual location for MCT1 (based on current knowledge of its function), nuclear MCT1 expression was present in more than half of the tumours (present 58.9%, absent 40.1%; Fig. 2j-k).

There was a wide range in the intensity and distribution of staining, which was scored as described in the methods section. Briefly, tumours were recorded as high expressers when their score was equal to or exceeded 200; tumours with scores below this were regarded as low expressers. Interestingly, for MCT1, using the score of 200 resulted in 53.9% of tumours scoring low and 46.1% of tumours scoring high. Using the same 200 score cut off high MCT4 expression was observed in 32.2% of tumours and high levels of CD147 expression were observed in 64.4% of the tumours. There was a significant association between expression of CD147 and MCT1 ($p = 0.003$) but not MCT4 ($p = 0.207$) in our cohort (Pearson correlation coefficients = 0.32 and 0.14, respectively). There was no significant association between MCT1 and MCT4 expression ($p = 0.93$).

Associations between metabolic markers and clinico-pathological data

There were no significant associations between the clinico-pathological characteristics of the tumours and expression levels of either MCT1 or MCT4 (Table 1). CD147 expression was significantly associated with FIGO 2009 stage (Pearson Correlation Coefficient = 0.24), although this association would not be considered significant if allowance was made for the number of characteristics tested.

MCT1 expression is associated with reduced overall survival in EC

When the expression of these three metabolic markers was correlated with patient survival parameters (recurrence free, cancer specific and overall survival), MCT1 was identified as a prognostic marker in EC. Using an unadjusted Log-rank test, patients with high MCT1 expression showed reduced recurrence free and cancer specific survival and a significantly reduced overall survival (Fig. 3a-c, respectively).

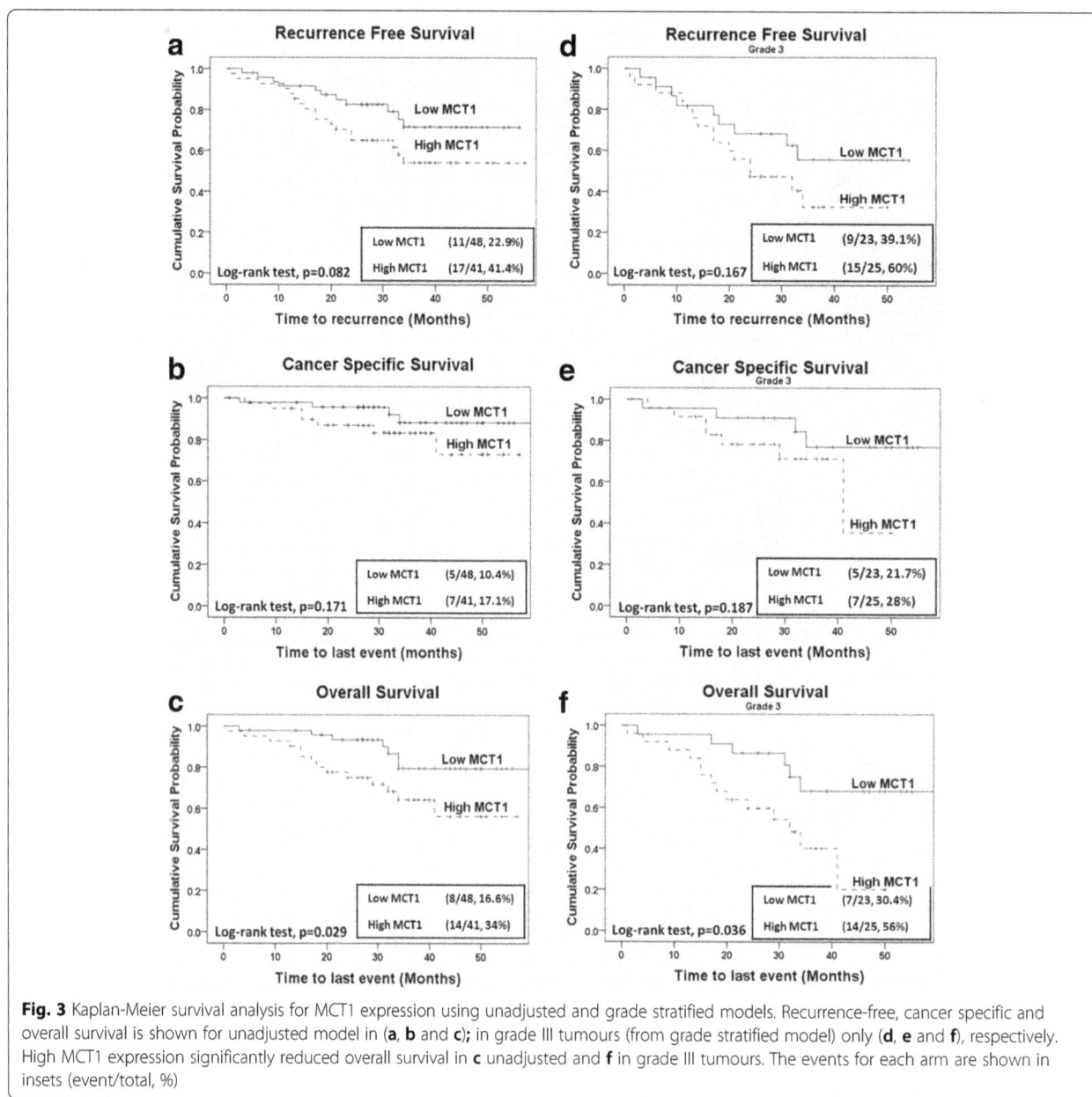

Fig. 3 Kaplan-Meier survival analysis for MCT1 expression using unadjusted and grade stratified models. Recurrence-free, cancer specific and overall survival is shown for unadjusted model in (**a**, **b** and **c**); in grade III tumours (from grade stratified model) only (**d**, **e** and **f**), respectively. High MCT1 expression significantly reduced overall survival in **c** unadjusted and **f** in grade III tumours. The events for each arm are shown in insets (event/total, %)

Amongst survival outcome covariates (grade, FIGO stage, tumour size, LVSI and depth of myometrial invasion), grade and FIGO 2009 stage were the most significant prognostic factors in our study (Table 2). In order to evaluate whether MCT1 expression was an independent prognostic factor, MCT1 expression was tested in a large adjusted model with all of the listed covariates and a simpler model with just the major predictors, grade and stage (Table 2). In these analyses, MCT1 remained statistically significant after adjustment for all six possible covariates as well as in the simpler stage and grade-adjusted model (Table 2).

Due to the limited number of events observed for recurrence free and cancer specific survival, full adjustment for

covariates was not possible for these endpoints. Therefore, we used a simpler adjustment for the most important predictor of survival in our cohort, which was grade, and fitted this as a stratified Log-rank test and Cox regression model.

When the overall cohort was stratified according to grade (I/II vs III), similar to the unadjusted model, an increased trend towards reduced recurrence free, cancer specific and overall survival was observed in patients with high MCT1 expressing grade III (mainly composed of Non-EEC) tumours (Fig. 3d-f). This effect reached statistical significance for overall survival (Table 3). There were too few events in patients with grade I/II tumours for meaningful statistical analysis (only composed

Table 2 Unadjusted and adjusted Cox proportional hazard analysis for overall survival

Overall survival	Unadjusted model Overall cohort			Large adjusted model Overall cohort			Simple adjusted model Overall cohort		
	HR	95% CI	p	HR	95% CI	p	HR	95% CI	p
MCT1	**1.622**	**1.030–2.554**	**0.037**	**2.123**	**1.145–3.937**	**0.017**	**1.963**	**1.199–3.214**	**0.007**
Grade	**4.684**	**1.715–12.79**	**0.003**	**3.210**	**1.136–9.076**	**0.028**	**3.797**	**1.372–10.50**	**0.010**
Stage	**2.288**	**1.500–3.489**	**<0.001**	**1.965**	**1.078–3.579**	**0.027**	**2.080**	**1.300–3.328**	**0.002**
Size	1.269	0.585–2.750	0.547	0.681	0.306–1.515	0.346	–	–	–
LVSI	2.347	0.935–5.891	0.069	1.185	0.378–3.718	0.771	–	–	–
MI	1.447	0.609–3.436	0.403	1.121	0.340–3.690	0.851	–	–	–

Grade categorised as Grade I/II and III tumours; Stage: FIGO 2009 stage categorised as 1, 2, 3 and 4; Size categorised as <2 cm, between 2 and 5 cm and bigger than 5 cm; LVSI: Lymphovascular space involvement categorised as "Yes" and "No"; MI: Depth of myometrial invasion categorised as <50% and more than 50%; HR: hazard ratio, CI: confidence interval. Bold text indicates statistically significant data at $p < 0.05$ level

of EEC tumours, shown in Additional file 1: Figure S1). Grade stratified Cox proportional hazard analysis performed on other markers (CD147 and MCT4) showed an increased risk of earlier time to event for patients with high CD147 expression but this effect did not reach statistical significance. There were no significant associations between these two metabolic markers and any of the survival parameters evaluated in this study (Table 3).

Discussion

This is the first study to evaluate the prognostic significance of MCT1, MCT4 and CD147 expression in EC. Using both unadjusted and adjusted analyses we found high MCT1 expression to be an independent factor predicting poor survival in patients with EC. This finding is consistent with previous studies examining the role of MCT1 in other cancer types [14, 20, 22, 34] and supports its development as a therapeutic target in EC and other malignancies.

Increased glucose uptake, glycolysis and adaptation to acidosis are key events during cancer progression [35].

MCT1 and MCT4 are important contributors to the regulation of tumour intracellular pH and induction of extracellular acidosis. Understanding the role of these transporters in tumours will clarify their contribution to tumour metabolism and the malignant phenotype. Recent efforts have been made to identify the prognostic significance of MCT1 [14, 15, 21, 23, 24, 34] and MCT4 (reviewed by [36]) in different tumour types, however none have studied their role in EC.

In EC, MCT1 and MCT4 were expressed in the cytoplasm, the plasma membrane or both. The observed cytoplasmic as well as membranous MCT1 and MCT4 staining suggests either the presence of alternative mechanisms that ensure acid efflux and maintenance of intracellular pH or the use of non-glycolytic metabolic pathways in EC. Interestingly, mitochondrial membrane expression of MCT1 [37] and MCT4 [13, 38–40] has been described in other tumour types. Moreover, an increased cytoplasmic (as well as plasma membrane) expression of MCT1 is reported in basal like breast cancers [15] suggesting it may have additional functions

Table 3 Cox proportional hazard analysis of recurrence free, cancer specific and overall survival in unadjusted and grade stratified model

		Unadjusted Model			Grade Stratified Model		
		HR	95% CI	p	HR	95% CI	P
MCT1	RFS	1.390	0.951–2.031	0.089	1.302	0.889–1.907	0.175
	CSS	1.518	0.820–2.809	0.184	1.508	0.805–2.826	0.199
	OS	**1.622**	**1.030–2.554**	**0.037**	**1.604**	**1.012–2.541**	**0.044**
MCT4	RFS	0.829	0.539–1.275	0.394	0.771	0.501–1.186	0.237
	CSS	0.685	0.318–1.474	0.333	0.641	0.279–1.381	0.256
	OS	0.905	0.563–1.453	0.679	0.846	0.526–1.359	0.489
CD147	RFS	1.309	0.853–2.008	0.217	1.331	0.867–2.044	0.191
	CSS	1.251	0.644–2.431	0.508	1.383	0.704–2.718	0.347
	OS	1.358	0.822–2.245	0.232	1.469	0.884–2.443	0.138

RFS recurrence free survival, OS overall survival, CSS cancer specific survival, HR hazard ratio, CI confidence interval. Bold text indicates statistically significant data at $p < 0.05$ level

such as transportation of lactate/pyruvate through the mitochondrial membrane. Further, in more than half of the tumours evaluated in this study, nuclear MCT1 expression was present. This is consistent with a previous study of soft tissue sarcomas [20]. To the best of our knowledge, this is the first study showing expression of nuclear MCT1 in EC. As the cellular localization does not fit with the classic role of this protein as a transmembrane transporter, this finding suggests an additional, not yet described, role for MCT1. We found no statistically significant association between nuclear MCT1 expression and recurrence free, overall or cancer-specific survival.

Based on their functional differences, both MCT1 and MCT4 display tissue specific patterns of distribution. MCT1 and MCT4 are variably expressed in tumours originating from the breast, colon, lung and ovary (reviewed by [41]). In addition, different MCTs are known to transport lactic acid between different cell types within the same tumour tissue. It has been proposed that hypoxic and glycolytic tumour cells distant from functional blood vessels use MCT4 to export lactic acid, which is then absorbed by the peripheral oxidative tumour cells through MCT1 [42]. Indeed, in some of the tumours studied here, MCT1 and MCT4 were expressed independently in different epithelial zones of the same tumour, suggesting that metabolic needs varied according to the precise location of cells expressing different transporters. This observation is consistent with the metabolic heterogeneity described by Sonveaux et al. [42] and in a recent study of urothelial bladder cancer [43]. Moreover, differential expression of MCT1 and MCT4 were observed in the stromal compartment of these tumours. A meta-analysis performed by Bovenzi et al. [36], showed that MCT4 expression in the tumour stromal compartment was associated with reduced overall and disease free survival, however, there was not sufficient information to perform a similar analysis on MCT1. Nevertheless, this finding suggests that the differential stromal expression of MCT1 and 4 observed in our EC cohort might be due to a metabolic symbiosis established between the tumour and its microenvironment supporting highly proliferative epithelial cancer cells [44].

CD147 plays an important role in cancer progression [29, 30] and the regulation of MCT1 and MCT4 activity and expression [45]. In this study, we observed CD147 to be primarily associated with the plasma membrane and often co-localizing with MCT1. This association was not seen with MCT4 expression. This is consistent with other cancer types such as ovarian and oral cavity tumours [23, 40] and provides evidence for the importance of CD147 in MCT1 localization and function in EC. Lack of significant association between membrane localization of MCT4 and CD147 leads us to speculate that MCT4 plasma localization in EC may depend on an additional protein such as CD44 [40, 46].

Conclusions

In summary, this is the first study evaluating the expression of MCT1, MCT4 and CD147 in EC. The results demonstrate MCT1 to be an important marker for overall survival in EC. The differential staining patterns for MCT1 in low grade EEC and non-EEC tumours indicate metabolic differences between the tumour types. Our data suggest that agents targeting MCT1 may have potential in the treatment of this disease and support the notion that exploitation of metabolic targets may pave the way for personalised EC prevention and therapy.

Abbreviations
BMI: Body mass index; CSS: Cancer-specific survival; DAB: Diaminobenzidine tetrahydrochloride; EC: Endometrial cancer; EEC: Endometrioid endometrial cancer; FIGO: Federation of Gynecology and Obstetrics; HRP: Horseradish peroxidase; Ig: Immunoglobulin; IHC: Immunohistochemistry; IQR: Interquartile range; LVSI: Lymphovascular space involvement; MCT: Monocarboxylate transporter; OS: Overall survival; RFS: Recurrence free survival

Acknowledgements
We would like to thank the women who kindly donated their tissues and clinical data for this research project.

Funding
This study was supported by National Institute for Health Research (NIHR) Research & Innovation Division, Strategic Project Funding 2013. This article presents independent research funded by the NIHR and facilitated by the Greater Manchester Local Clinical Research Network. In part of this study AL was supported by a Manchester Pharmacy School Fellowship. VNS is funded through a Wellcome Trust/ Wellbeing of Women Research Training Fellowship (098670/Z/12). EJC and SJK are funded through an NIHR Clinician Scientist fellowship (NIHR-CS-012-009). The views expressed are those of the authors and not necessarily those of the NHS, the NIHR or the Department of Health.

Authors' contributions
AL performed scoring for all markers, collated scoring and clinical data, designed and performed statistical analysis and prepared the manuscript. ALC conceived funding, co-ordinated IHC and performed scoring for all markers. HJG performed IHC for MCT1, MCT4 and CD147. SK and VS collected the clinico-pathological data. SAR oversaw the statistical analysis and interpretation. RM and JB performed pathologic examination of tumours. EJC and IJS conceived and secured funding for the project; provided overall supervision of the work and helped draft the manuscript. KMM and KJW helped interpret the data. All authors reviewed and agreed the final version of the manuscript.

Competing interests
The authors declare that they have no competing interests.

Author details
[1]Division of Pharmacy and Optometry, Faculty of Biology, Medicine and Health, University of Manchester, Manchester, UK. [2]Gynaecological Oncology

Research Group, Division of Cancer Sciences, Faculty of Biology, Medicine and Health, University of Manchester, Level 5 – Research, St Mary's Hospital, Oxford Road, Manchester M13 9WL, UK. [3]Department of Histopathology, Central Manchester University Hospitals NHS Foundation Trust, Manchester Academic Health Science Centre, Manchester, UK. [4]Division of Population Health, Health Services Research and Primary Care, Faculty of Biology, Medicine and Health, University of Manchester, Manchester, UK. [5]Department of Obstetrics and Gynaecology, St Mary's Hospital, Central Manchester University Hospitals NHS Foundation Trust, Manchester Academic Health Science Centre, Manchester, UK.

References

1. Cancer Research UK Statistics. http://www.cancerresearchuk.org/health-professional/cancer-statistics.

2. Thigpen JT, Brady MF, Alvarez MD, Adelson RD, Homesley HD, Manetta A, et al. Oral medroxyprogesterone acetate in the treatment of advanced or recurrent endometrial carcinoma: a dose-response study by the gynecologic oncology group. J Clin Oncol. 1999;17:1736–44.

3. Ma BB, Oza A, Eisenhauer E, Stanimir G, Carey M, Chapman W, et al. The activity of letrozole in patients with advanced or recurrent endometrial cancer and correlation with biological markers–a study of the National Cancer Institute of Canada clinical trials group. Int J Gynecol Cancer. 2004; 14:650–8.

4. Bellone S, Shah HR, McKenney JK, Stone PJ, Santin AD. Recurrent endometrial carcinoma regression with the use of the aromatase inhibitor anastrozole. Am J Obstet Gynecol. 2008;199:e7–e10.

5. Friberg E, Orsini N, Mantzoros CS, Wolk A. Diabetes mellitus and risk of endometrial cancer: a meta-analysis. Diabetologia. 2007;50:1365–74.

6. Crosbie EJ, Zwahlen M, Kitchener HC, Egger M, Renehan AG. Body mass index, hormone replacement therapy, and endometrial cancer risk: a meta-analysis. Cancer Epidemiol Biomark Prev. 2010;19:3119–30.

7. Renehan AG, Tyson M, Egger M, Heller RF, Zwahlen M. Body-mass index and incidence of cancer: a systematic review and meta-analysis of prospective observational studies. Lancet. 2008;371:569–78.

8. Algire C, Amrein L, Zakikhani M, Panasci L, Pollak M. Metformin blocks the stimulative effect of a high-energy diet on colon carcinoma growth in vivo and is associated with reduced expression of fatty acid synthase. Endocr Relat Cancer. 2010;17:351–60.

9. Warburg O, Wind F, Negelein E. The metabolism of tumors in the body. J Gen Physiol. 1927;8:519–30.

10. Halestrap AP. The SLC16 gene family - structure, role and regulation in health and disease. Mol Asp Med. 2013;34:337–49.

11. Halestrap AP, Price NT. The proton-linked monocarboxylate transporter (MCT) family: structure, function and regulation. Biochem J. 1999;343:281–99.

12. Nakayama Y, Torigoe T, Inoue Y, Minagawa N, Izumi H, Kohno K, et al. Prognostic significance of monocarboxylate transporter 4 expression in patients with colorectal cancer. Exp Ther Med. 2012;3:25–30.

13. Pinheiro C, Longatto-Filho A, Scapulatempo C, Ferreira L, Martins S, Pellerin L, et al. Increased expression of monocarboxylate transporters 1, 2, and 4 in colorectal carcinomas. Virchows Arch. 2008;452:139–46.

14. Pinheiro C, Longatto-Filho A, Pereira SM, Etlinger D, Moreira MA, Jube LF, et al. Monocarboxylate transporters 1 and 4 are associated with CD147 in cervical carcinoma. Dis Markers. 2009;26:97–103.

15. Pinheiro C, Albergaria A, Paredes J, Sousa B, Dufloth R, Vieira D, et al. Monocarboxylate transporter 1 is up-regulated in basal-like breast carcinoma. Histopathology. 2010;56:860–7.

16. Doyen J, Trastour C, Ettore F, Peyrottes I, Toussant N, Gal J, et al. Expression of the hypoxia-inducible monocarboxylate transporter MCT4 is increased in triple negative breast cancer and correlates independently with clinical outcome. Biochem Biophys Res Commun. 2014;451:54–61.

17. Pertega-Gomes N, Vizcaino JR, Miranda-Goncalves V, Pinheiro C, Silva J, Pereira H, et al. Monocarboxylate transporter 4 (MCT4) and CD147 overexpression is associated with poor prognosis in prostate cancer. BMC Cancer. 2011;11:312.

18. Froberg MK, Gerhart DZ, Enerson BE, Manivel C, Guzman-Paz M, Seacotte N, et al. Expression of monocarboxylate transporter MCT1 in normal and neoplastic human CNS tissues. Neuroreport. 2001;12:761–5.

19. Miranda-Goncalves V, Honavar M, Pinheiro C, Martinho O, Pires MM, Pinheiro C, et al. Monocarboxylate transporters (MCTs) in gliomas: expression and exploitation as therapeutic targets. Neuro-Oncology. 2013; 15:172–88.

20. Pinheiro C, Penna V, Morais-Santos F, Abrahao-Machado LF, Ribeiro G, Curcelli EC, et al. Characterization of monocarboxylate transporters (MCTs) expression in soft tissue sarcomas: distinct prognostic impact of MCT1 sub-cellular localization. J Transl Med. 2014;12:118.

21. Pinheiro C, Longatto-Filho A, Simoes K, Jacob CE, Bresciani CJ, Zilberstein B, et al. The prognostic value of CD147/EMMPRIN is associated with monocarboxylate transporter 1 co-expression in gastric cancer. Eur J Cancer. 2009;45:2418–24.

22. de Oliveira AT, Pinheiro C, Longatto-Filho A, Brito MJ, Martinho O, Matos D, et al. Co-expression of monocarboxylate transporter 1 (MCT1) and its chaperone (CD147) is associated with low survival in patients with gastrointestinal stromal tumors (GISTs). J Bioenerg Biomembr. 2012;44:171–8.

23. Simoes-Sousa S, Granja S, Pinheiro C, Fernandes D, Longatto-Filho A, Laus AC, et al. Prognostic significance of monocarboxylate transporter expression in oral cavity tumors. Cell Cycle. 2016;15:1865–73.

24. Choi JW, Kim Y, Lee JH, Kim YS. Prognostic significance of lactate/proton symporters MCT1, MCT4, and their chaperone CD147 expressions in urothelial carcinoma of the bladder. Urology. 2014;84:245.e249–15.

25. Eilertsen M, Andersen S, Al-Saad S, Kiselev Y, Donnem T, Stenvold H, et al. Monocarboxylate transporters 1-4 in NSCLC: MCT1 is an independent prognostic marker for survival. PLoS One. 2014;9:e105038.

26. Kirk P, Wilson MC, Heddle C, Brown MH, Barclay AN, Halestrap AP. CD147 is tightly associated with lactate transporters MCT1 and MCT4 and facilitates their cell surface expression. EMBO. 2000;19:3896–904.

27. Wilson MC, Meredith D, Fox JE, Manoharan C, Davies AJ, Halestrap AP. Basigin (CD147) is the target for organomercurial inhibition of monocarboxylate transporter isoforms 1 and 4: the ancillary protein for the insensitive MCT2 is EMBIGIN (gp70). J Biol Chem. 2005;280:27213–21.

28. Deora AA, Philp N, Hu J, Bok D, Rodriguez-Boulan E. Mechanisms regulating tissue-specific polarity of monocarboxylate transporters and their chaperone CD147 in kidney and retinal epithelia. Proc Natl Acad Sci U S A. 2005;102: 16245–50.

29. Gabison EE, Hoang-Xuan T, Mauviel A, Menashi S. EMMPRIN/CD147, an MMP modulator in cancer, development and tissue repair. Biochimie. 2005; 87:361–8.

30. Nabeshima K, Iwasaki H, Koga K, Hojo H, Suzumiya J, Kikuchi M. Emmprin (basigin/CD147): matrix metalloproteinase modulator and multifunctional cell recognition molecule that plays a critical role in cancer progression. Pathol Int. 2006;56:359–67.

31. Riethdorf S, Reimers N, Assmann V, Kornfield JW, Terracciano L, Sauter G. High incidence of EMMPRIN expression in human tumors. Int J Cancer. 2006;119:1800–10.

32. Gallagher SM, Castorino JJ, Wang D, Philp NJ. Monocarboxylate transporter 4 regulates maturation and trafficking of CD147 to the plasma membrane in the metastatic breast cancer cell line MDA-MB-231. Cancer Res. 2007;67:4182–9.

33. Nakamura K, Kodama J, Hongo A, Hiramatsu Y. Role of emmprin in endometrial cancer. BMC Cancer. 2012;12:191.

34. Kim Y, Choi JW, Lee JH, Kim YS. Expression of lactate/H(+) symporters MCT1 and MCT4 and their chaperone CD147 predicts tumor progression in clear cell renal cell carcinoma: immunohistochemical and the cancer genome atlas data analyses. Hum Pathol. 2015;46:104–12.

35. Gatenby RA, Gillies RJ. Why do cancers have high aerobic glycolysis? Nat Rev Cancer. 2004;4:891–9.

36. Bovenzi CD, Hamilton J, Tassone P, Johnson J, Cognetti DM, Luginbuhi A, et al. Prognostic indications of elevated MCT4 and CD147 across cancer types: a meta-analysis. Biomed Res Int. 2015;2015:242437.

37. Hashimoto T, Hussien R, Brooks GA. Colocalization of MCT1, CD147, and LDH in mitochondrial inner membrane of L6 muscle cells: evidence of a mitochondrial lactate oxidation complex. American J Physiol Endocrinol Metab. 2006;290:E1237–44.

38. Hussien R, Brooks GA. Mitochondrial and plasma membrane lactate transporter and lactate dehydrogenase isoform expression in breast cancer cell lines. Physiol Genomics. 2011;43:255–64.

39. Koukourakis MI, Giatromanolaki A, Bougioukas G, Sivridis E. Lung cancer: a comparative study of metabolism related protein expression in cancer cells and tumor associated stroma. Cancer Biol Ther. 2007;6:1476–9.

40. Pinheiro C, Reis RM, Ricardo S, Longatto-Filho A, Schmitt F, Baltazar F. Expression of monocarboxylate transporters 1, 2, and 4 in human tumours and their association with CD147 and CD44. J Biomed Biotechnol. 2010; 2010:427694.

41. Pinheiro C, Longatto-Filho A, Azevedo-Silva J, Casal M, Schmitt FC, Baltazar F. Role of monocarboxylate transporters in human cancers: state of the art. J Bioenerg Biomembr. 2012;44:127–39.

42. Sonveaux P, Vegran F, Schroeder T, Wergin MC, Verrax J, Rabbani ZN, et al. Targeting lactate-fueled respiration selectively kills hypoxic tumor cells in mice. J Clin Invest. 2008;118:3930–42.

43. Afonso J, Santos LL, Morais A, Amaro T, Longatto-Filho A, Baltazar F. Metabolic coupling in urothelial bladder cancer compartments and its correlation to tumor aggressiveness. Cell Cycle. 2016;15:368–80.

44. Curry JM, Tuluc M, Whitaker-Menezes D, Ames JA, Anantharaman A, Butera A, et al. Cancer metabolism, stemness and tumor recurrence: MCT1 and MCT4 are functional biomarkers of metabolic symbiosis in head and neck cancer. Cell Cycle. 2013;12:1371–84.

45. Marchiq I, Le Floch R, Roux D, Simon MP, Pouyssegur J. Genetic disruption of lactate/H+ symporters (MCTs) and their subunit CD147/BASIGIN sensitizes glycolytic tumor cells to phenformin. Cancer Res. 2015;75:171–80.

46. Slomiany MG, Grass GD, Robertson AD, Yang XY, Maria BL, Beeson C, et al. Hyaluronan, CD44, and emmprin regulate lactate efflux and membrane localization of monocarboxylate transporters in human breast carcinoma cells. Cancer Res. 2009;69:1293–301.

19

Mycetoma in a non-endemic area: a diagnostic challenge

Boubacar Efared[1*], Layla Tahiri[1], Marou Soumana Boubacar[2], Gabrielle Atsam-Ebang[1], Nawal Hammas[1], El Fatemi Hinde[1] and Laila Chbani[1]

Abstract

Background: Mycetoma is a chronic granulomatous infectious disease caused by filamentous bacteria or by fungi. The disease is endemic in certain tropical and subtropical areas of the world but can be found elsewhere posing sometimes a diagnostic challenge for clinicians.

Case presentation: A 65-year- old man presented with a right foot swelling evolving for 25 years. During that time, several diagnosis and treatments have been made without any improvement. The disease spread to bones, and misdiagnosed as Kaposi's sarcoma. Transtibial amputation has been performed, and the histopathological examination revealed finally the diagnosis of eumycotic mycetoma. The patient recovered well after surgery and orthopedic prosthesis was prescribed for him.

Conclusion: Mycetoma in non endemic areas is usually misdiagnosed and mismanaged leading to unnecessary and inappropriate surgery. Health practitioners should be aware of that fact in order to provide an accurate management.

Keywords: Actinomycetoma, Eumycetoma, Misdiagnosis, Pathology

Background

Madura foot or mycetoma is a chronic granulomatous disease of the subcutaneous tissue, that can progress to deeper structures like muscles or bones [1–3]. It is caused either by fungi (eumycetoma) or by aerobic filamentous bacteria (actinomycetoma) [1, 4]. It affects mostly lower extremities of the body, especially foot and leg but can affect any part of the body, such us head and neck, arms, the chest wall or the abdominal wall [1, 2, 5]. The disease often occurs in tropical and subtropical regions of the world, in the zone called "mycetoma belt", extending between latitudes 15° south and 30° north [1, 3, 6]. Mexico, Senegal, India, Sudan, are the most affected countries [1–4]. Sudan seems to be the most endemic country where eumycetoma represents the main aetiologic type of the disease. This country hosts an important research center for mycetoma where large studies on the topic were performed [5]. But, in temperate climate, cases of mycetoma have been reported, mostly imported cases from immigrants

[7–10]. In 2014, Buonfrate et al. had reported 42 cases of mycetoma acquired in Europe, through a literature review, suggesting that Europeans without travel history can be affected by the disease [11]. Typically, mycetoma is encountered in rural areas in poor people working in agricultural sector [1, 3, 5]. In 2013, the World Health Organisation (WHO) listed the disease among neglected tropical disease [12]. Several causative fungal or bacterial agents are responsible for the disease. The treatment is based on the type of causative agent, bacterial or fungal, and on the extent of the disease. Unfortunately, the diagnosis of the disease and the identification of the etiological agent is a very challenging issue, especially in non-endemic areas [13–16].

We report herein, a case of Madura foot evolving for more than 2 decades, that had escaped all diagnostic tools, misdiagnosed as cancer and leading finally to amputation. The final diagnosis has been achieved by the histopathological examination of the resected specimen.

Case presentation

A 65-year-old man was referred for evaluation of the right foot tumor diagnosed recently as Kaposi's sarcoma. The patient was a shopkeeper living in the town of Fès

* Correspondence: befared2013@gmail.com
[1]Departement of Pathology, Hassan II Teaching Hospital, Fès, Morocco
Full list of author information is available at the end of the article

and did not report any trip to an endemic area of myce- toma. He had a right foot chronic lesion for 25 years, with several repeated histological biopsies revealing, ke- loid scar, non specific inflammation, or Kaposi's Sar- coma. The Physical examination showed chronic skin changes on the right foot and leg, with multiple scars and hard abscessed ulcerations on the plantar face of the foot. There were no grain discharge and the patient did not report such information. The culture of the abscess showed *Staphylococcus aureus* species. X-ray of the right foot was performed and showed extensive de- struction of the tarse, metatarse and phalanges (Fig. 1). Other radiological evaluation did not found further lesions. The diagnosis of locally invasive Kaposi's Sarcoma was suspected and a right trans-tibial amputa- tion was performed.

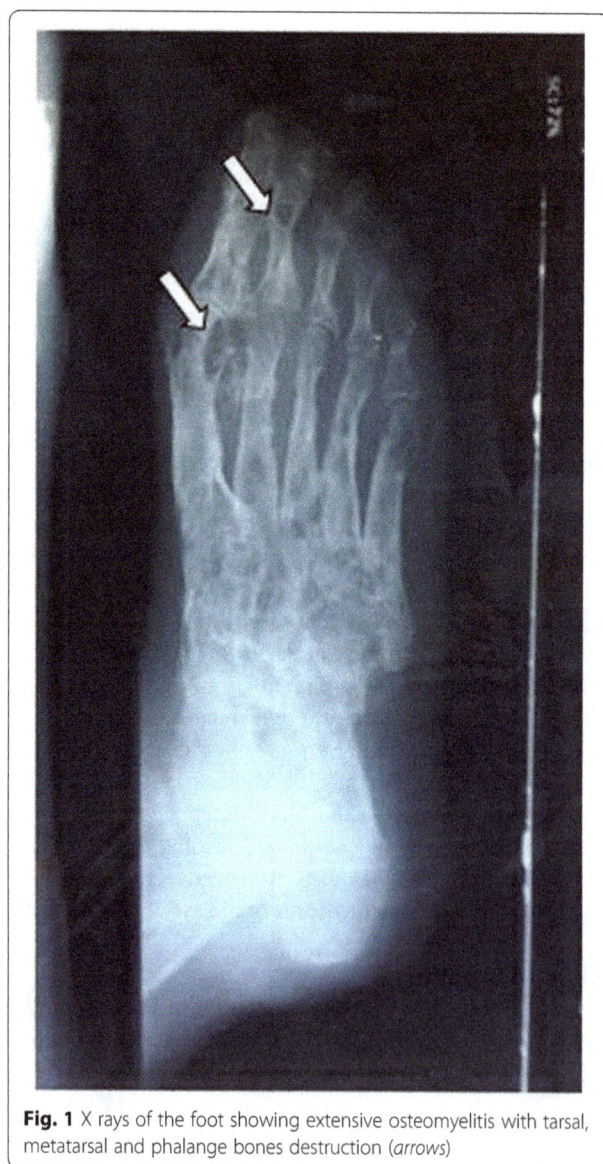

Fig. 1 X rays of the foot showing extensive osteomyelitis with tarsal, metatarsal and phalange bones destruction (*arrows*)

Histopathological findings

On macroscopic evaluation, the leg measured 30x11cm, the foot measured 27x10cm. The foot showed an indu- rated skin with some areas of hard abscess without any disharges. The initial sampling from these lesions showed a non specific inflammation without any tu- moral lesion. Then, the remaining bone was submitted to decalcification by nitric acid. Some weeks later, after the process of decalcification, the macroscopic evalu- ation found a deep soft tissue and bone destruction consisted of round cavitis filled of yellowish crumbly material (Fig. 2). The histological examination on hematoxylin-eosine-safran (HES) stained sections re- vealed several multilobulated colonies surrounded by granulomatous inflammation composed of plasma cells, epithelioid cells, macrophages and some multinucleated cells. The colonies had deeply basophilic outer layers with branching filaments (Figs. 3 and 4); some colonies were fractured and had a pale center. They stained posi- tive for PAS (Periodic Acid-Schiff) (Fig. 5). These histo- logical aspects were strongly consistent with eumycotic mycetoma. The post-operative course was uneventful and the patient was discharged from the hospital. Two months after surgery, the patients had no signs of the disease and orthopedic prosthesis was prescribed for him.

Discussion

Mycetoma is one of the neglected infectious diseases that is endemic in tropical and subtropical areas of the world [1, 5, 6]. The disease affects typically poor people living in rural areas and usually working in farms. Myce- toma affects all age groups, but it is more common in 20 – 40 year old men; this epidemiological feature suggests that young men are more exposed to the disease because they are supposed to be the more productive age group in developping countries [1, 3, 4]. The low prevalence of the disease in women could be due to hormonal factors as in rural areas women take part in agricultural and other activities that expose to mycetoma [1]. But, in countries out of the "mycetoma belt", in temperate cli- mate regions, cases of mycetoma have been reported from immigrants [7–10]. Also, cases from autochtonous patients without history of travelling to endemic regions, have been reported [11]. Health practitionners in these areas are not familiar to the disease, thus cases were usually misdiagnosed and mismanaged leading to serious consequences for patients. In fact, our case, is from Morocco, a country that is out of the "mycetoma belt", where no more than 100 cases have been reported.

Several causative micro-organisms (more than 56), ei- ther fungi or bacteria, are known to date to be linked to mycetoma [1, 4, 6]. They are found in the environnment in plants thorns or in the soil. People become infected

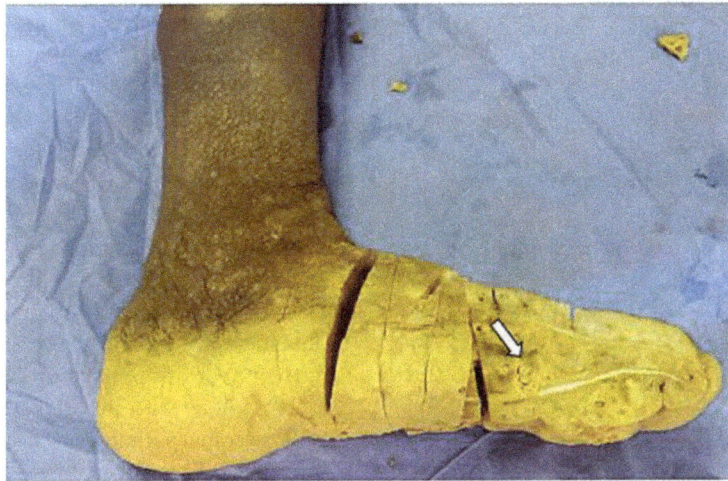

Fig. 2 The resected specimen showing cavitis filled of yellowish materiel (*arrow*) corresponding to mycetoma grains

by the disease after injury by plants thorns or when walking bearfoot [4, 6]. The prevalence of causative agents vary in the world. In Sudan, the main causative agents are fungi, while in latin America, in countries like Mexico, bacterial agents are predominant. One recent review and meta-analysis, found that the species like *Actinomadura madurae, Streptomyces somaliensis, Actinomadura pelletieri, Nocardia brasiliensis* and *Nocardia asteroides* were considered to be common causative agents of actinomycetoma, while *Madurella mycetomatis* was the main causative agent of eumycetoma [1].

The clinical presentation of mycetoma is similar whether the causative agent is a fungi or a bacteria, however actinomycetoma has more agressive course and invades deeper structures earlier than eumycetoma [1]. Typically, patients present with a classical triad consisted of a painless firm subcutaneous mass, multiple sinus formation, and a purulent or seropurulent discharge containing grains. The disease pursues a long course, because of the indolor feature or the lack of appropriate health information about the disease, hence it occurs in poorly educated patients. Another factor that explains the long evolution of the disease, is the misdiagnosis especially in non endemic regions, as illustrated by our case that has disease for more than 20 years, repeatdly misdiagnosed, leading to leg amputation. Similarly,

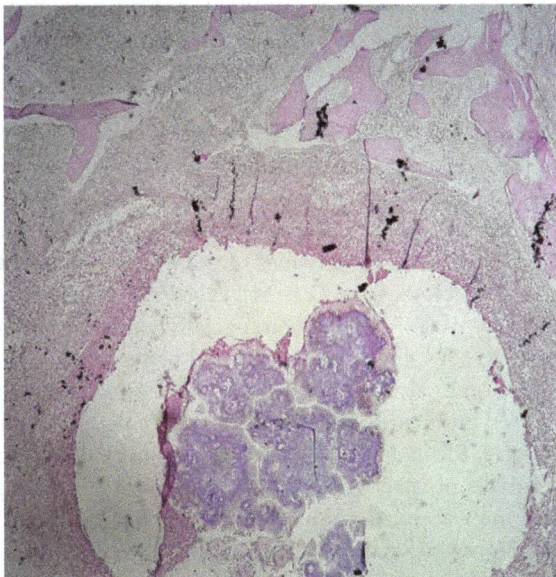

Fig. 3 Histological aspects (HES stained section) with a fractured colony destroying the bone tissue

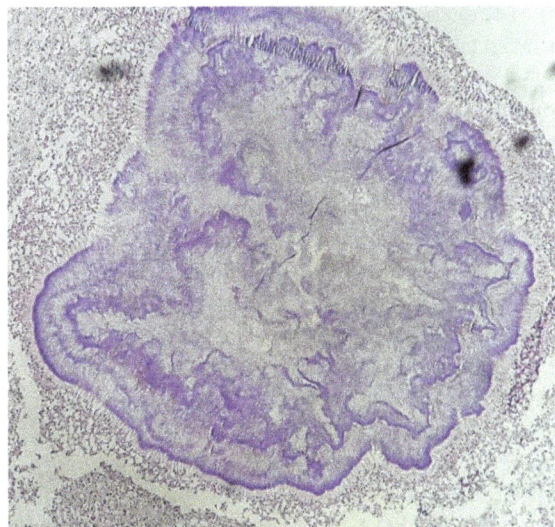

Fig. 4 The histological image (HES stained section) showing a mycetoma colony with deeply basophilic outer layer and a pale center

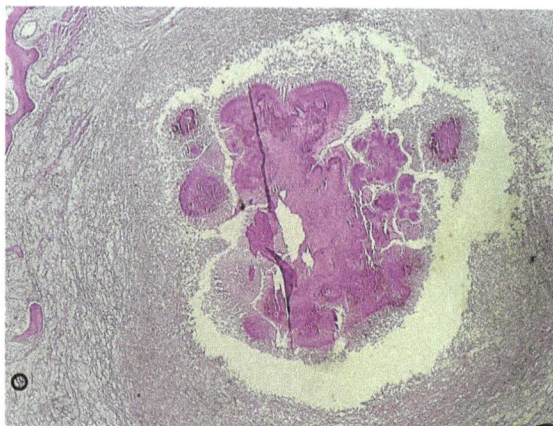

Fig. 5 Histological image (PAS stained section) showing a positive staining colony

mycetoma cases have been reported in Europe, with long course and subsequent amputation [11].

The more challenging issue with mycetoma is the diagnosis in early stage of the disease before complications that could lead to aggressive therapeutic option such as amputation. The issue becomes even more challenging when it comes to identification of the causative agent. In fact, the treatment depends on the type of the causative microorganism and on the severity and extension of the disease. The imaging technics such as X-rays, ultrasonography, computed tomography (CT Scan) and magnetic resonance imaging (MRI) allow easily to assess the extension of mycetoma especially invasion of deeper structures like muscles or bones [13, 14, 16].

To identify the causative agents, culture methods are considered the gold standard as they allow the identification of the wide species linked to mycetoma [1, 13, 16]. However cultures methods are time consuming, certain species are difficult to identify, and contaminations are common. [1, 13, 14] The culture failed to identify the causative agent in our case, it only has identified *stapyloccocus aureus species.* Similarly, skin tests or serology could be used to identify the causative agents at species level, but these technics are not fully reliable [1, 13, 16]. Currently, molecular technics are the only reliable diagnostic tool to identify the exact species of the causative organisms. The main drawback of molecular technics is their high cost for developing countries where mycetoma is mostly endemic [1, 13]. Histopathology is another diagnostic tool that can aid to identify the causative agent. The main merits of pathology is to differentiate eumycetoma from actinomycetoma, identification at species level is not reliable, almost impossible [13–17]. Grains of the causative agent can be obtained by cotton swab from sinuses, by fine needle aspiration or by biopsy [1, 6, 16, 17]. Superficial grains from sinuses

are often non viable and contaminated with other organisms, ideally deep-seated grains provide more diagnostic informations. The macroscopic examination of grains do not provide any specific diagnostic orientation. Eumycetoma could have black, white or yellow grains, whereas actinomycotic grains could have yellow, white, red or pink color. However, in a long standing disease, fibrotic lesions can be so extensive that discharge from sinuses becomes scarce or completely inapparent [14]. Biopsy from these lesions are always non conclusive or misleading, showing non specific inflammation or mimic certain malignancies, as commonly reported in the literature. In fact, the important population of reactive fibroblasts and histiocyts, along with fibrotic and haemorrhagic changes, may lead some pathologists to think about Kaposi sarcoma. The long course of the disease and its extension to adjacent structures may also play a role in the misdiagnosis of malignancies. Recently, in Morocco, another case has been reported where the patient had been misdiagnosed as Kaposi's sarcoma, and given chemotherapy before the correct diagnosis of mycetoma [18]. Typically, our case illustrated also the diagnostic challenge posed by mycetoma especially in non endemic areas. The patient had several biopsies that showed non specific inflammation, the latest has concluded to Kaposi's sarcoma invading bone structures, justifying amputation. The histopathological diagnostic approch uses hemateineosin-safran (HES) stain combined with other special stain such as PAS, Gram stain, Ziehl Nielson stain (ZN), Grocott satin,...etc. [1, 13–17]. With HES stain, the grains represent colonies of the causative agent, surrounded by granulomatous inflammation composed of plasma cells, polymorphonuclear cells, macrophages and giant cells. Colonies from actinomycetoma have different size, often round or multilobulated, with deeply stained basophilic outer border and slightly paler center [14, 15, 18]. Sometimes, an eosinophilic hyaline-like material surrounds the colonies, this aspect is referred to as Splendore-Hoeppli Phenomenon [14]. The colonies may also show fractured aspect [1, 14, 15]. The filaments are thin, their thickness is no more than 1 μm [13–17]. Typically, actinomycotic colonies are Gram positive and negative for PAS stain [13, 14]. *Nocardia* species stain positively to ZN [1, 14]. Histologically, our case stained postive to PAS, the fact that allowed us to rule out actinomycetoma although colonies were multilobulated, fractured and had basophilic outer layers with pale centers, at HES stain. Colonies from eumycetoma show several histological aspects that can have overlapping appearence with actinomycetoma colonies, but their filaments are thicker, 2-6 μm [13, 14]. They stain positive for PAS, negative for Gram stain or ZN stain. In fact, as cultures are time-consuming, and sometimes negative, pathology provides useful aid to discriminate between actinomycotic and eumycotic causative agents, by using HES stain combined with other special stains [13–17]. Pathology also rule out any malignancy or specific granulomatous inflammations such us tuberculosis. Thus, treatment can be adjusted.

The treatment of mycetoma depends on the causative agent, either fungal or bacterial, hence the necessary determination of the type of causative organism. Both eumycetoma and actinomycetoma are treated with antifungal or antibacterial drugs, sometimes combined with surgery. The treatment of eumycetoma uses antifungal drugs belonging to the azole class, such as ketoconazole, itranonazole, terbinafine or voriconazole. But since 2013, there was some restrictions of the use of ketoconazole by the US Food and Drug Administration, followed latter by the European Medicines Agency, because of several side effects [1]. These drugs are used for months, and associated with surgical debridement. Recurrences are frequent, and compliance to treatment seems difficult [1, 4]. Actinomycetoma is treated by a combination of trimethoprim and sulfamethoxazole with aminosids (amikacin or netilmicine), for weeks. The prognosis of actinomycetoma seems to be better compared to eumycetoma [1, 6, 18]. Table 1 summarizes some different charactristics of eumycetoma and actinomycetoma.

Despite the long-term treatment and recurrences observed in medical treatment, aggressive surgery is not the first line of treatment [1, 6, 19]. Amputations are generally due to misdiagnosis or a long-standing disease that spreads to deeper structures of the body [5, 7, 11, 18]. In fact, our patient should have been treated medically, rather than surgically, but the misdiagnosis due to the fact that clinicians were not familiar to mycetoma here in Morocco, as it is not an endemic area of mycetoma. Misdiagnosis and mismanagement are common in non endemic regions.

Conclusion

We have reported a case of mycetoma in a non endemic area, that evolved for more than 2 decades, misdiagnosed as a cancer and leading to an unnecessary and aggressive surgery. This case illustrated well the diagnostic challenge of mycetoma in certain areas of the world where the disease is not endemic; health practitioners should be aware of that in order to provide early diagnosis and appropriate treatment.

Abbreviations
HES: hematoxyline-eosine-safran; PAS: periodic acid-Schiff; WHO: World Health Organisation; ZN: Ziehl Nielson stain

Acknowledgements
Not applicable.

Funding
The authors received no specific funding for this study.

Authors' contributions
BE wrote the article, made substantial contributions to conception and design of the article; LT, MSB, GAE, NH and EFH made critical assessement of the article; LC has been involved in drafting the manuscript and revising it critically for important intellectual content. All authors read and approved the final version of the manuscript.

Competing interests
The authors declare that they have no competing interests.

Author details
[1]Departement of Pathology, Hassan II Teaching Hospital, Fès, Morocco.
[2]Departement of Parasitology, Hassan II Teaching Hospital, Fès, Morocco.

References
1. Zijlstra EE, van de Sande WW, Welsh O, Mahgoub ES, Goodfellow M, Fahal AH. Mycetoma: a unique neglected tropical disease. Lancet Infect Dis. 2016; 16:100–12.
2. Zijlstra EE, van de Sande WW, Fahal AH. Mycetoma: A Long Journey from Neglect. PLoS Negl Trop Dis. 2016;10(1):e0004244.
3. Schwartz E, Shpiro A. Madura Foot or Philoctetes Foot? Isr Med Assoc J. 2015;17(7):442–4.
4. Rattanavang S, Vongthonchit S, Bounphamala K, Vongphakdy P, Gubler J, Mayxay M, et al. Actinomycetoma in SE Asia: the first case from Laos and a review of the literature. BMC Infect Dis. 2012;12(12):349.
5. Fahal A, Mahgoub el S, El Hassan AM, Abdel-Rahman ME. Mycetoma in the Sudan: an update from the Mycetoma Research Centre, University of Khartoum,Sudan. PLoS Negl Trop Dis. 2015;9(3):e0003679.
6. van de Sande WW. Global Burden of Human Mycetoma: A Systematic Review and Meta-analysis. PLoS Negl Trop Dis. 2013;7(11):e2550.
7. Pickert AJ, Nguyen X. Madura foot. N Engl J Med. 2012;366(1):e2.
8. Viguier M, Lafaurie M. Actinomycetoma. N Engl J Med. 2015;372(3):264.
9. Brufman T, Ben-Ami R, Mizrahi M, Bash E, Paran Y. Mycetoma of the Foot Caused by Madurella Mycetomatis in Immigrants from Sudan. Isr Med Assoc J. 2015;17(7):418–20.
10. Mestre T, Vieira R, Coutinho J. Mycetoma of the Foot-Diagnosis of the Etiologic Agent and Surgical Treatment. Am J Trop Med Hyg. 2015;93(1):1–2.
11. Buonfrate D, Gobbi F, Angheben A, Marocco S, Farina C, Van Den Ende J, et al. Autochthonous cases of mycetoma in Europe: report of two cases and review of literature. PLoS One. 2014;9(6):e100590.
12. Hay RJ, Fahal AH. Mycetoma: an old and still neglected tropical disease. Trans R Soc Trop Med Hyg. 2015;109(3):169–70.
13. van de Sande WW, Fahal AH, Goodfellow M, Mahgoub el S, Welsh O, Zijlstra EE. Merits and pitfalls of currently used diagnostic tools in mycetoma. PLoS Negl Trop Dis. 2014;8(7):e2918.
14. Chufal SS, Thapliyal NC, Gupta MK. An approach to histology-based diagnosis and treatment of Madura foot. J Infect Dev Ctries. 2012;6(9):684–8.
15. Ibrahim AI, El Hassan AM, Fahal A, van de Sande WW. A histopathological exploration of the Madurella mycetomatis grain. PLoS One. 2013;8(3): e57774.

Table 1 Differential characteristics between eumycetoma and actinomycetoma

	Eumycetoma	Actinomycetoma
Epidemiology	Africa, India	Latin America
Clinical course	Less aggressive	More aggressive
Grain	Black, yellow, white	Yellow, white, red, pink
PAS	Positive	Negative
Gram	Negative	Postive/Negative
Ziehl Nielson	Negative	Positive/Negative
Filaments	2-5 µm	<1 µm
Treatment	Antifungal (azole) + surgery	Antibacterials

20

The use of dielectric blood coagulometry in the evaluation of coagulability in patients with peripheral arterial disease

Kimihiro Igari[*], Toshifumi Kudo, Takahiro Toyofuku and Yoshinori Inoue

Abstract

Background: Platelets and coagulation proteins contribute to the development of peripheral arterial disease, especially atherosclerotic disease. Several experimental studies have proven a significant correlation between hypercoagulability and atherosclerosis. We used dielectric blood coagulometry, which was initially designed to evaluate the coagulable status, to examine the coagulability of peripheral arterial disease patients, and investigated the factors that were significantly correlated with the results.

Methods: We performed dielectric blood coagulometry in 49 peripheral arterial disease patients. In addition, we recorded the patients' demographic information, including the presence of comorbidities, hemodynamic status, and laboratory findings. To investigate coagulability, we calculated the T_{max} value, which indicates the time from recalcification to maximum normalized permittivity.

Results: The T_{max} values of diabetes mellitus patients were significantly lower than those of non-diabetic patients (1 MHz, $P = 0.010$; 10 MHz, 0.011). Furthermore, the T_{max} value was statistically correlated with the activated partial thromboplastin time (1 MHz, $\rho = 0.286$, $P = 0.048$; 10 MHz, $\rho = 0.301$, $P = 0.037$).

Conclusions: Dielectric blood coagulometry detected the hypercoagulable status in diabetes mellitus patients, and reflected their level of coagulability, which was also evaluated by the activated partial thromboplastin time.

Keywords: Peripheral arterial disease, Dielectric blood coagulometry, Blood coagulation, Diabetes mellitus, Activated partial thromboplastin time

Background

Peripheral arterial disease (PAD), especially atherosclerotic obliterans, is usually characterized by chronic inflammatory disease [1]. The inflammatory reaction, which is affected by local inflammation due to leukocytes, monocytes and macrophages, leads to endothelial dysfunction [2]. Although platelets have been shown to contribute to the development of atherosclerotic disease [3], the potential role of coagulation proteins remains to be proven. However, several experimental studies have shown a significant association between hypercoagulability and the development of atherosclerosis [4].

A number of measures are used to evaluate coagulability, including the prothrombin time, the international normalized ratio (PT-INR), and the activated partial thromboplastin time (APTT). Even though these tests might evaluate the bleeding tendency, they do not properly reflect the actual hypercoagulable status in vivo [5]. Furthermore, several enzymatic factors in the plasma components and blood cells have shown to affect hypercoagulability, which are not taken into account in the PT-INR and APTT tests [6].

Dielectric blood coagulometry (DBCM), is a recently developed method of evaluating coagulability [7, 8]. DBCM calculates the temporal changes in whole blood dielectric permittivity, and evaluates the coagulable status. Hasegawa et al. [9] reported the application of DBCM in the evaluation of hypercoagulability in patients with several risk factors for atherosclerosis; however, no studies have used DBCM to investigate coagulability in PAD patients.

* Correspondence: igari.srg1@tmd.ac.jp
Division of Vascular and Endovascular Surgery, Department of Surgery, Tokyo Medical and Dental University, 1-5-45, Yushima, Bunkyo-ku, Tokyo 113-8519, Japan

In the present study, we conducted the DBCM test for the patients with PAD. Furthermore, we investigated the relationships between the DBCM results and various parameters.

Methods
Patient selection
Between September 2014 and June 2015, 49 patients with PAD due to atherosclerosis who were treated at the outpatient clinic of Tokyo Medical and Dental University Hospital were recruited for the present study. All of the patients provided their written informed consent, then we enrolled. This study was approved by the ethics committee of Tokyo Medical and Dental University (No. 701).

PAD was diagnosed based on the presence of >50% vessel stenosis due to lesions in the lower limbs. We mainly assessed the vessel stenosis by computed tomography angiography. In the cases with contraindication of using contrast media, such as chronic kidney disease and allergy, we evaluated the stenosis using magnetic resonance angiography and/or duplex ultrasound sonography. In this study, PAD of all patients was due to the atherosclerosis. Furthermore, in the present study, we included patients who previously underwent revascularization procedures to treat PAD lesions. We excluded the patients who had a history of recent malignant disease, systemic inflammatory disease, treatment with anticoagulants, or abnormal bleeding.

We retrospectively obtained the patients' demographics, medications, and medical histories using a dedicated database. The patients' medical records were reviewed as described below. Hypertension was defined as a systolic blood pressure of >130 mmHg, a diastolic blood pressure of >80 mmHg, or a history of treatment for hypertension. Dyslipidemia was defined as a serum low-density lipoprotein cholesterol level of >140 mg/dl, a high-density lipoprotein cholesterol level of <40 mg/dl, a triglyceride level of >150 mg/dl, or a history of treatment for dyslipidemia. Coronary arterial disease (CAD) was defined as the presence of angina pectoris, myocardial infarction or both, as documented on coronary angiography or based on a history of having undergone any coronary artery revascularization procedures. Cerebrovascular disease (CVD) was defined as a history of stroke, transient ischemic attacks, carotid artery revascularization, or cerebral hemorrhage. Chronic kidney disease (CKD) was defined as an estimated glomerular filtration rate of <60 ml/min/1.73 m^2, which was calculated by the serum creatinine level, age, and gender. Diabetes mellitus (DM) was defined as a fasting blood glucose level of >126 mg/dl, a hemoglobin A1c level of >6.5%, or the use of antidiabetes medication. The severity of PAD was assessed by the measurement of the ankle brachial pressure index (ABI), which was calculated as the ankle systolic blood pressure divided by the brachial

systolic blood pressure using a VasoGuard P84™ system (SciMed Ltd., Bristol, UK). Furthermore, the clinical severity of PAD was assessed by the Rutherford classification [10].

The measurement of the collected blood samples
After the patients had fasted for at least 12 h, we collected blood samples by venipuncture. The samples were kept in tubes containing 3.13% sodium citrate. Complete blood cell counts, biochemistry examinations, and coagulation tests were conducted via standard laboratory methods in our hospital. The blood samples that were used for DBCM were kept at room temperature and were examined at 3–5 h after collection.

Dielectric blood coagulometry
We performed DBCM using a prototype dielectric coagulometer (Sony Corp., Tokyo, Japan) in accordance with the methods of previous studies [7, 8, 11]. In summary, we kept the blood samples at 37 °C, and DBCM was completed at 60 min after recalcification. The measurement frequency at which DBCM measured the dielectric permittivity was ranged from 100 Hz to 10 MHz, the sampling intervals were 1 min. DBCM was performed using a 180-μl citrated whole blood sample, and blood coagulability was assessed by recalcification using 15 μl of 308 mM $CaCl_2$. A typical DBCM result is shown in a 3D plot of permittivity against the time and frequency in Fig. 1a. Hayashi et al. [8] reported that the time of dielectric coagulation obtained from the time-dependent permittivity has been well correlated with the coagulation time which was evaluated by the rheologic measurement. Then, coagulability was evaluated as the normalized permittivity according to the time series and frequency. Hayashi et al. [7] reported that the monitoring of the dielectric response at 1 MHz made it possible to obtain the clotting time, while Hasegawa et al. [9] evaluated the temporal change in the dielectric permittivity at 10 MHz, and showed a significant correlation with a hypercoagulable status. We therefore measured the change of permittivity at both 1 and 10 MHz, and evaluated the coagulability. DBCM showed a gradual increase in dielectric permittivity, which indicated the temporal acceleration of the coagulation. We therefore defined "T_{max}," which represents the time from recalcification to maximum normalized permittivity, as a parameter of coagulability (Fig. 1b). The repuroducibility of this DBCM test has been already evaluated by previous study [9].

Statistical analysis
The continuous variables are expressed as the median and interquartile range (IQR), and the categorical variables are expressed as the frequency and percentage. Statistical significance was assessed using the Mann-Whitney U test for comparisons between two groups.

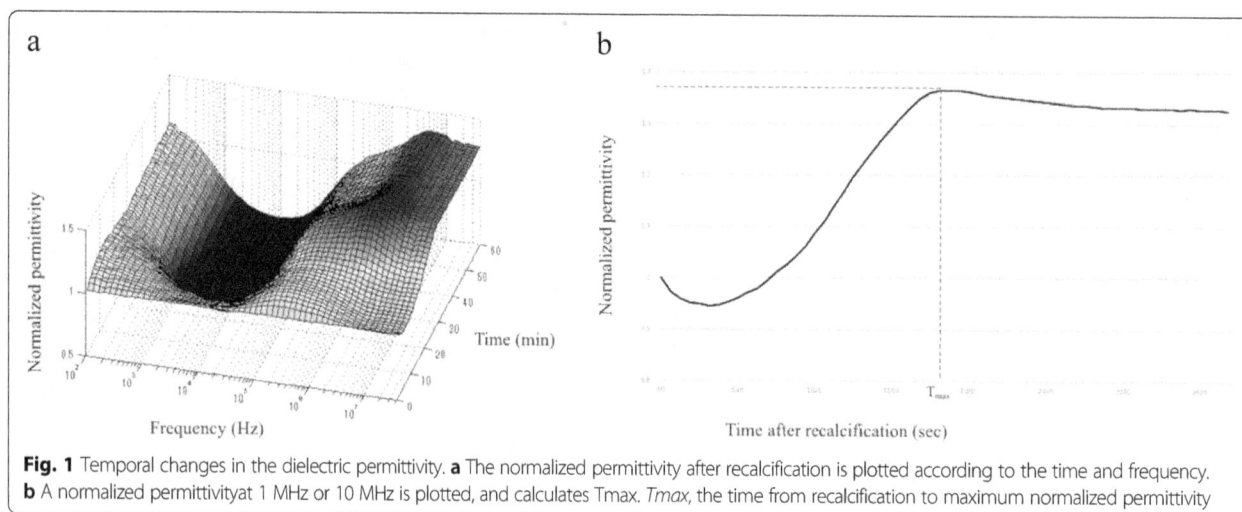

Fig. 1 Temporal changes in the dielectric permittivity. **a** The normalized permittivity after recalcification is plotted according to the time and frequency. **b** A normalized permittivity at 1 MHz or 10 MHz is plotted, and calculates Tmax. *Tmax*, the time from recalcification to maximum normalized permittivity

Correlation was assessed using Spearman's rank correlation coefficient, which reflects the degree of correlation between variables. P values <0.05 were considered to indicate statistical significance. The statistical analyses were performed using the Stat View software program (version 5, Abacus Concept Inc., Berkley, CA, USA).

Results

Patient demographics

We evaluated 49 (41 males and 8 females) PAD patients in the present study. The median age was 70 years (IQR, 63–77), and the median body mass index was 22.7 kg/m^2 (IQR, 20.8–25.1). The documented comorbidities included smoking history (85.7%), hypertension (65.3%), dyslipidemia (51.0%), CKD (22.4%), CVD (18.4%), and CAD (10.2%). All patients with DM (44.9%) were diagnosed due to the medication of antidiabetes. The patient's medications included Ca-blockers, n = 24 (49.0%); β-blockers, n = 6 (12.2%); angiotensin converting enzyme inhibitors, n = 2 (4.1%); angiotensin II receptor blockers, n = 20 (40.8%); statins, n = 22 (44.9%); and antiplatelet drugs, n = 44 (89.8%). None of the patients took anticoagulant drugs. By the Rutherford classification, 21 patients were classified as category 1, 14 patients as category 2, 8 patients as category 3, and 6 patients were divided in category 4.

Comparisons according to the patient demographics

We performed DBCM and calculated the T_{max} at 1 MHz and 10 MHz. The median T_{max} values at 1 MHz and 10 MHz were 1320 s (IQR, 1140–1620 s) and 1560 s (IQR, 1380–1920 s), respectively. We assessed the DBCM tests according to the patients' comorbidities and demographics (Table 1). The patients with DM showed significantly shorter T_{max} values than those without DM (P = 0.010 at 1 MHz, and P = 0.011 at 10 MHz, respectively). Interestingly, the T_{max} values of the patients who were receiving antiplatelet therapy did not differ to a

statistically significant extent from those of the patients who did not receive antiplatelet therapy.

The correlations between T_{max} and the other parameters

The correlations between T_{max} and each of the parameters are shown in Table 2. With the exception of the APTT (ρ = 0.286, P = 0.048 at 1 MHz, and ρ = 0.301, P = 0.037 at 10 MHz, respectively), none of the factors was significantly correlated with the T_{max} value.

Discussion

A comprehensive test that can evaluate the coagulable status is essential for the effective control of coagulability. DBCM might meet these necessities by measuring the changes in the permittivity [7]. In the present study, we evaluated the changes in permittivity at 1 MHz and 10 MHz. The dielectric permittivity of blood mainly changes at frequencies that range from hundreds of kilohertz to 10 MHz. The change occurs due to the accumulation of charge at the interface between the cytoplasm and the erythrocyte membrane [12]. Hayashi et al. [11] reported that the temporal changes in permittivity at 1 MHz reflected the clotting time. On the other hand, Hasegawa et al. [9] reported that DBCM represented a gradual increase in the dielectric permittivity from 2.5–16 MHz, and they focused on the temporal change in the dielectric permittivity at 10 MHz. Thus, both 1 and 10 MHz might be reasonable frequencies for evaluating coagulability based on the temporal changes in the permittivity. Moreover, Hayashi et al. [7] reported that the T_{max} parameter, which was referred to as "$T_{i(DS)}$" in their report, was useful for evaluating the coagulability. In our study, we evaluated the temporal changes in permittivity at frequency of 1 and 10 MHz, and calculated the 'T_{max}' value. We showed the significant correlation with the T_{max} and APTT, which represented the coagulable status, and DBCM might indicate the coagulability.

Table 1 Patient demographics and comparisons

Variables	Number	1 MHz, Tmax		10 MHz, Tmax	
		Median	P-value	Median	P-value
Gender (Male: Female)	41: 8	1320: 1260	0.569	1620: 1500	0.705
Smoking history (+: -)	42: 7	1320: 1320	0.841	1560: 1800	0.852
Hypertension (+: -)	32: 17	1290: 1440	0.338	1500: 1740	0.152
Dyslipidemia (+: -)	25: 24	1260: 1440	0.173	1500: 1650	0.652
Coronary artery disease (+: -)	5: 44	1320: 1320	0.987	1740: 1560	0.741
Cerebrovascular disease (+: -)	9: 40	1200: 1410	0.1473	1500: 1650	0.224
Chronic kidney disease (+: -)	11: 38	1080: 1380	0.167	1260: 1710	0.052
Diabetes mellitus (+: -)	22: 27	1170: 1500	0.010	1470: 1800	0.011
Ca-blocker (+: -)	24: 25	1320: 1320	0.711	1500: 1680	0.331
β-blocker (+: -)	6: 43	1500: 1320	0.492	1680: 1560	0.783
ACE-I (+: -)	2: 47	1440: 1320	0.667	1620: 1560	0.859
ARB (+: -)	20: 29	1290: 1320	0.714	1500: 1680	0.154
Statin (+: -)	22: 27	1260: 1440	0.487	1620: 1560	0.840
Antiplatelet (+: -)	44: 5	1350: 1320	0.620	1560: 1620	0.408

IQR interquartile range; ACE-I angiotensin converting enzyme – inhibitor; ARB angiotensin II receptor blocker

Our study showed a statistically significant correlation between the T_{max} and APTT values. Shortened APTTs are generally considered to be laboratory artifacts that arise from problematic venipuncture. However, there is increasing evidence to support that shortened APTT values may in some cases reflect a hypercoagulable state, which is potentially associated with an increased risk of thromboembolism [13, 14]. Tripodi et al. [15] reported that hypercoagulability, as detected by a shortened APTT value, was significantly associated with the occurrence of venous thromboembolism (VTE). In line with these reports, Hayashi et al. [8] found that DBCM allows quantitative monitoring of blood coagulability and that it is promising technique for the evaluation of VTE. Even though this mechanism has been uncertain, Hasegawa et al. [9] reported that the APTT was positively correlated with the end of acceleration time, which is almost the same as the T_{max}. The APTT might reflect the intrinsic pathways of coagulation cascade [16]. Therefore, the T_{max} might also be affected by the intrinsic pathways,

Table 2 Correlations with several parameters

Variables	Median, [IQR]	1 MHz, Tmax	10 MHz, Tmax
		ρ, P-value	ρ, P-value
Age (years)	70, [63-77]	−0.219, 0.129	−0.219, 0.130
BMI (kg/m²)	22.7, [20.8-25.1]	0.080, 0.577	0.035, 0.807
ABI	0.95, [0.78-1.07]	0.019, 0.895	0.036, 0.803
White blood cell (/μl)	6400, [5100-7600]	−0.184, 0.202	−0.162, 0.262
Hemoglobin (g/dl)	13.9, [12.9-15.1]	0.203, 0.159	0.255, 0.078
Platelet (×10⁴/μl)	22.7, [20.2-26.9]	−0.126, 0.382	−0.060, 0.678
PT-INR	0.98, [0.94-1.01]	0.223, 0.122	0.125, 0.385
APTT (sec)	28.9, [27.5-31.6]	0.286, 0.048	0.301, 0.037
Fibrinogen (mg/dl)	302, [269-339]	−0.207, 0.151	−0.058, 0.688
Albumin (g/dl))	4.1, [3.8-4.4]	0.213, 0.189	0.212, 0.192
Creatinine (mg/dl)	0.89, [0.75-1.0]	−0.104, 0.472	−0.107, 0.457
Total cholesterol (mg/dl)	185, [166.3-207.8]	−0.057, 0.697	0.048, 0.741
Triglycerides (mg/dl)	118, [80.5-165]	0.061, 0.681	0.100, 0.500
LDL (mg/dl)	106, [94.5-121.8]	0.195, 0.224	0.182, 0.256

BMI body mass index; ABI ankle brachial pressure index; APTT activated partial thromboplastin time; LDL low-density lipoprotein; IQR interquartile range; PT-INR Prothrombin time – International normalized ratio

and potentially be used to assess the coagulable status as same as the APTT.

Patients with DM showed significantly shorter T_{max} values at 1 and 10 MHz than those without DM in the present study. This is because hyperglycemia contributes to the hyperfibrinogemia and activates the coagulative cascade, leading to an increase in thrombin formation and in the levels of fibrinogen degradation products [17]. However, the exact mechanisms of the development of the hypercoagulable state in diabetic patients is likely to multifactorial and is not yet completely understood. Lippi et al. [18] reported that the APTT values were significantly shortened in DM patients. Similarly, Zhao et al. [19] found that the DM patients showed statistically shortened APTT values in comparison to patients without DM. Similarly, we revealed that DM patients showed significantly shortened APTT values (median, 28.5 s) in comparison to patients without DM (29.4 s) ($P < 0.001$). Thus, the present study shows that the T_{max} values yielded by DBCM are significantly correlated with both the coagulable state (as reflected by the APTT) and a hyperglycemic status, which leads to hypercoagulability.

There were no significant differences in the T_{max} values of patients who were treated with/without anti-platelet drugs. The same result was shown in a previous report [9]. In addition to DBCM, several modalities, including thromboelastography and rotational throm-boelastometry, can be used to assess whole blood coagu-lability. These modalities can be used to evaluate the effects of antiplatelet treatment [20]. Even though we theoretically evaluated the effects of antiplatelet drugs, which led to an increased T_{max} value, we did not observe any differences. This might be due to the small sample size, which was one of the limitations associated with the present study. Both the APTT value and the pres-ence of DM might have affected the association between the T_{max} and the use of antiplatelet drugs. Although the platelet counts of diabetic patients are normal, multiple studies have shown evidence of enhanced activation or increased platelet activity in DM patients [21]. Our study included 15 patients who received sarpogrelate hydrochlor-ide as antiplatelet therapy. The drug, which is a selective 5-hydroxytryptaminen 2A receptor antagonist that is used in the treatment of diabetic patients with PAD, suppresses platelet aggregation [22]. It was very interesting that anti-platelet drugs, including aspirin, clopidogrel, and cilostazol did not significantly affect the patients' T_{max} values, but that patients who were treated with sarpogrelate hydro-chloride showed increased T_{max} values at 1 and 10 MHz in comparison to patients who did not receive the drug (1 MHz: median T_{max}, 1500 vs. 1260, $P = 0.044$; 10 MHz: 1860 vs. 1500, $P = 0.027$). These discrepancies might be due to the small number of subjects and/or a bias associ-ated with the inclusion criteria. Future studies in a larger

population might reveal the effects of antiplatelet drug by DBCM.

Conclusions

We herein demonstrated that the measurement of the T_{max} value by DBCM detected a change in the coagulable status according to the APTT value and the presence of DM. Even though the use of DBCM did not reveal the exact effects of antiplatelet drugs in the present study, the T_{max} values of patients who received sarpogrelate hydro-chloride, an antiplatelet drug, were increased in comparison to those of patients who did not receive the drug. A more sensitive measurement with DBCM might therefore be successful in elucidating the effects of antiplatelet drugs.

Abbreviations
ABI: Ankle brachial pressure index; APTT: Activated partial thromboplastin time; CAD: Coronary arterial disease; CKD: Chronic kidney disease; CVD: Cerebrovascular disease; DBCM: Dielectric blood coagulometry; DM: Diabetes mellitus; IQR: Interquartile range; PAD: Peripheral arterial disease; PT-INR: Prothrombin time, the international normalized ratio; VTE: Venous thromboembolism

Acknowledgements
Not applicable.

Funding
This research did not receive any specific grant from funding agencies in the public, commercial, or not-for-profit sectors.

Authors' contributions
KI participated in study design, and data analysis and interpretation, and writing and final approval. TK and TT participated in data analysis and interpretation. YI participated in study design, and final approval. All authors read and approved the final manuscript.

Competing interests
All of the authors declare that they have no competing interests.

References
1. Hasson GK. Inflammation, atherosclerosis, and coronary artery disease. N Engl J Med. 2005;352:1685–95.
2. Libby P. Inflammation in atherosclerosis. Nature. 2002;420:868–74.
3. Davi G, Patrono C. Platelet activation and atherothrombosis. N Engl J Med. 2007;357:2482–94.
4. Loeffen R, Spronk HM, ten Cate H. The impact of blood coagulability on atherosclerosis and cardiovascular disease. J Thromb Haemost. 2012;10:1207–16.
5. Park MS, Martini WZ, Dubick MA, Salinas J, Butenas S, Kheirabadi BS, et al. Thromboelastography as a better indicator of hypercoagulable state after injury than prothrombin time or activated partial thromboplastin time. J Trauma. 2009;67:266–75.
6. Mackman N. Role of tissue factor in hemostasis, thrombosis, and vascular development. Arterioscler Thromb Vasc Biol. 2004;24:1015–22.
7. Hayashi Y, Brun MA, Machida K, Nagasawa M. Principle of dielectric blood coagulometry as a comprehensive coagulation test. Anal Chem. 2015;87:10072–9.
8. Hayashi Y, Katsumoto Y, Omori S, Yasuda A, Asami K, Kaibara M, et al. Dielectric coagulometry: a new approach to estimate venous thrombosis risk. Anal Chem. 2010;82:9769–74.
9. Hasegawa Y, Hamada S, Nishimura T, Sasaki T, Ebana Y, Kawabata M, et al. Novel dielectric coagulometer identifies hypercoagulability in patients with a high CHADS$_2$ score without atrial fibrillation. PLoS One. 2016;11:e0156557.

10. Rutherford RB, Baker JD, Ernst C, Johnston KW, Porter JM, Ahn S, et al. Recommended standards for reports dealing with lower extremity ischemia: revised version. J Vasc Surg. 1997;26:517–38.

11. Hayashi Y, Oshige I, Katsumoto Y, Omori S, Yasuda A, Asami K. Dielectric inspection of erythrocyte morphology. Phys Med Biol. 2008;53:2553–64.

12. Livshits L, Caduff A, Talary MS, Lutz HU, Hayashi Y, Puzenko A, et al. The role of GLUT1 in the sugar-induced dielectric response of human erythrocytes. J Phys Chem B. 2009;113:2212–20.

13. Mina A, Favaloro EJ, Mohammed S, Koutts J. A laboratory evaluation into the short activated partial thromboplastin time. Blood Coagul Fibrinolysis. 2010;21:152–7.

14. Korte W, Clarke S, Lefkowitz JB. Short activated partial thromboplastin time are related to increased thrombin generation and an increased risk for thromboembolism. Am J Clin Pathol. 2000;113:123–7.

15. Tripodi A, Chantarangkul V, Martineli I, Bucciarelli P, Mannucci PM. A shortened activated partial thromboplastin time is associated with the risk of venous thromboembolism. Blood. 2004;104:3631–4.

16. Bombeli T, Spahn DR. Updates in perioperative coagulation: physiology and management of thromboembolism and haemorrhage. Br J Anaesth. 2004;93:275–87.

17. Barazzoni R, Zanetti M, Davanzo G, Kiwanuka E, Carraro P, Tiengo A, et al. Increased fibrinogen production in type 2 diabetic patients without detectable vascular complications: correlation with plasma glucagon concentrations. J Clin Endocrinol Metab. 2000;85:3121–5.

18. Lippi G, Franchini M, Targher G, Montagnana M, Salvagno GL, Guidi GC, et al. Epidemiological association between fasting plasma glucose and shortened APTT. Clin Biochem. 2009;42:118–20.

19. Zhao Y, Zhang J, Zhang J, Wu J. Diabetes mellitus is associated with shortened activated partial thromboplastin time and increased fibrinogen values. PLoS One. 2011;6:e16470.

20. Swallow RA, Agarwala RA, Dawkins KD, Curzen NP. Thromboelastrography: potential bedside tool to assess the effects of antiplatelet therapy? Platelets. 2006;17:385–92.

21. Carr ME. Diabetes mellitus: a hypercoagulable state. J Diabetes Complicat. 2001;15:44–54.

22. Nakayama D, Ohira M, Saiki A, Shirai K, Tatsuno I. Sarpogrelate hydrochloride decreases cardio-ankle vascular index accompanied by increased serum lipoprotein lipase mass in type 2 diabetic patients. Int Heart J. 2014;55:337–41.

Impending relapse of myelodysplastic syndrome after allogeneic transplant is difficult to diagnose and requires a multi-modal approach

Elizabeth L. Courville[1]*(ID), Megan Griffith[1], Celalettin Ustun[2], Sophia Yohe[1] and Erica Warlick[2]

Abstract

Background: The only potentially curative therapy for myelodysplastic syndrome is allogeneic hematopoietic cell transplant; unfortunately, there is a high relapse rate. The objective of this study was to perform a detailed clinicopathologic study of patients with relapsed myeloid neoplasm following allogeneic hematopoietic cell transplant for myelodysplastic syndrome.

Methods: Pre-transplant, post-transplant, and relapse bone marrow and peripheral blood morphologic features (including dysplasia) were retrospectively evaluated by study authors. Clinical features and results of cytogenetic analysis and engraftment/chimerism studies were obtained from the medical record.

Results: Our study describes 21 patients with a median time to relapse of 6 months (range 2–82). Ten of the patients relapsed with higher grade disease, including six with overt acute myeloid leukemia. Pre-transplant megakaryocyte dysplasia was associated with dysplastic megakaryocytes in the relapse specimen; however, neither erythroid dysplasia nor granulocytic dysplasia were associated with their counterpart in the relapse specimen. Relapse specimens had a lower marrow cellularity and higher blast percentage than pre-transplant disease. Cytogenetic comparisons before and after transplant showed variety, including clonal evolution (22%), the same abnormal clone (33%), or a different abnormal clone (22%).

Conclusions: Our detailed review of post-transplant marrow biopsies prior to relapse highlights the difficulty in diagnosing relapse and particularly impending relapse.

Keywords: Allogeneic stem cell transplant, Myelodysplastic syndrome, Relapse, Cytogenetic, Acute myeloid leukemia

Background

Myelodysplastic syndromes (MDS) are the most commonly diagnosed myeloid neoplasms in the United States. MDS are clonal hematopoietic neoplasms characterized by ineffective hematopoiesis and varying risk of transformation to acute myeloid leukemia (AML). According to the World Health Organization (WHO) [1], MDS are further subclassified based on the number of dysplastic lineages, the number of cytopenic lineages, the percentage of ring sideroblasts, the bone marrow and peripheral blood blast percentages, the presence or absence of Auer rods, and cytogenetic findings. This heterogeneous group has variable prognoses and treatments ranging from supportive care only to chemotherapy (hypomethylating agent based therapy or intensive AML-type induction chemotherapy) to possible subsequent allogeneic hematopoietic cell transplant (HCT) [2, 3]. Therapy choice is guided by risk stratification based on the International Prognostic Scoring System (IPSS) and revised IPSS (IPSS-R) [4, 5], as well as other patient factors including age, performance status, transfusion needs, and response to first-line therapy, and donor options.

* Correspondence: ecourvil@umn.edu
[1]Department of Laboratory Medicine and Pathology, University of Minnesota, 420 Delaware St SE, MMC 609, Minneapolis, MN 55455, USA
Full list of author information is available at the end of the article

The only potentially curative therapy for MDS is allogeneic HCT. Unfortunately, relapse remains a concern with rates in the 20–50% range [6–8]. The relapse risk likely depends on multiple factors including the preparative regimen (myeloablative versus non-myeloablative or reduced-intensity), stem cell and donor source (umbilical cord blood versus sibling or adult unrelated bone marrow/peripheral blood), and pre-transplant MDS disease burden as well as MDS disease characteristics. The optimal method or combination of methods to detect impending relapse following transplant is not clear nor is the optimal therapeutic intervention for impending relapse [7].

In this study, we performed a detailed assessment of 21 patients with relapsed myeloid neoplasm following allogeneic HCT. We evaluated diagnostic MDS characteristics (IPSS, WHO classification, cytogenetics) as well as a comparison of pre-transplant and relapsed disease morphology, cytogenetics, and flow cytometry. Intervening (post-transplant, pre-relapse) data was also reviewed. Late relapse cases arising >6 months after transplant were compared to early relapse cases.

Methods

This retrospective study was approved by the University of Minnesota Institutional Review Board (Study Number 1312 M46725) and performed according to the ethical standards of our institution. As part of the approval process by the University of Minnesota IRB, it was determined that informed consent was not required for this retrospective research study. Patients were identified by search of the bone marrow transplant database. Adult patients (≥18 years old) were included if they received their first allogeneic HCT for MDS at the University of Minnesota between 2000 and 2015. Patients were excluded if their pre-transplant bone marrow biopsy slides were not reviewed at our institution, if no post-transplant biopsy was obtained, or if there was persistent marrow disease post-transplant. The electronic medical record was used to extract clinical information. Pathology reports from the following specimens were reviewed for all patients: [1] original MDS diagnosis, [2] pre-transplant MDS diagnosis, [3] immediate pre-transplant biopsy (following cytoreductive therapy), [4] post-transplant biopsy specimens interpreted at our institution up to and including [5] the post-transplant relapse biopsy. The information extracted included the bone marrow cellularity and blast percentage, peripheral blood counts, and circulating blast percentages. The post-transplant cases, [4], were categorized as "negative" or "indeterminate" for morphologic evidence of myeloid neoplasm based on review of the original pathology report.

Available slides from the pre-transplant MDS diagnosis [2] (slides available for 15 patients) and post-transplant relapse marrow [5] (slides available for 20

patients) were reviewed by study author EC and scored for dysplasia in a semi-quantitative manner modified from the system used by Weinberg, et al. [9]. Reviewed slides included H&E stained slides of the trephine core, immunohistochemical stains performed at the time of diagnosis, Wright-Giemsa stained marrow aspirate and peripheral blood slides, and Dacie (iron) stained marrow slides. Dysplasia was scored in each lineage in increments of 10%. Specific dysplastic features in the megakaryocyte lineage were: micromegakaryocytes, hypolobated or monolobated megakaryocytes of normal size, megakaryocytes with two or more separated rounded nuclear lobes. Specific dysplastic features in the erythroid lineage were: megaloblastoid change, multinucleation, nuclear irregularities, pyknosis, and basophilic stippling. Ring sideroblast percentage was documented. Specific dysplastic features in the granulocyte lineage were: abnormal nuclear shape and hypogranulation. A lineage was only evaluated if sufficient cells were available for analysis.

To evaluate for morphologic features of impending relapse, slides from the bone marrow biopsy specimen immediately prior to the relapse specimen were reviewed by study author SY, who was blinded to the original pathology interpretation and the results of corresponding ancillary studies. The presence or absence of dysplasia, and affected lineages, was documented, and blasts were evaluated as increased or decreased. Based on the morphology alone, the specimens were re-interpreted as "negative", "positive", or "indeterminate" for relapsed myeloid neoplasm.

Flow cytometric studies and cytogenetic analysis were performed using standard techniques at the time of diagnosis, with the interpretive reports reviewed for this study. Flow cytometry studies evaluated for aberrant antigen expression on myeloid blasts using either 4-color or 10-color panels. Antigens evaluated included CD3, CD7, CD10, CD13, CD14, CD15, CD19, CD33, CD34, CD45, CD56, CD117, and HLA-DR. Myeloid maturation patterns by flow cytometry were not evaluated. Engraftment/chimerism analysis was performed as previously described [10], with interpretive reports reviewed for this study.

Statistical analysis was performed using the IBM SPSS Statistics program version 22. A two-tailed Fisher's exact test was used for categorical data and a Mann-Whitney U test (for independent samples) or Wilcoxon signed-ranks test (for related samples) was used for continuous data.

Results

Our patient cohort included 10 males and 11 females. The median age at transplant was 59 years (range 34 to 71). Three patients had a medication history compatible with therapy-related myeloid neoplasm. One patient received cyclophosphamide for scleroderma/interstitial lung disease for 2 years ending 3 years prior to MDS diagnosis, one patient received multi-agent chemotherapy for breast cancer (including paclitaxel, doxorubicin, and cyclophosphamide) 4 years prior to MDS diagnosis, and one patient was treated with doxorubicin and cyclophosphamide for breast cancer 10 years prior to MDS diagnosis.

Eighteen patients were treated with a non-myeloablative/reduced intensity conditioning regimen prior to transplant (cytarabine, fludarabine, and total body irradiation with or without anti-thymocyte globulin, $n = 17$, or busulfan/fludarabine, $n = 1$) and three were treated with a myeloablative conditioning regimen (busulfan and cytarabine or cytarabine and fractionated total body irradiation). Graft-versus-host-disease prophylaxis included cyclosporine and mycophenolate mofetil ($n = 17$), cyclosporine and methotrexate ($n = 3$) or methotrexate and tacrolimus ($n = 1$). Source of donor stem cells included umbilical cord blood ($n = 10$), sibling ($n = 9$), and unrelated donor ($n = 2$).

Pre-transplant MDS versus relapse characteristics

Patient were most commonly transplanted for refractory anemia with excess blasts (RAEB-1 or 2, $n = 13$) and refractory cytopenias with multilineage dysplasia (RCMD, $n = 3$). In eight patients, disease prior to transplant included ring sideroblasts, with five having a ring sideroblast percentage $\geq 15\%$. Of the relapses, six cases relapsed with overt AML and one additional case (Case 75) progressed to AML 2 months after initial relapse (only withdrawal of immunosuppression prior to progression). Two cases relapsed as MDS with increased blasts where the pre-transplant disease lacked excess blasts, and an additional case lacked an increase in blasts in both the pre-transplant and relapse specimens but progressed to RAEB-1 2 months after initial relapse despite a reduction in immunosuppression in the intervening time.

The presence of dysplastic megakaryocytes in the pre-transplant specimen showed a statistically significant association with the presence of dysplastic megakaryocytes in the relapse specimen ($p = 0.018$) with increased significance ($p = 0.001$) when a dysplastic megakaryocyte threshold of 50% was applied. In contrast, neither erythroid dysplasia/ring sideroblasts in the pre-transplant specimen nor granulocytic dysplasia in the pre-transplant specimen was associated with their counterpart in the relapse specimen ($p = 0.520/1.0$, and 0.070, respectively).

There was a significant difference between the pre-transplant and relapse bone marrow cellularity [pre-transplant median of 73% (range 15–95%) and relapse median of 45% (range 10–90%), $p = 0.003$] and blast percentage [pre-transplant median of 5% (range 1–19%) and relapse median of 10% (range 0.2–51%), $p = 0.023$] but there was no significant difference between the pre-transplant and relapse peripheral blood blast percentage.

There was a significant difference between the pre-transplant and relapse platelet count [pre-transplant median of 73×10^9/L (range 5–1242) and relapse median 38×10^9/L (range 7–189), $p = 0.028$] and a borderline significant difference between the pre-transplant and relapse white blood cell count [pre-transplant median 3.3×10^9/L (1–33 range) and relapse median 2.5×10^9/L (0.6–7.6 range) $p = 0.054$]. No statistically significant difference was seen between the pre-transplant and relapse hemoglobin, mean corpuscular volume (MCV) or absolute neutrophil count.

The majority (18/21, 86%) of cases had an abnormal karyotype in the myeloid neoplasm before and/or after transplant. Pre- and post-transplant cytogenetic comparisons were categorized as follows: same abnormal relapse clone (6/18, 33%), relapse clone with some similarities (4, 22%), relapse clone showing clonal evolution (4, 22%), and different relapse clone (4, 22%). Some cases were placed in the "relapse clone with some similarities" category because only targeted FISH analysis and not a full karyotype was performed at the time of relapse.

Flow cytometry data was available for a subset of specimens. Of the nine pre-transplant flow cytometry studies, three showed an increase in blasts and three showed an abnormal immunophenotype on blasts (heterogeneous/partial CD7 expression or homogenous expression of antigens/discrete cluster). The majority of relapse disease flow cytometry specimens (15/19, 79%) had increased blasts. In those cases without increased blasts, immunophenotypic abnormalities noted but not considered definitive included heterogenous or partial CD7 expression or homogenous expression of myeloid markers such as CD13 and CD33. A single pair of pre-transplant and relapse flow cytometry studies showed immunophenotypic similarities with partial CD7 expression in both.

Early versus late relapse (Table 1)

The median time to relapse after transplant was 6 months (range 2–82). Eleven patients had a late relapse, defined as >180 days (6 months) after transplant, with a median time to relapse of 15.4 months (range 6–81.6 months). The ten patients with early relapse had a median time to relapse of 3 months (range 2.2–5.8). Table 1 compares the patients with early versus late relapse.

To summarize, patients with late relapse had a younger median age at transplant and had a higher median bone marrow blast percentage at relapse. Donor source (umbilical cord blood versus non-umbilical cord blood), conditioning regimen (myeloablative versus non-myeloablative), and IPSS risk score were not associated with timing of relapse, although the number of patients in each category was small. All three therapy-related MDS cases were late relapses, occurring 6, 19, and

Table 1 Comparison of Hematologic and Morphologic Features Between Early and Late Relapse Patients

	Early Relapse (<6 months) n = 10	Late Relapse (>6 months) n = 11	p-value
Age at transplant, years, median (range)	67 (34–71)	58 (46–61)	**0.013**
Gender, M:F	5:5	6:5	NS
Time to relapse from transplant, months, median (range)	3 (2–6)	15 (6–82)	**<0.001**
Pre-transplant MDS specimen, peripheral blood and bone marrow characteristics			
Hgb, g/dL, median(range)	9.0 (7.6–12.7)	9.3 (5.6–12.9)	NS
MCV, fL, median (range)	89 (73–109)	101 (86–107)	**0.023**
WBC, $\times 10^9$/L, median (range)	3.0 (1.1–10.2)	3.3 (1–33)	NS
ANC, $\times 10^9$/L, median (range)	0.9 (0.1–7.8)	1.1 (0.4–24.1)	NS
Platelets, $\times 10^9$/L, median (range)	36 (10–1242)	89 (5–206)	NS
Blood blasts, %, median (range)	1 (0–16)	0.5 (0–13)	NS
Dysgranulopoiesis[a]	4/7	3/8	NS
Dyserythropoeisis[a]	5/7	6/8	NS
Dysmegakaryopoiesis[a]	4/6	5/3	NS
Ring sideroblasts[a]	4/8	4/9	NS
Marrow cellularity, %, median (range)	90 (15–95)	43 (30–95)	0.075
Bone marrow blasts, %, median (range)	4 (1–19)	7 (2–14)	NS
Increased marrow blasts (>5%)	7/10 (70%)	8/11 (72%)	NS
Relapse myeloid neoplasm specimen, peripheral blood and bone marrow characteristics			
Hgb, g/dL, median(range)	10.0 (8.6–12.2)	9.8 (8.1–13)	NS
MCV, fL, median (range)	88 (80–105)	99 (87–113)	0.051
WBC, $\times 10^9$/L, median (range)	2.2 (0.6–7.6)	2.5 (1.5–3.4)	NS
ANC, $\times 10^9$/L, median (range)	1.3 (0.2–5.9)	1.2 (0.2–2.5)	NS
Platelets, $\times 10^9$/L, median (range)	20 (7–128)	66 (10–189)	0.061
Blood blasts, %, median (range)	0.3 (0–15)	2 (0–38)	NS
Dysgranulopoiesis[a]	3/9	2/11	NS
Dyserythropoeisis[a]	5/9	6/11	NS
Dysmegakaryopoiesis[a]	7/8:5/8	6/10:3/10	NS
Ring sideroblasts[a]	6/6	1/3	**0.033**
Marrow cellularity, %, median (range)	48 (20–90)	45 (10–90)	NS
Bone marrow blasts, %, median (range)	5 (0.2–30)	14 (4–51)	**0.029**
Increased marrow blasts (>5%)	5/10 (50%)	10/11 (91%)	0.063

Bold indicates statistical significance

[a]Any degree of dysplasia ≥10% of a lineage. See text (materials and methods section) for specific dysplastic features included for this study; "n" for dysplasia and ring sideroblast evaluation varies for each category depending on the slides and number of precursors in each lineage available for review

49 months after transplant. Dysplasia characteristics in the pre-transplant or relapse specimens did not show a statistically significant association with timing of relapse, nor did the cytogenetic comparison. There was no association between relapse as overt AML (>20% blasts) and timing of relapse.

Pre-relapse marrow evaluation

Post-transplant bone marrow biopsy specimens evaluated at our institution up to and including the relapse specimen are presented in Tables 2 and 3 (divided into early and late relapse cases) including morphologic interpretation,

engraftment results, and cytogenetics results. There was no significant association between a morphologic interpretation of indeterminate and subsequent morphologic interpretation of relapse (6 of 15 specimens interpreted as indeterminate and 14 of 48 specimens interpreted as negative had morphologic relapse in the subsequent marrow biopsy, p = 0.528).

For this study, we retrospectively reviewed, blinded to the original interpretation and time-point, slides from the bone marrow biopsy immediately prior to the relapse specimen. The morphologic conclusion at the time of original interpretation and at the time of review for this

Table 2 Early Relapse Cases

Study No	Age at transplant/ IPSS score	Original MDS Diagnosis — Diagnosis/CG	Pre-transplant MDS Diagnosis — Diagnosis/CG	Immediate pre-transplant Marrow Biopsy (following cytoreductive therapy) — Diagnosis/CG	Post-transplant Assessment 1 — Morphologic Conclusion/ Engraftment[a]/CG	Post-transplant Assessment 2 — Morphologic Conclusion/ Engraftment[a]/CG	Post-transplant Assessment 3 — Morphologic Conclusion/ Engraftment[a]/CG	Post-transplant Assessment 4 — Morphologic Conclusion/ Engraftment[a]/CG	Follow-up — Status/Relapse Treatment	Cytogenetics Comparison
7	61/INT-1	RARS /46,XX,del(12)(p11.2p13)[7]/46,XX [13]	RARS /46,XX,del(12)(p11.2p13)[3]/46,XX [17]	No intervening marrows pre-transplant	Indeterminate /6 /Neg by FISH	**MDS with dyserythropoiesis and numerous ring sideroblasts, no increase in blasts[c] /88 /46,XX[49]//46,XY[1]**			Deceased of invasive aspergillus lung infection with persistent MDS/ reduction in immunosuppression then DLI for subsequent RAEB-1	Some similarities between clones
Days[b]		-699			23	100			237/137 (post-relapse)	
27	69/Unknown	RCMD-RS	RCMD-RS/45,XY,-7,del(20q)(q11.2q13.1) [3]	No intervening marrows pre-transplant	Indeterminate /30.6 / monosomy 7 by FISH (8% interphase cells)	Negative /0 /monosomy 7 by FISH (2.75%, slightly above normal control range)	Negative /0 /not performed	**MDS with dysmegakaryopoiesis, numerous ring sideroblasts, no increase in blasts /12.6 /45,XY,-7,del(20q)(q11.2q13.3)[3]/46,XY[12]**	Unknown/ Unknown	Same abnormal clone
Days[b]			-15		22	60	98	155		
32	62/INT-1	RAEB-1	RAEB-2/clone with trisomy 8	Hypercellular marrow with no increase in blasts; 3.25% by FISH with extra chromosome 8	Indeterminate /6.1 /Neg by FISH	Indeterminate /11.8 /Neg by FISH and karyotype	AML /41.8 /46,XX,t(2:3)(q23;q26-27)[4]/46,XX[14]		Unknown/ Unknown	Different abnormal clone
Days[b]		-111	-31	-29	21	63	98			
34	49/HIGH	RAEB-1 /complex karyotype including deletion of 5q	Same specimen as original MDS diagnosis	Normocellular marrow with no increase in blasts/cytogenetics not performed	Negative /57.4 /Neg by FISH	Negative /29.6 /loss of chromosome 5 by FISH (6.75% interphase cells) and complex karyotype	MDS with dysgranulopoiesis, borderline increased marrow blasts, and rare circulating blasts / 20.3/FISH: 19.5% had a signal pattern indicative of loss of both 5p15.2 and q31		Unknown/ Unknown	Some similarities between clones
Days[b]		-376	-141		33	36	65			
58	67/LOW	MDS with isolated del(5q) /46,XY,del(5)(q13q33) [18]/46,XY [2]	RAEB-2/46,XY,del(5)(q22q33)[18]/46,XY [2]	No intervening marrows pre-transplant	Indeterminate /0 /Neg by FISH	Indeterminate /3 /Neg by FISH	RAEB-1 /38 /46,XY,del(5)(q22q35)[11*]/46,XY[7]/46,XX[2]		Unknown/ Unknown	Same abnormal clone
Days[b]		-200		-25	21	98	137			
63	68/INT-2	RCMD-RS /45~46,XY,add(4)(q31),del(5)(q15q33),del(7)(q22q34),+8,del(11)(q14q23),add(12)(p11.2),add(12)(p11.2),dic(14;15)P(11.2p11.2),-18,+2mar[cp5]	RAEB-2/44-46,XY,-3,del(4)(q31q35),del(5)(q15q33),del(7)(q22q36),+8,del(11)(q21q23),add(12)(p11.2),add(12)(p11.2),dic(14;15)(p11.2p11.2),-17,-18,+2mar[cp5]	Normocellular marrow with no increase in blasts/ Negative by FISH	Negative /2.9 /Neg by FISH	**RAEB-2 /91.8 /FISH: 83% had a signal pattern consistent with deletion of the long arm of one chromosome 5**			Unknown/ azacitidine	Some similarities between clones
Days[b]		-458			21	98				

Table 2 Early Relapse Cases (Continued)

Case	Age / IPSS	Diagnostic marrow (Days)	Pre-transplant / intervening marrow (Days)	Post-transplant marrow (Days)	Later marrow (Days)	Relapse marrow (BOLD) (Days)	Survival (engraftment/post-relapse)[a]	Outcome	Comment
(cont.)						8,01mar[cp18]/46,XY [2]			
78	69/LOW	RARS-T /46,XY,dup(1)(q21q43) [14]/46,XY,der(15)t(1;15)(q12p11.2) [3]/46,XY [3] (−298)	Same specimen as original MDS diagnosis[d] (−126); No intervening marrows pre-transplant (−15)	Indeterminate/0 /Neg by FISH (21)	Negative/7 /Neg by FISH (90)	**Abnormal with 5% ring sideroblasts /14 /46,XY,dup(1)(q21q43)[2]/46,XY,der(15)t(1;15)(q12p11.2)[1*]/46,XY[17]**	129/39 (post-relapse)	Deceased with steroid refractory late acute GVHD/No intervention	Same abnormal clone
79	70/INT-2	RAEB-1 /43–44,XX,−5,−7,−19,−22,+12mar [3]/42,45,sl,−18,+14[11]/46,XX [6] (−21)	Persistent MDS with 3% marrow blasts/44,XX,−5,−7,−18,−19,−22,+3mar [2]/46,XX [19]	Negative/ not performed /Neg by FISH (23)	(100)	**Suspicious for myeloid neoplasm with slight trilineage dyspoiesis and 4% to 5% blasts /23 /44,XX,−5,−7,−19,−22,+mar1,+mar2[3]/43,idem,−18[2]/46,XY[15]** (174)	232/58 (post-relapse)	Alive currently undergoing treatment for relapse (as AML) that occurred 2 years after DLI/ immunosuppression withdrawal	Same abnormal clone
81	71/INT-1	RAEB-1; RAEB-1/Normal karyotype (−70)	No evidence of residual disease/cytogenetics not performed (−28)	Negative[e] /38 /normal karyotype (20)		**RAEB-1 / 26/ 46,XX[19]** (90)	625/535 (post-relapse)	Deceased with persistent disease/withdrawal of immunosuppression then ALT-803 trial	No clonal abnormality pre-transplant disease and relapse
82[f]	34/INT-1	RCMD /46,XY,add(6)(7p21.2) [18]/46,XY [2] (−735/−230); RCMD /46,XY add(6)(7p21.1) [20] (−165)	No intervening marrows pre-transplant (−38/−35)	Indeterminate /0 /normal karyotype (21/62)	Indeterminate /1 /not performed (98/99)	**AML /66 /46,XY ,add(6)(p21.1) [4]/46,idem,t(9;14)(q34;q24)[14]/46,X,t(Y;1)(p11.3;q21),del(4)(q11), der(13)t(4;13)(q11.p13),add(6)[2]** (139)	465/367; 374/235 (post-relapse)	Deceased with persistent disease/ 7 + 3 induction, ALT-803, GCLAC chemotherapy, azacitidine, DLI	Clonal evolution

RELAPSE MARROWS in BOLD

Abbreviations: IPSS International prognostic scoring system, MDS myelodysplastic syndrome, CG cytogenetics, INT-1 Intermediate-1, INT-2 Intermediate-2, RARS Refractory anemia with ring sideroblasts, RCMD refractory cytopenias with multilineage dysplasia, RCMD-RS refractory cytopenias with multilineage dysplasia and ring sideroblasts, RAEB refractory anemia with excess blasts, AML acute myeloid leukemia, FISH fluorescence in-situ hybridization, DLI donor lymphocyte infusion, GCLAC G-CSF priming, cloraribine, and high dose cytarabine, ALT-803 trial IL-15 Superagonist Clinical Trial, GVHD graft versus host disease

[a] Engraftment is reported as % recipient
[b] Days are relative to transplant date unless otherwise noted
[c] Bone marrow biopsy 2 months after showed RAEB-1
[d] Patient carries diagnosis of RARS-T since 2007, reason for transplant is clonal progression and development of transfusion requirements
[e] Case 81 was called positive on study review due to increased blasts
[f] Received myeloablative chemotherapy pre-transplant

Table 3 Late Relapse Cases

Study No	Age at transplant/ IPSS score	Original MDS Diagnosis	Pre-transplant MDS Diagnosis	Immediate pre-transplant Marrow Biopsy (following cytoreductive therapy)	Post-transplant Assessment 1	Post-transplant Assessment 2	Post-transplant Assessment 3	Post-transplant Assessment 4	Post-transplant Assessment 5	Post-transplant Assessment
		Diagnosis/CG	Diagnosis/CG	Diagnosis/CG	Morphologic Conclusion/Engraftment[a]/CG	Morphologic Conclusion/Engraftment[a]/CG	Morphologic Conclusion/Engraftment[a]/CG	Morphologic Conclusion/Engraftment[a]/CG	Morphologic Conclusion/Engraftment[a]/CG	Morpho Conclus Engraftm /CG
10[b,c]	51 /INT-2	RCMD/45,XX,-5,add(7)(q11.2) [8]/41-43,XX,-5,add(7)(q11.2),-12,-16,-18,-20[cp4]/46,XX [9]	RCMD/45,XX,-5,add(7)(q11.2) [4]/42,idem,-12,-16, -20[6]/49XX [10]	No intervening marrows pre-transplant	Negative /0 /Neg by karyotype	**AML /47.6 /Abn by FISH. 36% with loss of the long arm of one chromosome 5 and 41.5% had a signal pattern consistent with loss of the long arm of chromosome 7**				
Days[d]		−129	−17		95	1477				
17	50 /INT-1	RCMD/ 46,XX,+1,der(1;7)(q10:p10) [15]/46,XX [5]	RCMD/46,XX,+1,der(1;7)(q10p10) [5]/46,XX,-7,+21[11]/46,XX [4]	No intervening marrows pre-transplant	Negative /0 /Neg by FISH	Negative /0 /not performed	Negative /0 /not performed	Negative /0 /not performed	Negative /0 /Neg by FISH	Negative Neg by
Days		−849	−17		21	61	98	182	367	733
33	46 /INT-2	RAEB-2/46,XX [20]	Same specimen as original MDS diagnosis	Normocellular marrow with no dysplasia and no increase in blasts/ normal karyotype	Negative /37.5 /not performed	Negative /0 /not performed	Negative /0 /not performed	Indeterminate[e] /0 /46,XX,t(6;12)(p22;p13) [3]/46,XX [11]/46,XX[16]	**AML /26.1 /46,XX,t(6;12)(p22;p13)[9]/46,XX[11]**	
Days		−90	−17		21	101	182	364	410	
39	59 /INT-1	RAEB-1/46,XY,add(11)(q13)	RAEB-1/46,XY,der(11)t(3;11)(q13.2;q13)[15]/46,XY [5]	No intervening marrows pre-transplant	Negative /72.5 /derivative 11 in 2 of 6 male (recipient) metaphases	Negative /70.7 derivative 11 in 7 of 12 male metaphases	Negative /12.4 /derivative 11 in 2 of 2 male metaphases	Negative /13.2 /derivative 11 in 4 of 4 male metaphases and 2 with additional t(1;7;13)(p31;q22;q13)	Negative /42.7 /derivative 11 in 9 of 9 male metaphases with and 2 with additional t(1;7;13)	**RAEB-1 XY,der(2q13)[(1;7;13)[3]/46,X**
Days		−244	−15		21	66	170	352	546	658
61	58 /INT-2	RAEB-2/Normal karyotype	Same specimen as original MDS diagnosis	Slightly hypocellular marrow with no dysplasia and no increase in blasts/normal karyotype	Negative /41 /not performed	Negative /0 /not performed	Indeterminate /0 /Neg by karyotype	Negative /0 /Neg by karyotype	**RAEB-2 /48 /46,XY[15]/46,XY[5] chimerism based on G-band polymorphisms**	
Days		−244	−15		21	66	170	352	546	

Table 3 Late Relapse Cases (Continued)

Case 66 — 61 / unknown

Days	−106	−14	20	101	178	392	722
	RAEB-2/46,X,idic(X)(q13)[17]/46,XX [3]	Hypocellular marrow with slight dysgranulopoiesis and 4% blasts/46,X,idic(X)(q13) [16]/46,XX [4]	Negative /5.1 /Neg by karyotype	Indeterminate[e] /0 / Negative by karyotype	**AML /60.9 /45,XX,−7[2]/46,idem,+21[8]/46,XX [10]**	Negative /0 /not performed	Negative /4.4 /Neg by karyotype

Case 67 — 60 / High

Days	−243	−107	−30	21	152	310	364
	MDS-U/unknown	MDS-U with <5% marrow blasts/47,X,Y,+8,inv.(12)(p13q13) [7]/46,XY [13]	No intervening marrows pre-transplant	Negative /4.8 /Neg by karyotype	Negative /2 /Neg by FISH	**RAEB-1 8,t(8;17)(q24.1;p1…)(12)(p1…**	Indeterminate /0 /Neg by karyotype

Case 74[b] — 59 / INT-2

Days	−84	−15	7	57	88	172	252	583
	RAEB-1/45,XY,−7[19]/46,XY [1]	Same specimen as original MDS diagnosis	Normocellular marrow with no increase in blasts/Negative by FISH	Negative /3 /Neg by FISH	Negative /0 /Neg by FISH	Negative /0 /Neg by FISH	Negative /0 /Neg by FISH and karyotype	**AML /n… /45,XY,−…**

Case 75[b] — 58 / INT-2

Days	−161	−27	20	99	127	192	358
	T-MDS/normal karyotype	Slightly hypocellular marrow with minimal dysplasia and no increase in blasts/unknown	Negative /0 /Not performed	Negative /0 /not performed	**Early relapsed myeloid neoplasm with slight trilineage dyspoiesis, borderline increased marrow blasts, and rare circulating blasts[f] /9 /46,XX[20]**	Negative /0 /not performed	

Case 76 — 46 / INT-1

Days	−205	−130	−30	21	96	181		
	RAEB-2/46,XY,inv.(3)(q21q26.6) [6]/46,sl,+…	Same specimen as original MDS diagnosis	Slightly hypocellular marrow with mild…	Indeterminate /6 /46,XY,inv.(3)(q21q26.2) [1]/46,XY [18],nuc ish	Negative /6 /Neg by FISH and karyotype	Negative /2 /Negative by FISH and normal karyotype	Negative /0 / Neg by FISH	Negative /7 /Negative by FISH and normal karyotype

RELAPSE MARROWS in BOLD

Abbreviations: IPSS International prognostic scoring system, MDS myelodysplastic syndrome, CG cytogenetics, INT-1 Intermediate-1, INT-2 Intermediate-2, RCMD refractory cytopenias with multilineage dysplasia, RAEB refractory anemia with excess blasts, MDS-U myelodysplastic syndrome, unclassifiable, AML acute myeloid leukemia, T-MDS therapy related myelodysplastic syndrome, FISH fluorescence in-situ hybridization, DLI donor lymphocyte infusion, GCLAC G-CSF priming, cloarabine, and high dose cytarabine, ALT-803 trial IL-15 Superagonist Clinical Trial, GVHD graft versus host disease, LYF73636 clinical trial

[a] Engraftment is reported as % recipient [b] Patient has a history of cytotoxic chemotherapy [c] Received myeloablative transplant [d] Days are relative to transplant date unless otherwise noted [e] Case 33 was called positive on study review due to identification of rare blasts with Auer rods; Case 66 was called positive on study review due to trilineage dysplasia including abnormal lobation of granulocytes, small and hypolobated megakaryocytes, and ring sideroblasts [f] Progressed to AML 2 months after with only withdrawal of immunosuppression in intervening time [g] Institutional review reports as MDS associated with myelofibrosis versus RAEB-1

Table 3 Late Relapse Cases (Continued)

Days	-102	-34	20	65	132	206	311	328
80c	14,i(14)(q10) [3]/46,XY [11]	dysplasia and no increase in blasts/normal karyotype	(EVI1x2)(5'EVI1 sep 3' EVI1x1)[4/800]	Negative /0 /Neg by FISH	Negative /0 /Neg by FISH			FISH and normal karyotype

Days	-375	-166	-18	21	100	183	370
55 /INT-1	MDS associated with myelofibrosis/46,XX, t(3;8)(q26.2;q24.1) [17]/46,XX [3]	MDS associated with myelofibrosis/46,XX,t(3;8)(q26.2;q24.1) [3]/46,XX [17]	Hypocellular marrow with slight dysgranulopoiesis and borderline increased blasts/not performed				**RAEB-2 /45 /46,XX,t(3;8)(q26.2;q24.1), del(5)(q11.2), del(11)(p11.2 p15),der(12)t(5;12)(q11.2; p11.2)[cp7] /46,XX[12]**

RELAPSE MARROWS in BOLD

Abbreviations: IPSS International prognostic scoring system, *MDS* myelodysplastic syndrome, *CG* cytogenetics, *INT-1* Intermediate-1, *INT-2* Intermediate-2, *RCMD* refractory cytopenias with multilineage dysplasia, *RAEB* refractory anemia with excess blasts, *MDS-U* myelodysplastic syndrome, unclassifiable, *AML* acute myeloid leukemia, *T-MDS* therapy related myelodysplastic syndrome, *FISH* fluorescence in-situ hybridization, *DLI* donor lymphocyte infusion, *GCLAC* G-CSF priming, cloarabine, and high dose cytarabine, *ALT-803 trial* IL-15 Superagonist Clinical Trial, *GVHD* graft versus host disease, *LYF73636* clinical trial

a Engraftment is reported as % recipient

b Patient has a history of cytotoxic chemotherapy

c Received myeloablative transplant

d Days are relative to transplant date unless otherwise noted

e Case 33 was called positive on study review due to identification of rare blasts with Auer rods; Case 66 was called positive on study review due to trilineage dysplasia including abnormal lobation of granuloccytes, small and hypolobated megakaryocytes, and ring sideroblasts

f Progressed to AML 2 months after with only withdrawal of immunosuppression in intervening time

g Institutional review reports as MDS associated with myelofibrosis versus RAEB-1

study varied for nine of the cases, mainly between negative and indeterminate (six cases). Three cases (cases 81, 66, and 33) were re-interpreted as positive for myeloid neoplasm. Case 81 had dysplastic granulocytes, rare ring sideroblasts, atypical monocytes, and increased blasts. Case 66 showed trilineage dysplasia including abnormal lobation in granulocytes, small and hypolobate megakaryocytes, and ring sideroblasts. Case 33 lacked dysplasia and did not have an increase in blasts; however rare blasts with Auer rods were seen in the peripheral blood and bone marrow aspirate slides.

Outcomes post relapse

Four of the five patients with early relapse and known follow-up were deceased, with a median survival of 306 days post-transplant (range 232 to 465 days) and 186 days post-relapse (range 58 to 367 days). The one patient (Case 79) alive at last follow-up of 625 days post-transplant/535 days post-relapse was treated for relapse with withdrawal of immunosuppression and donor lymphocyte infusion and achieved complete remission for approximately 2 years followed by relapse as AML for which she is undergoing treatment.

Eight of the ten patients with late relapse and known follow-up were deceased, with a median survival of 608 days post-transplant (range 298–2604 days) and 120 days post-relapse (range 40–583 days). Treatment protocols following disease relapse varied and are detailed in Table 3. Two patients were alive at last follow-up, 539 and 1892 days post-relapse, both in complete remission. Case 33 was 46 years old at the time of transplant and relapsed with AML for which she was treated with induction chemotherapy followed by HaploNK therapy with transplant. Case 76, also 46 years old at the time of transplant, had graft failure within a year of transplant for which he received a stem cell boost; subsequent relapsed disease (characterized by dyspoiesis in two lineages and 4% to 7% blasts) was treated with a second allogeneic sibling transplant.

Discussion

Our study highlights the challenges of predicting MDS relapse post allogeneic HCT. Our patient cohort showed varied morphologic findings between pre-transplant disease and relapse with a large percentage of patients relapsing with a higher grade/higher blast MDS or frank AML. We found the presence of pre-transplant megakaryocyte dysplasia to correspond with the presence of megakaryocyte dysplasia in the relapse specimen but no consistency with erythroid or granulocytic dysplasia between pre- and post-transplant specimens. Similar to previous studies [11], cytogenetic abnormalities in the pre-transplant and relapse disease showed variability, including substantial proportions with clonal evolution

pre-transplant to relapse or emergence of a previously undetected/undetectable clone. While the available flow cytometric data was too sparse in our cohort, studies on the immunophenotype of neoplastic blasts and maturing myeloid lineage cells in MDS pre-transplant and at relapse using modern and reproducible parameters (such as outlined by the European LeukemiaNet Working Group [12]) is needed. Our data highlight the need for additional more objective and quantitative measures of disease such as genetic profiling for common MDS mutations [13–15] for assessment of efficacy of interventions for relapse/impending relapse, such as that presented by Woo et al. [16].

Previous work by our group focusing on patients transplanted for MDS evaluated features of the marrow in the immediate pre-transplant biopsy, including blast percentage and the percentage of cytogenetically abnormal cells, and correlated with outcomes (survival and relapse). The Trottier study [17] evaluated patients from 1995 to the end of 2012 and only included those patients with abnormal cytogenetics in the diagnostic MDS sample. In contrast, in our current study, we performed a detailed retrospective evaluation of blood and marrow features prior to any preparative or cytoreductive therapy performed in anticipation of transplant and contrasted to blood and marrow features of the relapse specimen. In addition, our study includes only those patients with known relapse and we include all relapse patients and not those only with abnormal cytogenetics at MDS diagnosis. In reviewing the cases in common, 15 of the cases in the current analysis are in common with the Trottier report, which included 82 MDS patients. The current work expands on prior work in an attempt to identify features of impending relapse.

Our relapse patterns were consistent with the literature that describes the majority of relapses after allogeneic transplant for MDS occurring within the first year post transplant. Thirteen (62%) of the relapses in our cohort occurred within a year of transplant. There was a near even division of our patient cohort between those that relapsed before and after 6 months, defined as early and late relapse for this study. We found no specific features that differed between patients with late versus early relapse, with the exception of age and marrow blast percentage, likely correlating with myeloablative conditioning. Perhaps counter-intuitive to the usual poor prognosis attributed to therapy-related myeloid neoplasms, all three t-MDS cases were late relapses occurring 6, 19, and 49 months after transplant. Eighteen months has been used previously in the literature to define late versus early relapse [11]. In our cohort, the five patients who relapsed more than 18 months after transplant (patients 10, 17, 39, 61, and 74) did not show distinguishing features.

Relapse and impending relapse are difficult to define in the context of post-allogeneic stem cell transplant for MDS, particularly for low-grade MDS. Relapsed MDS does not always have increased blasts and dysplasia alone may be the only feature suggesting impending relapse. Unfortunately, the specificity of dysplasia in the post-transplant setting is low, even with published criteria for the definition and enumeration of ring sideroblasts and morphologic dysplasia [18, 19]. Dyspoiesis is described following bone marrow transplant in the erythroid lineage (including ring sideroblasts), granulocytic lineage, and megakaryocytes [20–22]. Granulocytic dysplasia can be seen in the context of immunosuppressive medication such as tacrolimus or mycophenylate mofetil [23]. Borderline increased blasts can also be seen with recombinant growth factor therapy (G-CSF and GM-CSF) administration and early robust marrow regeneration. In addition, a graft-versus leukemia effect may suppress persistent disease/impending relapse without additional intervention. Due to these factors, there is variability in the interpretation and clinical significance assigned to morphologic dysplasia in the post-transplant context. Our morphologic re-review of pre-relapse biopsies emphasizes the inter-observer variability in interpretation of dysplasia, with a different morphologic conclusion from the original interpretation in nine cases. Thus additional criteria beyond morphologic dysplasia are needed to help identify impending relapse.

Cytogenetic analysis is a valuable tool for detecting impending relapse. However, as a subset of MDS lack a cytogenetic abnormality and sampling may be a source of false negatives, results of cytogenetic analysis do not always yield the final answer. In addition, the relapse clonal abnormality may vary from the pre-transplant disease limiting the utility of directed FISH analysis. Genetic mutation analysis holds promise in detection of impending relapse, even in cases without cytogenetic abnormalities, although sampling and limits of detection are potentials for false-negatives and clonal heterogeneity within an MDS [24, 25] can create complexity in interpretation. Engraftment/chimerism studies can aid in identification of impending relapse; however, donor-cell derived MDS after allogeneic stem cell transplant [26] is a well described entity.

Conclusions

A pragmatic approach to detection of MDS relapse and more importantly impending relapse following transplant is needed. Such an approach includes incorporation of morphologic, cytogenetic, and molecular data (including engraftment/chimerism studies). As with the initial diagnosis of MDS [27], it may take multiple sequential biopsies to make a definitive diagnosis of relapsed MDS. Detection of impending relapse is more difficult in cases with normal cytogenetics as morphologic

features of dysplasia overlap with post-transplant changes and the dysplastic lineage(s) of the relapse disease may not correspond to those of the pre-transplant disease; molecular mutational analysis may prove very beneficial in these cases. While the appropriate intervention(s) for relapse and impending relapse is not well established, identifying definitive impending relapse and early relapse may allow for targeted interventions that may prevent a full blown relapse and improve patient survival. The pathologist's role in diagnosis of impending relapse/relapse includes not only accurate morphologic identification of dysplasia and blast percentage, but an appreciation and knowledge of the multimodal approach to an MDS relapse diagnosis.

Abbreviations
AML: Acute myeloid leukemia; HCT: Hematopoietic cell transplant; IPSS: International prognostic scoring system; MDS: Myelodysplastic syndrome; RAEB: Refractory anemia with excess blasts; WHO: World Health Organization

Acknowledgements
Not applicable

Funding
Research reported in this publication was supported by NIH grant P30 CA77598 utilizing the Biostatistics and Bioinformatics Core shared resource of the Masonic Cancer Center, University of Minnesota and by the National Center for Advancing Translational Sciences of the National Institutes of Health Award Number UL1TR000114. The content is solely the responsibility of the authors and does not necessarily represent the official views of the National Institutes of Health.

Authors' contributions
EC devised the study design, collected and analyzed data, and wrote the manuscript; MG collected and analyzed data and edited the manuscript; CU collected data and edited the manuscript; SY collected data and edited the manuscript; EW collected data and wrote the manuscript. All authors have read and approved the manuscript.

Competing interests
The authors have no relevant competing interests or financial disclosures.

Author details
[1]Department of Laboratory Medicine and Pathology, University of Minnesota, 420 Delaware St SE, MMC 609, Minneapolis, MN 55455, USA. [2]Division of Hematology, Oncology, and Transplantation, Department of Medicine, University of Minnesota, Minneapolis, MN, USA.

References

1. Arber DA, Orazi A, Hasserjian R, Thiele J, Borowitz MJ, Le Beau MM, Bloomfield CD, Cazzola M, Vardiman JW. The 2016 revision to the World Health Organization classification of myeloid neoplasms and acute leukemia. Blood. 2016;127(20):2391–405.
2. Fenaux P, Ades L. How we treat lower-risk myelodysplastic syndromes. Blood. 2013;121(21):4280–6.
3. Sekeres MA, Cutler C. How we treat higher-risk myelodysplastic syndromes. Blood. 2014;123(6):829–36.
4. Greenberg P, Cox C, LeBeau MM, Fenaux P, Morel P, Sanz G, Sanz M, Vallespi T, Hamblin T, Oscier D, et al. International scoring system for evaluating prognosis in myelodysplastic syndromes. Blood. 1997;89(6):2079–88.
5. Greenberg PL, Tuechler H, Schanz J, Sanz G, Garcia-Manero G, Sole F, Bennett JM, Bowen D, Fenaux P, Dreyfus F, et al. Revised international prognostic scoring system for myelodysplastic syndromes. Blood. 2012;120(12):2454–65.
6. Kindwall-Keller T, Isola LM. The evolution of hematopoietic SCT in myelodysplastic syndrome. Bone Marrow Transplant. 2009;43(8):597–609.
7. Christopeit M, Kroger N, Haferlach T, Bacher U. Relapse assessment following allogeneic SCT in patients with MDS and AML. Ann Hematol. 2014;93(7):1097–110.
8. Warlick ED, Cioc A, Defor T, Dolan M, Weisdorf D. Allogeneic stem cell transplantation for adults with myelodysplastic syndromes: importance of pretransplant disease burden. Biol Blood Marrow Transplant. 2009;15(1):30–8.
9. Weinberg OK, Pozdnyakova O, Campigotto F, DeAngelo DJ, Stone RM, Neuberg D, Hasserjian RP. Reproducibility and prognostic significance of morphologic dysplasia in de novo acute myeloid leukemia. Mod Pathol. 2015;28(7):965–76.
10. Thyagarajan B, Young S, Floodman S, Peterson R, Wang X. Systematic analysis of interference due to stutter in estimating chimerism following hematopoietic cell transplantation. J Clin Lab Anal. 2009;23(5):308–13.
11. Yeung CC, Gerds AT, Fang M, Scott BL, Flowers ME, Gooley T, Deeg HJ. Relapse after Allogeneic hematopoietic cell transplantation for Myelodysplastic syndromes: analysis of late relapse using comparative Karyotype and chromosome genome Array testing. Biol Blood Marrow Transplant. 2015;21(9):1565–75.
12. Westers TM, Ireland R, Kern W, Alhan C, Balleisen JS, Bettelheim P, Burbury K, Cullen M, Cutler JA, Della Porta MG, et al. Standardization of flow cytometry in myelodysplastic syndromes: a report from an international consortium and the European LeukemiaNet working group. Leukemia. 2012;26(7):1730–41.
13. Bejar R, Levine R, Ebert BL. Unraveling the molecular pathophysiology of myelodysplastic syndromes. J Clin Oncol. 2011;29(5):504–15.
14. Bejar R, Stevenson K, Abdel-Wahab O, Galili N, Nilsson B, Garcia-Manero G, Kantarjian H, Raza A, Levine RL, Neuberg D, et al. Clinical effect of point mutations in myelodysplastic syndromes. N Engl J Med. 2011;364(26):2496–506.
15. Ciabatti E, Valetto A, Bertini V, Ferreri MI, Guazzelli A, Grassi S, Guerrini F, Petrini I, Metelli MR, Caligo MA, et al. Myelodysplastic syndromes: advantages of a combined cytogenetic and molecular diagnostic workup. Oncotarget. 2017;8(45):79188–9200.
16. Woo J, Howard NP, Storer BE, Fang M, Yeung CC, Scott BL, Deeg HJ. Mutational analysis in serial marrow samples during azacitidine treatment in patients with post-transplant relapse of acute myeloid leukemia or myelodysplastic syndromes. Haematologica. 2017;102(6):e216–8.
17. Trottier BJ, Sachs Z, DeFor TE, Shune L, Dolan M, Weisdorf DJ, Ustun C, Warlick ED. Novel disease burden assessment predicts allogeneic transplantation outcomes in myelodysplastic syndrome. Bone Marrow Transplant. 2016;51(2):199–204.
18. Brunning RD, Orazi A, Germing U, Le Beau MM, Porwit A, Baumann I, Vardiman JW, Hellstrom-Lindberg E. Myelodysplastic syndromes/neoplasms, overview. In: Swerdlow SH, Campo E, Harris NL, Jaffe ES, Pileri SA, Stein H, Thiele J, Vardiman JW, editors. WHO classification of tumours of haematopoietic and lymphoid tissues. 4th ed. Lyon: IARC; 2008. p. 88–93.
19. Mufti GJ, Bennett JM, Goasguen J, Bain BJ, Baumann I, Brunning R, Cazzola M, Fenaux P, Germing U, Hellstrom-Lindberg E, et al. Diagnosis and classification of myelodysplastic syndrome: international working group on morphology of myelodysplastic syndrome (IWGM-MDS) consensus proposals for the definition and enumeration of myeloblasts and ring sideroblasts. Haematologica. 2008;93(11):1712–7.
20. Reichard KK, Foucar K. Bone marrow morphologic changes after chemotherapy and stem cell transplantation. In: Orazi A, Foucar K, Knowles D, Weiss LM, editors. Knowles' Neoplastic Hematopathology. 3rd ed. Philadelphia, PA: Lippincott Williams & Wilkins; 2014.
21. van Marion AM, Thiele J, Kvasnicka HM, van den Tweel JG. Morphology of the bone marrow after stem cell transplantation. Histopathology. 2006;48(4):329–42.
22. van den Berg H, Kluin PM, Vossen JM. Early reconstitution of haematopoiesis after allogeneic bone marrow transplantation: a prospective histopathological study of bone marrow biopsy specimens. J Clin Pathol. 1990;43(5):365–9.
23. Bain BJ, Clark DM, Wilkins BS. Bone marrow pathology. 4th ed. West Sussex: Wiley-Blackwell; 2010.
24. Bejar R, Abdel-Wahab O. The importance of subclonal genetic events in MDS. Blood. 2013;122(22):3550–1.
25. Papaemmanuil E, Gerstung M, Malcovati L, Tauro S, Gundem G, Van Loo P, Yoon CJ, Ellis P, Wedge DC, Pellagatti A, et al. Clinical and biological implications of driver mutations in myelodysplastic syndromes. Blood. 2013;122(22):3616–27. quiz 3699
26. Dietz AC, DeFor TE, Brunstein CG, Wagner JE. Donor-derived myelodysplastic syndrome and acute leukaemia after allogeneic haematopoietic stem cell transplantation: incidence, natural history and treatment response. Br J Haematol. 2014;166(2):209–12.
27. Malcovati L, Hellstrom-Lindberg E, Bowen D, Ades L, Cermak J, Del Canizo C, Della Porta MG, Fenaux P, Gattermann N, Germing U, et al. Diagnosis and treatment of primary myelodysplastic syndromes in adults: recommendations from the European LeukemiaNet. Blood. 2013;122(17):2943–64.

22

Dried blood spot omega-3 and omega-6 long chain polyunsaturated fatty acid levels in 7–9 year old Zimbabwean children: a cross sectional study

Grace Mashavave[1*], Patience Kuona[2], Willard Tinago[3], Babill Stray-Pedersen[4], Marshall Munjoma[5] and Cuthbert Musarurwa[1]

Abstract

Background: Omega-3 long chain-polyunsaturated fatty acids (LC-PUFAs)–docosahexaenoic acid (DHA), docosapentaenoic acid (DPA) and eicosapentaenoic acid (EPA)– and omega-6 LC-PUFA arachidonic acid (ARA), are essential for optimum physical and mental development in children. Prior to this study, the blood omega-3 LC-PUFA levels were unknown in Zimbabwean children, particularly in those aged 7–9 years, despite the documented benefits of LC-PUFAs. Documentation of the LC-PUFA levels in this age group would help determine whether interventions, such as fortification, are necessary. This study aimed to determine dried whole blood spot omega-3 and omega-6 LC-PUFA levels and LC-PUFA reference intervals among a selected group of Zimbabwean children aged 7–9 years old.

Methods: We conducted a cross sectional study from September 2011 to August 2012 on a cohort of peri-urban, Zimbabwean children aged 7–9 years. The children were born to mothers enrolled at late pregnancy into an HIV prevention program between 2002 and 2004. Dried whole blood spots were sampled on butylated hydroxytoluene antioxidant impregnated filter papers and dried. LC-PUFAs were quantified using gas liquid chromatography. Differences in LC-PUFAs between groups were compared using the Kruskal Wallis test and reference intervals determined using non-parametric statistical methods.

Results: LC-PUFAs levels were determined in 297 Zimbabwean children of whom 170 (57.2 %) were girls. The study determined that LC-PUFAs (wt/wt) ranges were EPA 0.06–0.55 %, DPA 0.38–1.98 %, DHA 1.13–3.52 %, ARA 5.58–14.64 % and ARA: EPA ratio 15.47–1633.33. Sixteen participants had omega-3 LC-PUFAs levels below the determined reference intervals, while 18 had higher omega-6 LC-PUFAs. The study did not show gender differences in omega-3 and omega-6 LC-PUFAs levels (all $p > 0.05$). EPA was significantly higher in the 8 year age group compared to those aged 7 and 9 years (median; 0.20 vs 0.17 vs 0.18, respectively, $p = 0.049$). ARA: EPA ratio was significantly higher in the 7 year age group compared to those aged 8 and 9 years (median; 64.38 vs 56.43 vs 55.87 respectively, $p = 0.014$).

Conclusions: In this cohort of children, lower EPA levels and higher ARA: EPA ratios were observed compared to those reported in apparently healthy children elsewhere. The high ARA: EPA ratios might increase the vulnerability of these children to inflammatory pathologies. Identification and incorporation into diet of locally produced foodstuffs rich in omega-3 LC-PUFAs is recommended as well as advocating for dietary supplementation with omega-3 fish oils and algae based oils.

Keywords: Omega-3 long chain-polyunsaturated fatty acids, Docosahexaenoic acid, Eicosapentaenoic acid, Docosapentaenoic acid, Arachidonic acid, Dried blood spot, Children, 7–9 year old

* Correspondence: gracemashavave@yahoo.com
[1]Department of Chemical Pathology, College of Health Sciences, University of Zimbabwe, PO BOX A178, Avondale, Harare, Zimbabwe
Full list of author information is available at the end of the article

Background

Omega-3 long chain-polyunsaturated fatty acids (LC-PUFAs)—docosahexaenoic acid (DHA), eicosapentaenoic acid (EPA) and docosapentaenoic acid (DPA)—are essential for growth, development and general health [1]. Omega-6 LC-PUFA arachidonic acid (ARA) is essential for brain development [2]. DHA is especially critical for optimal brain [2], cognitive [3] and behavior development. EPA is a precursor of anti-inflammatory eicosanoids (prostaglandins (3 series), leukotrienes (5 series) and thromboxanes (TXA$_3$)) [4], and adequate intake of EPA is closely related to positive immunological [5], inflammatory [6] and metabolic [7] outcomes. DPA has been reported to have beneficial effects which include inhibiting platelet aggregation, stimulating endothelial cell migration and regulating gene expression [8]. Though Arachidonic acid (ARA) is a precursor of pro-inflammatory eicosanoids (prostaglandins (2 series), leukotrienes (4 series) and thromboxanes(TXA$_2$)) [4]; it produces some metabolites that are required for systemic homeostasis [9]. ARA and its metabolite lipoxin A$_4$ have been shown to function as endogenous anti-diabetic molecules [10]. ARA together with LC-PUFAs and their anti-inflammatory products: lipoxins, resolvins, protectins and maresins suppress production of pro-inflammatory eicosanoids, limit inflammation, enhance wound healing, resolve inflammation thus restoring normal cellular, tissue and organ function [10].

Supplementation with omega-3 LC-PUFAs in cardiovascular diseases (CVD) [11], diabetes mellitus [12], hypertension [13], sickle cell anemia [14], inborn errors of metabolism [15, 16], non-alcoholic fatty liver disease [17, 18], attention-defect/hyperactivity disorder [19] autism [20] and asthma [21] has been reported to prevent or alleviate symptoms in children, though other studies have reported conflicting results [22–25].

The above disorders are due to deficiencies in omega-3 fatty acids. Deficiencies in omega-3 fatty acids may result from factors that affect availability of omega-3 LC-PUFAs and influence the metabolism of essential fatty acids (EFA) to LC-PUFAs. These include, imbalances in metabolic pathways [26], genetics [27], imbalances in ARA: EPA ratios [28] and sex hormones [29]. The imbalances in the metabolic pathway may result from linoleic acid (LA) competing with α-linolenic acid (ALA) for the endogenous conversion of ALA to the long chain derivatives EPA and DHA and also inhibition of incorporation of DHA and EPA into tissues [26]. Therefore high levels of LA in the diet result in low ALA and low omega-3 LC-PUFA levels. This in turn affects the omega-6: omega-3 (ARA: EPA) ratios which are critical in human health outcomes [20, 28]. The high levels of LA lead to increased activity of the ARA metabolic pathway [4], which has deleterious effects such as neurological and neurodevelopmental disorders [30]. High concentrations of ARA

compete with EPA for incorporation into cell membrane phospholipid leading to high ARA: EPA ratios [28]. The low omega-3 LC-PUFA levels can be due to deficiencies and defects in the Δ6 or Δ5 desaturase enzyme [31] or mutations in the fatty acid desaturase (FADS) gene [27]. Protein malnutrition, carnitine and α-tocopherol enzyme deficiency as well as excess oxygen free radical production in chronic diseases also affect LC-PUFA availability [32]. Oestrogen and testosterone, have been reported to affect EFA metabolism hence availability of long chain metabolites, leading to higher levels in females compared to males [29]. The conversion of EFA into their long chain metabolites is stimulated by oestrogen and inhibited by testosterone [29].

Despite the reported benefits of omega-3 LC-PUFAs in children, most studies demonstrating the nutritional importance of omega-3 LC-PUFAs in children have been carried out in developed countries [2, 3, 11–13], [15–17, 19, 21] with a limited number of studies on African children [14, 33–35]. In most of sub-Saharan Africa healthcare facilities, omega-3 LC-PUFA levels are not on clinical laboratories test menus because the laboratories lack the expertise and technology to perform the tests [36]. In the past the assessment of omega-3 LC-PUFAs has been hindered by difficult methodology [37] and sample instability [38, 39]. Analysis has since been revolutionized by the use of minimally invasive dried blood spots (DBS) [40], which allow the estimation of fatty acid composition of red blood cells and plasma phospholipids that are more reflective of the nutritional status [41]. To date, only a few studies have developed protocols for testing LC-PUFAs in DBS [37–40, 42], with none being carried out in Africa.

In Southern Africa, a region with high prevalence of childhood infectious diseases [43], the levels of omega-3 LC-PUFAs in children are unknown, except in South Africa where the positive effects of omega-3 LC-PUFA supplementation on cognitive development were reported in children aged between 6 and 11 years [33–35]. There is paucity of data on omega-3 LC-PUFA levels in the rest of African countries, including Zimbabwe, especially in children whose adequate intake of LC-PUFAs should be ensured for cognitive development and other positive health outcomes [44].

Monitoring of fatty acid levels and results interpretation in individual patients or in populations require availability of reference intervals obtained from apparently healthy individuals [45]. Fatty acids reference intervals have been established for glycerophospholipids in German children aged 2 and 6 years, for whole blood in apparently healthy European children aged 3–8 years [46] and in apparently healthy Spanish children who were on a normal diet for their age elsewhere [15] but these may not be transferable to a different population. However, scanty studies have been done in low income settings particularly in African children and none in Zimbabwe. At present no reference intervals for LC-PUFAs have been established in these settings.

In this study, the levels of omega-3 LC-PUFAs were determined in Zimbabwean children aged between 7 and 9 years using DBS and reference intervals for LC-PUFAs were determined. The LC-PUFAs were compared between groups by gender and by age.

Methods

Study design and setting

From September 2011 to August 2012 we conducted a cross sectional study at three peri-urban primary health care clinics around Harare, the capital city of Zimbabwe. Children aged 7 to 9 years born between 2002 and 2004 to a cohort of mothers previously recruited at late pregnancy from a national HIV prevention of mother to child transmission (PMTCT) program [47], were invited to participate in the study. These children were also eligible if they had no major chronic diseases. Children who were not born to the specified cohort, or who were siblings to the original cohort or whose care givers declined to allow them to take part in the study were excluded as well as those who were HIV-infected, those with inflammatory pathologies and other chronic diseases like diabetes mellitus that may influence the fatty acid composition. All the children were tested for HIV infection at birth, at 6 weeks and subsequently after 18 months.

The study protocol and consent forms were approved by the Joint Research Ethics Committee: (JREC/170/12), and the Medical Research Council of Zimbabwe: (MRCZ/B/359). The consent forms were also approved by the Norwegian Research Ethics Committee. Permission to ship participant samples abroad for laboratory analysis was granted by the Research Council of Zimbabwe. Written informed consent to participate in the study and for long term specimen storage and shipping was obtained from parents or legal guardians and written assent was also obtained from all the children.

Blood collection

After cleaning, warming and punching a fingertip with an automatic lancing device equipped with a sterile lancet, a drop of non-fasting capillary whole blood sample (~50 μl) from each participant was spotted onto each of the four pre-defined circles on a Whatman 903 (Lot number 6833909/82) filter paper cards (GE Healthcare, UK), which was impregnated with anti-oxidant (butylated hydroxytoluene (BHT; 50 mg/100 ml in ethanol) (Sigma Aldrich Limited, Gillingham Dorset, UK)), for the determination of omega-3 LC-PUFA levels [39].

BHT in Ethanol was prepared at a concentration of 0.05 %. Each spot on the Whatman 903 filter paper card to be used for blood collection was impregnated with the BHT in ethanol solution, by fully covering each collection spot with the solution (by adding two drops). The cards were air-dried for an hour and placed in a sealed polyethylene bag overnight. The filter paper cards were treated with the BHT antioxidant to prevent the polyunsaturated fatty acids losses due to oxidation. The samples were air-dried for 3 h and stored at –25 °C in a zip lock foil paper (Whatman, Maidstone/Banbury UK) with a desiccant (Whatman, Maidstone/Banbury UK) [39].

Preparation of fatty acid methyl esters (FAMEs) in DBS, extraction, purification and detection

Fatty acid extraction and detection

Analysis of PUFAs was carried out at the Nutrition Group Laboratories, Institute of Aquaculture at the University of Stirling, Scotland UK, using a fingertip rapid method that was evaluated by Marangoni et al. [40], and validated by Bell et al. [39]. One DBS circle (per sample), one DBS circle (internal standard), and one DBS circle (control) were cut out from the main DBS filter paper cards using a pair of scissors and forceps and were placed each in a pre-labeled 10 ml screw cap vial which was loaded on the CTC-PAL machine carousel. At the beginning and end of each batch of samples or once a week, a marinol FAME secondary reference material and the Supelco 37 controls were run simultaneously with each run/batch of participants to ensure reproducibility of the known control values. The fatty acids from participants' samples, standards and quality control samples were transesterified to fatty acid methyl esters (FAMEs) using 1.25 M HCL/Methanol and incubated in dry heating block at 70 °C for 1 h [39]. This was a modification of the one step direct transmethylation method described by Lepage and Roy [48]. The FAMEs were extracted into iso-hexane (Fisher Scientific, Loughborough, UK) and precipitated with saturated potassium chloride (Fisher Scientific, Loughborough, UK) before purification [39]. Purification was done by passing the extract through a preconditioned solid phase extraction (SPE) cartridge (Clean-Up Extraction Columns, UCT, Bristol, USA) (prewashed with iso-hexane) and eluted with iso-hexane—diethyl ether (95:5 v/v) (Fisher Scientific, Loughborough, UK) [39]. The FAME extracts were dried under nitrogen (BOC Gases, Guildford, UK) using a nitrogen evaporator (N-EVAP™ 111, Organomation Associates, Berlin USA) at room temperature, re-dissolved in 0.2 ml iso-hexane and placed in an autosampler vial (Chromacol, Herts, UK) prior to gas liquid chromatography (GLC) (Thermo Fisher Trace, Hertfordshire UK) analysis [39]. The stability of the fatty acid analytes in whole wet blood and in the dried whole blood samples at different temperatures (room temperature, 4 and −20 °C) and at different times periods ((3 h post drying) and subsequent samples were removed for analysis after 48 h, 7 days, 14 days and 28 days in storage) was investigated by Bell et al. [39].

The GLC was calibrated using duplicate injections of standard mixtures of known composition (Supelco AOCS No. 37 standards containing 14:0 to 22:6n-3). A second standard, a Supelco custom mix containing 14:0, 16:0, 16:In-7, 18:0, 18:In-7, 18:2n-6, 10:0, 10:5n-3, 22:In-9, 22:5n-3 and 22-6n-3, was used to check calibration and replication by making three consecutive analyses. FAMEs (1 μl) were injected, separated and quantified by GLC using a 60 m × 0.32 mm × 0.25 μm film thick capillary column (ZB Wax; Phenomenex, Macclesfield, Cheshire, UK). Hydrogen gas (BOC Gases, Guildford, UK) was used as a carrier gas at a flow rate of 4.0 ml/min and the temperature program was from 50 to 150 °C at 40 °C/min then to 195 °C at 2 °C/min and finally to 215 °C at 0.5 °C/min [39]. The FAMEs were detected by a flame ionization detector. The FAMEs were compared to well-characterized in-house standards as well as commercial FAME mixtures (Supelco™ 37 FAME mix; Sigma Aldrich Limited, Gillingham Dorset, UK). Fatty acids ranging from C14:0 to C22:6 carbons were detected. The fatty acid data was collected from the GLC and processed using the Chromocard software computer package for Windows (version 2.1) (Thermoquest Italia S. p. A., Milan, Italy). The FAMEs results were expressed as percent weight of individual fatty acids in total fatty acids (% weight/weight (% wt/wt)). Precision and coefficient of variation were done by Bell et al. using the same analytical method, on same instrumentation and in the same establishment as the work published in this manuscript.

The total omega-6 LC-PUFAs measured included; Dihomo-gamma-linolenic acid (DGLA), ARA and Docosapentaenoic acid (DPA) (n-6) whereas the total omega-3 LC-PUFAs included; EPA, DPA (n-3) and DHA. Omega-6 LC-PUFAs were included in the results since they compete with omega-3 LC-PUFAs for the same enzymes for desaturation. The results of EPA, DPA (n-3), DHA, ARA, and the calculated total omega-3 PUFAs, total omega-3 LC-PUFA: total omega LC-PUFAs, ARA: EPA, total omega-6 LC-PUFA: total omega-3 LC-PUFA ratios were selected for data analysis.

Statistical analysis

Participants' characteristics were summarized using percentages for categorical variables and median [interquartile ranges (IQR)] for continuous non-normal variables. Differences in median omega-3 LC-PUFAs by age group and by gender were compared using the Kruskal-Wallis test. To account for multiple comparisons, we applied the Bonferroni correction which lowers

(adjust) the α value (type1 error) to account for the number of comparisons being performed simultaneously, thereby avoiding a lot of spurious positives. Non-parametric statistical methods from Reference Value Advisor v1.3 [49] were used to determine the central 95 % reference interval limits, with the lower limit defined as the 2.5 percentile and the upper limit defined as the 97.5 percentile, together with the 90 % confidence intervals (CI) of the distribution of omega-3 LC-PUFAs. For all statistical comparisons α (p value) was set at 0.05. Data entry and analysis was conducted using Statistical Package for Social Scientists (SPSS, New York, USA).

Results

A total of 319 of the available children from the original cohort participated in the study. Of these children, one had a DBS collected on a non BHT treated filter paper and 21 (6.6 %) were HIV-infected. Those who were HIV infected were all excluded from further analysis. Of the remaining 297, the median age (range) was 9 (7–9) years and 170 (57.2 %) were girls (Table 1).

Distribution and comparison of LC-PUFA levels

Sixteen (5.39 %) of the children had EPA, DPAn-3, DHA levels that were below the determined reference intervals and 18 (6.06 %) had ARA levels, ARA: EPA and total omega-6 PUFA: Total omega-3 PUFA ratios that were above the determined reference intervals. The LC-PUFAs (% wt/wt) ranges were as follows: EPA 0.06–0.55 %, DPA 0.38–1.98 %, DHA 1.13–3.52 %, ARA 5.58–14.64 % and ARA: EPA ratio 15.47–1633.33 (Table 2).

The median LC-PUFA levels between boys and girls were not significantly different (p > 0.05).

EPA levels were significantly elevated in the 8 year age group compared to those aged 7 and 9 years (0.17 vs 0.20 vs 0.18, respectively, p = 0.049). The median ARA: EPA ratio was significantly elevated in the 7 year age group compared to the other age groups (p = 0.014) (Table 2). Distribution of median ARA: EPA ratio was significantly different between age groups after being corrected using the Bonferoni test (Fig. 1).

Table 1 Age and gender of the children

Variable	Frequency $n = 297$
Gender of the children	
Boys	127 (42.8 %)
Girls	170 (57.2 %)
Children age group (years)	
7	21 (7.1 %)
8	93 (31.3 %)
9	183 (61.6 %)

p-values calculated using Bonferroni test. Statistically Significance (p < 0.05) (2-tailed)

Table 2 Distribution of median (IQR) LC-PUFA levels (% wt/wt) by gender and age group of 297 Zimbabwean children

Variables		LC-PUFAs (% wt/wt)				Total Omega-3 LC-PUFA	% Omega LC-PUFA: Total LC-PUFA	ARA: EPA	Total n-6 PUFA: Total n-3 PUFA
		EPA	DPA	DHA	ARA				
	Median (IQR) (n = 297)	0.18 (0.15–0.23)	0.79 (0.70–0.89)	2.14 (1.87–2.42)	10.62 (9.77–11.38)	3.13 (2.83–3.49)	18.42 (17.10–19.92)	57.47 (44.72–72.24)	10.82 (9.83–11.79)
	Mean (SD) (n = 297)	0.20 (0.071)	0.81 (0.17)	2.15 (0.40)	10.56 (1.26)	3.55 (0.53)	18.11 (2.27)	61.31 (23.64)	10.91 (1.62)
	Range All (n = 297)	0.06–0.55	0.38–0.198	1.13–3.52	5.58–14.64	1.73–5.95	13.34–28.11	15.47–163-33	5.94–16.03
Children's gender median IQR	Boys (n = 127)	0.19 (0.15–0.23)	0.81 (0.72–0.91)	2.11 (1.91–2.46)	10.55 (9.80–11.32)	3.25 (2.62–3.42)	18.38 (17.32–19.94)	57.16 (45.24–71.82)	10.71 (9.78–11.68)
	Girls (n = 170)	0.18 (0.15–0.24)	0.78 (0.70–0.89)	2.15 (1.84–2.36)	10.67 (9.73–11.46)	3.10 (2.82–3.47)	18.44 (16.94–19.89)	57.72 (44.09–72.91)	10.95 (9.88–11.97)
Children's Age group median (IQR)	(7) (n = 21)	0.17 (0.13–0.18)	0.78 (0.74–0.86)	2.27 (2.03–2.48)	10.89 (10.68–11.75)	3.18 (2.92–3.53)	18.20 (16.69–19.52)	64.38 (59.71–91.04)	10.60 (9.93–11.89)
	(8) (n = 93)	0.20 (0.16–0.24)	0.81 (0.70–0.93)	2.16 (1.93–2.51)	10.63 (9.61–11.39)	3.18 (2.87–3.57)	18.64 (17.35–20.18)	56.43 (41.39–72.02)	10.55 (9.68–11.45)
	(9) (n = 183)	0.18 (0.15–0.23)	0.79 (0.70–0.89)	2.10 (1.83–2.35)	10.48 (9.76–11.35)	3.09 (2.80–3.40)	18.34 (16.94–19.88)	55.87 (44.90–70.64)	10.94 (9.87–12.01)
p-values		P = 0.049[a]						P = .014[a]	

p-values calculated using Kruskal Wallis Test Asterisks: Significance tests: [a]Statistically Significance (*p* < 0.05) (2-tailed)

Key to Tables 2-3

EPA (20:5n-3):	Eicosapentaenoic acid;
DPA (22:5n-3):	Docosapentaenoic acid (n-3);
DHA (22:6n-3):	Docosahexaenoic acid
ARA (20:4n-6)	Arachidonic acid
Total Omega-3 PUFA	(EPA + DPA + DHA)
Total Omega-6 PUFA	(DGLA + ARA + AA + DPA (n-6))
% Omgea-3 LC-PUFA: Total LC-PUFA	[(EPA + DPA + DHA)]: [(DGLA + ARA + AA + DPA (n-6)) + (EPA + DPA + DHA)]
Total n-6 PUFA: Total n-3 PUFA	(DGLA + ARA + AA + DPA (n-6)): (EPA + DPA + DHA)
ARA: EPA	Arachidonic acid: Eicosapentaenoic acid
DGLA (20:3n-6)	Dihomo-gamma-linolenic acid
AA (22:4n-6)	Adrenic acid
DPA (22:5n-6)	Docosapentaenoic acid (n-6)

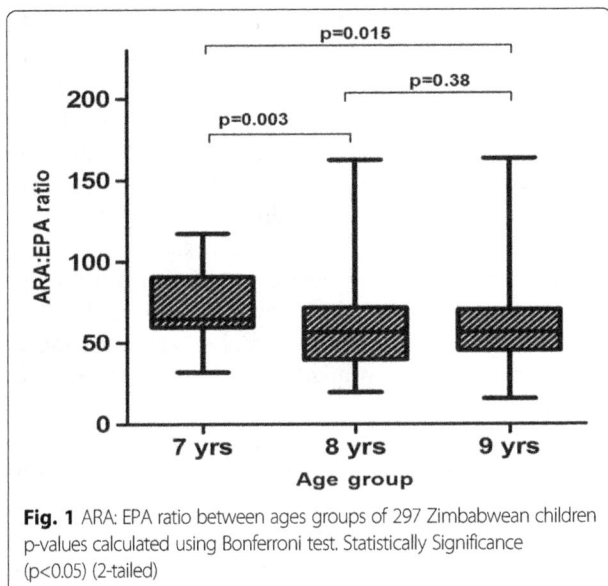

Fig. 1 ARA: EPA ratio between ages groups of 297 Zimbabwean children p-values calculated using Bonferroni test. Statistically Significance (p<0.05) (2-tailed)

Reference intervals of LC-PUFAs

Reference intervals were determined for the 297 7–9 year old Zimbabwean children. Five children (1.7 %) had EPA levels below the 2.5 percentile (0.09 % wt/wt), while 6 (2.0 %) had EPA levels above the 97.5 percentile (0.37 % wt/wt). Five children (1.7 %) had DPA levels below the 2.5 percentile (0.53 % wt/wt) and 6 (2.0 %) were above the 97.5 percentile (1.15 % wt/wt). Six children (2.0 %) had DHA levels below the 2.5 percentile

(1.35 % wt/wt) and 6 (2.0 %) were above the 97.5 percentile (2.93 % wt/wt). Six children (2.0 %) had ARA levels below the 2.5 percentile (7.85 % wt/wt) and 7 (2.4 %) were above the 97.5 percentile (12.92 % wt/wt). The LC-PUFA reference intervals with 90 % CI as determined from the results of the 7–9 year old Zimbabwean children are shown in Table 3.

Discussion

To our knowledge, this is the first study to report blood levels of omega-3 and omega-6 LC-PUFAs and to determine LC-PUFA reference intervals in 7–9 year old Zimbabwean children.

The levels for omega-3 LC-PUFAs (EPA, DPAn-3 and DHA) of the children in this study were strikingly low, while those of omega-6 LC-PUFA (ARA) were surprisingly high compared to the determined reference intervals and to the results obtained from a UK study on similar age groups and biomarker [42] (EPA 0.20 v 0.56, DPAn-3 0.81 v 1.03, DHA 2.15 v 1.9, ARA 10.56 v 8.17). Generally, these children had very low omega-3 PUFAs and very high saturated fats, monounsaturated and omega-6 fatty acids. The essential omega-3 fatty acid, α-linolenic acid, which is the precursor of the omega-3 LC-PUFAs (EPA, DPA and DHA), mainly found in seeds, nuts and some vegetable oils, was also low in the children under study (median level 0.38 % wt/wt) compared to results obtained from a study on similar age groups and biomarker [42]. The highest EPA value

Table 3 Reference Intervals of LC-PUFAs (% wt/wt) in Zimbabwean children aged 7–9 years

LC-PUFAs (% wt/wt)	Median (IQR) (n = 297)	Reference Intervals 7–9 years old n = 297	
		2.5th Percentile (90 % CI)	97.5th Percentile (90 % CI)
Omega-3 fatty acids			
ALA (18:3n-3)	0.38 (0.29–0.47)	0.17 (0.16 0.20)	0.73 (0.67 0.86)
EPA (20:5n-3)	0.18 (0.15–0.23)	0.09 (0.08 0.10)	0.37 (0.33 0.45)
DPA (22:5n-3)	0.79 (0.70–0.89)	0.53 (0.49 0.57)	1.15 (1.07 1.26)
DHA (22:6n-3)	2.14 (1.87–2.42)	1.35 (1.26 1.46)	2.93 (2.86 3.16)
Total n-3 PUFA	3.55 (3.22–3.87)	2.55 (2.39 2.64)	4.64 (4.45 5.10)
Omega-6 fatty acids			
ARA (20:4n-6)	10.62 (9.77–11.38)	7.85 (6.86 8.32)	12.92 (12.57 13.55)
Total n-6 PUFA	38.10 (36.72–39.39)	33.18 (31.72 33.91)	41.74 (41.14 42.41)
Other fatty acids			
Total saturated	38.55 (37.45–39.74)	35.82 (35.51 36.12)	42. 71 (41.50 43.18)
Total monounsaturated	16.20 (15.33–17.61)	13.75 (13.37 14.07)	21.39 (20.23 22.04)
Total DMA	3.29 (3.00–3.62)	2.44 (1.99 2.62)	4.15 (3.96 4.38)
ARA: EPA	57.47 (44.72–72.24)	26.51 (21.58 28.26)	110.83 (104.50 144.63)
% n-3LC-PUFA: Total LC-PUFA	18.42 (17.10 19.92)	14.54 (14.06 14.98)	24.56 (23.00 26.34)
Total n-3 LC-PUFA	3.13 (2.83–3.49)	2.14 (1.98 2.28)	4.29 (4.03 4.71)
Total n-6 PUFA: Total n-3 PUFA ratio	10.82 (9.83–11.79)	7.91 (7.42 8.48)	14.48 (14.04 15.13)

Fatty Acids Acronyms: ALA "α-Linolenic acid", EPA "Eicosapentaenoic acid", DPA "Docosapentaenoic acid", ARA Arachidonic acid", DMA Dimethylacetal

obtained in this study of 0.55 % *wt/wt* was lower than the mean values obtained from a study on similar age groups and biomarker [42]. Results of the present study also demonstrated the lowest EPA value of 0.06 % *wt/wt* reported in apparently healthy children compared to results obtained from a study on similar age groups and biomarker [42]. This might be a reflection of the different geographical backgrounds, diet and genetic make-up of the children in the different studies.

The low EPA and high ARA levels are of health concern because they lead to very high ARA: EPA ratios, which are pro-inflammatory, and to very high total omega-6 PUFA: total omega-3 PUFA ratios [30]. The high ratios observed in this study reflect possible imbalances in the dietary intake of omega-6 and omega-3 rich foods. The imbalances could be as a result of contemporary changes in human nutrition caused by increased consumption of diets rich in saturated fats (rich in beef), monounsaturated and omega-6 fatty acids including the use of cooking oils, vegetable oils and bread spreads rich in omega-6 PUFAs, accompanied by a decreased intake of omega-3 PUFA-rich foods [50]. Deficiencies in DHA exposes children between the ages of 7 and 9 to impaired brain development during the 7–9 year old "Brain Spurt" [44], possibly leading to compromised intellectual development, academic performance, low verbal learning ability, memory and learning difficulties [33, 34].

The LC-PUFA levels of all parameters except DHA were lower in the present study compared to the expected values from the University of Stirling Aquaculture laboratory [39] that used the same method of analysis and sample type (DBS) as the present study (EPA 0.20 v 0.91, DPA 0.81 v 2.47, DHA 2.15 v 2.47, ARA 10.56 v 13.88). The median EPA level in the present study was similar to that obtained by Mohammed et al. on pregnant Zimbabwean black women [36], indicating a general view of the dietary intake of foods poor in omega-3 LC-PUFAs and α-linolenic acid in the population.

Our findings of no differences by gender in median LC-PUFAs levels were in agreement with those of Glaser et al. on a paediatric population [45]. However, another study on a paediatric population reported a more pronounced low omega-3 and omega-6 LC-PUFA status in girls than boys [42], while another study reported slightly higher omega-6 ARA in boys than in girls [46]. Yet another study, reported that sex hormones (testosterone and oestrogen) influence the enzymatic synthesis of LC-PUFAs, leading to gender related differences in LC-PUFA status with higher levels occurring in adult females [29]. The reason for the lack of gender differences in LC-PUFA levels observed in this study was perhaps due to the younger age of the participants.

The observed differences in median EPA and ARA: EPA ratio across and between the children's age groups is probably due to differences in dietary content. The 7 year old children had lower EPA and higher ARA

values leading to high ARA: EPA ratio. The low EPA values observed in the children understudy are however constrained by the lower sample size in this particular age group; hence the results should be interpreted with caution. These findings were similar to UK study on similar age groups and biomarker [42] and also similar to the study with European children though with no age dependence for ARA [46]. An Italian study with differences in fatty acids by age groups concluded that the differences resulted either from lower intakes or the rates of utilization and resulting physiological requirements which are higher in younger age groups compared to older age groups [51].

The study also determined DBS LC-PUFA reference intervals for the apparently healthy 7–9 year old Zimbabwean children. However, these DBS LC-PUFA reference intervals cannot be generalised to the rest of the population since the LC-PUFA results were from children from a select group born to a cohort residing in a peri-urban setting, which did not include rural and urban children. The determined LC-PUFA reference intervals were not comparable to those of three other studies which determined LC-PUFA reference intervals perhaps due to methodological differences [15, 45, 46].

Our results showed generally low values across the omega-3 LC-PUFA range. The levels of these LC-PUFAs could be improved by identifying and encouraging the intake of locally available omega-3 LC-PUFA rich foods. Supplementation with EPA and DHA omega-3 fish oils and algae based oils to balance ARA levels is recommended in the children since low omega-3 LC-PUFA levels are recognized confounders of general health. Limited intake of ARA-rich foods is also recommended if the desirable total omega-6 PUFA: total omega-3 PUFA ratio of 1–4:1 [6] is to be achieved. There is need for a public awareness campaign on food sources rich in omega-3 LC-PUFAs and the benefits of omega-3 LC-PUFAs throughout life. We recommend further studies on children under the age of 5 years and inclusion of children from rural and urban Zimbabwe to ascertain their omega-3 LC-PUFA levels. Results from such studies could be used as the basis for establishing reference intervals that can be generalized to the whole Zimbabwean paediatric population, as well as the basis for food fortification and the implementation of omega-3 LC-PUFA supplementation policies.

The study has a number of limitations. Firstly no dietary intake assessment was done during specimen collection to ascertain the practices that could explain the low omega-3 LC-PUFA levels, hence, the causes of low omega-3 LC-PUFA levels are assumption based. Secondly, the determined reference intervals are limited to the children born to the specified cohort as a limited age group was used for this study. The study population was also restricted to children in a peri-urban setting that may not be truly reflective of the Zimbabwean population. The determined DBS reference intervals could also not be compared to those from other populations because of analytical method differences [15, 45, 46]. Lastly, the three age groups were unequal and this could distort the distribution of omega-3 LC-PUFAs findings by age.

Conclusion

Nevertheless, this is an important study that observed very low EPA levels and very high ARA: EPA and total omega-6 PUFA: total omega-3 PUFA ratios ever reported in apparently healthy children. The findings of this research could be the basis for future omega-3 LC-PUFA intervention studies in Zimbabwe. The techniques learnt for LC-PUFA analysis could the basis of technology transfer to Zimbabwe.

Abbreviations

% wt/wt, % weight to weight; ALA, α-linolenic acid; ARA, arachidonic acid; BHT, butylated hydroxytoluene; CI, confidence intervals; CVD, cardiovascular diseases; DBS, dried blood spot; DGLA, dihomo-gamma-linolenic acid; DHA, docosahexaenoic acid; DPA, docosapentaenoic acid; EFA, essential fatty acids; EPA, eicosapentaenoic acid; FADS, fatty acid desaturase; FAME, fatty acid methyl ester; GLC, gas liquid chromatography; IQR, inter-quartile ranges; LA, linoleic acid; LC-PUFA, long chain polyunsaturated fatty acids; PMTCT, prevention of mother to child transmission; SPE, solid phase extraction; TXA_2, thromboxanes; TXA_3, thromboxanes

Acknowledgements

This study was funded by the Letten Foundation (Oslo, Norway). We would like to thank the Letten Research Center for access to samples, the participants, their parents and legal guardians without whom this study would not have been possible. We would like to express our gratitude to Professor Bell of the Institute of Aquaculture University of Stirling Scotland UK, for training the first author in the analysis of the fatty acids, James Dick, Elizabeth MacKinlay and Irene Younger for hands on training and analysis of the samples.

Funding

This research was funded by the Letten Foundation (Oslo, Norway). The funders had no role in study design, data collection and analysis, decision to publish, or preparation of the manuscript.

Authors' contributions

GM Conception of the study, designed the study, coordinated the study, processed the sample, analyzed the samples, acquisition of data, drafting of the manuscript, interpretation of laboratory data, performed statistical analysis, data interpretation, manuscript review final manuscript write up. PK participated in study design and coordination, clinical examination of the children, sample collection and manuscript review. WT helped in statistical analysis review, interpretation of data and manuscript review. BS-P conception of the study, participated in study design and coordination and manuscript review. MM assisted in study conception, participated in study design and coordination, assisted in sample processing, helped to draft the manuscript and manuscript review. CM participated in study design, coordination, assisted to draft the manuscript and critical manuscript review. All authors read and approved the final manuscript.

Authors' information

Grace Mashavave (gracemashavave@yahoo.com)
MSc Clinical Biochemistry (UZ), Department of Chemical Pathology, University of Zimbabwe College of Health Sciences.

Patience Kuona (patiekuona@gmail.com)
MMED Paediatrics (UZ), Department of Paediatrics and Child Health, University of Zimbabwe College of Health Sciences.
Willard Tinago (wtinago@gmail.com)
PhD, Medical Statistics (University College Dublin, Ireland), Department of Community Medicine, University of Zimbabwe College of Health Sciences.
Babill Stray-Pedersen (babill.stray-pedersen@medisin.uio.no)
PhD, Division of Women and Children, Rikshospitalet, Oslo University Hospital and Institute of Clinical Medicine, University of Oslo, Norway.
Marshall Munjoma (marshall@uz-ucsf.co.zw)
PhD, Epidemiology and Diagnosis of Sexually Transmitted Infections (University of Oslo, Norway), Department of Obstetrics and Gynaecology, University of Zimbabwe College of Health Sciences.
Cuthbert Musarurwa (curtbertm@yahoo.com)
MSc Clinical Biochemistry (UZ), MSc Clinical Epidemiology (UZ), Department of Chemical Pathology, University of Zimbabwe College of Health Sciences.

Competing interests

The authors declare that they have no competing interests.

Ethics approval and consent to participate

The study protocol and consent forms were approved by the Joint Research Ethics Committee: (JREC/170/12), and the Medical Research Council of Zimbabwe: (MRCZ/B/359). The consent forms were also approved by the Norwegian Research Ethics Committee. Permission to ship participant samples abroad for laboratory analysis was granted by the Research Council of Zimbabwe. Written informed consent to participate in the study and for long term specimen storage and shipping was obtained from parents or legal guardians and written assent was also obtained from all the children.

Author details

[1]Department of Chemical Pathology, College of Health Sciences, University of Zimbabwe, PO BOX A178, Avondale, Harare, Zimbabwe. [2]Department of Paediatrics and Child Health, College of Health Sciences, University of Zimbabwe, Harare, Zimbabwe. [3]Department of Community Medicine, College of Health Sciences, University of Zimbabwe, Harare, Zimbabwe. [4]Division of Women and Children, Oslo University Hospital and Institute of Clinical Medicine, University of Oslo, Oslo, Norway. [5]Department of Obstetrics and Gynaecology, College of Health Sciences, University of Zimbabwe, Harare, Zimbabwe.

References

1. Mozurkewich E, Berman DR, Chilmigras J. Role of Omega-3 Fatty Acids in Maternal, Fetal, Infant and Child Wellbeing. Expert Rev Obstet Gynecol. 2010;5(1):125–38.
2. Schuchardt JP, Huss M, Stauss-Garbo M, Hahn A. Significance of long-chain polyunsaturated fatty acids (PUFAs) for the development and behaviour of children. Eur J Pediatr. 2010;169(2):149–64.
3. Richardson AJ, Burton JR, Sewell RP, Spreckelsen TF and Montgomery P. Docosahexaenoic Acid for Reading, Cognition and behavior in Children Aged 7-9 Years: A Randomized, Control Trial (the DOLAB Study). PLoS ONE 2012;7(9):e43909. doi: 10.1371.
4. Das UN. Essential fatty acids: biochemistry, physiology and pathology. Biotechnol J. 2006;1:420–39.
5. Bailey N. Immunonutrition: the role of long chain omega-3 fatty acids. The Nutrition Practitioner Spring 2010;11(1):24-26.
6. Patterson E, Wall R, Fitzgerald GF, Ross RP, Stanton C. Health Implications of High Dietary Omega-6 Polyunsaturated Fatty Acids. J Nutr Metab. 2012. doi:10.1155/2012/539426.
7. Poudyal H, Panchal SK, Diwan V, Brown L. Omega-3 fatty acids and metabolic syndrome: Effects and emerging mechanisms of action. Prog Lipid Res. 2011;50:372–87.
8. Gunveen K, Cameron-Smith D, Garg M, Sinclair AJ. Docosapentaenoic acid (22:5n-3): A review of its biological effects. Prog Lipid Res. 2011;50:28–34.

9.   Kidd PM. Omega-3 DHA and EPA for Cognition, Behaviour, and Mood: Functional Synergies with Cell Membrane, Phospholipids. Altern Med Rev. 2007;12(3):207–27.

10. Das UN. Arachidonic acid and lipoxin A4 as possible endogenous anti-diabetic molecules. Prostaglandins Leukot Essent Fatty Acids. 2013;88:201–10.

11. Engler MM, Engler MB, Malloy M, Chiu E, Besio D, Paul S, Stuehlinger M, et al. Docosahexaenoic acid restores endothelial function in children with hyperlipemia: results from the EARLY Study. Int J Clin Pharmacol Ther. 2004;42(12):672–9.

12. Norris JM, Yin X, Lamb MM, Barriga K, Sifert J, Hoffman M, et al. Omega-3 Polyunsaturated Fatty Acid intake and Islet Autoimmunity in Children at Increased Risk for Type 1 Diabetes. J Am Med Assoc. 2007;298(12):1420–8.

13. Forsyth JS, Willatts P, Agostoni C, Bissenden J, Casaer P, Boehm G. Long chain polyunsaturated fatty acid supplementation in infant formula and blood pressure in later childhood: follow up of a randomized controlled trial. Br Med J. 2003;953-doi:10.1136/bmj.326.7396.953-955.

14. Daak AA, Ghebremeskel K, Hassan Z, Attallah B, Azan B, Elbashir MI, Crawford M. Effect of omega-3 (n-3) fatty acid supplementation in patients with sickle cell anemia: randomized, double-blind, placebo-controlled trial. Am J Clin Nutr. 2013;97:37–44.

15. Vilaseca MA, Gomez-Lopez L, Lambruschini N, Gutiérrez A, García R, Meavilla S, et al. Long-chain polyunsaturated fatty acid concentration in patients with inborn errors of metabolism. Nutr Hosp 2011;26(1):128–136.

16. Beblo S, Reinhardt H, Demmelmair H, Muntau AC, Koletzko B. Effect of Fish Oil Supplementation of Fatty Acid Status, Coordination and Fine Motor Skills in Children with Phenylketonuria. J Pediatr. 2007;150:479–84.

17. Janczyk W, Socha P, Lebeneszstein D, Wierzbicka A, Mazur A, Neuhoff-Murawska J, Matusik P. Omega-3 fatty acids treatment of non-alcoholic fatty liver disease: design and rationale of randomised controlled trial. BMC Pediatr. 2013;13:85.

18. Nobili V, Alisi A, Corte CD, Risé P, Galli C, Agostoni C, Bedogni G. Docosahexaenoic acid for the treatment of fatty liver: Randomised controlled trial in children. Nutr Metab Cardiovasc Dis. 2013;23(11):1066–70.

19. Belanger SA, Vanasse M, Spahis S, Sylvester MP, Lippe S, L'heureux F, Ghadirian P, Vanasse CM, Levy E. Omega-3 fatty acid treatment of children with attention-deficit hyperactivity disorder: a randomized, double-blind, placebo-controlled study. Paediatr Child Health. 2009;14:89–98.

20. Bell JG, Miller D, MacDonald DJ, MacKinlay EE, Dick JR, Cheseldine S, et al. The fatty acid compositions of erythrocyte and plasma polar lipids in children with autism, developmental delay or typically developing controls and the effect of fish oil intake. Br J Nutr. 2010;103:1160–7.

21. Biltagi MA, Baset AA, Bassiouny M, Attia M. Omega-3 fatty acids, vitamin C, and Zn supplementation in asthmatic children: A randomized self-controlled study. Acta Paediatr. 2009;98:737–42.

22. Chalasani N, Younossi Z, Lavine JE, Diehl AM, Brunt EM, Cusi K, Charlton M, Snayal AJ. The diagnosis and management of non-alcoholic fatty liver disease: Practice guideline but the American Association for the liver diseases, American College of Gastroenterology, and the American Gastroenterological Association. Hepatology. 2012;55(6):2005–23.

23. Hodge L, Salome CM, Hughes JM, Liu-Brennan D, Rimmer J, Allman M, Pang D, Armour C, Woolcock AJ. Effect of dietary intake of omega-3 and omega-6 fatty acids on severity of asthma in children. Eur Respir J. 1998;11:361–5.

24. Miller MR, Yin X, Seifert J, Clare-Salzler M, Eisenbarth GS, Rewers M, Norris JM. Erythrocyte membrane omega-3 fatty acid levels and omega-3 fatty acid intake are not associated with conversion to type 1diabetes in children with islet autoimmunity: the Diabetes Autoimmunity Study in the Young (DAISY). Paediatr Diabetes. 2011;12:669–75.

25. Mankad DA, Dupuis A, Smile S, Roberts W, Brian J, Lui T, Genore L, Zaghloul D, laboni A, Marcon PMA, Anagnostou E. A randomized, placebo controlled trial og omega-3 fatty acids in the treatment of young children with autism. Molecular Autism. 2015;6(18). doi:10.1186/s13229-015-0010-7.

26. Gibson RA, Muhlhausler B, Makrides M. Conversion of Linolenic acid and alpha-linolenic acid to long chain polyunsaturated fatty acids, with focus on pregnancy, lactation and the first 2 years of life. Matern Child Nutr. 2011;Suppl 2:17–26.

27. Glaser C, Lattka E, Rzehak P, Steer C, Koletzko B. Genetic variation in polyunsaturated fatty acid metabolism and its potential relevance for human development and health. Matern Child Nutr. 2011;7 Suppl 2:27–40.

28. Simopoulos AP. The importance of the ratio of omega-6/omega-3 essential fatty acids. Biomed Pharmacother. 2002;56:365–79.

29. Decsi T, Kennedy K. Sex-specific differences in essential fatty acids metabolism. Am J Clin Nutr. 2011;94(Suppl):1914s–1919S.

30. Richardson AJ, Ross MA. Fatty acid metabolism in neurodevelopment disorder: a new perspective on associations between attention-deficit/hyperactivity disorder, dyslexia, dyspraxia, and the autism spectrum. Prostaglandins Leukot Essent Fatty Acids. 2000;63:1–9.

31. Das UN. A defect in Delta6 and Delta5 desaturases may be a factor in the initiation and progression of insulin resistance, the metabolic syndrome and ischemic heart disease in South Asians. Lipids Health Dis. 2010;9:130.

32. Infante JP, Huszagh VA. Secondary carnitine deficiency and impaired docosahexaenoic (22:6n-3) acid synthesis: a common denominator in the pathophysiology of disease of oxidative phosphorylation and beta-oxidation. FEBS Lett. 2000;468:1–5.

33. Dalton A, Wolmarans P, Witthuhn RC, van Stuijvenberg ME, Swanevelder SA, Smuts CM. A randomised control trial in school children showed improvement in cognitive function after consuming a bread spread, containing fish flour from a marine source. Prostaglandins Leukot Essent Fat Acids. 2009;80:143–9.

34. Tichelaar HY, Smuts CM, Kvalsvig JD, et al. Randomised study of cognitive effects of omega-3 fatty acid supplementation in undernourished rural school children. S Afr J Clin Nutr. 2000;13:100. abstr.

35. Baumgartner J, Smuts CM, Malan L, Kvalsvig J, van Stuijvenberg ME, Hurrell RF, Zimmermann MB. Effects of iron and n-3 fatty acid supplementation, alone and in combination, on cognition in school children: A Randomized double-blind, placebo-controlled intervention in South Africa. Am J Clin Nutr. 2012;96(6):1327-38. doi: 10.3945/ajcn.112.041004.

36. Mahomed K, Williams MA, King IB, Mudzamiri S, Woelk GB. Erythrocyte omega-3, omega-6 and trans fatty acids in relation to risk of preeclampsia among women delivering at Harare Maternity Hospital, Zimbabwe. Physiol Res. 2007;56(1):37–50.

37. Bailey-Hall E, Nelson EB, Ryan AS. Validation of a rapid measure of blood PUFA levels in humans. Lipids. 2008;43(2):181–6.

38. Ichihara K, Waku K, Yamaguchi C, Saito K, Shibahara A, Miyatani S, Yamamoto K: A convenient method for determination of the C 20-22 PUFA composition of glycerolipids in blood and breast milk. Lipids 2002;37(5):523–6

39. Bell JG, Mackinlay EE, Dick JR, Younger I, Lands B, Gilhooly T. Using a fingertip whole blood sample for rapid fatty acid measurement: method validation and correlation with erythrocyte polar lipid compositions in UK subjects. Br J Nutr. 2011;106:1408–15.

40. Marangoni F, Colombo C, Galli C. A method for the direct evaluation of the fatty acid status in a drop of blood from a fingertip in humans: applicability to nutritional and epidemiological studies. Anal Biochem. 2004;326:267–72.

41. Baylin A, Campos H. The use of fatty acid biomarkers to reflect dietary intake. Curr Opin Lipidol. 2006;17(1):22–7.

42. Montgomery P, Burton JR, Sewell RP, Spreckelsen TF, Richardson AJ. Low blood long chain omega-3 fatty acids in UK children are associated with poor cognitive performance and behavior: a cross-sectional analysis from the DOLAB study. PLoS One. 2013;8(6):e66697.

43. Taborda-Barats L, Potter PC. Socio-epidemiological Aspects of Respiratory Allergic Diseases in Southern Africa. World Allergy Organization J. 2012;5:1–8.

44. Thatcher RW. Maturation of the human frontal lobes. Physiological evidence for staging. Dev Neuropsychol. 1991;1:397–419.

45. Glaser C, Demmelmair H, Sausenthaler S, Herbarth O, Heinrich J, Koletzko B. Fatty acid composition serum glycophospholipids in children. J Pediatr. 2010;157:826–31.

46. Wolters MSH, Foraita R, Galli C, Risé P, Moreni LA, Molnár D, Russo P, Veidebaum T, Tornaritis M, Vyncke K, Eiben G, Lacoviello L, Ahrens W. Reference values of whole-blood fatty acids by age and sex from European children aged 3–8 years. Int J Obes. 2014;38:S86–98.

47. Kurewa NE, Munjoma MW, Chirenje ZM, Rusakaniko S, Hussain A, Stray-Pedersen B. Compliance and loss to follow up of HIV negative and positive mothers recruited from a PMTCT programme in Zimbabwe. Cent Afr J Med. 2007;53(5–8):25–30.

48. Lepage G, Roy CC. Direct transesterification of all classes of lipids in a one-step reaction. J Lipid Res. 1986;27:114–20.

49. Geffré A, Concordet D, Braun J-P, Trumel C. Reference Value Advisor: a new freeware set of macroinstructions to calculate reference intervals with Microsoft Excel. Vet Clin Pathol. 2011;40(1):107–12.

23

Evaluation of SD BIOLINE *H. pylori* Ag rapid test against double ELISA with SD *H. pylori* Ag ELISA and EZ-STEP *H. pylori* Ag ELISA tests

Markos Negash[1*], Afework Kassu[2], Bemnet Amare[3], Gizachew Yismaw[2] and Beyene Moges[1*]

Abstract

Background: *Helicobacter pylori* antibody titters fall very slowly even after successful treatment. Therefore, tests detecting *H. pylori* antibody lack specificity and sensitivity. On the other hand, *H. pylori* stool antigen tests are reported as an alternative assay because of their reliability and simplicity. However, the comparative performance of *H. pylori* stool antigen tests for detecting the presence of the bacterium in clinical specimens in the study area is not assessed. Therefore, in this study we evaluated the performance of SD BIOLINE *H. pylori* Ag rapid test with reference to the commercially available EZ- STEP ELISA and SD BIOLINE *H. pylori* Ag ELISA tests.

Methods: Stool samples were collected to analyse the diagnostic performance of SD BIOLINE *H. pylori* Ag rapid test kit using SD *H. pylori* Ag ELISA kit and EZ- STEP ELISA tests as a gold standard. Serum samples were also collected from each patient to test for the presence of *H. pylori* antibodies using dBest *H. pylori* Test Disk. Sensitivity, specificity, predictive values and kappa value are assessed. *P* values < 0.05 were taken statistically significant.

Results: Stool and serum samples were collected from 201 dyspeptic patients and analysed. The sensitivity, specificity, positive and negative predictive values of the SD BIOLINE *H. pylori* Ag rapid test were: 95.6% (95% CI, 88.8–98.8), 92.5% (95%CI, 89–94.1%), 86.7% (95% CI, 80.5–89.6), and 97.6% (95% CI, 993.9–99.3) respectively.

Conclusion: The performance of SD BIOLINE *H. pylori* Ag rapid test was better than the currently available antibody test in study area. Therefore, the SD BIOLINE Ag rapid stool test could replace and be used to diagnose active *H. pylori* infection before the commencement of therapy among dyspeptic patients.

Keywords: *Helicobacter pylori*, SD BIOLINE Ag rapid test, Stool antigen, Ethiopia

Background

Helicobacter pylori, a curved gram negative bacillus, has been etiologically associated with several pathogenic conditions of the stomach ranging from gastritis to gastric cancer [1–3]. Prevalence of *Helicobacter pylori* (*H. pylori*) infection varies based on several factors globally [4–6]. In developing countries more than 80% of the population is infected with *H. pylori* [7, 8].

According to the 2010 World Gastroenterology Organization report the prevalence of *H. pylori* in Ethiopia among the age groups 2–4 years, 6 years, and adults was 48%, 80% and > 95%, respectively [9]. It has been reported that dyspepsia is one of the commonest complaints in any Ethiopian outpatient department [10–12]. It is also reported to account 10% of hospital admissions in the country [13].

According to the American college of Gastroenterology, patients with un-investigated dyspepsia [14] can be diagnosed using different approaches [15–18]. Serology is a widely available and inexpensive test but with low diagnostic accuracy. On the other hand, the *H. pylori* stool antigen (HpSA) test has been put in the market as optional technique because of its reliability and simplicity.

* Correspondence: markosnegash@yahoo.com; beyemoges@gmail.com
[1]Department of Immunology and Molecular Biology, School of Biomedical and Laboratory Sciences, College of Medicine and Health Sciences, University of Gondar, P.O.BOX 196, Gondar, Ethiopia
Full list of author information is available at the end of the article

However, the comparative performance of HpSA tests for detecting presence of *H. pylori* in clinical specimens is not tested at the study area. Therefore, in this study, we determined the performance characteristics of the SD BIOLINE *H. pylori* Ag kit against the SD *H. pylori* Ag ELISA and commercial EZ-STEP *H. pylori* Ag ELISA tests by using stool specimen among dyspeptic patients attending the University of Gondar Hospital in Northwest Ethiopia, Gondar.

Methods

Study design, period and area
This facility based cross sectional study was conducted on clients with dyspepsia from February to March 2015 attending the medical outpatient department of the University of Gondar Hospital.

Study participants
After informed consent was taken all dyspeptic patients with no prior eradication therapy were included in the current study.

Sample collection and processing
Stool and blood specimens were collected from each patient for serologic tests. The blood was centrifuged until serum was separated and stored at -20°c. The stool specimens were also stored at -20°c until the lab tests were performed.

SD BIOLINE H. pylori Ag test
[Principle] The SD BIOLINE *H. pylori* Ag Rapid test kit result window has 2 pre-coated lines, "T" (Test Line) and "C" (Control Line). Both the Test Line and the Control Line in result window are not visible before applying any samples. The "T"" window coated with monoclonal anti-*H. pylori* will form a line after the addition of stool specimen (if there is *H. pylori* antigen). The Control window is used for procedural control and a line should always appear if the test procedure is performed correctly and the test reagents are working.

Stool specimens were subjected for the rapid test according to the manufacturer's instruction (STANDARD DIAGNOSTIC, INC. Korea). In brief, after taking a portion of stool (about 50 mg) with sterile swab it was inserted into a specimen tube containing assay diluents to dissolve the sample. Next, 1 ml of sample diluents was added in a clean test tube. We waited for 5–10 min and used the upper layer for the test. Three drops (about 80 μl) were put into the sample wells of the test device. Test results were interpreted within 10–15 min. No interpretation was performed after 15 min.

A colour band will appear on the left section of the result window (control/"C" band and/or test/"T" band). The presence of only one band ("C" band) within the result window indicates a negative result while the presence of two colour bands ("T" band and "C" band) within the result window indicates a positive result. In case where the purple colour band was not visible within the result window (of the "C" window) after performing the test, the result was considered invalid and the specimen were re-tested using a new test kit.

SD H. pylori Ag ELISA
[Principle] Stools from patients are used as a source of sample for the determination of *H. pylori* antigen. Micro plates are coated with a cocktail of affinity purified monoclonal antibodies directed to the *H. pylori* antigens. In the 1st incubation, the solid phase is treated with the sample and simultaneously with a mixture of monoclonal antibodies to *H. pylori* conjugated with peroxidase (HRP). After washing out, in the 2nd incubation the bound enzyme specifically present on the solid phase generates an optical signal that is proportional to the amount of *H. pylori* antigens present in the sample.

The test was performed according to the manufacturer's (STANDARD DIAGNOSTIC, INC., Republic of Korea (17099)) instruction. In brief, we prepared strip wells for negative control 3 wells, positive control 2 wells and sample wells. We pipette 100 μl of controls and patient's stool samples to each well. Then we added 25 μl of Enzyme Conjugate (mixture of monoclonal antibodies to *H. pylori* and horse reddish peroxidase) to each well. The micro plates was covered with adhesive plate sealer and mixed well on vibrating mixer. The wells were incubated at 37 ± 1 degree centigrade for 60 min. The wells were washed 5 times with 350 μl of diluted washing solution and then mixed with 100 μl TBM Substrate A and 100 μl TBM Substrate B and incubated in the dark at room temperature for 10 min. A blue color will develop. Then 100 μl of Stopping Solution was added into each well in the same sequence and timing as the TMB addition. The blue color will change to yellow.

The absorbance of each well was read within 30 min at a wavelength of 450 nm with a reference filter of 620 nm. The individual values of the absorbance for the control were used to calculate the mean value if $0.005 \leq$ A (neg.) ≤ 0.100 and A (pos.) ≥ 1.000. When one of the absorbance value of the negative controls was outside the specification, this value was neglected while both absorbance values of the positive control must comply with the specification. When these specifications were not met, the test was repeated. The mean absorbance of the negative controls was calculated to calculate the cut-off value by adding 0.100 [A (neg.) + 0.100 = cut-off value]. Based on the criteria of the test, the samples were classed as follows: A (sample) < cut-off≡*H. pylori* antigen negative; A (sample) ≥ cut-off≡*H. pylori* antigen positive. Samples with a test result greater or equal to the cut-off value were in duplicate. The test results were interpreted as follows:

Negative result: no detectable *H. pylori* antigen; Positive result: presence of detectable *H. pylori* antigen.

EZ-STEP H. pylori Ag ELISA

[Principle] the EZ-STEP *H. pylori* stool antigen test utilize polyclonal anti-*H. pylori* capture antibody adsorbed to micro wells. An aliquot of diluted patient samples is added to the micro well and incubated simultaneously with peroxidase conjugated polyclonal antibody, resulting in the *H. pylori* antigens being sandwiched between the solid phase and enzyme conjugate. After incubation at room temperature, the sample well is washed to remove unbound samples and enzyme labeled antibodies. Substrate is added and result can be read in 10 min. Any bound enzyme conjugate in the wells converts the colorless substrate to a blue color. Spectrophotometer determination will be done with the addition of stop solution. This commercially available *H. pylori* stool antigen test (DINONA, Inc., Seoul, Korea) was performed as per the manufacturer. In brief: 8 drops (about 400 µl) of sample diluents were added to a clean test tube. Using the sample collection stick provided, a portion of feces (about 0.1 g) was taken and inserted into the test tube containing Sample Diluents. The stick was sworn until the sample has been dissolved into the Sample Diluents.

Next, 3 drops (100 µl) of negative control in 2 wells, 3 drops (100 µl) of positive control in 2 wells, and 3 drops (100 µl) of samples prepared in each well were added using dropper provided. Then 3 drops (100 µl) of conjugate solution were added onto each negative control, positive control, and sample well. Then the plate was shaken on vibrating mixer for 15 s. The plate was sealed with the tape provided and incubated at room temperature for 60 min. Then plates were then washed with the diluted washing solution for 6 times (300 µl/well/cycle). Then 3 drops (100 µl) of substrate solution were added onto each well and shaken on vibrating mixer for 15 s and incubated at room temperature for 10 min in dark.

Next, 3 drops (100 µl) of Stopping Solution was added on wells before reading the absorbance for negative and positive controls using air blank. Absorbance was read in 15 min after adding the stopping solution at 450 nm with reference wavelength at 650 nm. The absorbance of positive control was all between 0.500 and 2.500 and the absorbance of two negative controls was between – 0.005 and 0.100. When the absorbance was – 0.005-0.000, then it may was calculated as 0.000. When it was out of the range, the test was repeated.

To calculate the mean absorbance of negative controls we used the following formula:

The mean absorbance of negative controls (NCx) = (N1 + N2)/2.

To calculate the mean absorbance of positive controls use the following formula:

The mean absorbance of positive controls (PCx) = (1.599 + 1.601)/2 = 1.600.

To calculate Cut off Value we used the following formula:

Cut off Value = NCx + 0.100.

Samples with absorbance higher than the cut off Value were considered positives while those lower than cut off Value were taken as negatives. When the result was interpreted as positive, test was repeated on 3 wells and a positive result in more than 1 well was interpreted as positive.

dBest H. pylori test disk

[Principle] This test contains a membrane strip, which is pre-coated with *H. pylori* capture antigen on test band region. The *H. pylori* antigen–colloid gold conjugate and serum sample moves along the membrane chromatographically to the test region (T) and forms a visible line as the antigen-antibody-antigen gold particle complex forms. This test device has a letter of T and C as "Test Line" and "Control Line" on the surface of the case. Both the Test Line and Control Line in result window are not visible before applying any samples. The Control Line is used for procedural control. Control line should always appear if the test procedure is performed properly and the test reagents of control line are working.

The dBest *H. pylori* Test Disk (Ameritech diagnostic reagent co ltd, Tongxiang, Zhejiang, China) test was performed according to the manufacturer's instruction. In brief: The test disk was removed from the foil pouch and placed on a flat, dry surface. A drop (20–30 µl) of serum/plasma was applied on to the sample well. Then two drops of the buffer were added on the sample well. As the test began to work, purple colour was seen moving across the result window in the centre of the test disk. Test results were interpreted within ten minutes. The presence of two colour bands, 'T' and 'C', meant the test was positive while the presence of only one band (only on 'C') was interpreted as negative. If no band or single band only on 'T' was formed after 10 min, the result was considered invalid and the experiment was repeated.

Statistical analysis

The data was cleaned and double entered on excel spread sheet and transported to SPSS version 20. Java Stat-two way contingency table analysis software (http://statpages.org/ctab2x2.html) was also used to calculate sensitivity, specificity, predictive and kappa values. In this study the results of SD BIOLINE *H. pylori* Ag test were compared with results of the reference methods (EZ- STEP ELISA

Table 1 Serology results of the SD BIOLINE *H. pylori* Ag rapid test, SD *H. pylori* Ag ELISA test, and ZE-STEP *H. pylori* Ag ELISA at University of Gondar Hospital, 2015

		SD BIOLINE *H. pylori* Ag		
		Positive N (%)	Negative N (%)	Total N (%)
SD *H. pylori* Ag ELISA	Positive	72(96.0%)	20 (15.9%)	92 (45.8%)
	Negative	3 (4.0%)	106 (84.1%)	109 (54.2%)
EZ- STEP ELISA	Positive	65 (86.7%)	16 (12.7%)	81 (40.3%)
	Negative	10 (13.3%)	110 (87.3%)	120 (59.7%)
EZ-STEP + SD *H.pylori* ELISA	Positive	65 (86.7%)	3 (2.4%)	68 (33.8%)
	Negative	10 (13.3%)	123 (97.6%)	133 (66.2%)

Ag Antigen, *ELISA* Enzyme Linked Immunosorbent Assay, *N* number, *SD* Standard Diagnostics

and SD *H. pylori* Ag ELISA test). *P* values < 0.05 were taken statistically significant.

Results

A total of 201 dyspeptic patients were included in the study of which 140 (69.7%) were males and the rest 60 (30.3%) were females. The age of the participants ranged from 7 to 85 years with a mean (±SD) of 29.5 years (±14.85). Stool samples from all participants were collected and analyzed by the three tests, namely: SD BIO-LINE *H. pylori* Ag test, SD *H. pylori* Ag ELISA, and EZ-STEP *H. pylori* Ag ELISA. Accordingly, 75 (37.1%) of the participants were positive by the SD BIOLINE *H. pylori* Ag rapid test while 92 (45.8%) were positive by the SD *H. pylori* Ag ELISA. The EZ-STEP *H. pylori* Ag ELISA detected 81 (40.3%) of the samples as positives for *H. pylori* infection. On the other hand, 68 (33.8%) were positive using both ELISA tests (Table 1). The dBest *H. pylori* Test disk detected 143(71.1%) of the samples as positive.

The performance characteristics of the SD BIOLINE *H. pylori* Ag rapid test against the SD *H. pylori* Ag ELISA and EZ-STEP *H. pylori* Ag ELISA was summarized in Table 2. Only those samples which were positive/negative for both ELISA tests were considered as positive/negative and used for the calculation of the performance activity of the rapid test. The sensitivity, specificity, positive and negative predictive values of the SD BIOLINE *H. pylori* Ag rapid test were: 95.6% (95% CI, 88.8–98.8), 92.5% (95%CI, 89–94.1%), 86.7% (95% CI, 80.5–89.6), and 97.6% (95% CI, 993.9–99.3), respectively. The kappa value was 0.859 (95% CI, 0.759–0.906).

Discussion

H. pylori infection can be diagnosed using either of the invasive and noninvasive approaches [17]. Among noninvasive techniques serology is the most widely used because it is cheap, simple and quick. However, it is unreliable to differentiate active and previous infection. Due to this its application especially to initiate and monitor eradication therapy has been in question. On the other hand, new noninvasive diagnostic test based on the detection of *H. pylori* stool antigen (HpSA) has been developed and made available to the market.

In the current study, the sensitivity of the SD BIO-LINE *H. pylori* Ag rapid test was 95.6% (95%CI, 88.8–98.8%). The sensitivity of the test is generally comparable with other HpSA tests [19–22], higher than some [23–25] and a little bit lower than others [26–28]. In any way, the high sensitivity of this rapid test could improve the detection of active infections and enhance the confidence of physicians to prescribe eradication therapy.

The specificity of the test was also very high, 92.5% (95%CI, 89–94.1%). It was generally comparable with previous HpSA reports [20, 29], higher than some [25–27] and slightly lower than others [23, 24]. This high specificity could increase the reliability of the rapid test in identifying an active infection and easy discrimination from a previous exposure.

The positive predictive value (PPV) of the test in the current study was also high 86.7% (95%CI, 80.5–89.6%). It was comparable [30], higher [25, 26] and lower [23, 24] when compared to other studies. Likewise, the negative predictive value (NPV) was also very high, 97.6% (95%CI,

Table 2 Performance result of the SD BIOLINE *H. pylori* Ag rapid test and dBest *H. pylori* Test Disk rapid Antibody test using EZ- STEP ELISA and SD *H. pylori* Ag ELISA test as standard at University of Gondar Hospital, 2015

Type of test	Sensitivity %(95%CI)	Specificity %(95%CI)	PPV %(95%CI)	NPV %(95%CI)	Kappa value N(95%CI)	P value
Ag rapid test (SD BIOLINE)	95.6 (88.8–98.8)	92.5 (89–94.1)	86.7 (80.5–89.6)	97.6 (93.9–99.3)	0.859 (0.759–0.906)	< 0.001
Antibody rapid test (dBest)	75 (65.3–83.5)	30.8 (25.9–35.1)	35.7 (31.1–39.7)	70.7 (59.4–80.6)	0.046 (−0.069–0.147)	0.416

Ag Antigen, *CI* confidence interval, *ELISA* Enzyme Linked Immunosorbent Assay, *N* number, *NPV* negative predictive value, *PPV* positive predictive value, *SD* Standard Diagnostics

93.9–99.3%). It was comparable [19, 25], higher [23, 24] and lower [26, 27] when compared to previous studies. The high positive predictive value (PPV) and NPV values could show the higher accuracy of the rapid test. In addition, the kappa value of the target test was very high, 0.859 (95%CI, 0759–0.906), which shows an excellent agreement between the rapid test and the reference standard used.

While a performance characteristic is typically compared against a gold standard test, we evaluated the SD BIOLINE H. pylori Ag rapid test kit against an already commercialized antigen tests, EZ-STEP H. pylori Ag test (DINONA, Inc., Korea) and SD H. pylori ELISA Ag tests (double ELISA) because of the lack of gold standard test in the study area. In addition, it is important to make note that the various tests compared above are based on their use of HpSA. They have also used different techniques as gold standards.

The sensitivity of the antibody test was 75% (95% CI, 65.3–83.5) which was much lower than the sensitivity of the SD BIOLINE H. pylori Ag test. Similarly, the specificity of the antibody test was also much lower than for the SD BIOLINE H. pylori Ag test, 30.8% (95% CI, 25.9–35.1%). H. pylori immunoglobulin G (IgG) serology detects an immune response, which could represent either a current infection or a previous exposure. Using such antibody tests may then predispose to an overuse of this drugs which could have a negative economic impact, increased risk of drug resistance, and exposure to unnecessary drug adverse effects.

Conclusion

The SD BIOLINE H. pylori Ag rapid test has a much better sensitivity, specificity and predictive values compared to the currently available antibody test in the market, in Ethiopia. Therefore, the SD BIOLINE H. pylori Ag rapid stool test could be used to diagnose active H. pylori infection before the commencement of eradication therapy. However, further studies are required on how to use this HpSA rapid test for monitoring of therapeutic response or test of cure.

Abbreviations
AUC: Area under curve; CIs: Confidence intervals; H. pylori: Helicobacter pylori; HpSA: H. pylori stool antigen; IgG: Immunoglobulin G; IRB: Institutional Review Board; NPV: Negative predictive value; PPV: Positive predictive value

Acknowledgements
We would like to acknowledge our technical assistants, Mr. Amare Kifle and Mr. Getnet Ayalew, for their excellent technical support during the conduct of the study. Our gratitude also goes to the University of Gondar Hospital and the staff for their unreserved support during the study.

Funding
This work was not supported by any governmental or nongovernmental foundations.

Authors' contributions
BM, AK and BA conceived the study concept and designed the study; MN, GY and BA carried out data collection and laboratory analysis; BM, GY, MN and BA supervised the data collection and laboratory analysis; BM, GY and BA analyzed the data and prepared the first manuscript draft; BM, AK, GY and BA reviewed the draft; all authors read and approved the final manuscript.

Ethics approval and consent to participate
This project was ethically cleared by the Institutional Review Board (IRB) of the University of Gondar. Participation was voluntary and informed verbal consent was taken from all adult participants and from the next of kin, caretakers, or guardians on behalf of the minors/children before inclusion to the study. Initially, participants were briefly explained about the objectives of the study, risks and benefits of the procedures, and on voluntary participation and the right to withdraw at any stage of the study using their local language. Participants were then asked if they understood what has been explained to them. If and only if they understand the facts, implications, and future consequences of their action on themselves or their children would like to be part of the study. Written consent wasn't acquired because all the participants were recruited from the outpatient department laboratory of the Gondar University Hospital where all the participant patients were sent to undergo H. pylori antibody test. The additional stool antigen test was a non-invasive procedure with minimal or no risk associated to it. Besides, patients were benefited from the stool antigen test as it added further information on whether to commence eradication therapy by the attending physician. The result from the antibody test was collected from the laboratory record book. Official permission was also obtained from the University of Gondar Hospital before access to the record book and the conduct of the study. Therefore, considering all these facts only verbal agreement was acquired to be included in the study. The IRB has also evaluated the consent procedure and cleared it as sufficient. Participants who were diagnosed as positive to H. pylori stool antigen test were immediately linked to the medical outpatient department of the University of Gondar Hospital for appropriate treatment and follow up.

Competing interests
The authors declare that they have no competing interests.

Author details
[1]Department of Immunology and Molecular Biology, School of Biomedical and Laboratory Sciences, College of Medicine and Health Sciences, University of Gondar, P.O.BOX 196, Gondar, Ethiopia. [2]Department of Medical Microbiology, School of Biomedical and Laboratory Sciences, College of Medicine and Health Sciences, University of Gondar, P.O.BOX 196, Gondar, Ethiopia. [3]Department of Biochemistry, School of Medicine, College of Medicine and Health Sciences, University of Gondar, P.O.BOX 196, Gondar, Ethiopia.

References
1. Goodwin CS, Worsley BW. Microbiology of helicobacter pylori. Gastroenterol Clin N Am. 1993;22:5.
2. Johannes G, Arnoud H, Ernst J. Pathogenesis of Helicobacter pylori infection. J Clin Microbiol. 2006;19(Suppl 3):449–90.
3. Nurgalieva Z, Malaty H, Graham D, Almuchambetova R, Machmudova A, Kapsultanova D, Osato M, Hollinger F, Zhangabylov A. Helicobacter pylori infection in Kazakhstan: effect of water source and household hygiene. Am J Trop Med. 2002;67(Suppl 2):201–6.
4. Ahmed KS, Khan AA, Ahmed I, Tiwari SK, Habeeb A, Ahi JD, Abid Z, Ahmed N, Habibullah CM. Impact of household hygiene and water source on the prevalence and transmission of helicobacter pylori: a south Indian perspective. Singap Med J. 2007;48(Suppl 6):543–9.
5. Amini M, Karbasi A, Khedmat H. Evaluation of eating habits in dyspeptic patients with or without Helicobacter pylori infection. J Trop Gastroenterol. 2009;30(Suppl 3):142–4.

6. Malaty HM, Graham DY. Importance of childhood socioeconomic status on the current prevalence of helicobacter pylori infection. Gut. 1994;35:742–5.

7. Perez-Perez GI, Rothenbacher D, Brenner H. Epidemiology of helicobacter pylori infection. Helicobacter. 2004;9(Suppl 1):1–6.

8. Fiedorek SC, Malaty HM, Evans DL, Pumphrey CL, Casteel HB, Evans DJ, Graham DY. Factors influencing the epidemiology of helicobacter pylori infection in children. Pediatrics. 1991;88:578–82.

9. World Gastroenterology Organization (WGO) (2010) *Helicobacter pylori* in developing countries. Accessed 22 Sept 2014.

10. Tsega E. Analysis of fibreoptic gastroduodenoscopy in 1084 Ethiopians. Trop Geog Med. 1980;33:149–54.

11. Tsega E. Non-ulcer dyspepsia and gastritis in Ethiopia. Addis Ababa: Artistic Printers; 1983. p. 5–7.

12. Zein ZA, Kloos H. The ecology of health and disease in Ethiopia. Addis Ababa: Ministry of Health; 1988.

13. Asrat D, Nilsson I, Mengistu Y, Ashenafi S, Ayenew K, Abu Al-Soud W, Wadstrom T, Kassa E. Prevalence of *Helicobacter pylori* infection among adult dyspeptic patients in Ethiopia. Annals Trop Med Parasitol. 2004;98:181–9.

14. Chey WD, Wong BC. Practice parameters Committee of the American College of gastroenterology guideline on the management of helicobacter pylori infection. Am J Gastroenterol. 2007;102:1808.

15. Vaira D, Malfertheiner P, Megraud F, Axon AT, Deltenre M, Hirschl AM, Gasbarrini G, O'Morain C, Garcia JM, Quina M, Tytgat GN. Diagnosis of helicobacter pylori infection with a new non-invasive antigen-based assay. Lancet. 1999;354:30–3.

16. Zagari RM, Bazzoli F, Pozzato P, Fossi S, De Luca L, Nicolini G, Berretti D, Roda E. Review article: non-invasive methods for the diagnosis of helicobacter pylori infection. Ital J Gastroenterol Hepatol. 1999;31:408–15.

17. Vaira D, Holton J, Menegatti M, et al. Review article: invasive and non-invasive tests for *Helicobacter pylori* infection. Aliment Pharmacol Ther. 2000;14:13–22.

18. Vaira D, Ricci C, Menegatti M, Gatta L, Geminiani A, Miglioli M. Clinical role of fecal antigen determination in the diagnosis of *Helicobacter pylori* infection. Clin Lab. 2000;46:487–91.

19. Haindl E, Finck A, Muehlstein V, Leodolter A, Mafertheiner P, Cullmann G. A novel enzyme immunoassay for the direct detection of *H. pylori* antigens in stools. Gastroenterology. 2001;120:2506.

20. Agha-Amiri K, Mainz D, Peitz U, Kahl S, Leodolter A, Malfertheiner P. Evaluation of an enzyme immunoassay for detecting *Helicobacter pylori* antigens in human stool samples. Z Gastroenterol. 1999;37:1145–9.

21. Arents NL, van Zwet AA, Thijs JC, de Jong A, Pool MO, Kleibeuker JH. The accuracy of the *Helicobacter pylori* stool antigen test in diagnosing *H. pylori* in treated and untreated patients. Eur J Gastroenterol Hepatol. 2001;13:383–6.

22. Dore MP, Wengler G, Tadeu V, et al. A novel monoclonal antibody test to detect *H. pylori* antigens in human stool. Gut. 2002;51(Suppl 2):108.

23. Rothenbacher D, Bode G, Brenner H. Diagnosis of *Helicobacter pylori* infection with a novel stool antigen-based assay in children. Pediatr Infect Dis. 2000;19:364–6.

24. Sarker SA, Bardhan PK, Rahaman M, Beglinger C. Usefulness of the *Helicobacter pylori* stool antigen test for detection of *Helicobacter pylori* infection in young Banglasdeshi children. Gastroenterology. 2003;124:1231.

25. Shepherd AJ, Williams CL, Doherty CP, et al. Comparison of an enzyme immunoassay for the detection of *Helicobacter pylori* antigens in the faeces with the urea breath test. Arch Dis Child. 2000;83:268–70.

26. Masoero G, Lombardo L, Della Monica P, et al. Discrepancy between *Helicobacter pylori* stool antigen assay and urea breath test in the detection of *Helicobacter pylori* infection. Dig Liver Dis. 2000;32:285–90.

27. Mullan K, Cooke M, O'Connor FA. A study of the usefulness in clinical practice of the HPSA enzyme immunoassay for the detection of *Helicobacter pylori* in stool specimens. Gut. 1999;45:118.

28. Altindis M, Dilek ON, Demir S, Akbulut G. Usefulness of the *Helicobacter pylori* stool antigen test for detection *Helicobacter pylori* infection. Acta Gastroenterol Belg. 2002;65:74–6.

29. Agha-Amiri K, Peitz U, Mainz D, Kahl S, Leodolter A, Malfertheiner P. A novel immunoassay based on monoclonal antibodies for the detection of *Helicobacter pylori* antigens in human stool. Z Gastroenterol. 2001;39:555–60.

30. Bonamico M, Strappini PM, Crisogianni M, et al. Detection in children of *Helicobacter pylori* antigen in stools: a new non-invasive method for diagnosis of infection. Gut. 2000;47:98.

24

Diagnostic accuracy of touch imprint cytology for head and neck malignancies: a useful intra-operative tool in resource limited countries

Hania Naveed[1], Mariam Abid[1], Atif Ali Hashmi[2], Muhammad Muzammamil Edhi[3], Ahmareen Khalid Sheikh[4], Ghazala Mudassir[1] and Amir Khan[5*]

Abstract

Background: Intraoperative consultation is an important tool for the evaluation of the upper aerodigestive tract (UAT) malignancies. Although frozen section analysis is a preferred method of intra-operative consultation, however in resource limited countries like Pakistan, this facility is not available in most institutes; therefore, we aimed to evaluate the diagnostic accuracy of touch imprint cytology for UAT malignancies using histopathology of the same tissue as gold standard.

Methods: The study involved 70 cases of UAT lesions operated during the study period. Intraoperatively, after obtaining the fresh biopsy specimen and prior to placing them in fixative, each specimen was imprinted on 4-6 glass slides, fixed immediately in 95% alcohol and stained with Hematoxylin and Eosin stain. After completion of the cytological procedure, the surgical biopsy specimen was processed. The slides of both touch Imprint cytology and histopathology were examined by two consultant histopathologists.

Results: The result of touch imprint cytology showed that touch imprint cytology was diagnostic in 68 cases (97.1%), 55 (78.6%) being malignant, 2 cases (2.9%) were suspicious for malignancy, 11 cases (15.7%) were negative for malignancy while 2 cases (2.9%) were false negative. Amongst the 70 cases, 55 cases (78.6%) were malignant showing squamous cell carcinoma in 49 cases (70%), adenoid cystic carcinoma in 2 cases (2.9%), non-Hodgkin lymphoma 2 cases (2.9%), Mucoepidermoid carcinoma 1 case (1.4%), spindle cell sarcoma in 1 case (1.4%). Two cases (2.9%) were suspicious of malignancy showing atypical squamoid cells on touch imprint cytology, while 13 cases (18.6%) were negative for malignancy, which also included 2 false negative cases. The overall diagnostic accuracy of touch imprint cytology came out to be 96.7% with a sensitivity and specificity of 96 and 100%, respectively while PPV and NPV of touch imprint cytology was found to be 100 and 84%, respectively.

Conclusion: Our experience in this study has demonstrated that touch imprint cytology provides reliable specific diagnoses and can be used as an adjunct to histopathology, particularly in developing countries, where the facility of frozen section is often not available, since a rapid preliminary diagnosis may help in the surgical management planning.

Keywords: Touch imprint cytology, Frozen section, Head and neck malignances

* Correspondence: dramirkhan04@gmail.com
[5]Kandahar University, Kandahar, Afghanistan
Full list of author information is available at the end of the article

Background

Of all human cancers, upper aerodigestive tract (UAT) malignancies are the most distressing since it is the site of most complex functional anatomy in the human body. Its importance is due to the major functional responsibilities of this region which includes breathing, taste, swallowing, voice, endocrine and cosmetic etc. Cancers that occur in this area have a major impact on these important human functions leading to difficulty in respiratory-swallowing coordination [1, 2].

Upper aerodigestive tract malignancies constitute 4-5% of all malignancies. It is the sixth most common cancer worldwide and constitutes a significant global problem with half of a million new cases diagnosed every year resulting in an average mortality rate of 7.3 and 3.2 per 100,000 males and females respectively [3]. In South East Asia, it is the second most common cancer. Pakistan falls into a high-risk head and neck cancer geographical zone with a prevalence of 22% [4–6]. Database of Karachi Cancer Registry have shown oral cavity as the most commonly affected site. Oral cavity carcinomas is showing a rising incidence with the mucosa cheek as the most common sub-site, followed by tongue, palate, gum, lip and floor of mouth [7].

The exact cause of cancer in this area of body is not well understood, but it is usually related to environmental and certain preventable risk factors which are self-inflicted. These include tobacco, alcohol, diet, radiation, pollution, drugs, viral infections, and other unknown factors. Amongst these, tobacco (smoked or smokeless in the form of pan and gutka chewing) is the most important, especially in our country. The prevalence of tobacco smoking in Pakistan is 36% for males and 9% for females [5, 8, 9].

In Pakistan, tobacco use is not limited to cigarette smoking. Other common forms of tobacco include water-pipe tobacco, chewing tobacco and snuff. Smokeless tobacco, whether it's chewing tobacco or snuff, is not a safe alternative of tobacco smoking and is responsible for a higher percentage of cases of oropharyngeal carcinoma in Pakistan [10].

Intraoperative consultation remains an invaluable tool in the initial evaluation of the surgically resected specimens. It not only includes frozen section but also gross evaluation of the specimen, examination of cytology preparations taken on the specimen (e.g. touch imprints), and aliquoting of the specimen for special studies (e.g. molecular pathology techniques, flow cytometry) [11].

Intraoperative diagnosis includes frozen section and touch imprint cytology both of which provide rapid intra-operative pathologic consultation.

Frozen section procedure involves a rapid microscopic analysis of a specimen by thin slicing of tissue cut from a fresh specimen [12, 13]. Frozen section has several limitations often making the interpretation difficult. The most important limitations that interfere with the results are the technical problems which include freezing artifacts, poor quality sections, bloated cell morphology and poorly stained sections [14].

Although it is generally believed that the conventional frozen section is the best technique for intraoperative consultation, intraoperative cytology also has emerged as an accurate, simple, cheap and rapid diagnostic tool [15].

Different studies carried out in different regions of the world have proved its diagnostic accuracy. In one study imprint cytology was correlated with histological diagnosis of the corresponding biopsy from 174 patients with laryngeal and pharyngeal tumors. The imprint cytology showed a diagnostic accuracy, sensitivity, specificity, positive predictive value and negative predictive values of 97, 96, 100, 100 and 92% respectively [16].

There was another study conducted in which correlation between the biopsy specimens and touch imprint preparations in patients with 30 head and neck mass lesions were examined. The concordance between touch imprint and paraffin sections was 90%. The sensitivity and specificity of touch imprint cytology in detecting malignancy were 88 and 92%, respectively [17].

This technique has also proven its accuracy in diagnosing surgical specimens belonging to prostate, breast cancer margins and sentinel lymph nodes; however a study of this type in UAT has been lacking in Pakistan [18, 19]. Therefore we evaluated the importance of touch imprint cytology in the intraoperative consultation of UAT malignancies and this may help in avoiding a preoperative invasive procedure. Furthermore this study is of special value is countries like Pakistan where cryostat facility is not available at many centers.

Methods

The study was conducted in the Department of Pathology, in collaboration with the Department of Otolaryngology, PIMS, Islamabad, from 1st July 2015 to 30th march 2016 for a period of 9 months. Consecutive (non-probability) sampling was used and the sample size was calculated by using WHO sample size calculator taking:

Sensitivity = 96% [10], Specificity = 100% [10], Expected prevalence = 22% [3].

Desired Precision = 10%, Confidence level = 95%.

Sample size = 69 patients.

Inclusion criteria:

1. Patients of all ages and both genders, presenting with mass lesions or ulceration in upper aerodigestive tract as clinically or radiologically detected.
2. Patients with any duration of illness are included.

3. Patients with any co-morbid diseases (diabetes, hypertension etc. as mentioned in the history) will be eligible to be selected.

Exclusion criteria:

1. Obvious inflammatory lesions of the Upper Aerodigestive Tract as diagnosed on biopsy.

Data collection procedure

Approval from hospital ethics committee was taken prior to the start of study. Patients were selected by consecutive sampling. After the informed consent, patients were included in the study based on lesions of upper aerodigestive tract. Intraoperatively, after obtaining the fresh biopsy specimen and prior to placing them in fixative, each specimen was imprinted on 4-6 glass slides, fixed immediately in 95% alcohol and stained with Hematoxylin and Eosin stain. The Cytology results were evaluated as

i. Malignant (Squamous cell carcinoma: isolated cells or clusters of malignant cells showing keratinization. The cells have distinct cell borders, vesicular nuclei and prominent nucleoli. Adenocarcinoma: cells are usually arranged in cohesive groups of various sizes in the form of loose clusters or acini with central lumina. The individual cells may show eccentric nuclei, mostly with prominent nucleoli and evidence of mucin production in the form of cytoplasmic vacuolation.)

ii. Suspicious for malignancy (suggestive of malignancy but uncertain due to limited number of cells or degree of atypia)

iii. Negative for malignancy (no evidence of malignancy like high N/C ratio, pleomorphism, hyperchromasia, coarse chromatin, irregular nuclear outlines).

iv. Non-diagnostic (scant cellularity, air drying or distortion artifact, obscuring blood).

After completion of the cytological procedure, the surgical biopsy specimen was immediately fixed in 10% buffered formalin. Following gross examination, the tissue was paraffin embedded. This was followed by cutting, slide preparation & staining with Hematoxylin and Eosin (H&E) stain. The Histopathology results were evaluated as:

i. Malignant (squamous cell carcinoma: sheets or nests of atypical squamoid cells having intercellular bridges and/or keratinization. Adenocarcinoma shows infiltration by malignant cells forming glandular pattern with large mucus secreting cells)

ii. Negative for malignancy (no evidence of malignancy like high N/C ratio, pleomorphism, hyperchromasia, coarse chromatin, irregular nuclear outlines seen in the biopsy material)

iii. Non-diagnostic (biopsy material inconclusive due to cautery effect or necrosis or fibrosis)

The slides of both touch imprint cytology and histopathology were examined under light microscope according to the set criteria and recorded by two consultant histopathologists and the results were recorded in a proforma.

Data analysis

Data was analyzed using SPSS Version 10. Descriptive statistics were calculated for both qualitative and quantitative variables. Mean and standard deviation (SD) were calculated for numerical variables like age. Frequency and percentage were presented for categorical variables i.e.; gender (M: F), cytological findings and histopathological findings.

2×2 tables was used to determine sensitivity, specificity, positive predictive value, negative predictive value and diagnostic accuracy.

Results

This study includes seventy cases which were collected in a 9 months period from 1st July 2015 to 30th march 2016. Random cases were selected which presented in the ENT OPD with different complains depending on the site involved. Patients with nasal tumors most commonly presented with a painless growth, sinusitis, etc. Patients with oral cavity lesions usually have non-healing ulcers, increasing growth, and difficulty in chewing etc. Laryngeal lesions usually showed hoarseness of voice, stridor, and difficulty in breathing. The patients were referred to the operation theatre for biopsy of the lesion, informed consent was taken from all the patients and the procedure of biopsy was preformed. Touch imprint slides were prepared from the fresh tissue in operation theatre.

Age distribution of the patients showed the patients range from 16 years to 93 years with the mean age being 52.87 +/- 18.26. Figure 1 demonstrates the age distribution. Majority of the patients fall in the range of 60-69 years (24 cases), followed by 30-39 years (11 cases). Of the total 70 cases, 47 cases (67.1%) were male while 23 cases (32.9%) were female. The male to female ratio is 2: 1.

Of the total seventy cases, 59 cases (84.3%) were malignant, while 11 cases (15.7%) were benign. The histologic breakdown of these cases, as diagnosed on histopathology showed 52 cases (72.9%) out of 59 malignant were squamous cell carcinoma of different grades.

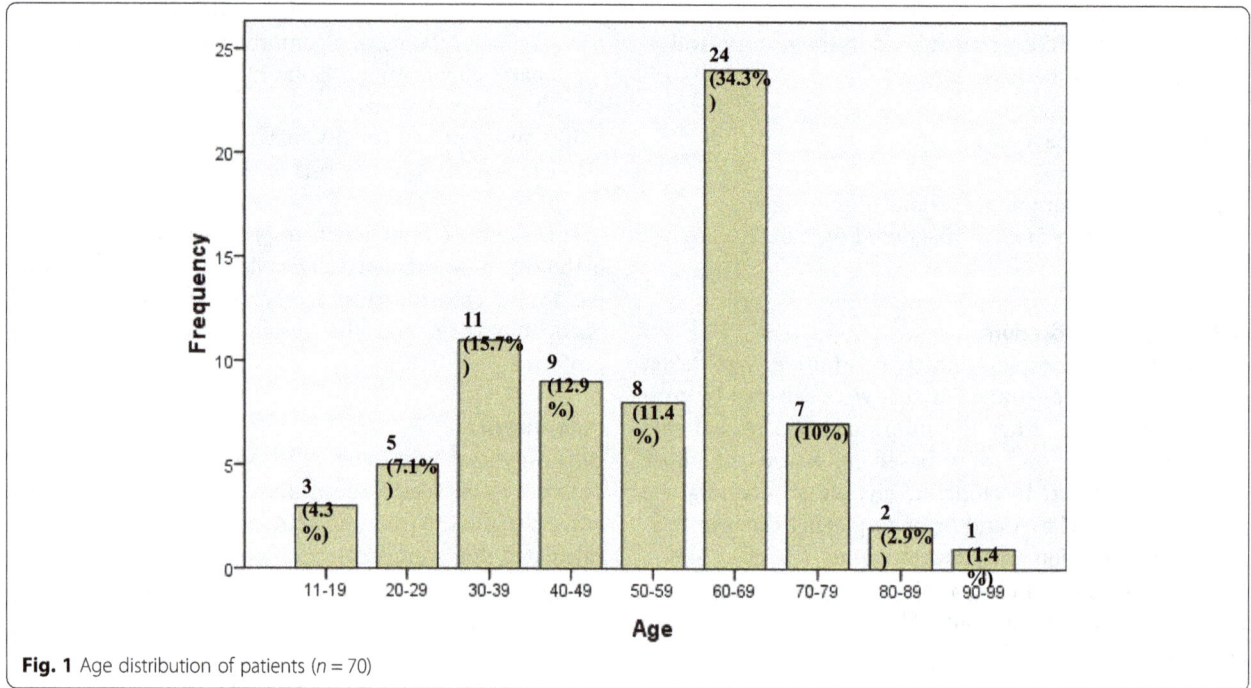

Fig. 1 Age distribution of patients (*n* = 70)

The remaining cases include malignant salivary gland tumors comprising of 3 cases (4.3%) which included 2 cases (2.9%) of adenoid cystic carcinoma and 1 case (1.4%) of Mucoepidermoid carcinoma, non-Hodgkin lymphoma 2 cases (2.9%), fibrosarcoma 1 case (1.4%) (Table 1). One case (1.4%) also included in the malignant category was of moderate dysplasia as diagnosed on biopsy. Frequency breakdown of these cases as diagnosed on histopathology is shown in Fig. 2.

The site breakdown of malignant tumors show oral cavity as the most common site of involvement, in 33 cases (47.1%), followed by larynx in 27 cases (38.6%).

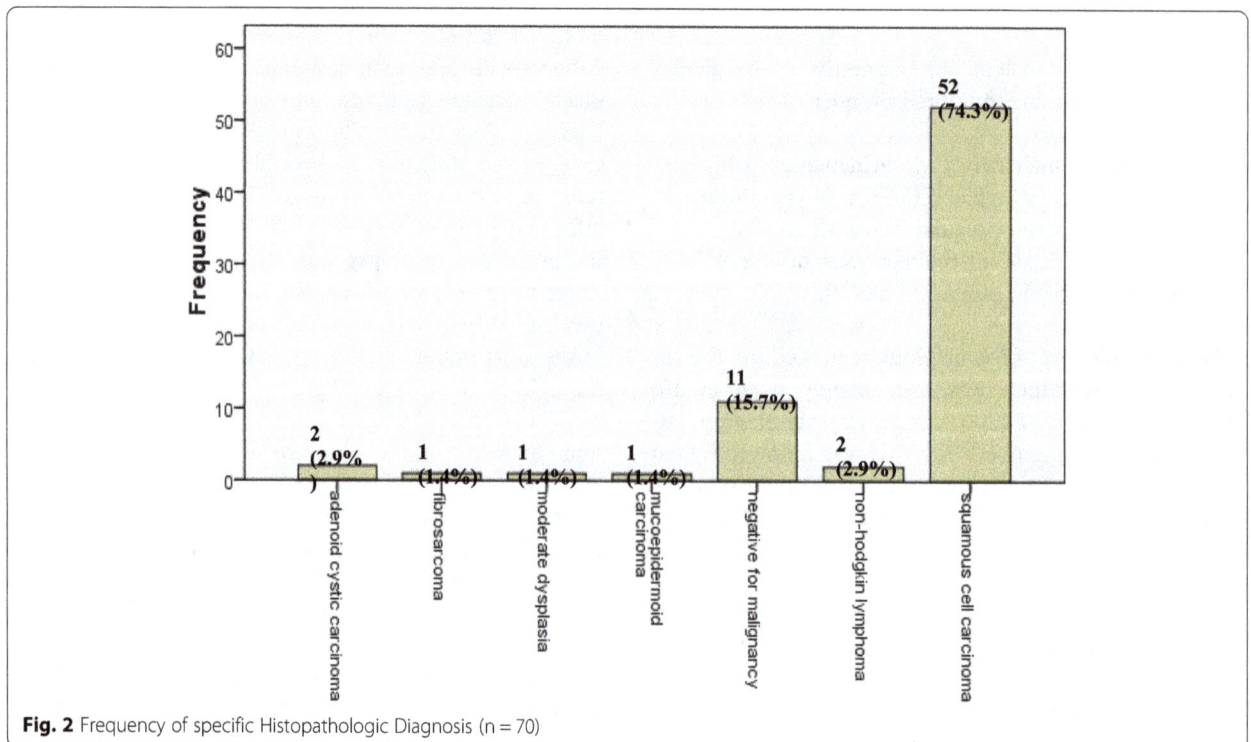

Fig. 2 Frequency of specific Histopathologic Diagnosis (n = 70)

The nasal cavity was involved in 2 cases (2.9%), naso-pharynx in 4 cases (5.7%), oropharynx in 1 case (1.4%) and laryngopharynx in 3 cases (4.3%). In the oral cavity, oral mucosa was the most commonly involved site, followed by tongue, hard palate, soft palate, tonsil, alveolar ridge and lower lip. In the larynx supraglottis is the most common site, followed by glottis, infraglottis, true vocal cord, pyriform fossa, false vocal cord and epiglottis. The site breakdowns of the cases are shown in Fig. 3.

The result of touch imprint cytology showed that touch imprint cytology was diagnostic in 68 cases (97.1%), 55 (78.6%) being malignant, 2 cases (2.9%) were suspicious for malignancy, 11 cases (15.7%) were negative for malignancy while 2 cases (2.9%) were false negative. Among the 70 cases, 55 cases (78.6%) were malignant showing squamous cell carcinoma in 49 cases (70%), adenoid cystic carcinoma in 2 cases (2.9%), non-Hodgkin lymphoma 2 cases (2.9%), Mucoepidermoid carcinoma 1 case (1.4%), spindle cell sarcoma in 1 case (1.4%). Two cases (2.9%) were suspicious of malignancy showing atypical squamoid cells on touch imprint cytology, while 13 cases (18.6%) were negative for malignancy, which also included 2 false negative cases. These statistics are shown in Fig. 4.

A strong correlation is found between the diagnosis made by touch imprint cytology and the final histopathological diagnosis as shown in Table 2. Of the 70 cases of head and neck tumors diagnosed on histopathology, complete correlation was seen in 68 cases (97.1%) cases and there was a lack of correlation in only two cases.

The overall diagnostic accuracy, sensitivity, specificity, positive predictive value and negative predictive value of touch imprint cytology were determined for all malignant

head and neck tumors. Separate statistics were calculated for squamous cell carcinoma as this was the predominant histologic type.

The overall diagnostic accuracy of Touch imprint cytology in diagnosing malignant head and neck lesions came out to be 96.7%, as shown in Table 3. The sensitivity and specificity of touch imprint cytology came out to be 96 and 100%, respectively. Whereas the PPV and NPV of touch imprint cytology was found to be 100 and 84%, respectively. 2×2 table for malignant aerodigestive tract lesions are shown in Table 4.

The sensitivity and specificity of touch imprint cytology in diagnosing squamous cell carcinoma came out to be 96.2 and 100% respectively, as shown in Table 5. The PPV and NPV was 100 and 84.6%, respectively with the diagnostic accuracy being 96.8%. 2×2 table for squamous cell carcinoma are shown in Table 6.

The sensitivity and specificity of touch imprint cytology in diagnosing malignant salivary gland neoplasm and non-hodgkins lymphoma came out to be 100 and 100% respectively.

Discussion
Touch imprint cytology is a well known rapid histopathological method of intraoperative analysis of biopsy specimens along with frozen section. Different studies have analyzed the importance of both procedures; however frozen sections have shown interpretational difficulties in the form of freezing artifacts, cost effectiveness, and expertise in operating the cryostat machine etc. Touch imprint cytology on the other hand is a very simple, cheap and easy to perform procedure requiring pathologist's expertise in the cytology interpretation [20, 21].

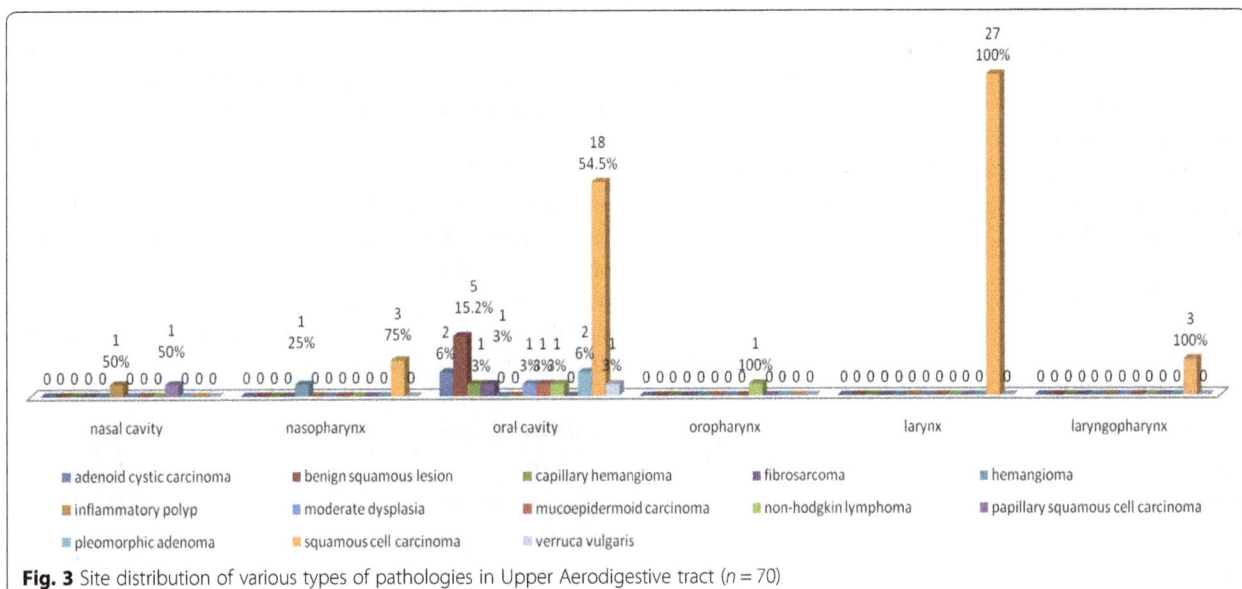

Fig. 3 Site distribution of various types of pathologies in Upper Aerodigestive tract (*n* = 70)

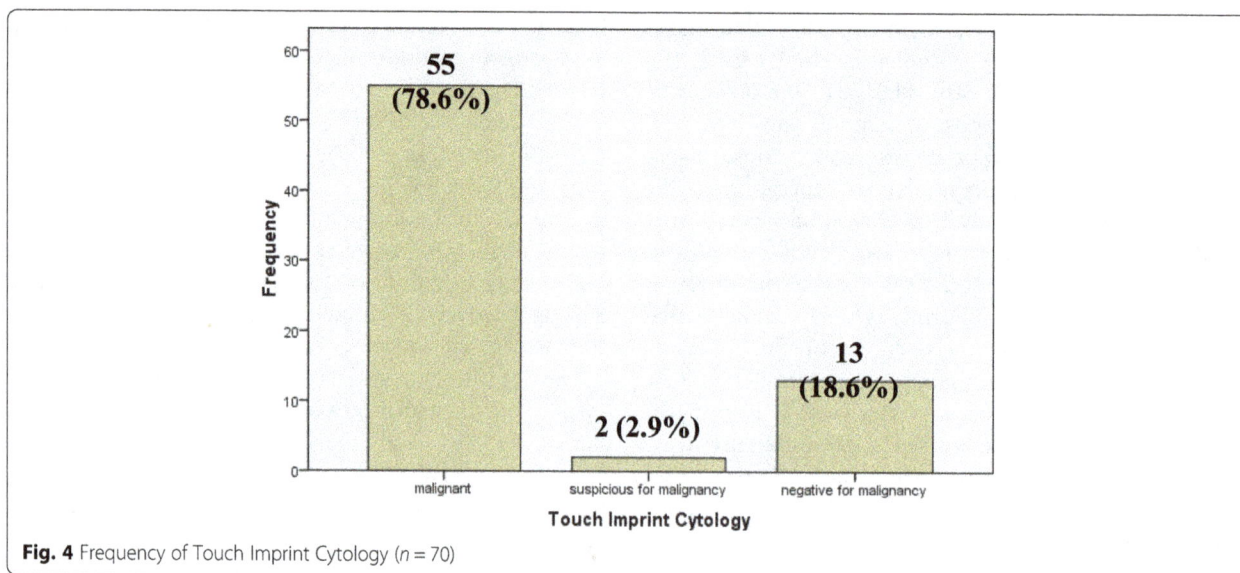

Fig. 4 Frequency of Touch Imprint Cytology (n = 70)

In this study a total of seventy cases were collected over a period of 9 months. Most of the patients were referred from the E.N.T. department to operation theatre for the biopsy procedure of patient with complaints of increasing growth lesion, a non-healing ulcer, difficulty in swallowing, hoarseness of voice and stridor etc. The aim of this study was to evaluate the diagnostic accuracy of touch imprint cytology of upper aerodigestive tract malignancies in all age groups. We found that touch imprint cytology is highly sensitive and specific intraoperative procedure [22].

Most of the patients in our study were in the age range of 60-69 years comprising of 24 patients, followed by a comparatively younger age group of 30-39 years comprising of 11 cases. There were 5 cases in the range of 20-29 years, while 51 cases were above 40 years. These results are comparable to the study done by Mehrota R, who showed a head and neck cancer predominance in adults, although majority of their patients were in the range of 50-59 yrs. [23].

Our study showed a male predominance comprising of 47 males (67.1%) and 23 (32.9%) females with a male to female ratio of 2:1. The results of our study are comparable to study done by Adeyami BF et al. who analyzed

Table 1 Frequency of specific Touch Imprint Cytology diagnosis (n = 70)

Diagnosis	Frequency	Percentage
Squamous cell carcinoma	49	72.8%
Adenoid cystic carcinoma	2	2.9%
Mucoepidermoid carcinoma	1	1.4%
Non-Hodgkin lymphoma	2	2.9%
Spindle cell sarcoma	1	1.4%
Suspicious for malignancy	2	2.9%

head and neck cancer in a Nigerian tertiary healthcare centre. They found a male predominance in the head and neck cancers with a male to female ratio of 1.8:1. Similar findings were reported by Alverenge Lde M et al.; they also found a male predominance in carcinomas of head and neck region [24, 25].

The patients in our study usually presented with lesions in the oral cavity comprising of 33 cases (47.1%), and the second most common site is larynx comprising of 27 cases (38.6%). In the oral cavity, the oral mucosa was the most commonly involved sub-type, comprising of 16 cases and the patients usually presented with non-healing ulcer at this site. After oral mucosa, tongue is the second commonly involved site in eight patients with ulceration as the most common presentation. These results are comparable to the study conducted by Mirbod SM et al. [26].

The sensitivity and specificity of touch imprint cytology for malignant upper aerodigestive tract lesion in our study was calculated as 96% and 100% respectively. Hussein et al. conducted a similar study of touch imprint cytological preparations and head and neck lesions and they found sensitivity and specificity in detecting malignancy was 88% and 92% respectively. Comparison of intraoperative cytology and frozen section in nose and paranasal tumors were also evaluated by Nigam J et al. and they found a sensitivity, specificity and positive predictive value of 100% [10, 20].

Table 2 Degree of Correlation

Degree of correlation	Frequency (%)
Complete correlation	55 (93%)
Correlation with category only	2 (3.3%)
No correlation	2 (3.3%)

Table 3 Diagnostic Accuracy of Touch imprint cytology in diagnosing Malignant Upper Aerodigestive Tract lesions (n = 70)

Touch Imprint Cytology in Upper Aerodigestive Tract lesions	
Sensitivity	96%
Specificity	100%
Positive predictive value	100%
Negative predictive value	84%
Diagnostic accuracy	96.7%

Table 5 Diagnostic Accuracy of Touch imprint cytology in diagnosing Squamous cell carcinoma (n = 52)

Touch Imprint Cytology in Squamous cell carcinoma	
Sensitivity	96.2%
Specificity	100%
Positive predictive value	100%
Negative predictive value	84.6%
Diagnostic accuracy	96.8%

There were a total of seventy cases, showing squamous cell carcinoma in 52 cases, which were accurately picked up by the touch imprint cytology in 50 cases. Twenty-four cases were well differentiated squamous cell carcinoma, 19 were moderately differentiated while 9 were poorly differentiated (Figs. 5 & 6).

The sensitivity and specificity of touch imprint cytology for squamous cell carcinoma in our study was 96.2 and 100% respectively. This is in accordance with the study conducted by Nieberler M et al. who evaluated the intraoperative cytology of bone resection margins in oral squamous cell carcinoma and found a high sensitivity and specificity of touch imprint cytology. Their study concluded the sensitivity and specificity of touch imprint cytology as 95.3% and 96% respectively. The positive predictive value, negative predictive value and diagnostic accuracy of their study came out to be 93.8, 96.9 and 95.7% respectively [27].

Three cases of malignant salivary gland neoplasm were also encountered. They included one intermediate grade Mucoepidermoid carcinoma and two cases of adenoid cystic carcinoma. Touch imprint cytology accurately picked up both cases with a sensitivity, specificity, positive predictive value, negative predictive value and diagnostic accuracy of 100%. On touch imprint cytology of Mucoepidermoid carcinoma there were cells with typical squamoid appearance mimicking a squamous cell carcinoma, however there were admixed large cells with abundant, mucin filled cytoplasm, thereby confirming a diagnosis of Mucoepidermoid carcinoma (Fig. 7). Adenoid cystic carcinoma on the other hand showed cells arranged in a cribriform architecture on touch imprint cytology. The neoplastic cells have hyperchromatic, angulated nuclei and scant cytoplasm (Fig. 8). All three cases aroused from the hard palate which is most common site for minor

salivary gland neoplasm. Jansisyanont P et al. in their experience of intraoral minor salivary gland tumors also found palate as the most frequently involved site by minor salivary gland neoplasms [28].

There were two cases of non-Hodgkin lymphoma, both involved the oral cavity. One case involved the tonsil while the other involved the oral cavity. Both cases on touch imprint cytology showed sheet of large atypical lymphoid cells having with increased nuclear size, vhirregular chromatin clumping, prominent nucleoli and scant cytoplasm. Atypical mitotic figures were also seen. On permanent sections both cases were diagnosed as non-Hodgkin lymphoma.

There was one case of spindle cell sarcoma, diagnosed as fibrosarcoma after the application of immunohistochemistry on histologic sections. The sarcoma involved the oral mucosa showed sheets of atypical spindle shaped cells having hyperchromatic, pleomorphic nuclei with irregular nuclear contours and chromatin on cytology smears. Frequent atypical mitoses were also seen. Resection specimen of the same case showed spindle cell sarcoma in a herring bone pattern, which on immunohistochemistry was negative for all specific lineage markers like smooth muscle actin, desmin, myogenin, pancytokeratin etc.

Two cases were given suspicious of malignancy, due to atypical nuclear features but the cellularity was too low to make a definitive diagnosis. One of the case had atypical cells admixed with benign squamoid cells misleading the diagnosis. On permanent sections well differentiated squamous cell carcinoma was diagnosed. The other case showed mature squamoid cells with mild nuclear changes in the form of hyperchromasia, nuclear

Table 4 2 × 2 table showing cases with diagnosis of Malignant Upper Aerodigestive Tract Lesions (n = 70)

Touch imprint cytology	Histopathological Diagnosis (Malignant Upper Aerodigestive Tract Lesions)	
	True positive (a) 57	False positive (b) 0
	False negative (c) 2	True negative (d) 11

Table 6 2 × 2 table showing cases with a diagnosis of Squamous cell carcinoma (n = 52)

Touch imprint cytology diagnosis (squamous cell carcinoma)	Histopathological diagnosis (Squamous cell carcinoma)	
	True positive (a) 50	False positive (b) 0
	False negative (c) 0	True negative (d) 2

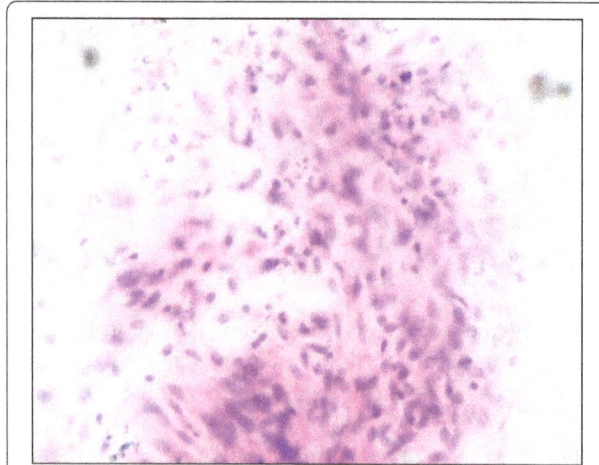

Fig. 5 Touch imprint cytology of well differentiated squamous cell carcinoma showing cluster of neoplastic cells have vesicular nuclei, slightly pleomorphic nuclei, prominent nucleoli and abundant cytoplasm (H&E ×400)

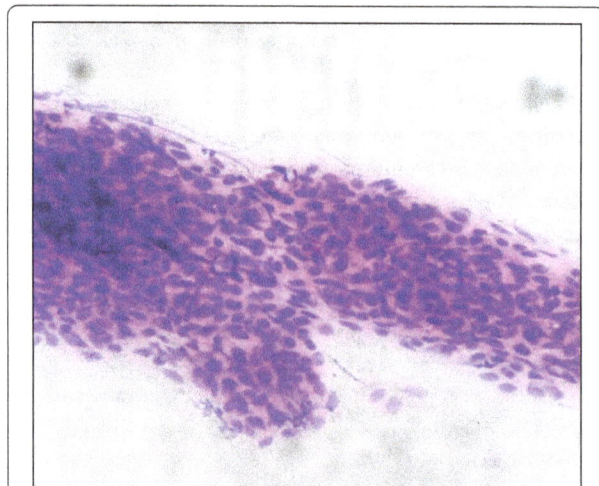

Fig. 7 Touch imprint cytology of Mucoepidermoid carcinoma showing intermediate cells and a mucin filled cell (H&E ×400)

membrane abnormalities, but the changes were not significant to diagnose it as a malignant smear. Permanent sections of the same case showed only moderate dysplasia of the lining epithelium. No invasive carcinoma was identified. Since touch imprint cytology shows only cytological features, architectural changes in the form of basement membrane invasion cannot be commented upon. This is the drawback of touch imprint cytology that invasion cannot be identified; however touch imprint cytology can detect dysplastic cytological changes.

There were two cases which showed benign morphology on touch imprint cytology, while the permanent sections showed malignant squamous cell carcinoma. One case on touch imprint cytology showed benign squamoid cells which

on permanent sections showed sections lined by stratified squamous epithelium with only a small focus showing dysplastic epithelial changes and invasion into the subepithelial tissue. This small focus was not sampled in touch imprint cytology giving a false negative diagnosis. The problem can be solved by making multiple smears from different biopsy sides so that all the cut surfaces are touched on the slides, minimizing the false negative results. The other case showed very hypocellular smears with mostly inflammatory cells. On permanent sections well differentiated squamous cell carcinoma was present along with ulceration of the epithelium.

Conclusion

Intraoperative consultation is an important tool for the evaluation of the lesions, specifically the nature of the

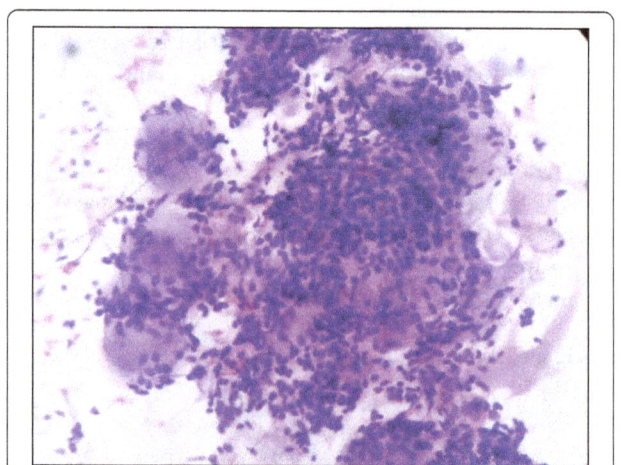

Fig. 6 Touch imprint cytology of poorly differentiated squamous cell carcinoma showing sheets of cells having vesicular, pleomorphic nuclei and high nuclear to cytoplasmic ratio (H&E ×400)

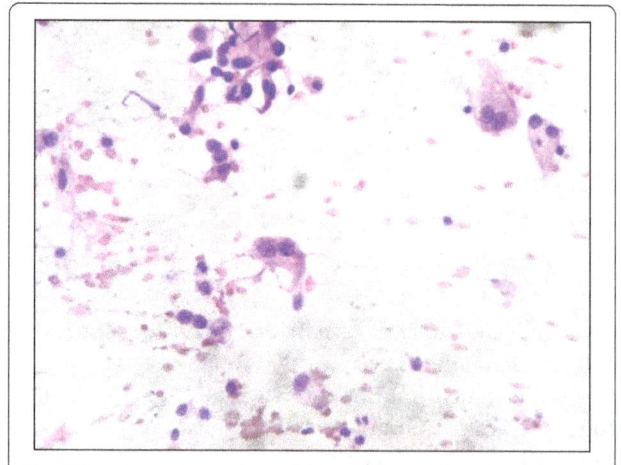

Fig. 8 Touch imprint cytology of adenoid cystic carcinoma showing cribriform arrangement of basaloid cells having hyperchromatic, angulated nuclei. Basophilic secretions characteristic of adenoid cystic carcinoma are also seen (H&E ×400)

lesion, adequacy of the biopsy, margin status etc. This study demonstrates that touch imprint cytology is an important tool for the evaluation of malignant upper aerodigestive tract lesions.

Although architectural features are subtle and focal in touch imprint cytology smears but the specific cytological features can help in avoiding diagnostic pitfalls. The smears should always be carefully interpreted by a trained cytopathologist to avoid misdiagnosis. Multiple smears should be made from the specimen after carefully dabbing the specimen surface to avoid blood obscuring artifacts and low cellularity etc. The clinical findings and other diagnostic modalities, like radiological imaging should always be known before interpretation of the lesion.

Our experience in this study has demonstrated that touch imprint cytology provides important diagnostic information that can play a significant role in patients management, especially by differentiating between neoplastic and reactive lesions. Moreover, in a majority of cases, it can provide reliable specific diagnoses and can be used as an adjunct to histopathology, particularly in developing countries like ours, where the facility of frozen sections is often not available, since a rapid preliminary diagnosis may help in surgical management planning.

Acknowledgments

We gratefully acknowledge all staff members of Pathology Department, Liaquat National Hospital, Karachi, Pakistan for their help and cooperation.

Funding

The funding helps in the design of the study and collection, analysis, and interpretation of data.

Authors' contributions

HN and MA: main author of manuscript, have made substantial contributions to conception and design of study. AAH, MME, AKS, HM AND AK have been involved in requisition, analysis of the data and gave final approval and revision of the manuscript. All authors read and approved the final manuscript.

Competing interests

The authors declare that they have no competing interests.

Author details

[1]Shifa Medical College, Islamabad, Pakistan. [2]Liaquat National Hospital and Medical College, Karachi, Pakistan. [3]Brown University, Providence, RI, USA. [4]Pakistan Institute of Medical Sciences, Islamabad, Pakistan. [5]Kandahar University, Kandahar, Afghanistan.

References

1. Uppaluri R, Dunn GP, Lewis JS Jr. Focus on TILs: prognostic significance of tumor infiltrating lymphocytes in head and neck cancers. Cancer Immun. 2008;8:16.
2. Givens DJ, Karnell LH, Gupta AK, Clamon GH, Pagedar NA, Chang KE, et al. Adverse events associated with concurrent chemoradiation therapy in patients with head and cancer. Arch Otolaryngol Head Neck Surg. 2009; 135(12):1209–17.
3. Masood N, Kayani MA. Mutational analysis of xenobiotic metabolizing genes (CYP1A1 and GSTP1) in sporadic head and neck cancer patients. Genet Mol Biol. 2011;34(4):533–8.
4. Chaudhry S, Khan AA, Mirza KM, Iqbal HA, Masood Y, Khan NR, et al. Estimating the burden of head and neck cancers in the public health sector of Pakistan. Asian Pac J Cancer Prev. 2008;9(3):529–32.
5. Goon PK, Stanley MA, Ebmeyer J, Steinstrasser L, Upile T, Jerjes W, et al. HPV and head and neck cancer a descriptive update. Head Neck Oncol. 2009;1:36.
6. Slootweg PJ, Richardson M. Squamous cell carcinoma of the upper aerodigestive system. In: Gnepp DR, editor. Diagnostic surgical pathology of head and neck. 2nd ed. Philadelphia: Elsevier Inc; 2009. p. 45–110.
7. Bhurgri Y, Bhurgri A, Usman A, Pervez S, Kayani N, Bashir I, et al. Epidemiological review of head and neck cancers in Karachi. Asian Pac J Cancer Prev. 2006;7(2):195–200.
8. Lee YC, Marron M, Benhamou S, Bouchardy C, Ahrens W, Pohlabeln H, et al. Active and involuntary tobacco smoking and upper aerodigestive tract cancer risks in a multicenter case-control study. Cancer Epidemiol Biomark Prev. 2009;18(12):3353–61.
9. hmed R, Rashid R, McDonald PW, Ahmed SW. Prevalence of cigarette smoking among young adults in Pakistan. JPMA. 2008;58(11):597–601.
10. Bile KM, Shaikh JA, Afridi HU, Khan Y. Smokeless tobacco use in Pakistan and its association with oropharyngeal cancer. East Mediterr Health J. 2010; 16 Suppl:S24-30.
11. Wenig BM. Intraoperative consultation (IOC) in mucosal lesions of the upper Aerodigestive tract. Head Neck Pathol. 2008;2(2):131–44.
12. Hashmi AA, Naz S, Edhi MM, Faridi N, Hussain SD, Mumtaz S, Khan M. Accuracy of intraoperative frozen section for the evaluation of ovarian neoplasms: an institutional experience. World J Surg Oncol. 2016;14:91.
13. Hashmi AA, Faridi N, Khurshid A, Naqvi H, Malik B, Malik FR, Fida Z, Mujtuba S. Accuracy of frozen section analysis of sentinel lymph nodes for the detection of Asian breast cancer micrometastasis - experience from Pakistan. Asian Pac J Cancer Prev. 2013;14(4):2657–62.
14. Thomson AM, Wallace WA. Fixation artifacts in an intra-operative frozen section: a potential cause of misinterpretation. J Cardiothorac Surg. 2007;2:45.
15. Khalid A, Haque AU. Touch imprint cytology versus frozen section as intraoperative consultation diagnosis. Int J Pathol. 2004;2(2):63–70.
16. Loncar B, Pajtler M, Milicić-Juhas V, Kotromanović Z, Staklenac B, Pauzar B. Imprint cytology in laryngeal and pharyngeal tumors. Cytopathology. 2007; 18(1):40–3.
17. Hussein MR, Rashad UM, Hassanein KA. Touch imprint cytological preparations and the diagnosis of head and neck mass lesions. Ann Oncol. 2005;16(1):171–2.
18. Aytac B, Atalay FO, Vuruskan H, Filiz G. Touch imprint cytology of prostate core needle biopsy specimens: a useful method for immediate reporting of prostate cancer. J Cytol. 2012;29(3):173–6.
19. Esbona K, Li Z, Wilke LG. Intraoperative imprint cytology and frozen section pathology for margin assessment in breast conservation surgery: a systematic review. Ann Surg Oncol. 2012;19(10):3236–45.
20. Jaafar H. Intra-operative frozen section consultation: concepts, applications and limitations. Malays J Med Sci. 2006;13(1):4–12.
21. Nigam J, Misra V, Dhingra V, Jain S, Varma K, Singh A. Comparative study of intra-operative cytology, frozen sections, and histology of tumor and tumor-like lesions of nose and paranasal sinuses. J Cytol. 2013;30(1):13–7.
22. Mehanna H, Paleri V, West CM, Nutting C. Head and neck cancer–part 1: epidemiology, presentation, and prevention. BMJ. 2010;341:c4684.
23. Mehrotra R, Singh M, Gupta RK, Singh M, Kapoor AK. Trends of prevalence and pathological spectrum of head and neck cancers in North India. Indian J Cancer. 2005;42(2):89–93.
24. Adeyemi BF, Adekunle LV, Kolude BM, Akang EE, Lawoyin JO. Head and neck cancer–a clinicopathological study in a tertiary care center. J Natl Med Assoc. 2008;100(6):690–7.

25. Alvarenga Lde M, Ruiz MT, Pavarino-Bertelli EC, Ruback MJ, Maniglia JV, Goloni-Bertollo M. Epidemiologic evaluation of head and neck patients in a university hospital of Northwestern São Paulo state. Braz J Otorhinolaryngol. 2008;74(1):68–73.
26. Mirbod SM, Ahing SI. Tobacco-associated lesions of the oral cavity: part II. Malignant lesions. J Can Dent Assoc. 2000;66(6):308–11.
27. Nieberler M, Häusler P, Drecoll E, Stoeckelhuber M, Deppe H, Hölzle F, et al. Evaluation of intraoperative cytological assessment of bone resection margins in patients with oral squamous cell carcinoma. Cancer Cytopathol. 2014;122(9):646–56.
28. Jansisyanont P, Blanchaert RH Jr, Ord RA. Intraoral minor salivary gland neoplasm: a single institution experience of 80 cases. Int J Oral Maxillofac Surg. 2002;31(3):257–61.

25

Prognostic significance of p16 & p53 immunohistochemical expression in triple negative breast cancer

Atif Ali Hashmi[1], Samreen Naz[1], Shumaila Kanwal Hashmi[2], Zubaida Fida Hussain[1], Muhammad Irfan[1], Erum Yousuf Khan[1], Naveen Faridi[1], Amir Khan[3]* (iD) and Muhammad Muzzammil Edhi[4]

Abstract

Background: p16 and p53 genes are frequently mutated in triple negative breast cancer & prognostic value of these mutations have been shown; however, their role as immunohistochemical overexpression has not been fully validated. Therefore we aimed to evaluate the association of p16 and p53 overexpression in triple negative breast cancer with various prognostic parameters.

Methods: Total 150 cases of triple negative breast cancers were selected from records of pathology department archives that underwent surgeries at Liaquat National hospital, Karachi from January 2008 till December 2013. ER, PR and Her2neu immunohistochemistry were re-performed to confirm triple negative status. p16 & p53 immunohistochemistry was performed on all cases and association with various clinicopathologic parameters was determined.

Results: Mean age of the patients involved in the study was 48.9 years. Most of the patients presented at stage T2 with a high mean ki67 index i.e. 46.9%. 42.7% of cases had nodal metastasis. Although 84% cases were of invasive ductal carcinoma; however a significant proportion of cases were of metaplastic histology (9.3%). Fifty-one percent (76 cases) of cases showed positive p53 expression while 49% (74 cases) were negative. Higher percentage of p53 expression was found to correlate with higher T stage, high ki67 index and higher nodal stage. On the other hand, strong intensity of p53 expression was positively correlated with higher tumor grade and ki67 index. Seventy-one percent (98 cases) of cases showed positive p16 expression, whereas 24.8% (34 cases) were negative and 3.6% (5 cases) showed focal positive p16 expression. However, no significant association was found between p16 expression and various clinical and pathologic parameters. Similarly, no significant association of either p16 or p53 over-expression was noted with recurrence status of patients.

Conclusion: On the basis of significant association of p53 over-expression with worse prognostic factors in triple negative breast cancer, therefore we suggest that more large scale studies are needed to validate this finding in loco-regional population. Moreover, high expression of p16 in triple negative breast cancer suggests a potential role of this biomarker in triple negative breast cancer pathogenesis which should be investigated with molecular based research in our population.

Keywords: p53, p16, Triple negative breast cancer

* Correspondence: dramirkhan04@gmail.com
[3]Kandahar University, North, Kandahar 3802, Afghanistan
Full list of author information is available at the end of the article

Background

Triple negative breast cancers (TNBC) comprise approximately 20% of breast cancers worldwide while a higher frequency of TNBC were noted in south – Asian population [1, 2]. American Society of Clinical Oncology (ASCO)/ College of American Pathologists (CAP) defines TNBC as those breast cancers which shows < 1% estrogen receptor (ER)/ progesterone receptor (PR) expression by immunohistochemistry (IHC) and either 0–1+ Her2neu by IHC or 2+ with negative fluorescent insitu hybridization (FISH) [3–5]. TNBC are typically high grade and associated with worse prognostic and predictive factors and are therefore focus of current clinical research [6, 7]. Moreover TNBC are not a single clinical entity and various subtypes of TNBC have been defined based on molecular studies including basal like subtypes, immunomodulatory, mesenchymal, mesenchymal stem-like, luminal androgen subtypes, claudin low and interferon rich subtypes [8, 9]. Basal like subtype of TNBC is a molecularly defined subtype of TNBC with high expression of basal cytokeratins (CK5/6) and epidermal growth factor receptor (EGFR) and it correlates with IHC expression of CK5/6, [10, 11].

p16 and p53 are proteins which are involved in two major cell cycle control pathways frequently targeted in human tumorigenesis. Virtually all human cancers show dysregulation of either p16 or p53 pathways [12–14]. Prognostic value of p16 and p53 mutations in breast cancer has been shown in various studies [15, 16] however their role as IHC overexpression in TNBC has not been fully understood. Therefore, we aimed to evaluate the association of p16 and p53 overexpression in TNBC with various prognostic parameters like tumor stage, tumor grade, nodal metastasis and lymphovascular invasion.

Methods

The study included 150 cases of TNBC that had their primary resection at Liaquat National hospital from January 2008 till December 2013 over duration of 6 years. Type of surgeries included wide local excisions and simple mastectomies with sentinel lymph node dissection or wide local excision with axillary dissection and modified radical mastectomies. The approval of the study was taken from institutional research and ethical review committee. At the time of surgery, an informed written consent was taken from each patient. Clinical records of all patients were evaluated and histopathological findings like tumor type, grade and stage were recorded after reviewing H & E slides. Moreover, representative sections of all tumors were re-cut for H & E and IHC staining. ER, PR, Her2neu, Ki67, CK5/6, p16 and p53 IHC were performed on representative sections.

ER, PR, Her2neu and Ki67 IHC were performed using DAKO antibodies as under, with EnVision™ FLEX, high pH DAKO kit according to manufacturer's protocol.

1. FLEX Monoclonal Rabbit Anti-human Estrogen Receptor alpha, Clone EP1.
2. FLEX Monoclonal Mouse Anti-human Progesterone receptor clone PgR 636
3. Polyclonal Rabbit Anti-human c-erbB-2 oncoprotein
4. FLEX Monoclonal mouse Anti-human Ki67 Antigen clone MIB-1

For ER and PR IHC, nuclear staining in more than 1% cancer cells was taken as positive expression [4]. For, her2-neu IHC, staining was scored as per CAP guidelines into 1 + (weak), 2+ (intermediate) and 3+ (strong) expression. Cases with intermediate (2+) expression were subjected to Fluorescent insitu hybridization (FISH) testing and results were reported as amplified or non-amplified as per CAP guidelines [5].

Ki67 IHC was interpreted on the basis of average percentage of positively stained cancer cells. Only nuclear expression was taken as positive. At-least 1000 cancer cells were counted in five different areas of tumor and average percentage of positively stained cancer cells were recorded and then categorized.

CK5/6 IHC was performed by using FLEX Monoclonal Mouse Anti-human Cytokeratin 5/6, clone D5/16 B4 by DAKO envision method according to manufacturers protocol. Moderate to strong cytoplasmic and membranous staining in more than 10% cells was taken as positive expression. Tumors with positive CK5/6 were labeled as basal phenotype and those with negative CK5/6 expression were called as non-basal phenotype.

p53 IHC was performed using DAKO EnVision method using DAKO anti-human p53 protein, clone DO-7 according to manufacturers protocol. Nuclear staining for p53 was both quantitatively and qualitatively evaluated. Intensity of staining was categorized into no staining (0), weak (1+), intermediate (2+), strong (3+) while percentage of positively stained cells were measured as continuous variable. Intermediate to strong staining in > 10% cancer cells was considered positive while no staining or weak staining in < 10% cancer cells was taken as negative (Fig. 1). Moreover, p53 immunostaining was also categorized according to percentage of staining cells into different groups.

p16 antibody was purchased from Roche Ventana and IHC was performed using antibody CINtec R p16INK4a, clone E6H4™ according to manufacturers protocol. Tonsils and carcinoma cervix was taken as positive controls. Both nuclear and cytoplasmic staining was evaluated. Intensity of staining was categorized into no staining (0),

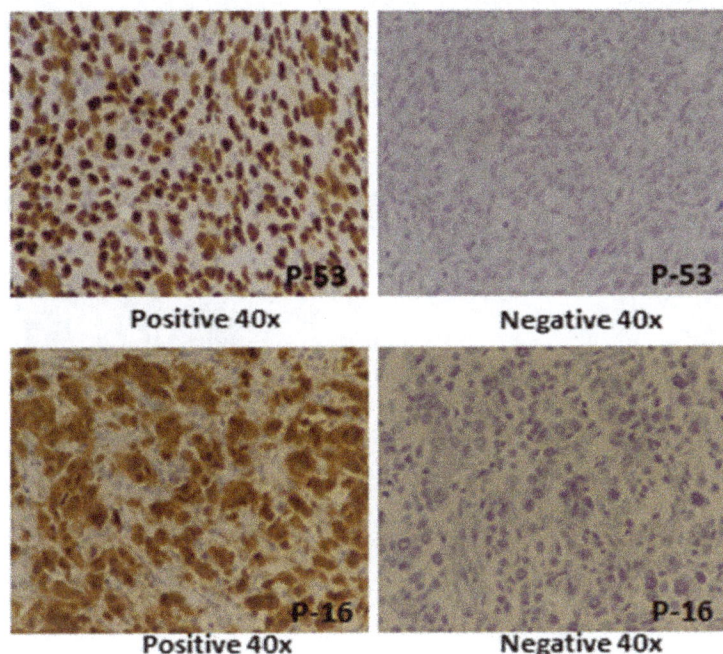

Fig. 1 p53 & p16 expression in triple negative breast cancer

weak (1+), intermediate (2+), strong (3+) while percentage of positively stained cells were measured as continuous variable. Intermediate to strong staining in > 10% cancer cells was considered positive while weak to intermediate staining in < 10% cancer cells was taken as focal positive (Fig. 1). Similarly, p16 immunostaining was also categorized according to percentage of staining cells into different groups.

Patient's clinical records were reviewed to evaluated recurrence and survival status. Time from surgery till death due to disease, local recurrence, distant metastasis or last follow was defined as disease free survival.

Statistical package for social sciences (SPSS 21) was used for data entry and analysis. We calculated mean and standard deviation for quantitative variables while, frequency and percentage were evaluated for qualitative variables. Chi-square was applied to determine association between the variables. Student t test or Mann witney test were applied to compare difference in means among groups where necessary. P-value of ≤0.05 was taken as significant. Survival curves were plotted using Kaplan- Meier method and the significance of difference between survival curves were evaluated using log-rank ratio.

A sample size of 150 achieves 79% power to detect an effect size (W) of 0.2994 using a 6 degrees of freedom Chi-Square Test with a significance level (alpha) of 0.05000.

Results

Mean age of the patients involved in the study was 48.9 years and most common age group was 31–50 years. Most of the patients presented at stage T2 with a high mean ki67 index i.e. 46.9%. 42.7% of cases had nodal metastasis. Although 84% cases were of conventional invasive ductal carcinoma, NST; however a significant proportion of cases were of metaplastic histology (9.3%). Majority cases were of high grade (86.7% grade III). Most tumors show lymphocytic infiltration and necrosis. Most of the tumors lack insitu component (61%) and only 10% cases were of basal phenotype (CK5/6 positive). Local recurrence or late distant metastasis was noted in 17.8% of cases (Table 1).

Fifty-one percent (76 cases) of TNBC showed positive p53 expression while 49% (74 cases) were negative. Further categorization on the basis of percentage of p53 expression revealed; 36% (54 cases) showed high p53 expression (> 70%), 12% (18 cases) revealed 51–70% p53 expression, 12% (18 cases) showed 11–50% p53 expression and 40% (60 cases) showed either no p53 expression or weak expression in less than 10% tumor cells. 30.7% (46 cases) showed no p53 expression while 14% (21 cases), 17.3% (26 cases) and 38% (57 cases) revealed weak, intermediate and strong 53 expression respectively. Correlation of percentage of p53 expression with various clinicopathologic variables revealed significant associations (Table 2). High p53 expression was found to correlate with higher T stage, high ki67 index and higher nodal stage. Although

Table 1 Clinicopathologic characteristics of triple negative breast cancer

	n (%)
Age(years)°	48.85 ± 11.49
Age groups	
≤ 30 years	5(3.3)
31–50 years	84(56)
> 50 years	61(40.7)
Tumor size(Unit)°	4.01 ± 1.99
Tumor stage/tumor size	
T1	7(4.7)
T2	116(77.3)
T3/T4	27(18)
Ki67 Index (%)	46.89 ± 23.88
ki67 index groups	
≤ 15%	17(11.3)
16–24%	8(5.3)
25–44%	45(30)
> 44%	80(53.3)
Nodal Status	
Positive	64(42.7)
Negative	86(57.3)
Nodal Stage	
No	88(58.7)
N1	30(20)
N2	13(8.7)
N3	19(12.7)
Histological Subtypes	
IDC	127(84.7)
Papillary	6(4)
Medullary	1(0.7)
Metaplastic	14(9.3)
Mixed	2(1.3)
Tumor Grade	
Grade-I	1(0.7)
Grade-II	19(12.7)
Grade-III	130(86.7)
Lymphocytic infiltration	
Absent	15(10)
Moderate	110(73.3)
Severe	25(16.7)
Lymhovascular Invasion	
Present	36(24)
Absent	114(76)
Dermal Lymphatic invasion	
Present	10(6.7)
Absent	140(93.3)

Table 1 Clinicopathologic characteristics of triple negative breast cancer *(Continued)*

	n (%)
Type of Surgery	
Modified radical mastectomy	94(62.7)
Simple mastectomy with sentinel lymph node dissection	42(28)
Wide local excision	14(9.3)
Necrosis	
Absent	21(14)
Moderate	90(60)
Severe	39(26)
Fibrosis	
Mild	42(28)
Moderate	88(58.7)
Severe	20(13.3)
Insitu component	
Present	58(38.7)
Absent	92(61.3)
Pagetoid Spread	
Present	2(1.3)
Absent	148(98.7)
Perinodal extension	
Present	30(20)
Absent	120(80)
Triple negative phenotype	
Basal	16(10.7)
Non-basal	134(89.3)
Adjuvant chemotherapy (*n* = 101)	
Yes	98(97)
No	3(3)
Adjuvant radiation(*n* = 101)	
Yes	69(68.3)
No	32(31.7)
Recurrence(*n* = 101)	
Yes	18(17.8)
No	83(82.2)

Mean ± SD

not statistically significant, but higher p53 expression was also noted in medullary and metaplastic cancers (*p*-value 0.06). On the other hand, intensity of p53 expression was positively correlated with tumor grade and ki67 index; however, correlation with other parameters was not significant (Table 3).

Seventy-one percent (98 cases) of TNBC showed positive p16 expression, whereas 24.8% (34 cases) were negative and 3.6% (5 cases) showed focal positive p16 expression. 24.8% (34 cases) revealed no p16 expression while 10.9% (15 cases), 28.5% (39 cases) and 35.8% (49 cases) showed weak, intermediate and strong p16 expression respectively. 28.5% (39 cases) revealed no expression or weak expression in < 10% cancer cells, 15.3% (21 cases) showed 11–50% expression, 13.1% (18 cases) showed 51–70% expression while 43.1% (59 cases) revealed > 70% p16 expression. However, no significant association was found between p16 expression and various clinical and pathologic parameters (Table 3). Similarly, no significant

Table 2 Association of percentage of p53 overexpression with various clinical & pathological parameters

	n (%)					p-Value
	≤10% (n = 60)	11–50% (n = 18)	51–70% (n = 18)	> 70% (n = 54)	Total (n = 150)	
Age groups						
≤ 30 years	2(3.3)	0(0)	0(0)	3(5.6)	5(3.3)	0.217
31–50 years	34(56.7)	7(38.9)	8(44.4)	35(64.8)	84(56)	
> 50 years	24(40)	11(61.1)	10(55.6)	16(29.6)	61(40.7)	
Tumor stage/tumor size						
T1(≤2 cm)	3(5)	6(33.3)	3(16.7)	14(25.9)	26(17.3)	0.020
T2(2.1–5.0 cm)	36(60)	6(33.3)	10(55.6)	27(50)	79(52.7)	
T3(> 5.0 cm)	21(35)	6(33.3)	5(27.8)	13(24.1)	45(30)	
ki67 index groups						
≤ 15%	6(10)	6(33.3)	4(22.2)	1(1.9)	17(11.3)	0.000
16–24%	2(3.3)	2(11.1)	3(16.7)	1(1.9)	8(5.3)	
25–44%	19(31.7)	6(33.3)	7(38.9)	13(24.1)	45(30)	
> 44%	33(55)	4(22.2)	4(22.2)	39(72.2)	80(53.3)	
Nodal Status						
Positive	30(50)	5(27.8)	10(55.6)	19(35.2)	64(42.7)	0.144
Negative	30(50)	13(72.2)	8(44.4)	35(64.8)	86(57.3)	
Nodal Stage						
No	32(53.3)	13(72.2)	8(44.4)	35(64.8)	88(58.7)	0.022
N1	15(25)	3(16.7)	2(11.1)	10(18.5)	30(20)	
N2	3(5)	1(5.6)	7(38.9)	2(3.7)	13(8.7)	
N3	10(16.7)	1(5.6)	1(5.6)	7(13)	19(12.7)	
Histological Subtypes						
IDC	51(85)	14(77.8)	12(66.7)	50(92.6)	127(84.7)	0.063
Papillary	1(1.7)	2(11.1)	2(11.1)	1(1.9)	6(4)	
Medullary	0(0)	0(0)	1(5.6)	0(0)	1(0.7)	
metaplastic	7(11.7)	2(11.1)	3(16.7)	2(3.7)	14(9.3)	
Mixed	1(1.7)	0(0)	0(0)	1(1.9)	2(1.3)	
Tumor Grade						
Grade-I	1(1.7)	0(0)	0(0)	0(0)	1(0.7)	0.118
Grade-II	6(10)	6(33.3)	1(5.6)	6(11.1)	19(12.7)	
Grade-III	53(88.3)	12(66.7)	17(94.4)	48(88.9)	130(86.7)	
Lymhovascular Invasion						
Present	13(21.7)	6(33.3)	7(38.9)	10(18.5)	36(24)	0.250
Absent	47(78.3)	12(66.7)	11(61.1)	44(81.5)	114(76)	
Perinodal extension						
Present	12(20)	2(11.1)	6(33.3)	10(18.5)	30(20)	0.436
Absent	48(80)	16(88.9)	12(66.7)	44(81.5)	120(80)	
Triple Negative phenotype						
Basal	6(10)	2(11.1)	2(11.1)	6(11.1)	16(10.7)	1.000
Non Basal	54(90)	16(88.9)	16(88.9)	48(88.9)	134(89.3)	

Chi-Square test applied
P-value≤0.05 considered as significant

Table 3 Association of intensity of p53 overexpression with various clinical & pathological parameters

	n (%)					P-Value
	Weak (n = 21)	Intermediate (n = 26)	Strong (n = 57)	Negative (n = 46)	Total (n = 150)	
Age groups						
≤ 30 years	0 (0)	0 (0)	3 (5.3)	2 (4.3)	5 (3.3)	0.347
31–50 years	8 (38.1)	14 (53.8)	34(59.6)	28 (60.9)	84 (56)	
> 50 years	13 (61.9)	12 (46.2)	20 (35.1)	16 (34.8)	61 (40.7)	
Tumor stage/tumor size						
T1 (≤2 cm)	6 (28.6)	5 (19.2)	14 (24.6)	1 (2.2)	26 (17.3)	0.023
T2 (2.1–5.0 cm)	9 (42.9)	12 (46.2)	29 (50.9)	29 (63)	79 (52.7)	
T3 (> 5.0 cm)	6 (28.6)	9 (34.6)	14 (24.6)	16 (34.8)	45 (30)	
ki67 index groups						
≤ 15%	5 (23.8)	8 (30.8)	1 (1.8)	3 (6.5)	17 (11.3)	0.006
16–24%	1 (4.8)	2 (7.7)	3 (5.3)	2 (4.3)	8 (5.3)	
25–44%	7 (33.3)	7 (26.9)	16 (28.1)	15 (32.6)	45 (30)	
> 44%	8 (38.1)	9 (34.6)	37 (64.9)	26 (56.5)	80 (53.3)	
Nodal Status						
Positive	9 (42.9)	13 (50)	21 (36.8)	21 (45.7)	64 (42.7)	0.675
Negative	12 (57.1)	13 (50)	36 (63.2)	25 (54.3)	86 (57.3)	
Nodal Stage						
No	12 (57.1)	13 (50)	36 (63.2)	27 (58.7)	88 (58.7)	0.357
N1	5 (23.8)	7 (26.9)	8 (14)	10 (21.7)	30 (20)	
N2	0 (0)	5 (19.2)	5 (8.8)	3 (6.5)	13 (8.7)	
N3	4 (19)	1 (3.8)	8 (14)	6 (13)	19 (12.7)	
Histological Subtypes						
IDC	17 (81)	21 (80.8)	50 (87.7)	39 (84.8)	127 (84.7)	0.620
Papillary	1 (4.8)	1 (3.8)	3 (5.3)	1 (2.2)	6 (4)	
Medullary	0 (0)	1 (3.8)	0 (0)	0 (0)	1 (0.7)	
metaplastic	2 (9.5)	3 (11.5)	3 (5.3)	6 (13)	14 (9.3)	
Mixed	1 (4.8)	0 (0)	1 (1.8)	0 (0)	2 (1.3)	
Tumor Grade						
Grade-I	1 (4.8)	0 (0)	0 (0)	0 (0)	1 (0.7)	0.041
Grade-II	6 (28.6)	4 (15.4)	6 (10.5)	3 (6.5)	19 (12.7)	
Grade-III	14 (66.7)	22 (84.6)	51 (89.6)	43 (93.5)	130 (86.7)	
Lymhovascular Invasion						
Present	7 (33.3)	6 (23.1)	15 (26.3)	8 (17.4)	36 (24)	0.516
Absent	14 (66.7)	20 (76.9)	42 (73.7)	38 (82.6)	114 (76)	
Perinodal extension						
Present	5 (23.8)	3 (11.5)	15 (26.3)	7 (15.2)	30 (20)	0.352
Absent	16 (76.2)	23 (88.5)	42 (73.7)	39 (84.8)	120 (80)	
Triple Negative phenotype						
Basal	3 (14.3)	3 (11.5)	5 (8.8)	5 (10.9)	16 (10.7)	0.913
Non Basal	18 (85.7)	23 (88.5)	52 (91.2)	41 (89.1)	89.3)	

Chi-Square test applied
P-value≤0.05 considered as significant

association of either p16 or p53 over-expression was noted with recurrence status of patients (Fig. 2).

Discussion

In the present study, high expression of p16 was noted in TNBC cases while a moderately high expression of p53 was also notable. Moreover, p53 over-expression significantly correlated with key prognostic factors of breast cancer like T-stage, N-stage, tumor grade and ki67 index.

Breast cancers are quite frequent in Southeast Asia and typically associated with adverse prognostic features [17–20]. Multiple studies investigated the prognostic significance of p53 mutations in breast cancer. Somatic mutations of p53 (TP53) are found in 20–30% of breast cancer [21], while germ-line mutations are relatively rare. Although, the predictive value of TP53 abnormalities is still unclear, somatic TP53 mutations signify worse prognosis independent of tumor size and nodal status [22]. A study involving 1800 patients of breast cancer revealed twice higher risk of death in tumors having TP53 mutations [23]. A similar association of p53 IHC expression with bad prognosis in breast cancer is debatable as cutoff values have not been defined and ASCO panel still don't advice routine p53 IHC expression testing in breast cancer. However, as mutated p53 protein is not digested quickly inside tumor cells as compared to wild type protein, and therefore accumulates inside tumor cells. Hence, it is reasonable to consider high p53 expression as a surrogate marker of TP53 mutation. Moreover, as various biomarker testing have now been shifted to IHC, therefore with the help of results of various ongoing research, p53 IHC may get incorporated in future ASCO/CAP recommendations. Furthermore, gene expression analysis studies revealed that p53 and other

tumor suppressor DNA repair gene mutation and aberrant expression in TNBC may have important clinical implications as they may effect sensitivity to platinum & other chemotherapeutic agents that are directly DNA damaging [24, 25].

Unlike p53, prognostic significance of p16 in TNBC is more controversial; however, high expression of p16 has been noted in various studies [26]. A study involving 60 TNBC cases revealed high ki67 index in p16 positive tumors regardless of p53 expression. As high ki67 index is a well defined prognostic factor in breast cancer [27], therefore they suggested a potential prognostic value of p16 over-expression in TNBC [28]; however, we didn't find any such association. Basal type phenotype of TNBC is a worse subtype of breast cancer with high expression of CK5/6 (Table 4). Frequency of basal subtype of TNBC in different areas of world is different; we found a low proportion of basal subtype in our study (10%). A study involving 85% of TNBC revealed a high expression of p16 in basal subtype as compared to non-basal phenotype (80% vs. 50.8% respectively) [29]; however, no such association was noted in our study.

One of the limitations of our study was that molecular testing of p16 & p53 was not performed, therefore we suggest molecular testing of p16 & p53 in TNBC of our population to establish mutation status and its correlation with IHC over-expression of these biomarkers. Moreover, we didn't find any significant correlation of recurrence status of TNBC with p53 &p16 over-expression; however it can't be concluded that there is no correlation of p53 expression with recurrence status, as other important factors determining recurrence like margin status of tumors was not taken into account.

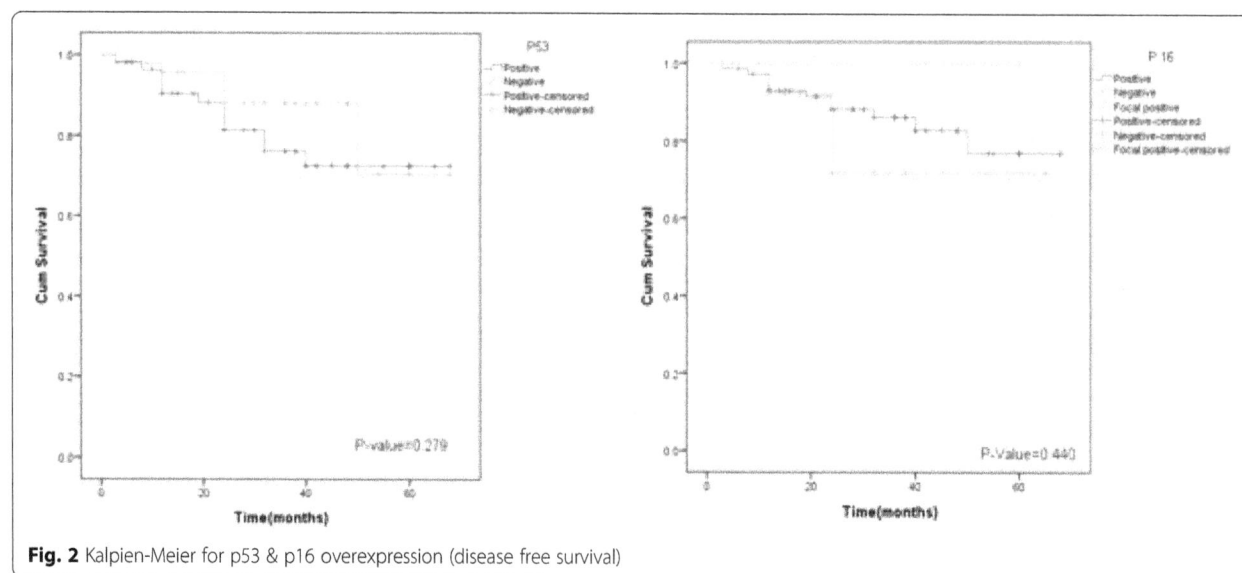

Fig. 2 Kalpien-Meier for p53 & p16 overexpression (disease free survival)

Table 4 Association of p16 overexpression with various clinical & pathological parameters

	n (%)				P-Value
	Positive (n = 98)	Negative (n = 34)	Focal Positive (n = 5)	Total (n = 137)	
Age groups					
≤ 30 years	3(3.1)	0(0)	0(0)	3(2.2)	0.460
31–50 years	59(60.2)	16(47.1)	3(60)	78(56.9)	
> 50 years	36(36.7)	18(52.9)	2(40)	56(40.9)	
Tumor stage/tumor size					
T1(≤2 cm)	16(16.3)	7(20.6)	1(20)	24(17.5)	0.964
T2(2.1–5.0 cm)	51(52)	17(50)	3(60)	71(51.8)	
T3(> 5.0 cm)	31(31.6)	10(29.4)	1(20)	42(30.7)	
ki67 index groups					
≤ 15%	10(10.2)	5(14.7)	2(40)	17(12.4)	0.345
16–24%	5(5.1)	3(8.8)	0(0)	8(5.8)	
25–44%	29(29.6)	11(32.4)	2(40)	42(30.7)	
> 44%	54(55.1)	15(44.1)	1(20)	70(51.1)	
Nodal Status					
Positive	42(42.9)	15(44.1)	2(40)	59(43.1)	1.000
Negative	56(57.1)	19(55.9)	3(60)	78(56.9)	
Nodal Stage					
No	58(59.2)	19(55.9)	3(60)	80(58.4)	0.907
N1	17(17.3)	8(23.5)	2(40)	27(19.7)	
N2	9(9.2)	3(8.8)	0(0)	12(8.8)	
N3	14(14.3)	4(11.8)	0(0)	18(13.1)	
Histological Subtypes					
IDC	83(84.7)	28(82.4)	5(100)	116(84.7)	0.633
Papillary	5(5.1)	0(0)	0(0)	5(3.6)	
Medullary	1(1)	0(0)	0(0)	1(0.7)	
metaplastic	8(8.2)	5(14.7)	0(0)	13(9.5)	
Mixed	1(1)	1(2.9)	0(0)	2(1.5)	
Tumor Grade					
Grade-I	0(0)	1(2.9)	0(0)	1(0.7)	0.165
Grade-II	11(11.2)	7(20.6)	0(0)	18(13.1)	
Grade-III	87(88.8)	26(76.5)	5(100)	118(86.1)	
Lymhovascular Invasion					
Present	25(25.5)	6(17.6)	1(20)	32(23.4)	0.788
Absent	73(74.5)	28(82.4)	4(80)	105(76.6)	
Perinodal extension					
Present	19(19.4)	9(26.5)	0(0)	28(20.4)	0.425
Absent	79(80.6)	25(73.5)	5(100)	109(79.6)	
Triple Negative phenotype					
Basal	10(10.2)	3(8.8)	1(20)	14(10.2)	0.532
Non Basal	88(89.8)	31(91.2)	4(80)	123(89.8)	

Chi-Square test applied
P-Value≤0.05, considerd as significant

Conclusion

On the basis of significant association of p53 IHC over-expression with worse prognostic factors in TNBC, therefore we suggest that more large scale studies are needed to validate this finding in loco-regional population. Moreover, high expression of p16 in TNBC suggests a potential role of this biomarker in TNBC pathogenesis which should be investigated with molecular based research in our population.

Acknowledgments
We gratefully acknowledge all staff members of Pathology, Liaquat National Hospital, Karachi, Pakistan for their help and cooperation.

Authors' contributions
AAH and SN: main author of manuscript, have made substantial contributions to conception and design of study. SKH, ZFH and MI: have been involved in requisition of data. EYK, NF, AK and MME have been involved in analysis of the data and revision of the manuscript. All authors read, revise and gave approval of the manuscript.

Competing interests
The authors declare that they have no competing interests.

Author details
[1]Liaquat National Hospital and Medical College, Karachi, Pakistan. [2]CMH Institute of Medical Sciences, Multan, Pakistan. [3]Kandahar University, North, Kandahar 3802, Afghanistan. [4]Brown University, Providence, RI, USA.

References
1. Swain S. Triple-negative breast Cancer: metastatic risk and role of platinum agents 2008 ASCO clinical science symposium, 2008. June 3, 2008.
2. Hashmi AA, Edhi MM, Naqvi H, Khurshid A, Faridi N. Molecular subtypes of breast cancer in South Asian population by immunohistochemical profile and Her2neu gene amplification by FISH technique: association with other clinicopathologic parameters. Breast J. 2014;20(6):578–85.
3. Hammond ME, Hayes DF, Dowsett M, et al. American Society of Clinical Oncology/College of American Pathologists guideline recommendations for immunohistochemical testing of estrogen and progesterone receptors in breast cancer (unabridged version). Arch Pathol Lab Med. 2010;134:e48.
4. Hammond ME, Hayes DF, Dowsett M, et al. American Society of Clinical Oncology/college of American pathologists guideline recommendations for immunohistochemical testing of estrogen and progesterone receptors in breast cancer. J Clin Oncol. 2010;28:2784.
5. Wolff AC, Hammond ME, Hicks DG, et al. Recommendations for human epidermal growth factor receptor 2 testing in breast cancer: American Society of Clinical Oncology/College of American Pathologists clinical practice guideline update. J Clin Oncol. 2013;31:3997.
6. Hashmi AA, Edhi MM, Naqvi H, Faridi N, Khurshid A, Khan M. Clinicopathologic features of triple negative breast cancers: an experience from Pakistan. Diagn Pathol. 2014;9:43.
7. Hashmi AA, Naz S, Hashmi SK, Hussain ZF, Irfan M, Bakar SMA, Faridi N, Khan A, Edhi MM. Cytokeratin 5/6 and cytokeratin 8/18 expression in triple negative breast cancers: clinicopathologic significance in South-Asian population. BMC Res Notes. 2018;11(1):372.
8. Lehmann BD, Bauer JA, Chen X, et al. Identification of human triple-negative breast cancer subtypes and preclinical models for selection of targeted therapies. J Clin Invest. 2011;121:2750.
9. Prat A, Parker JS, Karginova O, et al. Phenotypic and molecular characterization of the claudin-low intrinsic subtype of breast cancer. Breast Cancer Res. 2010;12:R68.
10. Livasy CA, Karaca G, Nanda R, et al. Phenotypic evaluation of the basal-like subtype of invasive breast carcinoma. Mod Pathol. 2006;19:264.
11. Nielsen TO, Hsu FD, Jensen K, et al. Immunohistochemical and clinical characterization of the basal-like subtype of invasive breast carcinoma. Clin Cancer Res. 2004;10:5367.
12. Montanari M, Boninsegna A, Faraglia B, Coco C, Giordano A, et al. Increased expression of geminin stimulates the growth of mammary epithelial cells and is a frequent event in human tumors. J Cell Physiol. 2005;202:215–22.
13. Zhang J, Pickering CR, Holst CR, Gauthier ML, Tlsty TD. p16INK4a modulates p53 in primary human mammary epithelial cells. Cancer Res. 2006;66:10325–31.
14. Hashmi AA, Hussain ZF, Hashmi SK, Irfan M, Khan EY, Faridi N, Khan A, Edhi MM. Immunohistochemical over expression of p53 in head and neck Squamous cell carcinoma: clinical and prognostic significance. BMC Res Notes. 2018;11(1):433.
15. Bartley AN, Ross DW. Validation of p53 immunohistochemistry as a prognostic factor in breast cancer in clinical practice. Arch Pathol Lab Med. 2002;126:456–8.
16. Hui R, Macmillan RD, Kenny FS, Musgrove EA, Blamey RW, et al. INK4a gene expression and methylation in primary breast cancer: overexpression of p16INK4a messenger RNA is a marker of poor prognosis. Clin Cancer Res. 2000;6:2777–87.
17. Hashmi AA, Mahboob R, Khan SM, Irfan M, Nisar M, Iftikhar N, Siddiqui M, Faridi N, Khan A, Edhi MM. Clinical and prognostic profile of Her2neu positive (non-luminal) intrinsic breast cancer subtype: comparison with Her2neu positive luminal breast cancers. BMC Res Notes. 2018;11(1):574.
18. Hashmi AA, Aijaz S, Mahboob R, Khan SM, Irfan M, Iftikhar N, Nisar M, Siddiqui M, Edhi MM, Faridi N, Khan A. Clinicopathologic features of invasive metaplastic and micropapillary breast carcinoma: comparison with invasive ductal carcinoma of breast. BMC Res Notes. 2018;11(1):531.
19. Hashmi AA, Aijaz S, Khan SM, Mahboob R, Irfan M, Zafar NI, Nisar M, Siddiqui M, Edhi MM, Faridi N, Khan A. Prognostic parameters of luminal A and luminal B intrinsic breast cancer subtypes of Pakistani patients. World J Surg Oncol. 2018;16(1):1.
20. Hashmi AA, Faridi N, Khurshid A, Naqvi H, Malik B, Malik FR, Fida Z, Mujtuba S. Accuracy of frozen section analysis of sentinel lymph nodes for the detection of Asian breast cancer micrometastasis - experience from Pakistan. Asian Pac J Cancer Prev. 2013;14(4):2657–62.
21. Petitjean A, Achatz MI, Borresen-Dale AL, et al. TP53 mutations in human cancers: functional selection and impact on cancer prognosis and outcomes. Oncogene. 2007;26:2157.
22. Bonnefoi H, Piccart M, Bogaerts J, et al. TP53 status for prediction of sensitivity to taxane versus non-taxane neoadjuvant chemotherapy in breast cancer (EORTC 10994/BIG 1-00): a randomised phase 3 trial. Lancet Oncol. 2011;12:527.
23. Olivier M, Langerød A, Carrieri P, et al. The clinical value of somatic TP53 gene mutations in 1,794 patients with breast cancer. Clin Cancer Res. 2006;12:1157.
24. Sørlie T, Perou CM, Tibshirani R, et al. Gene expression patterns of breast carcinomas distinguish tumor subclasses with clinical implications. Proc Natl Acad Sci U S A. 2001;98:10869.
25. Troester MA, Herschkowitz JI, Oh DS, et al. Gene expression patterns associated with p53 status in breast cancer. BMC Cancer. 2006;6:276.
26. Shan M, Zhang X, Liu X, Qin Y, Liu T, Liu Y, Wang J, Zhong Z, Zhang Y, Geng J, Pang D. P16 and p53 play distinct roles in different subtypes of breast cancer. PLoS One. 2013;8(10):e76408.
27. Haroon S, Hashmi AA, Khurshid A, Kanpurwala MA, Mujtuba S, Malik B, Faridi N. Ki67 index in breast cancer: correlation with other prognostic markers and potential in pakistani patients. Asian Pac J Cancer Prev. 2013;14(7):4353–8.
28. Sugianto J, Sarode V, Peng Y. Ki-67 expression is increased in p16-expressing triple-negative breast carcinoma and correlates with p16 only in p53-negative tumors. Hum Pathol. 2014;45(4):802–9.
29. Abou-Bakr AA, Eldweny HI. p16 expression correlates with basal-like triple-negative breast carcinoma. Ecancermedicalscience. 2013;7:317.

26

High expression of EphA3 (erythropoietin-producing hepatocellular A3) in gastric cancer is associated with metastasis and poor survival

Baongoc Nasri[1]* (iD), Mikito Inokuchi[2], Toshiaki Ishikawa[2], Hiroyuki Uetake[2], Yoko Takagi[3], Sho Otsuki[2], Kazuyuki Kojima[2] and Tatsuyuki Kawano[2]

Abstract

Background: As the major subfamily of receptor tyrosine, erythropoietin-producing hepatocellular (Eph) receptor has been related to progression and prognosis in different types of tumors. However, the role and mechanism of EPHA3 in gastric cancer is still not well understood.

Methods: Specimen were collected from 202 patients who underwent gastric resection for gastric adenocarcinoma. The expression of EphA3 was studied using immunohistochemistry. We analyzed the clinicopathological factors and prognostic relevance of EphA3 expression in gastric cancer.

Results: High expression of EphA3 was associated with male predominance ($p = 0.031$), differentiated histology ($p < 0.001$), depth of tumor ($p = 0.002$), lymph node metastasis ($p = 0.001$), distant metastasis ($p = 0.021$), liver metastasis ($p = 0.024$), advanced stage ($p < 0.001$), and high HER2 expression ($p = 0.017$). Relapse-free survival (RFS) was significantly worse in patients with high expression of EphA3 than in those with low expression of EphA3 ($p = 0.014$). Multivariate analysis for RFS showed that depth of tumor [hazard ratio (HR) 9.333, 95% confidence interval (CI) 2.183–39.911, $p = 0.003$] and lymph node metastasis [hazard ratio (HR) 5.734, 95% confidence interval (CI) 2.349–13.997, $p < 0.001$] were independent prognostic factors.

Conclusions: These findings suggest that high expression EphA3 may participate in metastasis and worse survival.

Keywords: Gastric cancer, Metastasis, Oncogenes

Background

Although a constant decrease in gastric cancer incidence and mortality rates has been reported, stomach cancer ranks as the fifth most common malignancy and the third leading cause of death worldwide [1]. Despite current advanced therapeutic options including surgical resection, chemotherapy, hormonal therapy, radiotherapy, the estimated 5-year survival rate is still poor, varying from 64% for early stage to 4% for advanced distant metastatic stage [2]. Although many receptor tyrosine kinases (RTKs) are related to invasion and metastasis of gastric cancer, only a human epidermal growth factor receptor (HER-2) blocker

has been accepted as molecular targeted therapy. Unfortunately, merely 10–20% of all patients with stomach cancer are HER-2 positive and the median survival time was only 16 months in HER-2 positive patients who underwent chemotherapy with trastuzumab [3, 4]. Hence, new diagnostic tools, novel therapeutic methods and new prognostic molecular markers for gastric cancer are urgently demanded.

Erythropoietin-producing hepatocellular carcinoma receptor (Eph) and their cell-associated ephrin ligands are associated with neoangiogenesis and invasive tumor progression, and are progressively being focused as new therapeutic targets in clinical trials [5]. Ephs and ephrins are abundantly found in multiple types of tumors, where their oncogenic roles often reflect their dichotomous

* Correspondence: pbngoc2001@yahoo.com
[1]Matsuzawa Hospital, Setagaya-ku, Tokyo, Japan
Full list of author information is available at the end of the article

developmental activities. Therefore, depending on tumor types and disease stages, high expression Ephs can stimulate or suppress tumor progression [6–8]. Recent papers have proven the prospective target therapy of EphA1 and EphA4 for gastric cancer. EphA3, a subclass of Ephs, is reported to relate to certain types of solid cancers [9, 10]. However the role and mechanism of EphA3 in gastric cancer is not well understood. We aim to elucidate the clinicopathological factors and prognostic importance of EphA3 role in gastric cancer.

Methods

Patients

Between January 2003 and March 2007, after excluding total 16 patients with distant metastasis at time of surgery or positive peritoneal lavage cytology for which were regarded as stage IV, there were total 202 patients undergoing gastrectomy for primary gastric tumor in the Department of Gastric Surgery of Tokyo Medical and Dental University. All participants received detailed explanation of the research, and well written informed consent was obtained. This study was designed in accordance with the Declaration of Helsinki and was authorized by the Institutional Review Board of Tokyo Medical and Dental University. All tumors were classified according to the 7th edition of tumor node metastasis classification. HER2

expression was also investigated. All patients were followed up every 3–6 months with multimodalities including computed tomography, abdominal ultrasonography, endoscopy, and tumor marker analysis. Positron emission tomography and bone scintigraphy, magnetic resonance imagings were considered as needed. Patients with recurrent disease received chemotherapy with TS-1 (Titanium silicate) as single regimen or combined chemotherapy. All patients were followed up for 5 years until July 2011. The mean follow up period was 61.4 ± 25.7 months. There were 60 deaths reported with 50 (83.3%) deaths from recurrence and 10 (16.7%) deaths due to other causes.

Immunohistocheminal Analysis of EphA3

All of the hematoxylin and eosin–stained samples were reviewed. Immunohistochemical staining was performed on 3- to 4-μM sections from formalin-fixed, paraffin-embedded tissue. After deparaffinization in xylene, the slides were rehydrated and treated with double-distilled water (DDW). Antigen retrieval by microwave pretreatment was performed for 15 min in 6 mmol/L sodium citrate buffer (pH 6.0) (Mitsubishi Chemical Medience Corporation, Tokyo, Japan) at 98 °C. Endogenous peroxidase was quenched by 15 minutes incubation in a mixture of 3% hydrogen peroxidase solution in 100% methanol. After treating with DDW and phosphate buffered saline

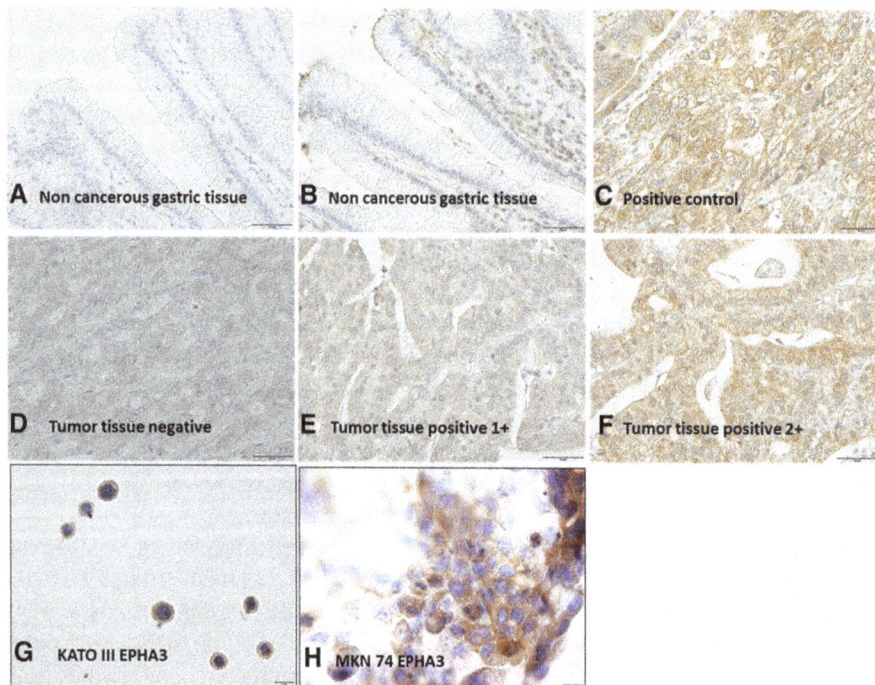

Fig. 1 Expression of EphA3 protein in gastric cancer. **a** Non-cancerous gastric tissue which was stained without 1st antibody, did not show immunostaining for EphA3. **b** Non-cancerous gastric tissue showed staining in the mesenchyme not in the mucosal layer. **c** Normal positive control showed strong immunostaining. Representative primary gastric carcinomas with intensity score of 0 (**d**), 1 (**e**), 2 (**f**). The images were captured under magnification 400x. Scale bar in the left lower corner is 50μm. **g** KATO III EphA3 (undifferentiated type) showed weak staining. **h** MKN 74 EphA3 (differentiated type) showed strong staining

(PBS), specimen was incubated with the primary antibody to EphA3 (dilution 1:500) (EphA3 (L-18): sc-920 SANTA CRUZ Biotechnology, USA) for 15 min at room temperature and then 16 h at 4 °C. Specimen was treated three times with 0.1% Tween 20/PBS and then was incubated with peroxidase-labelled anti-rabbit or anti-mouse antibodies (Histofine Simplestain Max PO; Nichirei) for 30 min at room temperature. Peroxidase activity was

Table 1 Correlation between EphA3 expression and clinicopathological features in gastric carcinoma

Variables	EphA3			
	n $n = 202$	Low $n = 111$ (n, %)	High $n = 91$ (n, %)	p value
Age				
< 65	97	60 (61.9)	37 (38.1)	0.067
≥ 65	105	51 (48.6)	54 (51.4)	
Gender				
Female	48	33 (68.8)	15 (31.3)	0.031
Male	154	78 (50.6)	76 (49.4)	
Main location				
Middle or Lower	160	93 (58.1)	67 (41.9)	0.084
Upper	42	18 (42.9)	24 (57.1)	
WHO pathological type				
Differentiated	99	39 (39.4)	60 (60.6)	<0.001
Undifferentiated	103	72 (69.9)	31 (30.1)	
Depth of invasion				
T1	87	59 (67.8)	28 (32.2)	0.002
T2/3/4	115	52 (45.2)	63 (54.8)	
Lymph node metastasis				
Negative	113	74 (65.5)	39 (34.5)	0.001
Positive	89	37 (41.6)	52 (58.4)	
Stage				
I	106	72 (67.9)	34 (32.1)	<0.001
II/III	96	39 (40.4)	57 (59.4)	
Distant recurrence				
Negative	152	91 (59.9)	61 (40.1)	0.021
Positive	50	20 (40)	30 (60)	
Liver recurrence				
Negative	194	110 (56.7)	84 (43.3)	0.024
Positive	8	1 (12.5)	7 (87.5)	
Peritoneal recurrence				
Negative	182	99 (54.4)	83 (45.6)	0.814
Positive	20	12 (60)	8 (40)	
HER2				
Negative	186	107 (57.5)	79 (42.5)	0.017
Positive	16	4 (25)	12 (75)	

$P < 0.05$, statistically significant

detected with diaminobenzidine (Nichirei). Sections were then counterstained with hematoxylin.

Interpretation of the immunostaining results

Staining intensity was classified into three grades: 0 (none), 1 (weakly positive), 2 (moderately or strongly positive). Staining extensity (positive frequency) was also classified into three grades according to the percentage of stained tumor cells: 0 (0–9%), 1 (10–49%), and 2 (50–100%). Samples with moderate positivity but staining extensity was less than 10% were graded as staining intensity of 1 (weakly positive). Composites score was the sum of the strongest intensity score and the total extensity score. For statistical analysis, composite scores ≥ 3 were classified as high expression and scores < 3 were classified as low expression. Two investigators (M.K and T.Y), who were blinded to patients' outcomes independently evaluated stained tumor cells in at least three field per section, including the deepest site invaded by tumor cells, the most superficial site of the lesion and the intermediate zone. Any differences between the two investigators were resolved by reassessment and consensus.

Statistical analysis

Chi-square test was utilized to analyze the hypothetical association between the expression of EphA3 and patient

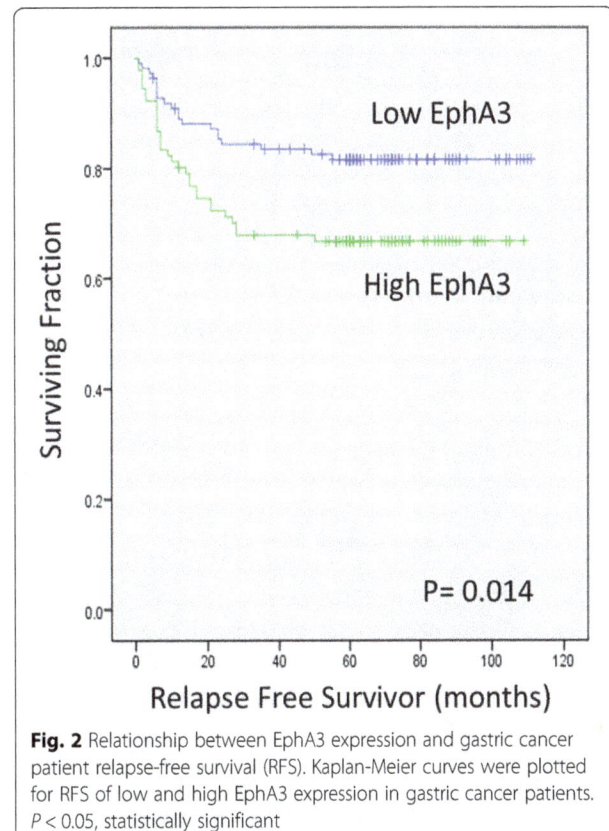

Fig. 2 Relationship between EphA3 expression and gastric cancer patient relapse-free survival (RFS). Kaplan-Meier curves were plotted for RFS of low and high EphA3 expression in gastric cancer patients. $P < 0.05$, statistically significant

clinicopathological factors. Overall survival (OS), and relapse-free survival (RFS) were used to evaluate the prognosis. Kaplan-Meier curves were plotted to assess the effect of EphA3 expression on overall survival (OS) and relapse-free survival (RFS). Differences between the curves were analyzed by the log-rank test. Multivariate Cox proportional-harzards regression models were utilized to analyze the prognostic significance of expression of EphA3 and other clinicopathological factors. Statistical analysis was performed using IBM SPSS Statistics 23 software (IBM, Inc., Armonk, NY, and U.S.A). A p value <0.05 was considered statistically significant.

Results
EPHA3 immunohistochemistry
Representative cases of each staining intensity are shown in Fig. 1. EphA3 expression was mainly located in the

Table 2 Univariate (log-rank) and multivariate (Cox proportional-harzards) analyses of the association between relapse free survival and clinicopathological factors including EphA3 expression

Variables	Univariate (log-rank)		Multivariate		
	5-years RFS (%)	p	HR	95% CI	p
Age					
< 65	75.5	0.809			
≥ 65	74.5				
Gender					
Female	77.1	0.655			
Male	74.4				
Main location					
Middle or Lower	80.1	0.001	1		
Upper	55.8		1.684	0.937–3.029	0.082
WHO pathological type					
Differentiated	84	0.03	1		
Undifferentiated	66.3		1.616	0.841–3.103	0.149
Depth of invasion					
T1	97.7	<0.001	1		
T2,3,4	58.1		9.333	2.183–39.911	0.003
Lymph node metastasis					
Negative	94.7	<0.001	1		
Positive	50.5		5.734	2.349–13.997	<0.001
EPHA3					
Low	82.0	0.014	1		
High	67.0		1.313	0.705–2.447	0.391
HER2					
Negative	75.5	0.538			
Positive	68.8				

RFS relapse-free survival, HR harzard ratio, CI confidence interval; P < 0.05, statistically significant

cytoplasm and at the cell membrane. High expression (composite score ≥ 3) of EphA3 was found in 91 sample (45%) and low expression (composite score < 3) of EphA3 was found in 111 samples (55%). Non-cancerous gastric tissue which was stained without 1st antibody did not show immunostaining for EphA3. Some non-cancerous gastric tissue showed staining in the mesenchyme not in the mucosal layer. We have two cell lines KATO III (undifferentiated type) which showed weak EphA3 staining and MKN 74 (differentiated type) which showed strong EphA3 staining. However staining in these cell lines is not known to express EphA3.

Relationship between EPHA3 expression and clinicopathological factors
The association between EphA3 expression and clinicopathological factors is summarized in Table 1. High expression of EphA3 was associated with differentiated histology ($p < 0.001$), depth of tumor ($p = 0.002$), lymph node metastasis ($p = 0.001$), stage ($p < 0.001$), recurrence ($p = 0.024$), especially liver recurrence ($p = 0.024$) and HER2 expression ($p = 0.017$).

Correlation between EPHA3 expression and survival
Kaplan-Meier curves were plotted to assess the effect of EphA3 expression on relapse free survival (RFS) and overall survival (OS). Survival analysis by log-rank test

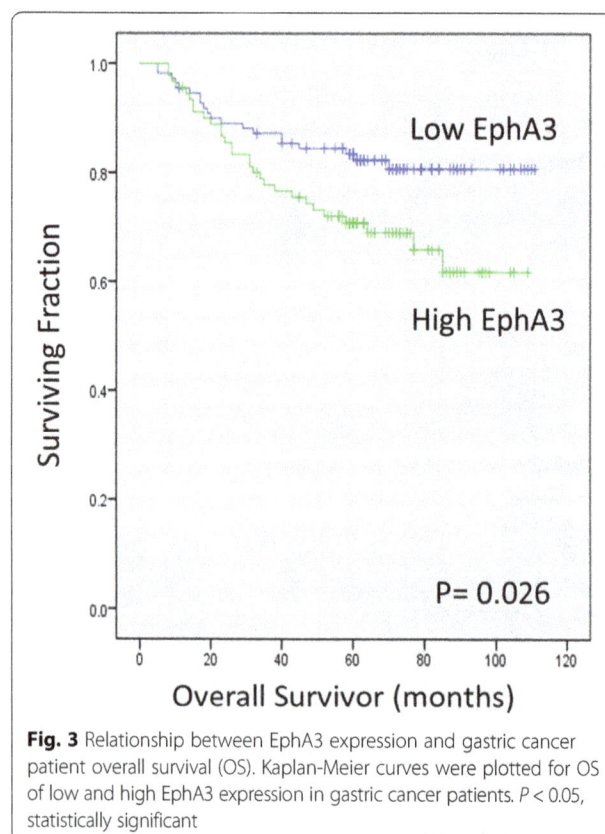

Fig. 3 Relationship between EphA3 expression and gastric cancer patient overall survival (OS). Kaplan-Meier curves were plotted for OS of low and high EphA3 expression in gastric cancer patients. P < 0.05, statistically significant

suggested that high EphA3 expression associated with a significantly shorter RFS (82% vs 67%) and OS (82% vs 68.1%) (Fig. 2; Table 2). Multivariate analysis for RFS showed that depth of tumor [hazard ratio (HR) 9.3, 95% confidence interval (CI) 2.183–39.911, $p = 0.003$] and lymph node metastasis [hazard ratio (HR) 5.7, 95% confidence interval (CI) 2.349–13.997, $p < 0.001$] were independent prognostic factors (Table 2). Similarly multivariate analysis for overall survival (OS) also showed that depth of tumor [hazard ratio (HR) 8.8, 95% confidence interval (CI) 2.038–37.881, $p = 0.004$] and lymph node metastasis [hazard ratio (HR) 5.9, 95% confidence interval (CI) 2.417–14.537, $p < 0.001$] were independent prognostic factors for OS (Fig. 3, Table 3).

Discussions

Our study suggests that high expression of EphA3 may play crucial roles in tumor development, metastasis, and survival in gastric cancer. To our best of knowledge, our study along with Xi et al is the only two articles regarding the clinical outcomes of the novel receptor EphA3 in gastric cancer [11].

EphA3 found abundantly in mesenchymal tissues of developing axial muscles, respiratory tract, kidney, and heart, is involved in mesoderm, neural patterning, and is crucial for endothelial-to-mesenchymal transition during heart development [12, 13]. There is very limited evidence for physiologic function, but EphA3 is overexpressed in solid and hematopoietic tumor cells [8, 11, 14]. The effect of EphA3 on human cancers is variable. High expression of EphA3 was related to lymph node metastasis and advanced stages in colorectal cancer [15] and was associated with higher Gleason score in prostate cancer [16]. In hepatocellular carcinoma, high EphA3 expression was related with tumor size, tumor grade, metastasis, venous invasion [9]. However, high expression of EphA3 was reported to suppress the growth of non-small cell lung cancer [10]. Eph receptor tyrosine kinases are crucial for intercellular communication during physiologic and oncogenic tissue patterning and tumor development [5, 17]. Differences in EphA3 are thought to generate certain morphological and

Table 3 Univariate (log-rank) and multivariate (Cox proportional-harzards) analyses of the association between overalls survival and clinicopathological factors including EphA3 expression

Variables	Univariate (log-rank)			Multivariate	
	5-years OS (%)	p	HR	95% CI	p
Age					
< 65	76.5	0.578			
≥ 65	74.5				
Gender					
Female	79.2	0.516			
Male	74.4				
Main location					
Middle or Lower	80.1	0.001	1		
Upper	58.1		1.654	0.907–3.017	0.101
WHO pathological type					
Differentiated	83	0.01	1		
Undifferentiated	68.3		1.475	0.766–2.842	0.246
Depth of invasion					
T1	97.7	<0.001	1		
T2,3,4	59		8.785	2.038–37.881	0.004
Lymph node metastasis					
Negative	94.7	<0.001	1		
Positive	51.6		5.928	2.417–14.537	<0.001
EPHA3					
Low	82.0	0.026	1		
High	68.1		1.147	0.603–2.181	0.677
HER2					
Negative	75.76.15	0.431			
Positive	68.8				

OS overall survival, *HR* harzard ratio, *CI* confidence interval; $P < 0.05$; statistically significant

biological characteristics, such as cell growth and viability, loss of cell adhesion to fibronectin, cell migration, and apoptosis. Abundant evidences show that aberrant regulation of EphA3 and its genetic variation are strongly related to the development and progression of many types of solid cancers [18–20]. Although the exact mechanism of how EphA3 regulates its downstream is not well understood, it is hypothesized that EphA subgroup stimulates tumor progression by activating Jak/Stat and Akt/PI3 K signals [21–24].

One of the limitations is that we do not have cell culture experiment results. Our study along with Xi et al [11] is the only two articles focusing on the newly discovered receptor EphA3. The recent study of Xi et al showed the higher expression of EphA3 in gastric adenocarcinoma than in normal tissue [11]. Although EphA3 failed to reach the statistical value for independent prognostic factor, our study showed that EphA3 overexpression was associated with depth of tumor, lymph node metastasis, stage, distant metastasis and recurrence of gastric cancer. These findings are in accord with Xi et al study. Other limitation is that our study mainly focused on immunohistochemical staining of EphA3. Further genetic evaluation or quantitative assessment is crucial to confirm the outcomes of this study, although mRNA expression level and Western blot of EphA3 was shown to be overexpressed in gastric cancer tissue than in normal tissue by Xi et al [11].

While Xi et al emphasized overexpression of EphA3 correlated with worse survival curve, our findings proved that high expression of EphA3 associated with poorer RFS of gastric cancer with higher rate of distant recurrence especially liver recurrence. Our study has suggested prospective investigation for the possibility of correlation between EphA3 and liver recurrence in gastric cancer.

Conclusions

This present study showed that EphA3 overexpression was associated with depth of tumor, lymph node metastasis, stage, distant recurrence, liver recurrence and poorer RFS of gastric cancer. These findings hypothesize that EphA3 can be a potential target of molecular targeted therapy of gastric cancer.

Abbreviations

CI: Confidence interval; DDW: Double-distilled water; EpHA3: Erythropoietin-producing hepatocellular A3; HER-2: Human epidermal growth factor receptor 2; HR: Hazard ratio; OS: Overall survival; PBS: Phosphate buffered saline; RFS: Relapse-free survival; RTKs: Receptor tyrosine kinases; TS-1: Titanium silicate

Acknowledgement

The authors deeply thank Ms. Junko Inoue for her exceptional technical assistance with the immunohistochemical staining of the present study.

Funding

There is no funding to be declared.

Authors' contributions

The paper was conceived by BN, MI and TI.The prediction model was created by HU, YT, SO, KK and TK provided insight into the validation cohort. All authors commented on initial drafts of the manuscript and approved the final version.

Competing interests

The authors declare that they have no competing interests.

Author details

[1]Matsuzawa Hospital, Setagaya-ku, Tokyo, Japan. [2]Department of Surgical Oncology, Graduate School, Tokyo Medical and Dental University, Bunkyo-ku, Tokyo, Japan. [3]Department of Translational Oncology, Graduate School, Tokyo Medical and Dental University, Bunkyo-ku, Tokyo, Japan.

References

1. Global Cancer Statistic. GLOBOCAN 2012: Estimated Cancer Incidence, Mortality and Prevalence Worldwide in 2012. http://globocan.iarc.fr/Default.aspx.
2. American Cancer Society's publication, Cancer Fact & Figures 2015.
3. Gravalos C, Jimeno A. HER-2 in gastric cancer: a new prognostic factor and a novel therapeutic target. Ann Oncol. 2008;19(9):1523–9.
4. Bang YJ, Van Cutsem E, Feyereislova A, et al. ToGA Trial Investigators. Trastuzumab in combination with chemotherapy versus chemotherapy alone for treatment of HER-2 positive advanced gastric or gastro-oesophageal junction cancer (ToGA): a phase 3, open-label, randomized controlled trial. Lancet. 2010;376:687–97.
5. Boyd AW, Bartlett PF, Lackmann M. Therapeutic targeting of EPH receptors and their ligands. Nat Rev Drug Discov. 2014;13:39–62.
6. Noren NK, Foos G, Hauser CA, Pasquale EB. The EphB4 receptor suppresses breast cancer cell tumorigenicity through an Abl-Crk pathway. Nat Cell Biol. 2006;8:815–25.
7. Genander M, Halford MM, Xu NJ, Eriksson M, Yu Z, Qiu Z, et al. Dissociation of EphB2 signaling pathways mediating progenitor cell proliferation and tumor suppression. Cell. 2009;139:679–92.
8. Day BW, Stringer BW, Al-Ejeh F, Ting MJ, Wilson J, Ensbey KS, et al. EphA3 maintains tumorigenicity and is a therapeutic target in glioblastoma multiforme. Cancer Cell. 2013;23:238–48.
9. Stephen LJ, Fawkes AL, Verhoeve A, Lemke G, Brown A. A critical role for the EphA3 receptor tyrosine kinase in heart development. Dev Biol. 2007;302:66–79.
10. Keane N, Freeman C, Swords R, Giles FJ. EPHA3 as a novel therapeutic target in the hematological malignancies. Expert Rev Hematol. 2012;5:325–40.
11. Nakagawa M, Inokuchi M, Takagi Y, Kato K, Sugita H, Otsuki S, Kojima K, Uetake H, Sugihara K. Erythropoietin-producing hepatocellular A1 is an Independent prognostic factor for gastric cancer. Ann Surg Oncol. 2015; 22(7):2329–35.
12. Miyazaki K, Inokuchi M, Takagi Y, Kato K, Kojima K, Sugihara K. EphA4 is a prognostic factor in gastric cancer. BMC Clin Pathol. 2013;13(1):19. Oates AC, Lackmann M, Power MA, Brennan C, Down LM, Do C, et al.
13. Lu CY, Yang ZX, Zhou L, Huang ZZ, et al. High levels of EphA3 expression are associated with high invasive capacity and poor overall survival in hepatocellular carcinoma. Oncol Rep. 2013;30(5):2179–86.
14. Zhuang G, Song W, Amato K, Hwang Y, et al. Effects of cancer-associated EPHA3 mutations on lung cancer. J Natl Cancer Inst. 2012;104(15):1182–97.
15. Xi H-Q, Wu X-S, Wei B, Lin C. Aberrant expression of EphA3 in gastric carcinoma: correlation with tumor angiogenesis and survival. J Gastroenterol. 2012;47(7):785–94.
16. Oates AC, Lackmann M, Power MA, Brennan C. An early developmental role for eph-ephrin interaction during vertebrate gastrulation. Mech Dev. 1999; 83:77–94.
17. Xi HQ, Zhao P. Clinicopathological significance and prognostic value of EphA3 and CD133 expression in colorectal carcinoma. J Clin Pathol. 2011;64(6):498–503.
18. Wu R, Wang H, Wang J, et al. EphA3, induced by PC-1/PrLZ, contributes to the malignant progression of prostate cancer. Oncol Rep. 2014;32(6):2657–65.
19. Pasquale EB. Eph receptors and ephrins in cancer: bidirectional signaling and beyond. Nat Rev Cancer. 2010;10:165–80.

27

Expression of podocalyxin-like protein is an independent prognostic biomarker in resected esophageal and gastric adenocarcinoma

David Borg*®, Charlotta Hedner, Björn Nodin, Anna Larsson, Anders Johnsson, Jakob Eberhard and Karin Jirström

Abstract

Background: Podocalyxin-like protein (PODXL) is a cell surface transmembrane glycoprotein, the expression of which has been associated with poor prognosis in a range of malignancies. The aim of this study was to investigate the impact of PODXL expression on survival in esophageal and gastric adenocarcinoma.

Methods: The study cohort consists of a consecutive series of 174 patients with esophageal (including the gastroesophageal junction) or gastric adenocarcinoma, surgically treated between 2006 and 2010 and not subjected to neoadjuvant treatment. Immunohistochemical expression of PODXL was assessed in tissue microarrays with cores from primary tumors, lymph node metastases, intestinal metaplasia and adjacent normal epithelium. Survival analyses were performed on patients with no distant metastases and no macroscopic residual tumor.

Results: In the majority of cases, expression of PODXL was significantly higher in cancer cells compared to normal epithelial cells and was significantly associated with lymph node metastases and high grade tumors. In esophageal adenocarcinoma, Kaplan-Meier analyses revealed that patients with PODXL negative tumors had a superior time to recurrence (TTR) and overall survival (OS) compared to patients with PODXL positive tumors. In gastric adenocarcinoma, patients with PODXL negative tumors had a superior TTR and a trend towards an improved OS. In esophageal and gastric adenocarcinoma combined, the prognostic significance of PODXL expression on TTR was confirmed in unadjusted Cox regression analysis (HR = 5.36, 95 % CI 1.68-17.06, $p = 0.005$) and remained significant in the adjusted model (HR = 3.39, 95 % CI 1.01-11.35, $p = 0.048$). Moreover, the impact of PODXL expression on OS was also confirmed in unadjusted analysis (HR = 2.52, 95 % CI 1.31-4.85, $p = 0.006$) and remained significant in the adjusted model (HR = 2.03, 95 % CI 1.04-3.98, $p = 0.039$).

Conclusions: In esophageal and gastric adenocarcinoma, PODXL expression is an independent prognostic biomarker for reduced time to recurrence and poor overall survival. This is the first report on the prognostic role of PODXL in esophageal adenocarcinoma and validates recent findings in gastric cancer.

Keywords: Esophageal neoplasms, Stomach neoplasms, Adenocarcinoma, Prognosis, *PODXL*

* Correspondence: david.borg@med.lu.se
Department of Clinical Sciences Lund, Division of Oncology and Pathology,
Lund University, Skåne University Hospital, SE-221 85 Lund, Sweden

Background

Esophageal and gastric cancers are among the most common types of cancer worldwide in terms of incidence and mortality [1]. Historically, the majority of esophageal cancers were squamous cell carcinomas, but in the last four decades there has been a drastic increase in the incidence of adenocarcinoma, especially in many Western countries, where it is now the most common subtype [2]. Adenocarcinoma in the esophagogastric (EG) junction is, since the 7th edition of the AJCC/UICC TNM staging system [3], classified as esophageal cancer. Proposed risk factors for esophageal and EG junction adenocarcinoma are gastroesophageal reflux disease, obesity and decreased prevalence of *Helicobacter pylori* infection [4, 5]. Regarding gastric adenocarcinoma, the incidence has been declining for several decades [6], possibly due to improved sanitary conditions and decreased prevalence of *Helicobacter pylori* infection [7], but globally it is still the 3rd leading cause of cancer death.

In resectable esophageal and gastric cancer, several phase III trials [8–13] have shown that the addition of neoadjuvant and/or adjuvant chemotherapy or chemoradiotherapy improves survival. However, the prognosis is still poor, especially in Western populations, with 5-year survival rates less than 40 %.

Hence, in addition to primary prevention and earlier detection, the key to improved outcome for patients with esophageal and gastric cancer is to find more effective treatments and also to personalize the treatment based on prognostic and response predictive factors.

Podocalyxin-like protein (PODXL) is a cell surface transmembrane glycoprotein, belonging to the CD34 family, that is encoded on chromosome 7q32-q33. It was first discovered in renal podocytes as an anti-adhesive protein [14] and has later been shown to be expressed in vascular endothelium [15] and to be involved in hematopoiesis [16] and neural development [17]. PODXL is expressed in a range of malignancies and overexpression has mostly been linked to poor prognosis, e.g. in glioblastoma multiforme [18], breast cancer [19], bladder cancer [20], periampullary and pancreatic adenocarcinoma [21, 22] and colorectal cancer [23–25]. Laitinen et al. [26] recently showed that in surgically treated gastric cancer, patients with PODXL negative tumors had a significantly better cancer-specific 5-year survival than patients with PODXL positive tumors.

The functional role of PODXL in tumorigenesis is largely unknown, but it has been demonstrated to promote cancer cell invasion and migration and to enhance metastatic potential [27–29]. Other proposed mechanisms are evasion of natural killer cell-mediated cytotoxicity [30] and maintaining and regulating the surface expression of glucose transporters [31]. In osteosarcoma cell lines, PODXL has been shown to promote chemoresistance to

cisplatin [32], which is particularly interesting since platinum compounds (cisplatin and oxaliplatin) are important cytotoxic drugs in the treatment of esophageal and gastric adenocarcinoma.

To our best knowledge, there are no reports on the prognostic value of PODXL expression in esophageal adenocarcinoma.

The aim of this study was to explore the expression of PODXL in both esophageal and gastric adenocarcinoma and to assess its impact on time to recurrence (TTR) and overall survival (OS) in a consecutive series of patients from southern Sweden, treated surgically between 2006 and 2010, prior to the wide implementation of neoadjuvant treatment.

Methods
Study design and participants

The study cohort consists of a consecutive series of 174 patients with chemo-/radiotherapy-naive esophageal (including EG junction) or gastric adenocarcinoma, subjected to surgical resection at the University Hospitals of Lund and Malmö between January 1, 2006 and December 31, 2010. This cohort has been examined in several previous biomarker studies [33–37]. Data on survival and recurrence were updated until December 31, 2014. Tumor location was based on endoscopy findings. Classification of tumor stage was done according to the 7th edition of the UICC/AJCC TNM classification [3]. Histotype according to Laurén [38] was denoted for all tumors as intestinal, mixed or diffuse growth pattern. This classification is generally applied on gastric cancer but can be used also for esophageal and EG junction adenocarcinoma. Residual tumor status was classified as: R0 = no residual tumor (free resection margins according to pathology report), R1 = possible microscopic residual tumor (narrow or compromised resection margins according to pathology report), R2 = macroscopic residual tumor (according to surgery report). The vast majority (98.7 %) of the patients were operated on with a curative intent but three patients with known distant metastases (M1-disease) were resected to palliate symptoms from the primary tumor. In 16 patients, M1-disease was revealed either during surgery or in the resected specimens. No patients received neoadjuvant oncological therapy and only a minority (7.5 %) of the patients received adjuvant treatment (chemo-/radiotherapy). Clinical data, recurrence status and vital status were obtained retrospectively from medical records. Clinicopathological factors and follow-up data are described in Additional file 1.

Tissue microarrays

Tissue microarrays (TMAs) were constructed using a semi-automated arraying device (TMArrayer™, Pathology

Devices, Westminster, MD, USA). From all 174 primary tumors, duplicate cores (1 mm) from separate donor blocks were obtained. In 81 cases lymph node metastases were sampled in duplicate cores (each from a separate metastasis if more than one). In addition 1–3 cores from areas with intestinal metaplasia (Barrett's esophagus or gastric intestinal metaplasia) were sampled in 73 cases. Single core samples from adjacent normal esophageal squamous epithelium (96 cases) and normal gastric columnar epithelium (131 cases) were also retrieved. All samples were paired.

Immunohistochemistry

For immunohistochemical analysis of PODXL expression, 4 μm TMA-sections were automatically pre-treated using the PT Link system and then stained in an Autostainer Plus (DAKO; Glostrup, Copenhagen, Denmark) with the rabbit polyclonal anti-PODXL antibody HPA002110 (Atlas Antibodies AB, Stockholm, Sweden) diluted 1:250. The same antibody was used by Laitinen et al. in their study on gastric cancer [26], and the specificity of the antibody has been validated previously [39]. Staining was assessed simultaneously by two different observers (KJ and DB) blinded to clinical and outcome data and scoring discrepancies were discussed to reach consensus. As in previous studies from our group [20, 21, 24, 25, 40], assessment of PODXL staining was registered as negative (0), weak cytoplasmic positivity in any proportion of cells (1), moderate cytoplasmic positivity in any proportion of cells (2), distinct membranous positivity in ≤50 % of cells (3) and distinct membranous positivity in >50 % of cells (4). For samples with duplicate cores the highest staining score was used.

Statistical analysis

For description of the cohort and in the analyses of the association between PODXL expression and clinicopathological factors, chi-square test (Fisher's exact for 2x2 tables and linear-by-linear association for tables with more than two rows) was used for categorical variables and Mann–Whitney U test for continuous variables. The Mann–Whitney U test was used to assess differences in PODXL expression between tissue types. In the analyses of the association between PODXL expression and clinicopathological factors and in the survival analyses, a dichotomized variable of negative (staining score 0) vs. positive (staining score 1–4) PODXL expression in the primary tumor and/or lymph node metastases was applied. The cut-off between negative and positive PODXL expression was the same as used in the study by Laitinen et al. in gastric cancer [26]. TTR was defined as time from diagnosis (date of result of the preoperative biopsy) to the date of biopsy or radiology proven recurrent disease. OS was defined as time from diagnosis (date of

result of the preoperative biopsy) to the date of death. TTR and OS were analyzed for resected patients with M0-disease and no macroscopic residual tumor (R0-1). Differences in Kaplan-Meier survival curves were computed using log-rank test. Unadjusted and adjusted hazard ratios (HR) for survival were determined using Cox proportional-hazards regression. For TTR we adjusted for T stage, N stage, R classification, differentiation grade and adjuvant treatment. For OS, the adjusted model included age, T stage, N stage, R classification and differentiation grade. All tests were 2-sided and a p-value <0.05 was considered significant. IBM® SPSS® Statistics version 22.0.0.1 for Mac was used for all statistical analyses.

Results

PODXL expression in normal epithelium, intestinal metaplasia, primary tumors and lymph node metastases

Immunohistochemical expression of PODXL could be assessed in 50/96 (52 %) samples with normal esophageal squamous epithelium, 79/131 (60 %) samples with normal gastric columnar epithelium, 51/73 (70 %) samples with intestinal metaplasia (Barrett's esophagus or gastric intestinal metaplasia), 170/174 (98 %) samples with primary tumors, and 76/81 (94 %) samples with lymph node metastases. PODXL staining was mainly detected in the cytoplasm, sometimes in a granular pattern, with or without an accentuation towards the membrane, and in some cases with a strong membranous component. Sample images are shown in Fig. 1. As expected there was a strong staining in endothelial cells, thus serving as an internal positive control. The distribution of immunohistochemical expression of PODXL in the different tissue types is shown in Fig. 2. Expression of PODXL was significantly higher in intestinal metaplasia (Barrett's esophagus or gastric intestinal metaplasia) compared to normal epithelium ($p < 0.001$) and PODXL expression was significantly higher in primary tumors and lymph node metastases compared to intestinal metaplasia ($p < 0.001$). PODXL expression was similar in Barrett's esophagus and gastric intestinal metaplasia ($p = 0.671$, data not shown). There was no significant difference in PODXL expression between primary tumors and lymph node metastases ($p = 0.645$) and PODXL expression in primary tumors and/or lymph node metastases did not differ significantly by primary tumor location ($p = 0.314$, data not shown).

Associations of PODXL expression with clinicopathological factors

As shown in Table 1, factors significantly associated with PODXL expression were N stage and high grade tumors. Negative PODXL expression was denoted in 14.2 % of the esophageal cancers and in 21.5 % of the gastric

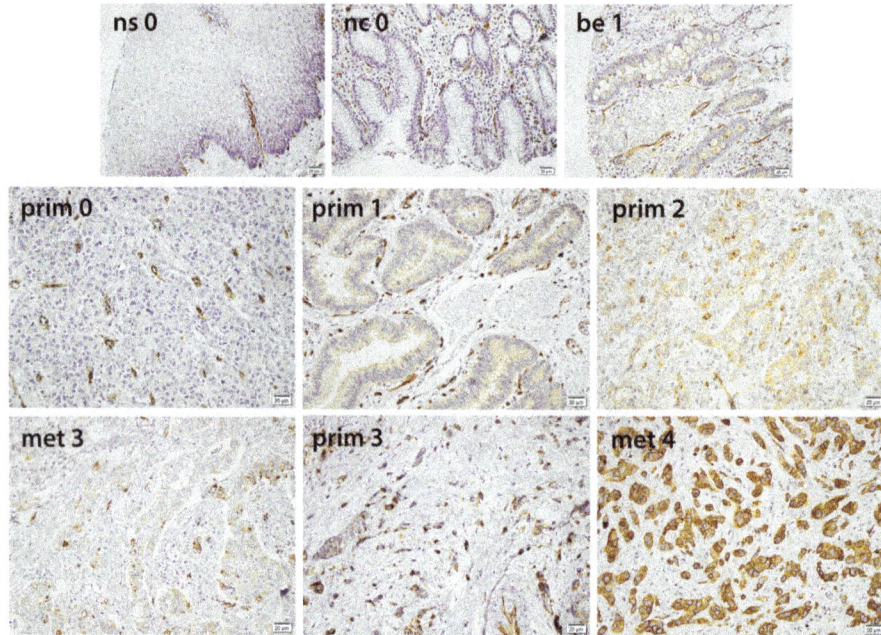

Fig. 1 Sample immunohistochemical images of PODXL expression (staining score 0–4), magnification x 20. *Top panel, from left*: Normal squamous epithelium (0). Normal columnar epithelium (0). Barrett's esophagus (1). *Middle panel, from left*: Primary gastric adenocarcinoma, diffuse subtype (0). Primary gastric adenocarcinoma, intestinal subtype (1). Primary gastric adenocarcinoma, intestinal subtype (2). *Bottom panel, from left*: Lymph node metastasis, intestinal subtype (3). Primary esophageal adenocarcinoma, diffuse subtype (3). Lymph node metastasis, intestinal subtype (4)

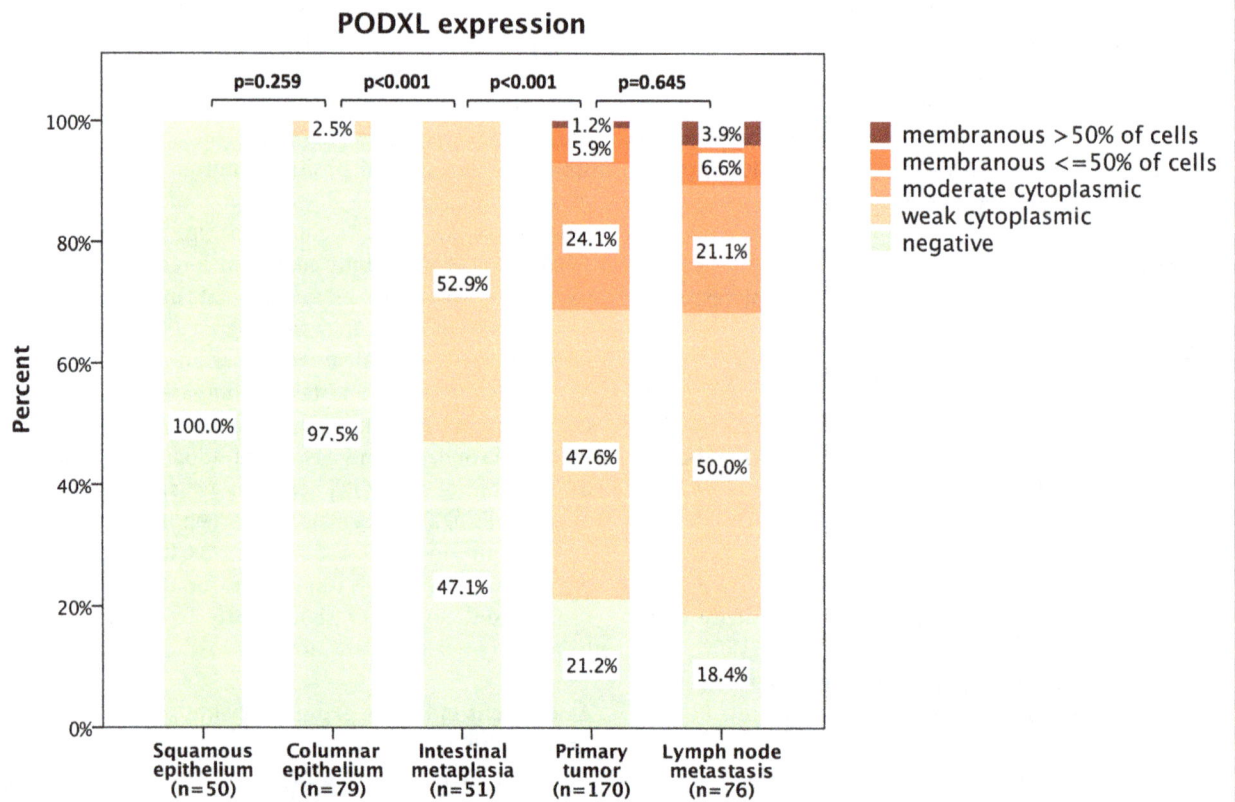

Fig. 2 Box plots visualizing the distribution of immunohistochemical expression of PODXL in normal squamous epithelium, normal gastric mucosa, intestinal metaplasia (Barrett's esophagus or gastric intestinal metaplasia), primary tumors and lymph node metastases in the entire cohort

Table 1 Associations of PODXL expression with clinicopathological factors

	Entire cohort n (%)	PODXL neg n (%)	PODXL pos n (%)	p-value
	171 (100.0)	29 (17.0)	142 (83.0)	
Age				
≤70	85 (49.7)	12 (41.4)	73 (51.4)	0.416
>70	86 (50.3)	17 (58.6)	69 (48.6)	
Sex				
Female	39 (22.8)	9 (31.0)	30 (21.1)	0.330
Male	132 (77.2)	20 (69.0)	112 (78.9)	
T stage				
T1	18 (10.5)	2 (6.9)	16 (11.3)	0.637
T2	32 (18.7)	6 (20.7)	26 (18.3)	
T3	94 (55.0)	16 (55.2)	78 (54.9)	
T4	27 (15.8)	5 (17.2)	22 (15.5)	
N stage				
N0	57 (33.3)	16 (55.2)	41 (28.9)	0.006
N1	29 (17.0)	4 (13.8)	25 (17.6)	
N2	41 (24.0)	6 (20.7)	35 (24.6)	
N3	44 (25.7)	3 (10.3)	41 (28.9)	
M stage				
M0	152 (88.9)	25 (86.2)	127 (89.4)	0.535
M1	19 (11.1)	4 (13.8)	15 (10.6)	
R classification				
R0	117 (68.4)	22 (75.9)	95 (66.9)	0.556
R1	45 (26.3)	5 (17.2)	40 (28.2)	
R2	9 (5.3)	2 (6.9)	7 (4.9)	
Differentiation grade				
Low grade	8 (4.7)	4 (13.8)	4 (2.8)	0.023
Intermediate grade	52 (30.4)	10 (34.5)	42 (29.6)	
High grade	111 (64.9)	15 (51.7)	96 (67.6)	
Lauren classification				
Intestinal	119 (69.6)	23 (79.3)	96 (67.6)	0.335
Mixed	9 (5.3)	0 (0.0)	9 (6.3)	
Diffuse	43 (25.1)	6 (20.7)	37 (26.1)	
Location				
Esophagus + EG junction	106 (62.0)	15 (51.7)	91 (64.1)	0.217
Stomach	65 (38.0)	14 (48.3)	51 (35.9)	

R0 = no residual tumor (free resection margins according to pathology report), R1 = possible microscopic residual tumor (narrow or compromised resection margins according to pathology report), R2 = macroscopic residual tumor (according to surgery report)
N1 = metastasis in 1–2 regional lymph nodes, N2 = metastasis in 3–6 regional lymph nodes, N3 = metastasis in 7 or more regional lymph nodes
The dichotomized variable for age is based on the mean/median age, as shown in Additional file 1

cancers, but the difference between locations was not statistically significant.

Impact of PODXL expression on prognosis

Survival analyses were performed on patients with M0-disease and no macroscopic residual tumor (R0-1). In esophageal adenocarcinoma the Kaplan-Meier analyses (Fig. 3a, c) revealed that patients with PODXL negative tumors had a superior TTR (estimated recurrence-free rate at 5 years 75 % vs. 35 %) and OS (estimated surviving rate at 5 years 69 % vs. 28 %) compared to patients with PODXL positive tumors. In gastric adenocarcinoma, patients with PODXL negative tumors had a superior TTR (estimated recurrence-free rate at 5 years 88 % vs. 45 %) and a trend towards an improved OS (estimated surviving rate at 5 years 55 % vs. 40 %) in the Kaplan-Meier analyses (Fig. 3b, d). In esophageal and gastric adenocarcinoma combined, as shown in Table 2, the prognostic significance of PODXL expression on TTR was confirmed in unadjusted Cox regression analysis (HR = 5.36, 95 % CI 1.68-17.06, $p = 0.005$) and remained significant in the adjusted model (HR = 3.39, 95 % CI 1.01-11.35, $p = 0.048$). Moreover, the impact of PODXL expression on OS was also confirmed in unadjusted analysis (HR = 2.52, 95 % CI 1.31-4.85, $p = 0.006$) and remained significant in the adjusted model (HR = 2.03, 95 % CI 1.04-3.98, $p = 0.039$).

Similar results were obtained when the survival analyses were stratified by primary tumor location (Additional file 2), and when considering PODXL expression in primary tumors and lymph node metastases separately (Additional file 3).

Discussion

In this study on resected esophageal and gastric adenocarcinoma we have shown that PODXL is expressed in the majority of cases and correlates with poor survival, but in the subgroup of patients with PODXL negative cancers the prognosis was excellent. This finding applies to both esophageal and gastric cancer with regard to both TTR and OS. To our best knowledge, this is the first report on the prognostic role of PODXL in esophageal adenocarcinoma. Furthermore, in gastric cancer, we have validated the recent findings from Laitinen et al. [26] of a negative prognostic impact of PODXL expression, even though the proportion of PODXL negative gastric cancer cases were lower in our study (21.5 % compared to 42.5 %). The reasons for this discrepancy are not clear, since we used the same polyclonal antibody and the same definition for negative vs. positive PODXL expression. However, whereas Laitinen et al. only examined primary tumors, we also included lymph node metastases in our analyses. This resulted in a non-significant ($p = 0.506$) decrease in PODXL negative gastric

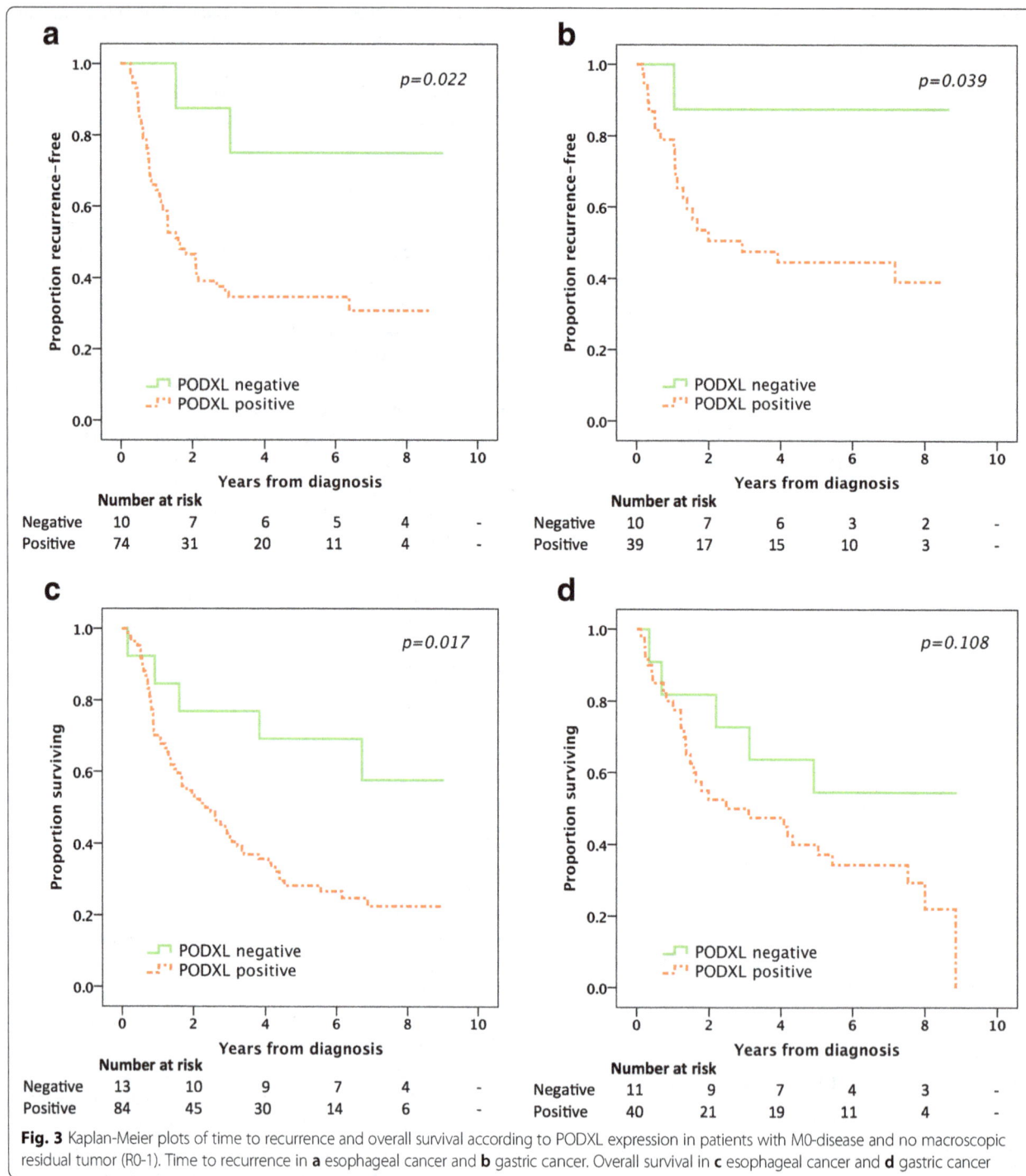

Fig. 3 Kaplan-Meier plots of time to recurrence and overall survival according to PODXL expression in patients with M0-disease and no macroscopic residual tumor (R0-1). Time to recurrence in **a** esophageal cancer and **b** gastric cancer. Overall survival in **c** esophageal cancer and **d** gastric cancer

cancer cases from 26.6 to 21.5 %. Another factor could be observer-dependent, such as setting the cut-off between negative and weak cytoplasmic staining. In other reports on PODXL as a prognostic marker in colo-rectal [23–25, 40], pancreatic and periampullary adenocar-cinoma [21, 22], using the same polyclonal antibody, the most evident prognostic cut-off was observed for mem-branous vs. non-membranous expression, with the former

being an independent factor of poor prognosis. However, in our study and in the report from Laitinen et al., the opti-mal prognostic cut-off was negative vs. positive, including membranous, PODXL expression. Hence, further studies are warranted to determine optimal cut-offs for prognosti-cation, which may well differ between different types of cancer. Of note, previous studies on colorectal [41] and pancreatic [22] cancer, using a monoclonal anti-PODXL

Table 2 Hazard ratios for recurrence and death (M0, R0-1)

	Time to recurrence					Overall survival				
	n (events)	Unadjusted HR (95 % CI)	p-value	Adjusted HR (95 % CI)	p-value	n (events)	Unadjusted HR (95 % CI)	p-value	Adjusted HR (95 % CI)	p-value
Age										
Continuous	136 (72)	1.00 (0.98–1.02)	0.610		0.610	151 (104)	1.04 (1.02–1.06)	<0.001	1.05 (1.03–1.07)	<0.001
Sex										
Female	27 (12)					30 (22)				
Male	109 (60)	1.18 (0.63–2.19)	0.610			121 (82)	0.81 (0.50–1.29)	0.370		
T stage			<0.001		0.043			0.010		0.511
T1	18 (3)					19 (7)				
T2	27 (8)	2.14 (0.57–8.06)	0.263	1.53 (0.39–5.96)	0.538	30 (19)	2.09 (0.88–4.97)	0.097	1.53 (0.62–3.78)	0.357
T3	77 (51)	6.92 (2.15–22.29)	0.001	3.72 (1.10–12.64)	0.035	86 (66)	3.27 (1.49–7.15)	0.003	1.79 (0.79–4.08)	0.164
T4	14 (10)	8.52 (2.33–31.16)	0.001	3.52 (0.92–13.56)	0.067	16 (12)	3.71 (1.45–9.48)	0.006	1.98 (0.74–5.31)	0.175
N stage										
N0	50 (7)					53 (26)				
N1-3	86 (65)	9.89 (4.51–21.72)	<0.001	7.78 (3.24–18.71)	<0.001	98 (78)	2.56 (1.63–4.00)	<0.001	2.79 (1.67–4.66)	<0.001
R classification										
R0	103 (46)					113 (69)				
R1	33 (26)	2.89 (1.76–4.74)	<0.001	1.38 (0.79–2.41)	0.253	38 (35)	2.75 (1.80–4.20)	<0.001	2.07 (1.29–3.31)	0.003
Differentiation grade										
Low/Intermediate grade	49 (18)					56 (31)				
High grade	87 (54)	2.22 (1.30–3.79)	0.004	1.93 (1.09–3.42)	0.025	95 (73)	1.73 (1.13–2.63)	0.011	1.40 (0.88–2.20)	0.153
Lauren classification										
Intestinal	94 (45)					106 (69)				
Diffuse/Mixed	42 (27)	1.57 (0.97–2.53)	0.064			45 (35)	1.35 (0.90–2.03)	0.149		
Adjuvant treatment										
No	126 (63)					138 (94)				
Chemo-/radiotherapy	10 (9)	2.12 (1.05–4.28)	0.036	0.96 (0.45–2.06)	0.924	13 (10)	1.20 (0.62–2.30)	0.589		
Location										
Esophagus + EG junction	86 (49)					99 (69)				
Stomach	50 (23)	0.74 (0.45–1.22)	0.239			52 (35)	0.90 (0.60–1.34)	0.592		
PODXL expression										
Negative	20 (3)					24 (10)				
Positive	113 (67)	5.36 (1.68–17.06)	0.005	3.39 (1.01–11.35)	0.048	124 (92)	2.52 (1.31–4.85)	0.006	2.03 (1.04–3.98)	0.039

R0 = no residual tumor (free resection margins according to pathology report), R1 = possible microscopic residual tumor (narrow or compromised resection margins according to pathology report)

antibody, demonstrated a correlation between cytoplasmic PODXL expression and poor survival.

A limitation of this study is its retrospective design. However, we have managed to access all the necessary clinical data, except for recurrence status in some cases, and the tissue specimens have been thoroughly re-examined. Due to heterogeneity within tumors there is always a risk of sampling bias with the TMA-technique. However, as we used duplicate cores from different donor blocks and, when available, also included cores from lymph node metastases when denoting the highest PODXL score for each case, the risk of overestimating the proportion of PODXL negative cancers should be reduced.

In current practice, most patients with resectable esophageal or gastric adenocarcinoma receive neoadjuvant and/or adjuvant chemotherapy or chemoradiotherapy, but only a minority (10-15 %) of the patients actually benefit from the oncological treatment [8–13]. For a biomarker to be really useful in clinical decision making it should not only be prognostic but also be able to predict whether a patient will benefit from a treatment or not. Further studies on PODXL in esophageal and gastric adenocarcinoma are warranted to validate its role as a prognostic biomarker and to explore whether it also may be useful as a treatment response predictive biomarker, as suggested in previous studies on colorectal [24] and periampullary cancer [21].

Conclusions

In summary, we have shown that PODXL is commonly expressed in esophageal and gastric adenocarcinoma and associated with lymph node metastases and high grade tumors. Furthermore, PODXL is an independent prognostic biomarker for reduced time to recurrence and poor overall survival, but in the subgroup of patients with PODXL negative tumors the prognosis appears to be excellent.

Abbreviations
CI, confidence interval; EG, esophagogastric; HR, hazard ratio; IHC, immunohistochemistry; OS, overall survival; PODXL, podocalyxin-like protein; TMA, tissue microarray; TTR, time to recurrence

Acknowledgements
None.

Funding
This study was supported by grants from the Knut and Alice Wallenberg Foundation, the Swedish Cancer Society, the Crafoord Foundation, the Olle Engkvist Foundation, Anna Lisa and Sven-Eric Lundgren's Foundation, the Swedish Government Grant for Clinical Research (ALF), Lund University Faculty of Medicine and Skåne University Hospital Funds and Donations.

Authors' contributions
DB evaluated the immunohistochemical stainings, re-examined clinicopathological data, updated survival data, performed the statistical analyses and drafted the manuscript. CH collected and re-examined clinicopathological data and assisted with the TMA construction. BN constructed the TMA and performed the IHC stainings. AL, AJ and JE contributed with intellectual input and contributed to the study design . KJ evaluated the immunohistochemical stainings and conceived of the study. All authors read and approved the final manuscript.

Authors' information
None.

Competing interests
The authors declare that they have no competing interests.

References
1. Ferlay J, Soerjomataram I, Ervik M, Dikshit R, Eser S, Mathers C, Rebelo M, Parkin D, Forman D, Bray F: GLOBOCAN 2012 v1.0, Cancer Incidence and Mortality Worldwide: IARC CancerBase No. 11. Lyon, France: 2013. http://globocan.iarc.fr, accessed on 6 Feb 2016.
2. Edgren G, Adami H-O, Weiderpass E, Nyrén O. A global assessment of the oesophageal adenocarcinoma epidemic. Gut. 2013;62:1406–14.
3. Sobin L, Gospodarowicz M, Wittekind C. TNM Classification of Malignant Tumours, 7th Edition. Wiley-Blackwell; 2009. http://eu.wiley.com/WileyCDA/WileyTitle/productCd-1444332414.html.
4. Carr JS, Zafar SF, Saba N, Khuri FR, El-Rayes BF. Risk factors for rising incidence of esophageal and gastric cardia adenocarcinoma. J Gastrointest Cancer. 2013;44:143–51.
5. Nie S, Chen T, Yang X, Huai P, Lu M. Association of Helicobacter pylori infection with esophageal adenocarcinoma and squamous cell carcinoma: a meta-analysis. Dis Esophagus. 2014;27:645–53.
6. Ferro A, Peleteiro B, Malvezzi M, Bosetti C, Bertuccio P, Levi F, Negri E, La Vecchia C, Lunet N. Worldwide trends in gastric cancer mortality (1980–2011), with predictions to 2015, and incidence by subtype. Eur J Cancer. 2014;50:1330–44.
7. Fuccio L, Eusebi L, Bazzoli F. Gastric cancer, Helicobacter pylori infection and other risk factors. World J Gastrointest Oncol. 2010;2:342.
8. Smalley SR, Benedetti JK, Haller DG, Hundahl SA, Estes NC, Ajani JA, Gunderson LL, Goldman B, Martenson JA, Jessup JM, Stemmermann GN, Blanke CD, Macdonald JS. Updated analysis of SWOG-directed intergroup study 0116: a phase III trial of adjuvant radiochemotherapy versus observation after curative gastric cancer resection. J Clin Oncol. 2012;30:2327–33.
9. Van Hagen P, Hulshof M, van Lanschot JJB, Steyerberg EW, Henegouwen M van B, Wijnhoven BPL, Richel DJ, Nieuwenhuijzen GAP, Hospers GAP, Bonenkamp JJ. Preoperative chemoradiotherapy for esophageal or junctional cancer. N Engl J Med. 2012;366:2074–84.
10. Cunningham D, Allum WH, Stenning SP, Thompson JN, Van de Velde CJ, Nicolson M, Scarffe JH, Lofts FJ, Falk SJ, Iveson TJ. Perioperative chemotherapy versus surgery alone for resectable gastroesophageal cancer. N Engl J Med. 2006;355:11–20.
11. Ychou M, Boige V, Pignon J-P, Conroy T, Bouche O, Lebreton G, Ducourtieux M, Bedenne L, Fabre J-M, Saint-Aubert B, Geneve J, Lasser P, Rougier P. Perioperative chemotherapy compared with surgery alone for resectable gastroesophageal adenocarcinoma: an FNCLCC and FFCD multicenter phase III trial. J Clin Oncol. 2011;29:1715–21.
12. Noh SH, Park SR, Yang H-K, Chung HC, Chung I-J, Kim S-W, Kim H-H. Adjuvant capecitabine plus oxaliplatin for gastric cancer after D2 gastrectomy (CLASSIC): 5-year follow-up of an open-label, randomised phase 3 trial. Lancet Oncol. 2014;15:1389–96.
13. Sasako M, Sakuramoto S, Katai H, Kinoshita T, Furukawa H, Yamaguchi T, Nashimoto A, Fujii M, Nakajima T, Ohashi Y. Five-year outcomes of a randomized phase III trial comparing adjuvant chemotherapy with S-1 versus surgery alone in stage II or III gastric cancer. J Clin Oncol. 2011;29:4387–93.
14. Kerjaschki D, Sharkey DJ, Farquhar MG. Identification and characterization of podocalyxin—the major sialoprotein of the renal glomerular epithelial cell. J Cell Biol. 1984;98:1591–6.
15. Horvat R, Hovorka A, Dekan G, Poczewski H, Kerjaschki D. Endothelial cell membranes contain podocalyxin—the major sialoprotein of visceral glomerular epithelial cells. J Cell Biol. 1986;102:484–91.

Expression of podocalyxin-like protein is an independent prognostic biomarker in resected esophageal...

229

16. Kerosuo L, Juvonen E, Alitalo R, Gylling M, Kerjaschki D, Miettinen A. Podocalyxin in human haematopoietic cells. Br J Haematol. 2004;124:809–18.

17. Vitureira N, Andrés R, Pérez-Martínez E, Martínez A, Bribián A, Blasi J, Chelliah S, López-Doménech G, De Castro F, Burgaya F, McNagny K, Soriano E. Podocalyxin is a novel polysialylated neural adhesion protein with multiple roles in neural development and synapse formation. PLoS One. 2010;5:e12003.

18. Binder ZA, Siu I-M, Eberhart CG, ap Rhys C, Bai R-Y, Staedtke V, Zhang H, Smoll NR, Piantadosi S, Piccirillo SG, DiMeco F, Weingart JD, Vescovi A, Olivi A, Riggins GJ, Gallia GL. Podocalyxin-like protein is expressed in glioblastoma multiforme stem-like cells and is associated with poor outcome. PLoS One. 2013;8:e75945.

19. Somasiri A, Nielsen JS, Makretsov N, McCoy ML, Prentice L, Gilks CB, Chia SK, Gelmon KA, Kershaw DB, Huntsman DG, et al. Overexpression of the anti-adhesin podocalyxin is an independent predictor of breast cancer progression. Cancer Res. 2004;64:5068–73.

20. Boman K, Larsson AH, Segersten U, Kuteeva E, Johannesson H, Nodin B, Eberhard J, Uhlén M, Malmström P-U, Jirström K. Membranous expression of podocalyxin-like protein is an independent factor of poor prognosis in urothelial bladder cancer. Br J Cancer. 2013;108:2321–8.

21. Heby M, Elebro J, Nodin B, Jirström K, Eberhard J. Prognostic and predictive significance of podocalyxin-like protein expression in pancreatic and periampullary adenocarcinoma. BMC Clin Pathol. 2015;15:10.

22. Saukkonen K, Hagström J, Mustonen H, Juuti A, Nordling S, Fermér C, Nilsson O, Seppänen H, Haglund C. Podocalyxin is a marker of poor prognosis in pancreatic ductal adenocarcinoma. PLoS One. 2015;10:e0129012.

23. Kaprio T, Hagström J, Fermér C, Mustonen H, Böckelman C, Nilsson O, Haglund C. A comparative study of two PODXL antibodies in 840 colorectal cancer patients. BMC Cancer. 2014;14:1.

24. Larsson A, Johansson ME, Wangefjord S, Gaber A, Nodin B, Kucharzewska P, Welinder C, Belting M, Eberhard J, Johnsson A, Uhlén M, Jirström K. Overexpression of podocalyxin-like protein is an independent factor of poor prognosis in colorectal cancer. Br J Cancer. 2011;105:666–72.

25. Larsson A, Fridberg M, Gaber A, Nodin B, Levéen P, Jönsson G, Uhlén M, Birgisson H, Jirström K. Validation of podocalyxin-like protein as a biomarker of poor prognosis in colorectal cancer. BMC Cancer. 2012;12:1.

26. Laitinen A, Böckelman C, Hagström J, Kokkola A, Fermér C, Nilsson O, Haglund C. Podocalyxin as a prognostic marker in gastric cancer. PLoS One. 2015;10:e0145079.

27. Flores-Téllez TNJ, Lopez TV, Vásquez Garzón VR, Villa-Treviño S. Co-expression of ezrin-CLIC5-podocalyxin is associated with migration and invasiveness in hepatocellular carcinoma. PLoS One. 2015;10:e0131605.

28. Snyder KA, Hughes MR, Hedberg B, Brandon J, Hernaez DC, Bergqvist P, Cruz F, Po K, Graves ML, Turvey ME, Nielsen JS, Wilkins JA, McColl SR, Babcook JS, Roskelley CD, McNagny KM. Podocalyxin enhances breast tumor growth and metastasis and is a target for monoclonal antibody therapy. Breast Cancer Res. 2015;17:46.

29. Lin C-W, Sun M-S, Wu H-C. Podocalyxin-like 1 is associated with tumor aggressiveness and metastatic gene expression in human oral squamous cell carcinoma. Int J Oncol. 2014;45:710–8.

30. Amo L, Tamayo-Orbegozo E, Maruri N, Buqué A, Solaun M, Riñón M, Arrieta A, Larrucea S. Podocalyxin-like protein 1 functions as an immunomodulatory molecule in breast cancer cells. Cancer Lett. 2015;368:26–35.

31. Schopperle WM, Lee JM, DeWolf WC. The human cancer and stem cell marker podocalyxin interacts with the glucose-3-transporter in malignant pluripotent stem cells. Biochem Biophys Res Commun. 2010;398:372–6.

32. Huang Z, Huang Y, He H, Ni J. Podocalyxin promotes cisplatin chemoresistance in osteosarcoma cells through phosphatidylinositide 3-kinase signaling. Mol Med Rep. 2015;12:3916–22.

33. Fristedt R, Gaber A, Hedner C, Nodin B, Uhlén M, Eberhard J, Jirstrom K. Expression and prognostic significance of the polymeric immunoglobulin receptor in esophageal and gastric adenocarcinoma. J Transl Med. 2014;12:83.

34. Jonsson L, Hedner C, Gaber A, Korkocic D, Nodin B, Uhlén M, Eberhard J, Jirström K. High expression of RNA-binding motif protein 3 in esophageal and gastric adenocarcinoma correlates with intestinal metaplasia-associated tumours and independently predicts a reduced risk of recurrence and death. Biomark Res. 2014;2:11.

35. Hedner C, Gaber A, Korkocic D, Nodin B, Uhlén M, Kuteeva E, Johannesson H, Jirström K, Eberhard J. SATB1 is an independent prognostic factor in radically resected upper gastrointestinal tract adenocarcinoma. Virchows Arch. 2014;465:649–59.

36. Hedner C, Tran L, Borg D, Nodin B, Jirström K, Eberhard J. Discordant human epidermal growth factor receptor 2 overexpression in primary and metastatic upper gastrointestinal adenocarcinoma signifies poor prognosis. Histopathology. 2016;68:230–40.

37. Hedner C, Borg D, Nodin B, Karnevi E, Jirström K, Eberhard J. Expression and prognostic significance of human epidermal growth factor receptors 1 and 3 in gastric and esophageal adenocarcinoma. PLoS One. 2016;11:e0148101.

38. Lauren P. The two histological main types of gastric carcinoma: diffuse and so-called intestinal-type carcinoma. An attempt at a histo-clinical classification. Acta Pathol Microbiol Scand. 1965;64:31–49.

39. The Human Protein Atlas. http://www.proteinatlas.org/ENSG00000128567-PODXL/antibody, accessed on 6 Feb 2016.

40. Larsson AH, Nodin B, Syk I, Palmquist I, Uhlén M, Eberhard J, Jirstrom K. Podocalyxin-like protein expression in primary colorectal cancer and synchronous lymph node metastases. Diagn Pathol. 2013;8:109.

41. Kaprio T, Fermér C, Hagström J, Mustonen H, Böckelman C, Nilsson O, Haglund C. Podocalyxin is a marker of poor prognosis in colorectal cancer. BMC Cancer. 2014;14:1.

28

Pelvic radiotherapy for cervical cancer affects importantly the reproducibility of cytological alterations evaluation

Fernanda A. Lucena[1] [ID], Ricardo F. A. Costa[1], Maira D. Stein[2], Carlos E. M. C. Andrade[3], Geórgia F. Cintra[3], Marcelo A. Vieira[3], Rozany M. Dufloth[4], José Humberto T. G. Fregnani[4] and Ricardo dos Reis[3*]

Abstract

Background: to evaluate the intraobserver and interobserver reproducibility of cervical cytopathology according to previous knowledge of whether patients received radiotherapy (RT) treatment or not.

Methods: The study analyzed a sample of 95 cervix cytological slides; 24 with cytological abnormalities (CA) and presence of RT; 21 without CA and presence of RT; 25 without CA and without previous RT; 25 with CA and without previous RT. Two cytopathology (CP) evaluations of the slides were carried out. For the first CP re-evaluation, the cytotechnologist was blinded for the information of previous RT. For the second CP re-evaluation, the cytotechnologist was informed about previous RT. The results were analyzed through inter and intraobserver agreement using the unweighted and weighted kappa.

Results: Post radiotherapy effects were identified in 44.4% of cases that undergone previous pelvic RT. The agreement for RT status was 66.32% (unweighted K = 0.31, 95%CI: 0.13; 0.49, moderate agreement). The intraobserver agreement, regarding the cytological diagnoses, regardless of radiotherapy status, was 80.32% (weighted K = 0.52, 95%CI: 0.34; 0.68). In no RT group, the intraobserver agreement was 70% (weighted K = 0.47, 95%CI: 0.27;0.65) and in patients that received RT, the intraobserver agreement was 84.09% (unweighted K = 0.37, 95%CI: 0.01;0.74). The interobserver agreement between cytopathology result (abnormal or normal) in the group with RT, considering normal and abnormal CP diagnosis was 14.0% and 12.5%, respectively. There was no association between the cytological alterations and the median time between the end of RT and the cytological diagnosis.

Conclusion: This study showed that RT has an important impact in CP diagnosis because the agreement, also in interobserver and intraobserver analysis, had high discrepancy in patients that received RT. Also, demonstrated that it is difficult to recognize the presence of RT in cytological slides when this information is not provided.

Keywords: Cervical cytology, Pelvic radiotherapy, Reproducibility, Cervical cancer, Post radiotherapy cells changes

Background

Radiotherapy (RT) is a necessary and frequently used procedure for the treatment of gynecological cancer [1]. However, RT may have adverse effects on the lower genital tract after maximal therapeutic doses. Squamous cells undergo major changes due to the effect of RT on the vagina and cervix, often leading to difficulties to obtain

proper diagnosis [2]. The Pap test is a useful tool for screening of precursor lesions detection prior to progression to invasive carcinoma forms, where the results are described through the Bethesda system [3, 4]. In contrast, cytology has limited sensitivity for detection of residual cervical cancer after radiotherapy [5, 6].

Some authors suggest that patients with a history of previous RT have Pap tests indicating an increase in the incidence of unsatisfactory sample slides, from 4.3 to 13.2% when evaluated using satisfactory cellularity criteria (> 8000 squamous cells and < 75% of the obscure epithelium) [7]. In

* Correspondence: drricardoreis@gmail.com
[3]Department of Gynecologic Oncology, Barretos Cancer Hospital, Rua Antenor Duarte Villela, 1331 - Dr. Paulo Prata, Barretos 14784-400, São Paulo, Brazil
Full list of author information is available at the end of the article

addition, the study by Shield et al. showed cytology presenting marked effects of RT in 29.2% of cases [2].

Some studies show that it is important to properly identify the types of abnormal cells present in smears under the influence of RT. This leads to determine how many of these modifications are due to a possible recurrence of the tumor or to a new neoplastic lesion [2, 8]. Actually, follow-up of patients treated for cervical cancer based on routine Pap smears does not permit earlier detection of recurrence and does not increase survival [9].

The literature is scarce regarding information on intraobserver performance and reproducibility in cytological exams after radiotherapy. On the other hand, its known that cytology has limited accuracy also in women not treated by radiotherapy [10, 11].It is observed the existence of a low interobserver agreement in the sample of patients who received RT, which is expected due to the bias induced by radiation, thus favoring the cytological categorization of uncertainty [12].

The objective of this study was to evaluate the intraobserver and interobserver reproducibility of cervical cytology exams according to the previous knowledge of whether the patient received RT or not.

Methods

The study was approved by the Research Ethics Committee of Barretos Cancer Hospital (BCH, Brazil) and designed to analyze intraobserver reproducibility of Pap smear result. The sample consisted initially of 100 slides of normal and abnormal cytological exams from patients treated at BCH in the Gynecology Oncology outpatient clinic and in the Prevention Department. This work did not include live subjects and also it was not necessary informed consent due to the design of the study. Demographic and diagnosis data (original cytopathology evaluation), type of CA and treatment length were collected from medical chart.

The samples were selected from a bank of slides – prepared using the method of liquid-based cytology in order to proceed to the cytological examination – and collected in 2010 and 2011. A sampling method stratified by Pap result (normal and abnormal) and radiotherapy status was adopted in order to select the slides.

Five slides were excluded from the study: one slide that had not been prepared on liquid-based cytology, and four slides that the cytotechnologist considered inadequate to perform the review. Therefore, the final sample consisted of 95 slides, 50 slides of cytological exams with abnormal (25) and normal (25) results in patients without previous pelvic RT and 45 slides of cytological exams with abnormal (24) and normal (21) results in patients who received previous pelvic RT for cervical cancer treatment. All patients received concomitant radiochemotherapy and the radiotherapy protocol was EBRT and Brachytherapy. The cytological changes were classified according to Bethesda system [4]. The Fig. 1 shows the difference between normal cytological findings: (a) Normal Squamous cells and (b) Radiotherapy changes: Nuclear enlargement and altered cytoplasmic staining. Both by Papanicolaou stain.

A senior cytotechnologist and a senior gynecologic oncology pathologist conducted the cytopathology (CP) re-evaluations, following the routine of the pathology department at BCH. The department's pathologist re-evaluated all slides that the cytotechnologist considered abnormal. In the first CP re-evaluation, 95 slides were evaluated with no information regarding the result of the original CP evaluation of the cytological exam (gold standard in this study) and the presence or absence of previous RT. Besides performing the CP evaluation, slides containing cells with signs of post radiotherapy effects were identified. At the second CP re-evaluation, conducted 6 months later, the same observers re-evaluated the 95 slides having no information on the result of the original diagnosis of the cytological exam, but knowing whether the patient received previous pelvic RT.

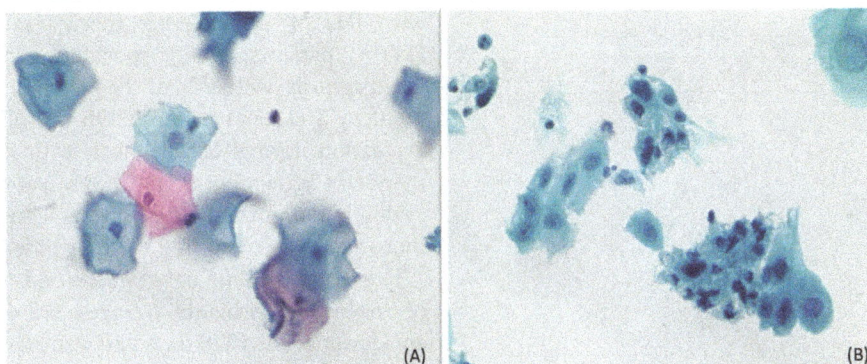

Fig. 1 a Cytological Findings: Normal Squamous cells by Papanicolaou stain. **b** Radiotherapy changes. The sheet shows nuclear enlargement and altered cytoplasmic staining by Papanicolaou stain

The agreement for RT status was calculated using unweighted kappa. For CP evaluation, three agreement analyses were conducted: considering all patients, patients with no RT and patients with RT. In the first analysis, the agreement (K^1) between the original CP evaluation and the first CP re-evaluation (blinded for RT information and cytological result) was evaluated. In the second analysis, the agreement (K^2) between the original CP evaluation and the second CP re-evaluation (blinded only for the cytological result, but not for RT status) was evaluated. K^1 and K^2 were considered interobserver assessment. In the third analysis, the intraobserver agreement (K^3) between the cytological result of the first CP re-evaluation and the second CP re-evaluation was evaluated. Weighted kappa was used to evaluate the agreement between the three evaluation phases; concordant results were given full credit [1], discordant results off by a single category were given half credit (0.5) and discordant results off by more than one category were given no credit (0). The values and the order of cytological results can be observed in Table 1. The agreement between the original CP evaluation and the first CP re-evaluation as well as between the second re-evaluation and the first re-evaluation considering the cytopathological diagnosis (normal and abnormal) and RT status (absence and presence), was evaluated using the unweighted kappa.

According to Landis and Koch [13], Kappa index is interpreted as follows: a range of 0.00–0.20 indicates slight agreement, a range of 0.21–0.40 indicates reasonable agreement, a range of 0.41–0.60 indicates moderate agreement, a range of 0.61–0.80 indicates substantial agreement, a range higher than 0.80 indicates near perfect agreement and 1.0 indicates perfect agreement. Chi-square test was used to evaluate the frequency and association of cytological abnormalities according to the time elapsed after RT and age. All analyzes were performed using Stata/MP 14.1 software. The level of statistical significance was set at 5%.

Table 1 Weight scheme for agreement analysis

	Negative	ASC-US	LSIL	AGC	ASC-H	HSIL	ADENO/CEC
Negative	1						
ASC-US	0.5	1					
LSIL	0	0.5	1				
AGC	0	0	0.5	1			
ASC-H	0	0	0	0.5	1		
HSIL	0	0	0	0	0.5	1	
ADENO/CEC	0	0	0	0	0	0.5	1

ADENO/CEC Adenocarcinoma, *AGC* Atypical Glandular cells, *ASC-H* Atypical Squamous Cells cannot exclude HSIL, *ASC-US* Atypical Squamous Cells of Undetermined Significance, *HSIL* High Grade Squamous Intraepithelial lesion, *LSIL* Low Grade Squamous Intraepithelial lesion

Results

In this study, 95 liquid-based cytology slides were analyzed. The median age was 51 years (17–91 years). Patients with abnormal cytology (49 individuals) were divided according to their age (below and above 50 years old). Of this group with abnormal cytology just one had histologically confirmed CIN2. Using Chi-square test, it was possible to verify that there was no association between age and types of CA ($p = 0.095$).

Of the 95 patients evaluated, 45 had undergone previous pelvic RT. In the first CP re-evaluation, post radiotherapy signs were identified in the cells of 27 slides (28.4%), of which 20 slides were from patients that actually undergone RT (74.1%). Therefore, the cytotechnologist was able to detect post radiotherapy effects in 44.4% (20/45) of cases that undergone previous pelvic RT. The agreement for RT status was 66.32% (unweighted K = 0.31, 95%CI: 0.13–0.49, moderate agreement).

Regarding the CP evaluations (original, 1st and 2nd re-evaluation), results are depicted in Table 2. The diagnoses with highest frequencies were: negative (48.4% in the original evaluation; 70.5% in the 1st re-evaluation and 57.4% in the 2nd re-evaluation), ASC-US (13.7% in the 1st re-evaluation; 26.6% in the 2nd re-evaluation) and ASC-H (18.9% in the original evaluation).

Table 3 shows the results of agreement values regarding the cytological diagnoses, considering all cases and RT status. Considering all patients, regardless of radiotherapy status, the intraobserver agreement was 80.32% (weighted K = 0.52, 95%CI: 0.34–0.68). In the patients that did not undergone RT, the intraobserver agreement was 70% (weighted K = 0.47, 95%CI: 0.27–0.65). In patients that undergone RT, the intraobserver agreement was 84.09% (unweighted K = 0.37, 95%CI: 0.01–0.74). An additional file with Additional file 1: Tables S1 to S9 show the values for the cytological diagnoses according to RT Status.

Table 4 demonstrates the agreement between cytopathology result (abnormal or normal) and post radiotherapy effect on the cells of the smear identified during 1st re-evaluation. Considering original normal CP diagnosis with RT, of 21 patients, there was agreement in 3 (14.0%) patients, while, considering original abnormal CP diagnosis with RT, of 24 patients, there was agreement in 3 (12.5%) patients. On the other hand, in 2nd evaluation normal CP diagnosis with RT, of 36 patients, there was agreement in 13 (36.0%) patients, while in 2nd evaluation abnormal CP diagnosis with RT, of 8 patients, there was agreement in 2 (25.0%) patients.

The length of time between the end of RT and the date of cytology abnormality averaged 848 days, with a standard deviation of 1278 days and a median of 364 days. No association between the cytological alterations and the median time between the end of RT and the cytological diagnosis was observed (Table 5).

Table 2 Results of analysis of slides, distributed by number and frequency

	Negative	ASC-US	LSIL	AGC	ASC-H	HSIL	ADENO/CEC	Total
Original evaluation	46	9	7	3	18	9	3	95
	48.4%	9.5%	7.4%	3.2%	18.9%	9.5%	3.2%	100%
1st Re-evaluation	67	13	5	1	6	3	0	95
	70.5%	13.7%	5.3%	1.1%	6.3%	3.2%	0%	100%
2nd Re-evaluation	54	25	3	2	6	4	0	94
	57.4%	26.6%	3.2%	2.1%	6.4%	4.3%	0%	100%

ADENO/CEC Adenocarcinoma, *AGC* Atypical Glandular cells, *ASC-H* Atypical Squamous Cells cannot exclude HSIL, *ASC-US* Atypical Squamous Cells of Undetermined Significance, *HSIL* High Grade Squamous Intraepithelial lesion, *LSIL* Low Grade Squamous Intraepithelial lesion

Discussion

The results suggest that radiotherapy has a strong influence in CP diagnosis also in normal or abnormal CP results. When we compared the interobserver agreement concerning CP diagnosis in patients that received RT, the agreement was only 14% and 12.5% in normal and abnormal CP diagnosis, respectively. This is one of the reasons that cytology is not recommended to use in follow-up of women treated with radiotherapy for cervical cancer [10].

In our study, the intraobserver evaluation (K^3), with presence of RT, demonstrated worst diagnostic agreement related to a decreased values of kappa (unweighted $K^3 = 0.37$) when compared to the same evaluation in all patients regardless RT status (weighted $K^3 = 0.52$) and patients without RT (weighted $K^3 = 0.47$). Also, Settakorn et al. [14] study, which compared interobserver agreement of two cytopathologists in cytologic interpretation of liquid based cytology preparations with conventional Papanicolaou smears, showed reasonable agreement (weighted $K = 0.37$, 95%CI = 0.31–0.44 and weighted $K = 0.40$, 95%CI = 0.33–0.46). In addition, the agreement about the presence of RT signals in the smear was low (44%). These findings corroborate that it is difficult to recognize the cytological RT signals in the cervical cells.

Regarding the interobserver agreement, Stein et al. [12] demonstrated that there was no difference in the

measurement of agreement between the observations (Kappa values) according to the status of radiotherapy and CA in the interpretation among cytotechnologists in manual and automated screening. The results of this work evidenced few differences in weighted kappa values when compared presence of RT ($K^1 = 0.016$ 95%CI: 0.03–0.06 e $K^2 = 0.041$ 95%CI: 0.01–0.09) and absence of RT ($K^1 = 0.149$ 95%CI: 0.02–0.32 e $K^2 = 0.120$ 95%CI: 0.04–0.31) in interobserver agreement between CP diagnosis. Nevertheless, this range of values keep in the same category of slight agreement. In spite of the similar conditions of slides analysis, our study demonstrated that the presence of radiotherapy influences the morphological classifications defined in the cytological diagnosis when evaluated by the same observer, which differs from the study by Stein et al., who evaluated only interobserver agreement.

According to the review undertaken for this article, this is the first study to correlate intraobserver reproducibility of cytological diagnosis with RT information. This work demonstrated that this agreement of the cytological diagnosis between two analysis conducted by the same cytotechnologist was moderate ($K = 0.52$) regarding the limits of the first and second CP re-evaluation. In evaluations by Tsilalis et al. [15], regarding telecytological diagnosis of cervical smears not related to RT, the intraobserver variability was near perfect among the five

Table 3 Values of agreements between cytopathological diagnosis

Patients	Evaluation	Exact Agreement	Expected Agreement	Weighted Kappa	95% Confidence Interval	N
	K^1	49.47%	45.74%	0.069	−0.05; 0.18	95
All	K^2	47.87%	44.11%	0.067	−0.05; 0.19	94
	K^3	80.32%	59.40%	0.515	0.34; 0.68	94
	K^1	51.00%	42.44%	0.149	−0.02;0.32	50
No	K^2	47.00%	39.78%	0.120	−0.04;0.31	50
RT	K^3	70.00%	43.18%	0.472	0.27;0.65	50
	K^1	47.78%	46.91%	0.016	−0,03;0.06	45
RT	K^2	48.86%	46.69%	0.041	−0.01;0.09	44
	K^3	84.09%	74.59%	0.374[a]	0.01;0.74	44

[a]Unweighted kappa, Less than three order categories

K^1: original vs first re-evaluation; K^2: original vs second re-evaluation; K^3: first re-evaluation vs second re-evaluation; *RT* radiotherapy

Table 4 Agreement between cytopathological diagnosis abnormal or not and presence or absence of RT in the cells of the smear

		1st re-evaluation					
		PAP(−) RT^1(−)	PAP(+) RT^1(−)	PAP(−) RT^1(+)	PAP(+) RT^1(+)	Total	Kappa (95%CI)
Original	PAP(−) RT(−)	14	9	2	0	25	0.098 (0.001;0.22)
	PAP(+) RT(−)	9	11	2	3	25	
	PAP(−) RT(+)	17	1	3	0	21	
	PAP(+) RT(+)	6	1	14	3	24	
	Total	46	22	21	6	95	
2nd re-evaluation	PAP(−) RT(−)	12	3	2	1	18	0.281 (0.14;0.41)
	PAP(+) RT(−)	11	17	2	2	32	
	PAP(−) RT(+)	21	1	13	1	36	
	PAP(+) RT(+)	2	1	3	2	8	
	Total	46	22	20	6	94	

PAP(−) Normal Pap test, *PAP(+)* Abnormal Pap test, *RT(−)* No radiotherapy, *RT(+)* Radiotherapy, *1* Identification of post radiotherapy effects in cells

cytopathologists and presented a gradual increase during the diagnostic evaluations with values for kappa ranging from 0.76 to 1.00. In a Norwegian study, the number of Pap smears evaluated as abnormal (ASC-US+) by the four pathologists varied from 61 to 85. The number of high-grade cytology (ASC-H+) varied from 26 to 50. There was moderate agreement (weighted kappa 0.45–0.58) between the observers [10]. In the ATHENA study, there were considerable differences among the laboratories both in overall cytological abnormal rates, ranging from 3.8 to 9.9%, and in sensitivity of cytology to detect CIN grade 2 or worse (CIN2+), from 42.0 to 73.0% [11].

The hypothesis here is that some patients who undergo RT may experience exfoliation of the epithelium over time (regeneration) and thus the cells under post radiotherapy effect may disappear giving rise to new cells without changes. This could explain the fact that patients in this study who underwent RT had no cytological changes from the radiation. In addition, some patients may have received vaginal hormone therapy with estrogen that could influence the disappearance of post radiotherapy CA.

It is relevant to note that this research includes an original methodology whose correlation of intraobserver reproducibility with prior RT information had not been studied to date. Although Stein et al. [16] point out that radiation produces a bias that favors the cytological categorization of uncertainty; this study emphasizes the need for cytotechnologists and cytopathologists to be able to recognize properly any type of abnormalities, regardless of whether they know the radiotherapy history of a slide. This is an important issue in order to improve the quality of the cytological interpretation and consequently reduce the errors of cytopathological classification.

The main limitation of this work was that the sample was small for the application of certain statistical tests, making it necessary to adapt some categories. However, the literature brings some studies with even smaller samples such as Lee et al. [17] with 50 randomized smear slides, as well as studies such as Stein with 10,165 cases of cervical cytology analyzed [16]. This study was conducted with only two cytopathologists and it is therefore difficult to generalize the findings to a broader population of cytopathologists. This could be a limitation for interobserver agreement, wherever the focus is in intraobserver reproducibility.

The strengths of this study lie in its prospective characteristic, in the use of liquid-based cytology that makes it possible to obtain a better smear with less unsatisfactory results, as well as in the evaluation of the intraobserver reproducibility. In addition, it is definitely a strength that the pathologist in the pathology department of BCH routinely reassessed all the dubious cytological diagnoses.

The intraobserver agreement was only moderate, suggesting there may have been influence of the knowledge of previous RT in the interpretation of the slides by the cytotechnologist. It was expected that this knowledge would lead to better agreement in the second CP

Table 5 List of the cytological abnormalities according to median time after end of radiotherapy

Cytological Abnormalities	Time < 364 days	Time ≥ 364 days	P-value*
ASC-US and LSIL	3 (60.0%)	2 (40.0%)	1.00
AGC, HSIL and ASC-H	9 (47.4%)	10 (52.6%)	1.00

*Fisher's exact test

AGC Atypical Glandular cells, *ASC-H* Atypical Squamous Cells cannot exclude HSIL, *ASC-US* Atypical Squamous Cells of Undetermined Significance, *HSIL* High Grade Squamous Intraepithelial lesion, *LSIL* Low Grade Squamous Intraepithelial lesion

re-evaluation, but this was not observed. Therefore, it has been shown that reproducibility is best when done by the same observer, since they are able to better identify proposed diagnoses.

The interobserver and intraobserver analysis concerning CP results agreement had high discrepancy in patients that received RT. Adequate knowledge about these abnormalities is imperative in order to avoid false positive diagnoses, since most of them are not associated with new intraepithelial/invasive lesions or tumor recurrence. Cytology and HPV cotesting increases the sensitivity and may reduce false positive diagnoses [18].

Conclusion

This study found that there is a difficulty on the part of the cytotechnologist to recognize cellular abnormalities due exclusively to RT when this information is not provided. It is important to emphasize, therefore, the importance of the personnel to inform at the time of the collection whether or not the patient received RT. The authors believe that cytology should not be indicated in follow-up after radiotherapy for cervical cancer treatment.

Abbreviations
AGC: Atypical Glandular Cells; ASC-H: Atypical Squamous Cells is not possible to exclude High-grade Intraepithelial Lesion; ASC-US: Atypical Squamous Cells of Undetermined Significance; BCH: Barretos Cancer Hospital; CA: Cytological Abnormalities; CP: Cytopathology; HSIL: High Grade Squamous Intraepithelial Lesion; RT: Radiotherapy

Funding
This work was supported by the FAPESP – Fundação de Amparo à Pesquisa do Estado de São Paulo. Process number: 2015/19964–5.

Authors' contributions
FL, RR, MD, JH, MA, CA, GF made contribution with the conception and design of the study.MD and RM made substantial contribution in the first evaluation, re-evaluation and interpretation of the slides. RF gave contribution in the statistical analysis and interpretation of the data results. RR, RF, FL,RM and MD agreed to be accountable for all aspects of the work in ensuring that questions related to the accuracy or integrity of any part of the work are appropriately investigated and resolved. FL, RR, CA, RM and JH been involved in drafting the manuscript or revising it critically for important intellectual content; All authors given final approval of the version to be published.

Competing interests
The authors declare that they have no competing interests.

Author details
¹Faculty of Health Science of Barretos Dr. Paulo Prata, Avenida Loja Maçônica Renovadora 68, N⁰ 100, Barretos 14785-002, São Paulo, Brazil. ²Department of Pathology, Barretos Cancer Hospital, Rua Antenor Duarte Villela, 1331 - Dr. Paulo Prata, Barretos 14784-400, São Paulo, Brazil. ³Department of Gynecologic Oncology, Barretos Cancer Hospital, Rua Antenor Duarte Villela, 1331 - Dr. Paulo Prata, Barretos 14784-400, São Paulo, Brazil. ⁴Post-Graduation Program in Oncology, Barretos Cancer Hospital, Rua Antenor Duarte Villela, 1331 - Dr. Paulo Prata, Barretos 14784-400, São Paulo, Brazil.

References

1. SOCIETY AC. Radiation therapy for cervical câncer 2014. Available from: http://www.cancer.org/cancer/cervicalcancer/detailedguide/cervical-cancer-treating-radiation
2. Shield PW. Chronic radiation effects: a correlative study of smears and biopsies from the cervix and vagina. Diagn Cytopathol. 1995;13(2):107–19.
3. Hatem F, Wilbur DC. High grade squamous cervical lesions following negative Papanicolaou smears: false-negative cervical cytology or rapid progression. Diagn Cytopathol. 1995;12(2):135–41.
4. Solomon D, Davey D, Kurman R, Moriarty A, O'Connor D, Prey M, Raab S, Sherman M, Wilbur D, Wright T Jr, Young N. The 2001 Bethesda system: terminology for reporting results of cervical cytology. JAMA. 2002;287(16):2114–9.
5. de Azevedo AEB, Carneiro FP, Neto FFC, Bocca AL, Teixeira LS, de Queiroz Maurício Filho MAF, de Magalhães AV. Association between human papillomavirus infection and cytological abnormalities during early follow-up of invasive cervical cancer. J Med Virol. 2012;84(7):1115–9.
6. Wright JD, Herzog TJ, Mutch DG, Gibb RK, Rader JS, Davila RM, Cohn DE. Liquid-based cytology for the postirradiation surveillance of women with gynecologic malignancies. Gynecol Oncol. 2003;91(1):134–8.
7. Lu CH, Chang CC, Ho ES, Chen SJ, Lin SJ, Fu TF, Chang MC. Should adequacy criteria in cervicovaginal cytology be modified after radiotherapy, chemotherapy, or hysterectomy? Cancer Cytopathol. 2010;118(6):474–81.
8. Levine PH, Elgert PA, Mittal K. False-positive squamous cell carcinoma in cervical smears: cytologic-histologic correlation in 19 cases. Diagn Cytopathol. 2003;28(1):23–7.
9. Morice P, Deyrolle C, Rey A, Atallah D, Pautier P, Camatte S, Thoury A, Lhomme C, Haie-Meder C, Castaigne D. Value of routine follow-up procedures for patients with stage I/II cervical cancer treated with combined surgery-radiation therapy. Ann Oncol. 2004 Feb;15(2):218–23.
10. Sørbye SW, Suhrke P, Revå BW, Berland J, Maurseth RJ, Al-Shibli K. Accuracy of cervical cytology: comparison of diagnoses of 100 pap smears read by four pathologists at three hospitals in Norway. BMC Clin Pathol. 2017;17(1):18.
11. Wright TC Jr, Stoler MH, Behrens CM, Sharma A, Sharma K, Apple R. Interlaboratory variation in the performance of liquid-based cytology: insights from the ATHENA trial. Int J Cancer. 2014;134(8):1835–43.
12. Stein MD, Fregnani JH, Scapulatempo-Neto C, Longatto-Filho A. Cervicovaginal cytology in patients undergoing pelvic radiotherapy using the Focalpoint system: results from the RODEO study. Diagn Pathol. 2015;10(1):1.
13. Landis JR, Koch GG. The measurement of observer agreement for categorical data. Biometrics. 1977;33(1):159–74.
14. Settakorn J, Rangdaeng S, Preechapornkul N, Nateewatana S, Pongsiralai K, Srisomboon J, Thorner PS. Interobserver reproducibility with LiquiPrep liquid-based cervical cytology screening in a developing country. Asian Pac J Cancer Prev. 2008;9:92–6.
15. Tsilalis T, Archondakis S, Meristoudis C, Margari N, Pouliakis A, Skagias L, Panayiotides I, Karakitsos P. Assessment of static telecytological diagnoses' reproducibility in cervical smears prepared by means of liquid-based cytology. Telemed J E Health. 2012;18(7):516–20.
16. Stein MD, Fregnani JH, Scapulatempo C, Mafra A, Campacci N, Longatto-Filho A, et al. Performance and reproducibility of gynecologic cytology interpretation using the FocalPoint system: results of the RODEO Study Team. Am J Clin Pathol. 2013;140(4):567–71.
17. Lee ES, Kim IS, Choi JS, Yeom BW, Kim HK, Han JH, et al. Accuracy and reproducibility of telecytology diagnosis of cervical smears. A tool for quality assurance programs. Am J Clin Pathol. 2003;119(3):356–60.
18. Wright TC Jr, Stoler MH, Aslam S, Behrens CM. Knowledge of Patients' human papillomavirus status at the time of Cytologic review significantly affects the performance of cervical cytology in the ATHENA study. Am J Clin Pathol 2016 Sep;146(3):391–398.

29

Traceability and distribution of *Neisseria meningitidis* DNA in archived post mortem tissue samples from patients with systemic meningococcal disease

Berit Sletbakk Brusletto[1,2]*, Bernt Christian Hellerud[4], Else Marit Løberg[3,2], Ingeborg Løstegaard Goverud[3,2], Åshild Vege[5,2], Jens Petter Berg[1,2], Petter Brandtzaeg[1,2] and Reidun Øvstebø[1]

Abstract

Background: The pathophysiology and outcome of meningococcal septic shock is closely associated with the plasma level of *N. meningitidis* lipopolysaccharides (LPS, endotoxin) and the circulating level of meningococcal DNA. The aim of the present study was to quantify the number of *N. meningitidis* in different formalin-fixed, paraffin-embedded (FFPE) tissue samples and fresh frozen (FF) tissue samples from patients with systemic meningococcal disease (SMD), to explore the distribution of *N. meningitidis* in the body.

Methods: DNA in FFPE and FF tissue samples from heart, lungs, liver, kidneys, spleen and brain from patients with meningococcal shock and controls (lethal pneumococcal infection) stored at variable times, were isolated. The bacterial load of *N. meningitidis* DNA was analyzed using quantitative real-time PCR (qPCR) and primers for the capsule transport A (ctrA) gene (1 copy per *N. meningitidis* DNA). The human beta-hemoglobin (HBB) gene was quantified to evaluate effect of the storage times (2-28 years) and storage method in archived tissue.

Results: *N. meningitidis* DNA was detected in FFPE and FF tissue samples from heart, lung, liver, kidney, and spleen in all patients with severe shock. In FFPE brain, *N. meningitidis* DNA was only detected in the patient with the highest concentration of LPS in the blood at admission to hospital. The highest levels of *N. meningitidis* DNA were found in heart tissue (median value 3.6×10^7 copies *N. meningitidis* DNA/µg human DNA) and lung tissue (median value 3.1×10^7 copies *N. meningitidis* DNA/µg human DNA) in all five patients. *N. meningitidis* DNA was not detectable in any of the tissue samples from two patients with clinical meningitis and the controls (pneumococcal infection). The quantity of HBB declined over time in FFPE tissue stored at room temperature, suggesting degradation of DNA.

Conclusions: High levels of *N. meningitidis* DNA were detected in the different tissue samples from meningococcal shock patients, particularly in the heart and lungs suggesting seeding and major proliferation of meningococci in these organs during the development of shock, probably contributing to the multiple organ failure. The age of archived tissue samples appear to have an impact on the amount of quantifiable *N. meningitidis* DNA.

Keywords: Systemic meningococcal disease, *Neisseria meningitidis*, FFPE, ctrA gene, Quality of archived tissue

* Correspondence: berit.brusletto@medisin.uio.no
[1]Blood Cell Research Group, Section for Research, Department of Medical Biochemistry, Oslo University Hospital HF, Ullevål Hospital, PO Box 4956 Nydalen, 0424 Oslo, Norway
[2]Institute of Clinical Medicine, University of Oslo, Oslo, Norway
Full list of author information is available at the end of the article

Background

Meningococcal infections remain a major public health problem worldwide with a case fatality rate (CFR) of 7-11% in sporadic cases increasing to 20-52% in outbreak situations in Europe and USA [1–3]. Approximately 30% of patients with systemic meningococcal disease (SMD) in Europe develop septic shock [2, 3]. Circulatory collapse is the primary cause of death owing to the combined effect of extreme vasodilation and septic cardiac failure resistant to treatment. The pathophysiology of SMD is closely associated with the ability of *N. meningitidis* to proliferate in the blood and subsequently invade the meninges, as documented by qPCR [2, 4–11]. Fulminant meningococcal septicemia, the most feared clinical presentation, is characterized by rapid progression of septic shock, large petechiae and ecchymoses, disseminated intravascular coagulation (DIC) and renal and pulmonary failure [1, 2, 9, 12, 13]. Post mortem examinations reveal hemorrhagic adrenals in the majority of the patients, "shock"-kidneys often with multiple thrombi in glomeruli, normal or congested lungs sometimes with thrombi and occasionally inflammatory foci in epi- and myocardium [10, 13]. The findings are in line with those described by Ferguson and Chapman [14].

Patients presenting with distinct symptoms of meningitis without shock is the most common presentation and have a much better prognosis than those with shock [1–3]. The number of meningococci and the LPS level in the plasma in these patients are low or undetectable [11] while the levels of meningococcal DNA, LPS and cytokines are 100- to 1000-fold higher in cerebrospinal fluid (CSF) than in blood [1, 2]. Death may be caused by brain edema and herniation of cerebellum.

The pathophysiology and outcome of meningococcal septic shock is closely associated with the plasma level of *N. meningitidis* lipopolysaccharides (LPS, endotoxin) and the circulating level of meningococcal DNA [4, 6, 11]. A rapid proliferation of *N. meningitidis* will result in huge amounts of LPS-containing material in plasma, and 95% of the patients with LPS levels in plasma above 10 endotoxin units (EU) /mL develop persistent shock with a detrimental activation of the innate immune system [1, 2, 9, 10, 12, 15, 16]. LPS, present in the membrane of the bacteria, are the most important but not the only meningococcal molecules that induce inflammation [17, 18].

A few studies have previously addressed detection and distribution of *N. meningitidis* DNA in FFPE human tissue [19, 20] but none has compared the results with FF tissue from the same post mortem examination. Recently, a porcine model of meningococcal septic shock, using the heat inactivated *N. meningitidis*, documented that large numbers of meningococci accumulated in the lungs, heart, liver, spleen and kidneys inducing a massive

organ inflammation [21]. Similar results were found in three patients with lethal meningococcal septic shock by examining fresh frozen (FF) tissue from the same organs [21]. As an extension of this study, we aimed to detect and quantify *N. meningitidis* DNA i.e. copy numbers using qPCR in tissue samples from different organs obtained by post mortem examination. The tissue samples were formalin-fixed, paraffin-embedded (FFPE) and stored at room temperature (20 – 25 °C) for up to 28 years. A human endogenous DNA control was included to evaluate the effect of storage time on degradation of tissue samples. Furthermore, we compared the qPCR results obtained from FFPE tissue stored at 20 – 25 °C with FF tissue stored at –80 °C for up to six years.

Methods
Clinical definitions
Systemic meningococcal disease (SMD) was present if *N.meningitidis* was cultivated or (–and) confirmed by polymerase chain reaction (PCR) in blood and/or (CSF) [4, 11].

Severe septic shock was defined as persistent hypotension because of bacterial infection, with an initial systolic blood pressure < 90 mmHg in adults (≥ 12 year) and <70 mmHg in children (< 12 year), that required fluid therapy and treatment with vasoactive drugs (dopamine, epinephrine, norepinephrine) for at least 24 h or until death [4].

Transient shock was defined as hypotension, as defined above, requiring volume treatment combined with vasoactive drugs for less than 6 h to stabilize the circulation.

Multiple organ failure was defined as: 1) reduced pulmonary function requiring artificial ventilation to maintain an adequate arterial oxygenation and 2) renal failure with reduced creatinine clearance (<60 mL /minute per 1.73 m^2 body surface) or pathologically elevated serum creatinine (related to age and collected within 12 h after admission).

Clinical meningitis was defined as nuchal and back rigidity with positive Kernig's and/or Brudzinski's signs and pleocytosis with ≥100 × 10^6 leukocytes/L CSF.

Subjects
Altogether seven patients were included in the study. Five patients (No 1 – 5) had severe shock without clinical meningitis whereas patient 6 had clinical meningitis without shock and patient 7 had clinical meningitis and transient shock (Table 1).

Formalin-fixed, paraffin-embedded (FFPE) tissue from patients with meningococcal shock and multiple organ failure (patient No 1 – 5): The formalin-fixed, paraffin-embedded tissues were selected according to histopathological findings; presence of neutrophilic inflammatory infiltrates or thrombi. Small tissue specimens from five

Table 1 Patients with systemic meningococcal disease and their clinical characteristics

Patient No Serogroup	Neisserial DNA; copy number of N.meningitidis/mL LPS (LAL); EU/mL at admission to hospital* not available	Age of tissue at isolation time of DNA (years)	Type of storage methods	Type of organ tissue	Findings at autopsy # no obviously pathological changes
1 Serogroup B	2.8x10^{8}copies/mL (plasma) 2100 EU/mL (plasma) No spinal puncture was performed	11	FFPE	Skin Adrenal glands Lungs Heart Liver Kidneys Spleen Brain	Skin hemorrhages Hemorrhage Edema Petechiae on epicard and endocard # Dark-red congested medulla and pale cortex (shock kidneys). Fibrin thrombi in glomeruli. # Fibrin thrombi in vessels in choroid plexus
2 Serogroup B	3.8x10^{7}copies/mL (plasma) 271 EU/mL (plasma) No spinal puncture was performed	10	FFPE	Skin Adrenal glands Lungs Heart Liver Kidneys Spleen Brain	Skin hemorrhages Hemorrhage An localized area with atelectasis, some neutrophils and small hemorrhages. Fibrin thrombi in vessels. Petechiae on epicard # Congested vessels in medulla and fibrin thrombi in glomeruli # Fibrin thrombi in some vessels
3 Serogroup B most likely	1.0x10^{8}copies/mL (serum) 2140 EU/mL (serum) Spinal puncture was performed post mortem. CSF contained 8 EU/mL	5 5	FFPE FF	Skin Adrenal glands Lungs Heart Liver Kidneys Spleen Brain	Skin hemorrhages Hemorrhage # Petechiae on epicard # Dark-red congested medulla and pale cortex (shock kidneys) # #
4 Serogroup C	3.0x10^{7}copies/mL (serum) 3800 EU/mL (serum) No spinal puncture was performed	2 2	FFPE FF	Skin Adrenal glands Lungs Heart Liver Kidneys Spleen Brain	Skin hemorrhages Hemorrhage Congestion Petechiae on epicard. Microabscess in myocard # Congested vessels in medulla and multiple fibrin thrombi in glomeruli # #
5 Serogroup C	* * *	6 6	FFPE FF	Skin Adrenal glands Lungs Heart Liver Kidneys Spleen Brain	Skin hemorrhages Hemorrhage # # # # # #
6 Serogroup B	0.25 EU/mL (plasma) *	28	FFPE	Lungs Heart Liver Kidneys Spleen Brain	Edema # # # # Edema, herniation of cerebellum, pus in meninges
7 Serogroup B	1.1x10^{5}copies/mL (plasma) 2.1 EU/mL (plasma) 4000 EU/mL (CSF)	28	FFPE	Lungs Kidneys Brain	Edema # Edema, herniation of cerebellum, pus in meninges

lungs, four hearts, four livers, four kidneys, three spleens and four brains were available.

The samples were collected during the routine post mortem examination within 24 h after the patient died. The storage times of the FFPE tissue samples were 11, 10, 6, 5 and 2 years (Table 1).

Fresh frozen (FF) tissue specimens from patients with meningococcal shock and multiple organ failure (patient No 3 – 5): Three lungs, three hearts, two livers, three kidneys, three spleens and one brain were collected in parallel with the routine post mortem examination and frozen at −80 °C for later analysis. The storage times of the FF tissue were 6, 5 and 2 years. The samples had been partially thawed once and examined before this analysis [21].

Formalin-fixed, paraffin-embedded (FFPE) tissue from patients with clinical meningitis and herniation of cerebellum (No 6 and 7): FFPE tissue from both patients were stored for 28 years. FFPE tissue samples from lungs, liver, spleen, kidneys and brain from patient No 6 and lung, kidney and brain from patient No 7 were analyzed.

Formalin-fixed, paraffin-embedded (FFPE) tissue from patients with lethal systemic pneumococcal infection (negative controls): FFPE tissue from two patients with microbiologically verified lethal pneumococcal infection with positive blood cultures served as negative controls. The storage time of the specimens was four and six years, respectively. Tissue from lungs, heart, liver, spleen, kidneys and brain were analyzed. The organ samples were collected at routine post mortem examination 24-48 h after death.

Autopsy procedure

The study was carried out at the Department of Pathology, Oslo University Hospital, Department of Pathology Stavanger University Hospital, and at the Section for Forensic Pediatric Pathology, Oslo University Hospital, Oslo, Norway (former: Department of Research and Development in Forensic Pathology, The Norwegian Institute of Public Health, Oslo, Norway). All the autopsies have been carried out by pathologists on duty and according to routine procedures (which include sterile equipment for microbiological sampling).

Fixation and paraffination procedure

All FFPE tissue samples were prepared according to routine procedures. The protocol for fixation of most tissue used in this study was as follows: The tissue samples were fixed in 4% buffered −neutral formalin, at room temperature for 6-48 h. Thereafter the tissue blocks were dehydrated, cleared and infiltrated with the embedding material in automated tissue processors ready for external embedding in paraffin.

The whole brain was fixed in unbuffered formalin for at least 3 weeks at room temperature before samples

from different regions of the brain were processed further in an automated tissue processor.

All tissue samples stored for 28 years before DNA isolating time (meningitis patients) had been fixed in unbuffered formalin, at room temperature for 6-24 h. Thereafter the tissue blocks were prepared as the other tissue samples.

Tissue staining

Tissue sections, 3 µm thick, were placed on slides, deparaffinized, and rehydrated through degraded alcohols and distilled water. Then the sections were stained with hematoxylin and eosin (HE) staining and Acid Fuchsin Orange K (AFOG) staining. All microscopy slides were examined by an experienced pathologist.

DNA extraction

DNA from freshly cut slices of five 10 µm-thick sections of archival FFPE blocks was isolated in parallel samples. The samples with the sections were immediately placed in 1 mL of Xylenes (cat.no: 534,056 Sigma −Aldrich) in a microcentrifuge tube for deparaffinization. The QIAamp DNA FFPE tissue kit (Qiagen, Hilden, Germany) was used for the extraction of DNA in the QIAcube robot www.qiagen.com/MyQIAcube according to manufacturer's instructions. RNase A was added to degrade RNA in the DNA samples. The DNA was eluted in 40 µL ATE buffer. Negative control (one sample without tissue sample) was subjected for isolation to check for contaminations. DNA samples were stored at −80 °C before further analysis.

DNA isolated in parallel from freshly cut sections of FFPE tissue gave almost similar yield and purity (260/280 ratio) for the parallel sections (data not shown). Therefore, only one of the samples from the parallel isolation of DNA from each tissue was used in the qPCR.

DNA from FF: 50 mg of frozen tissue was placed in 400 µL MagNA Pure DNA tissue lysis buffer (Roche Applies Science, Indianapolis, IN), then homogenized using a Xiril Dispomix (AH diagnostics, Aarhus, Denmark). Furthermore the samples were incubated for 30 min at room temperature for lysis, transferred to Nunc tubes and stored at −80 °C until analysis. The MagNA Pure LC DNA Isolation Kit II (Tissue kit) (Roche Applies Science, Indianapolis, IN) was used for extraction of DNA in the MagNA Pure LC Robot (Roche Applies Science, Indianapolis, IN) according to manufacturer's instructions. The DNA was eluted in 200 µL Elution Buffer and stored at -80 °C before further analysis. DNA concentration and purity (260/280 ratio) were determined with the NanoDrop ND-1000 Spectrophotometer (Thermo Fisher Scientific, Waltham, MA).

Quantitative real-time PCR

Quantitative real-time PCR (qPCR) with oligonucleotide primers for capsule transport A (ctrA) [22] (GenBank sequence M80593) [7], was used to quantify meningo-coccal DNA. A standard curve (range 10 ng to 0.01 pg, 7 standards) generated from known amount of DNA isolated from *N.meningitidis* was used for quantification. Each standard point was analyzed in triplicates and a new standard curve was included in every PCR analysis. The PCR efficiency and R^2 value were 92% and 0.996 ($n = 13$) respectively.

Sensitivity: The lower limit of detection (LLD) of the ctrA qPCR assay was 0.01 pg of genomic DNA. The coefficient of inter assay variation (CV %) based on an in house control, (DNA from *N.meningitidis*) was 2.4% measured as obtained cycle threshold (Ct) value and 31.9% when calculated from the standard curve. If no increase in the fluorescence signal was observed after 35 cycles, the sample was assumed to be negative. To rule out false negative results (due to inhibition) all samples were diluted from 100 to 0.01 ng DNA in the qPCR reaction.

Specificity: There were no cross-reaction using ctrA primers with human genomic DNA from negative controls, FFPE from patients with lethal pneumococcal infection or from patients suffering from a non-inflammatory disease (data not shown). A negative sample for ctrA had to simultaneously have a Ct value ≤35 for HBB. If not, the DNA in the sample was assumed to be too degraded to be included in the study.

Quality of isolated DNA from FFPE and FF tissue

To evaluate the quality of the DNA extraction and to verify the presence of amplifiable DNA, amplification of the human beta-hemoglobin (Human hemoglobin, beta HBB Hs00758889_s1, Thermo Fisher TaqMan® gene expression assay) [23–25] from every patient sample was analyzed. The inter assay variation (CV %) of an in house endogenous HBB control was 2.9% (Ct values). The association between storage time and Ct values was evaluated by quantification of HBB in lung tissue samples from FFPE and FF (Fig 1).

Quality of DNA to quantitative real-time PCR

To check for inhibition in the PCR reaction and to determine amount of input DNA, serial dilutions (ranging 100-0.1 ng) of DNA was used [20, 26]. DNA (5 µL) was amplified in 25 µL reaction volumes containing (Life technologies) 1.25 µL TaqMan® Gene expression assay (20X), 12.5 µL TaqMan® Universal Master Mix II (2X) and 6.25 µL RNase-free water.

Input of 100 ng DNA to the PCR reaction (quantified by the NanoDrop ND-1000 Spectrophotometer) was found appropriate for both *N. meningitidis* DNA and HBB quantification. The assays were carried out with the ViiA™ 7 Real-Time PCR systems (Applied Biosystems by Life Technologies, Carlsbad, CA 92008 USA) using the following cycling parameters: 50 °C for 2 min, then

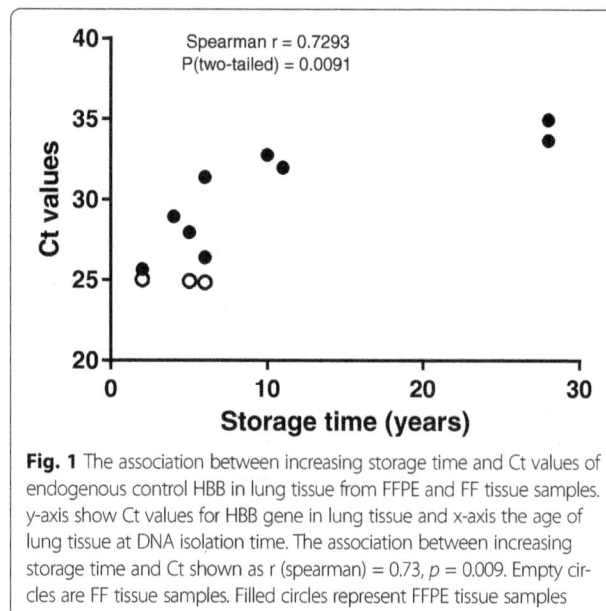

Fig. 1 The association between increasing storage time and Ct values of endogenous control HBB in lung tissue from FFPE and FF tissue samples. y-axis show Ct values for HBB gene in lung tissue and x-axis the age of lung tissue at DNA isolation time. The association between increasing storage time and Ct shown as r (spearman) = 0.73, p = 0.009. Empty circles are FF tissue samples. Filled circles represent FFPE tissue samples

95 °C for 10 min followed by 40 cycles of a 2-stage temperature profile of 95 °C for 15 s and 60 °C for 1 min. If no increase in the fluorescence signal was observed after 35 cycles, the sample was assumed to be negative. The final calculation of the bacterial load (copies *N. meningitidis* DNA/µg tissue DNA) and HBB gene (Ct) from samples and controls was performed by the software provided with the Applied Biosystems ViiA™ 7.

Only duplicate positive results for quantification of parallel samples from both *N. meningitidis* DNA and HBB were finally considered as positive. A no template control, a positive control for *N. meningitidis* DNA and a positive control for HBB were included in every run.

Quantification of *N.meningitidis* DNA and LPS in plasma/serum/CSF from patients with meningococcal disease in samples collected on hospital admission

The heparin-blood was collected, centrifuged, plasma pipetted off and aliquoted as described in detail earlier [4, 27]. Quantification of *N. meningitidis* DNA was performed as previously described in detail [11, 28]. The detection limit was 10^3 *N.meningitidis* DNA copies/mL.

Quantification of LPS in plasma/serum/CSF was initially performed with an in house developed limulus amebocyte lysate (LAL) assay and later with Chromo-LAL (Associates of Cape Cod, USA) with a detection limit of 0.2 EU/mL. The serum level is on average 63% of the plasma level [4, 27].

Statistical analysis

The GraphPad Prism Software Version 6.07 (GraphPad Software, San Diego, CA, USA) was used for all statistical analysis.

Results

DNA extraction: Yield and purity

DNA isolated from one to six different FFPE tissue samples from five patients with meningococcal shock disease ranged from 33.5 - 282.7 ng/µL, (n = 25 and median ng/µL = 83) in concentration and from 1.72-2.05 (260/280 ratio) in purity.

DNA isolated from FFPE tissue samples from patients with meningococcal meningitis ranged from 28.1-90.2 ng/µL, (n = 11 and median ng/µL = 60.3) in concentration and from 1.64-2.16 (260/280 ratio) in purity.

The DNA isolated from FFPE tissue samples from negative controls (*pneumococcal infection)* ranged from 48.3-214.3 ng/µL, (n = 12 and median ng/µL = 85.4) in concentration and from 1.38-1.94 (260/280 ratio) in purity.

DNA isolated from FF tissue from three patients with meningococcal disease ranged from 29.5-171.5 ng/µL, (n = 15 and median ng/µL = 74.3) in concentration and from1.73-1.98 (260/280 ratio) in purity.

Evaluation of the quality of isolated DNA from FFPE and FF tissue

The endogenous control HBB quantified in 100 ng FFPE and FF tissue showed variable Ct values dependent on age of storage and storage methods. In FF tissue we found Ct values around 25 (mean Ct value in lung tissue), range 24.84-25.03. In 28 years old FFPE tissue, Ct value was around 34.3 (mean Ct value in lung tissue), range 33.67-34.96. Storage time of tissue sample at DNA isolating time point was positively correlated to HBB Ct values, (Spearman r = 0.73, p = 0.009, n = 12) (Fig. 1).

Quantification of *N.meningitidis* DNA and LPS in plasma/serum or CSF from patients with severe shock and multiple organ failure

The number of *N.meningitidis*/mL in the circulation of the patients with meningococcal shock ranged from 3.0×10^7/mL to 2.8×10^8/mL (Table 1). LPS in plasma or serum ranged from 271 EU/mL to 3800 EU/mL (Table 1).

Patient 6 with clinical meningitis had LPS values in serum <0.25 EU/mL. CSF was not available for analysis. Patient 7 had *N. meningitidis* DNA 1.1×10^5 copies/mL and LPS 2.1 EU/mL in plasma and 4000 EU/mL of LPS in CSF. CSF for *N. meningitidis* DNA quantification was not available (Table 1).

Quantification of *Neisseria meningitidis* DNA in FFPE and FF tissue from patients with meningococcal shock and multiple organ failure

N.meningitidis DNA was detected in FFPE tissue in all patients with severe shock and multiple organ failure (Table 2 and Fig 2). The amount of *N. meningitidis*

DNA found in FFPE tissue from each patient showed large variability. For patient 1 and 2 the concentrations of *N. meningitidis* DNA in the organs ranged from $8,1 \times 10^4$ -$1,3 \times 10^6$ copies *N. meningitidis* DNA /µg human DNA. The storage time of these FFPE tissue was above 10 years. In patient 3, 4 and 5 with storage time of five, two and six years, the concentration of *N. meningitidis* DNA was above 1.3×10^6 copies *N. meningitidis* DNA /µg human DNA for most tissue, ranged from 1.1×10^5 -1.2×10^9 copies *N. meningitidis* DNA /µg human DNA (Table 2 and Fig 2).

Patient 4 had the highest concentration of *N. meningitidis* DNA in all organs of the five patients with severe shock and multiple organ failure, where the concentration ranged from 2.8×10^5-1.2×10^9 copies *N. meningitidis* DNA /µg human DNA. In this patient *N. meningitidis* DNA was also detected in the brain tissue with 2.8×10^5 copies *N. meningitidis* DNA /µg human DNA. Lung and liver tissue contained the highest concentration of *N. meningitidis* DNA as compared to the other organs. The storage time of these FFPE samples was only 2 years. This patient also had the highest concentration of LPS in the serum samples collected on hospital admission.

To evaluate the storage methods, we compared the levels of *N. meningitidis* DNA in FF tissue with FFPE tissue from three patients (3, 4 and 5) (Table 2 and Fig. 2). *N. meningitidis* DNA was present in all FF tissue. From patient 3, FF tissue from the brain was available and $5.2 \times 10e^7$ copies of *N. meningitidis* DNA /µg human DNA was detected. In general, we found higher levels of *N. meningitidis* DNA in FF tissue in patient 3 and 5 as compared with FFPE tissue. In patient 4, the amount of *N. meningitidis* DNA was higher in most FFPE tissue compared to FF tissue. The storage time of these samples was only 2 years.

The FF tissue results in patient 4 revealed the highest concentration of *N. meningitidis* DNA in lungs, liver and heart and were in accordance with the results obtained with FFPE tissue. The *N. meningitidis* DNA concentration in FFPE lung tissue however, was four times higher than in FF lung tissue (Table 2).

Quantification of *Neisseria meningitidis* DNA in FFPE tissue from patients with meningococcal meningitis and cerebellar herniation

N.meningitidis DNA was not detected in any FFPE tissue samples, including brain tissue, from the two patients with meningococcal meningitis (storage time 28 years) (Table 2).

Quantification of *Neisseria meningitidis* DNA in FFPE tissue from patients with lethal pneumococcal infection

N.meningitidis DNA was not detected in any of the tissue.

Table 2 Quantification of *N. meningitidis* DNA in FFPE and FF tissue from patients with systemic meningococcal disease

Patient No	Age of tissue at isolation time for DNA (years)	Type of organ	Copies *N. meningitidis* DNA/µg human DNA * not available	
			FFPE	FF
1	11	Lung	7.9x10e5	
		Heart	2.9x10e5	
		Liver	8.2x10e5	
		Kidney	5.3x10e5	
		Spleen	9.1x10e4	
		Brain	0	
2	10	Lung	1.0x10e6	
		Heart	1.3x10e6	
		Liver	2.2x10e5	
		Kidney	8.3x10e5	
		Spleen	8.1x10e4	
		Brain	0	
3	5	Lung	2.1x10e7	2.4x10e8
		Heart	4.6x10e7	4.2x10e6
		Liver	5.8x10e5	*
		Kidney	3.2x10e6	6.3x10e7
		Spleen	1.1x10e5	5.9x10e6
		Brain	0	5.2x10e7
4	2	Lung	1.2x10e9	2.3x10e8
		Heart	1.7x10e8	6.1x10e7
		Liver	3.3x10e8	1.2x10e8
		Kidney	1.4x10e7	8.3x10e7
		Spleen	*	4.3x10e7
		Brain	2.8x10e5	*
5	6	Lung	1.5x10e7	4.1x10e7
		Heart	*	3.5x10e7
		Liver	*	1.7x10e7
		Kidney	*	9.9x10e6
		Spleen	*	*
6	28	Lung	0	
		Heart	*	
		Liver	0	
		Kidney	0	
		Spleen	0	
		Brain	0	
7	28	Lung	0	
		Kidney	0	
		Brain	0	

Discussion

In this study, we detected *N. meningitidis* DNA in FFPE and FF tissue from the lungs, heart, liver, kidneys and spleen in five patients dying of severe meningococcal shock and multiple organ failure. The highest concentration of *N meningitidis* DNA was found in the lungs and hearts. In one patient (No 4), with the highest levels of meningococcal DNA and LPS in plasma, *N. meningitidis* DNA was also

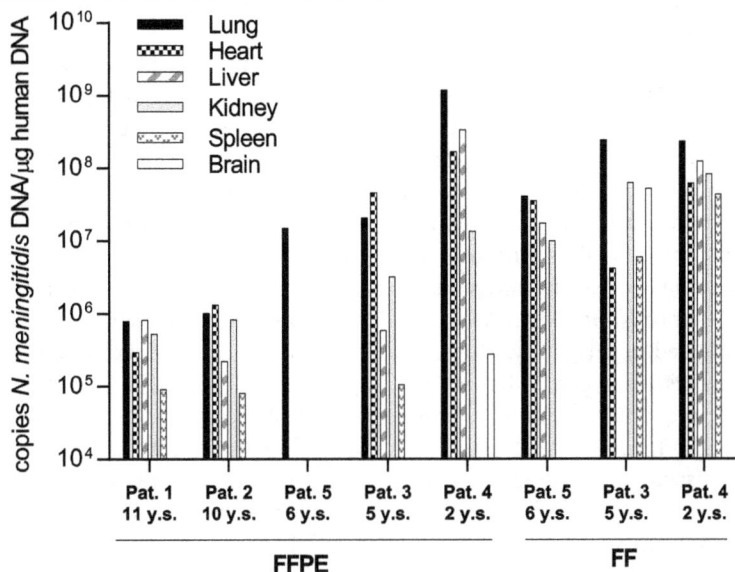

Fig. 2 Quantification of *N.meningitidis* DNA in FFPE and FF tissue from patients with systemic meningococcal disease. Input of 100 ng DNA from different tissue samples were quantified using specific *N.meningitidis* primers (capsule transport A) and quantitative PCR. The y-axis show the *N.meningitidis* DNA concentration, the x-axis show patients number (No 1-5), storage methods (FFPE and FF) and storage time at DNA isolating time (y.s)

detected in the brain FFPE tissue. In FF brain tissue from patient No 3 *N. meningitidis* DNA was also detected. Our results are in line with the current view that fulminant meningococcal septic shock and multiple organ failure is a compartmentalized infection with a massive proliferation of the bacteria in the circulation spreading to different large organs and the skin where they accumulate in large number. *N. meningitidis* can be detected in the CSF in shock patients but usually in much lower number as compared with patients with clinical symptoms of meningitis [4, 5, 11]. Our results are also in line with Fernández-Rodríguez et al. and Guarner et al. who detected *N. meningitidis* DNA in 81-100% of FFPE tissue from patients with meningococcal sudden deaths [19, 20]. Our previously published results also suggest that the majority of the nonviable bacteria could be disintegrated in various organs still exerting a powerful stimulus of the local innate immune system [21].

Brain tissue from two patients (6 and 7) dying of meningitis resulting in brain edema and cerebellar herniation, were without detectable *N. meningitidis* DNA in the brain and other organs. We know from previous studies that patients with meningitis as a group have high levels of LPS and inflammatory mediators as well as *N. meningitidis* DNA in CSF [1, 2, 5, 11, 29, 30]. In this study, the LPS level in CSF in one of two meningitis patients (No 7) was 4000 EU/mL, documenting a massive proliferation of meningococci in CSF. The storage time of tissue from brain and other organs, however, was 28 years at room temperature for both meningitis patients. We interpret our negative results in the brain tissue as a consequence

of gradual degradation of DNA due to storage time (over 28 years) at room temperature and fixation in unbuffered formalin [31, 32]. Quantitative measurements of HBB DNA suggest that human DNA is degraded over time as indicated in Fig. 1. We assume that the same is the case for bacterial DNA in human tissue stored at room temperature.

In the two patients (No 6 and 7) dying of cerebellar herniation all extracranial organs examined, were *N. meningitidis* PCR negative. In addition to degradation of DNA as discussed above, the negative results could reflect low seeding of the different organs. Both patients had low levels of LPS in plasma (Table 1) indicating a low bacterial load in the circulation and possibly tissue concentrations of *N. meningitidis* below detection level (true negative results) [2, 5, 11]. Since few patients with distinct clinical meningococcal meningitis without shock die, we did not have any recent post mortem tissues to verify this hypothesis.

The patients with lethal pneumococcal disease serving as negative controls, had as expected no detectable *N. meningitidis* DNA. We did not quantify the amount of *Streptococcus pneumoniae* DNA in the different tissue in these two control patients, however, in a recently published study, comprising 11 patients with systemic pneumococcal infections, FF tissue from the large organs contained $10^4 - 2 \times 10^6$ pneumococci per gram tissue, the highest levels detected in the lungs [21].

Does the copy number of *N. meningitidis* in the different tissues represent bacterial components located primarily in the capillaries of the different organs or do they indicate meningococcal molecules, primarily LPS, which trigger tissue macrophages and induce local inflammation? A histological case study of one patient with lethal meningococcal sepsis suggested that meningococci mainly adhered to capillaries located in low flow regions in the infected organs [33]. Presumably they proliferate in the capillary vascular bed [33]. The capillary density is known to vary anatomically and functionally in different organs as well as within a single organ [34, 35]. How capillary density and volume may influence the distribution of *N. meningitidis* in different organs is not investigated in this study. However, we have previously found massive organ inflammation by using multiplex assay and quantified tumor necrosis factor (TNF), interleukin (IL)-1β, IL-6 and IL-8 in homogenized fresh frozen tissue samples from lungs, heart, liver, spleen, kidneys and adrenals from patients 3,4 and 5 [21]. These observations suggest that LPS and other neisserial molecules are recognized by tissue macrophages in the different organs, implying that the bacterial components are located in the tissues and trigger a local immune response varying from organ to organ.

Pre-analytical factors that may have an influence on the DNA analysis of FFPE tissue can be: postmortem interval (PMI), cold ischemia time (time between biospecimen removal from the body and its preservation), specimen size, fixative buffer (unbuffered formalin or neutral buffered formalin), fixative delivery method, fixative temperature and duration, block storage, section thickness and section storage, and methods of nucleic acids isolation [36–41]. Several reports have shown that the FFPE method will lead to degradation of DNA over time due to the formalin fixation of tissue before paraffin embedding [38].

To monitor the quality of DNA extraction and to verify the presence of amplifiable DNA in our study, an endogenous DNA control gene HBB was quantified in FFPE and FF tissue (Fig1) [23, 42, 43]. Not surprisingly, the highest amount of HBB was found in the FF tissue, with Ct values of about 25 which indicates high amounts of high quality DNA as starting point for PCR amplification. When quantifying HBB in FFPE tissue, increasing Ct values, i.e. lower levels of intact DNA, were found with increasing storage time (storage time 28 years showed Ct values around 34) indicating degradation of DNA over time. In accordance with other studies this verifies that storage time of the FFPE tissue block has a major impact on the concentration of DNA found in the tissue [20, 31, 41, 44, 45]. Several reports show that amplification of DNA despite degradation of DNA may be possible [31, 41, 46]. The PCR products that are amplified in this study have amplicons under 100 base pairs. It is highly recommended to design the amplicons to be

as short as possible when carrying out the qPCR of DNA from FFPE [47].

Storage time of FFPE tissue and deposit temperature are two parameters that may influence the traceability of specific DNA [20, 31, 41, 44, 45]. We conclude that meningococcal DNA can be detected in different tissue with the present qPCR assay after storage at room temperature for 11 years in meningococcal patients with shock and multiple organ failure. Storage for 28 years at room temperature gave negative results also in brain tissue with expected high concentration of meningococci in CSF on hospital admission. These results are supported by finding a significant positive association ($r = 0.73$) between storage time of tissue and amount of amplifiable endogenous control (HBB). Detectable levels of HBB DNA decline over the years, and suggest a degradation over time. The results are also in line with the findings of Fernández-Rodríguez et al. [20].

To evaluate the storage methods, we compared the levels of *N. meningitidis* DNA in fresh frozen (FF) tissue with FFPE tissue from three patients (3, 4 and 5) (Table 2 and Fig. 2). The tissue were 5, 2 and 6 years old, respectively. *N. meningitidis* DNA was detected in all tissue. In patient 3 and 5, the results showed a greater amount of *N. meningitidis* DNA in most FF tissue samples compared to FFPE, which is in line with previous studies [48, 49]. Patient 4 showed more similar levels of *N. meningitidis* DNA in the FFPE tissue and in FF tissue for most of the samples compared with patient 3 and 5. An explanation might be that the patient samples were only 2 years old and in good quality with less degradation of DNA.

Conclusion

Important observations from this study are that detection of *N.meningitidis* DNA by qPCR is possible in both FF tissue and in the conventional FFPE tissue. However, fixation methods and storage times are issues that may affect the results. Inclusion of an endogenous DNA control in the assays will give trustworthy results.

This study suggests that *N. meningitidis* DNA is present in high concentrations in many of the major organs in meningococcal patients with shock and multiple organ failure [21]. *N. meningitidis* may induce a strong molecular inflammatory response in various tissues without distinct visible microscopical changes owing to the short duration of the infection before death [21].

Abbreviations
AFOG: Acid Fuchsin Orange K; CFR: Case fatality rate; CSF: Cerebrospinal fluid; Ct: Cycle threshold; CV: Coefficient of variation; DIC: Disseminated intravascular coagulation; EU: Endotoxin unit; FF: Fresh frozen; FFPE: Formalin-fixed, paraffin-embedded; HBB: Human beta-hemoglobin; HE: Hematoxylin and eosin; IL: Interleukin; LAL: Limulus amebocyte lysate; LLD: Lower limit of detection; LPS: Lipopolysaccharides; PCR: Polymerase

chain reaction; PMI: Postmortem interval; qPCR: Quantitative real-time PCR; SMD: Systemic meningococcal disease; TNF: Tumor necrosis factor

Acknowledgments

Hege Ulland Dirdal at Division of Medical Service, Department of Pathology, Stavanger University Hospital, Stavanger, Norway.
Anne-Marie Siebke Trøseid at Blood Cell Research Group, Section for Research, Department of Medical Biochemistry, Oslo University Hospital, Norway.
Marit S. Hellum at Blood Cell Research Group, Section for Research, Department of Medical Biochemistry, Oslo University Hospital and Institute of Clinical Medicine, University of Oslo, Norway.

Funding

This research was funded by South –Eastern Norway Regional Health Authority program.

Authors' contributions

Study concept and design (BSB, RØ, PB, BCH, JPB); contributed with patient data and paraffin blocks from their hospital (ÅV, EML, BCH); performed laboratory experiments (BSB, IGL, RØ); performed statistical analysis and drafted the manuscript (BSB, RØ and PB); critical revision of the manuscript (BSB, RØ, PB, JPB, BCH, ÅV, EML, IGL); supervision (RØ, PB). All authors read and approved the final manuscript.

Competing interests

The authors state that they have no competing interest.

Author details

[1]Blood Cell Research Group, Section for Research, Department of Medical Biochemistry, Oslo University Hospital HF, Ullevål Hospital, PO Box 4956 Nydalen, 0424 Oslo, Norway. [2]Institute of Clinical Medicine, University of Oslo, Oslo, Norway. [3]Department of Pathology, Oslo University Hospital, Oslo, Norway. [4]Institute of Immunology, Oslo University Hospital, Oslo, Norway. [5]Section for Forensic Pediatric Pathology, Department of Forensic Sciences, Oslo University Hospital, Oslo, Norway.

References

1. van Deuren M, Brandtzaeg P. Parents' and gps' key role in diagnosis of meningococcal septicaemia. Lancet (London, England). 2000;356(9234):954–5.
2. Brandtzaeg P, van Deuren M. Classification and pathogenesis of meningococcal infections. Methods in molecular biology (Clifton, NJ). 2012;799:21–35.
3. Stoof SP, Rodenburg GD, Knol MJ, Rumke LW, Bovenkerk S, Berbers GA, Spanjaard L, van der Ende A, Sanders EA. Disease burden of invasive meningococcal disease in the netherlands between june 1999 and june 2011: a subjective role for serogroup and clonal complex. Clinical infectious diseases: an official publication of the Infectious Diseases Society of America. 2015;61(8):1281–92.
4. Brandtzaeg P, Kierulf P, Gaustad P, Skulberg A, Bruun JN, Halvorsen S, Sorensen E. Plasma endotoxin as a predictor of multiple organ failure and death in systemic meningococcal disease. J Infect Dis. 1989;159(2):195–204.
5. Brandtzaeg P, Ovsteboo R, Kierulf P. Compartmentalization of lipopolysaccharide production correlates with clinical presentation in meningococcal disease. J Infect Dis. 1992;166(3):650–2.
6. Hackett SJ, Guiver M, Marsh J, Sills JA, Thomson AP, Kaczmarski EB, Hart CA. Meningococcal bacterial DNA load at presentation correlates with disease severity. Arch Dis Child. 2002;86(1):44–6.
7. Corless CE, Guiver M, Borrow R, Edwards-Jones V, Fox AJ, Kaczmarski EB. Simultaneous detection of neisseria meningitidis, haemophilus influenzae, and streptococcus pneumoniae in suspected cases of meningitis and septicemia using real-time pcr. J Clin Microbiol. 2001;39(4):1553–8.
8. Darton T, Guiver M, Naylor S, Jack DL, Kaczmarski EB, Borrow R, Read RC. Severity of meningococcal disease associated with genomic bacterial load. Clinical infectious diseases: an official publication of the Infectious Diseases Society of America. 2009;48(5):587 94.
9. Ovstebo R, Hellerud BC, Coureuil M, Nassif X, Brandtzaeg P. Pathogenesis of invasive disease. In: Feavers I, Pollard A, Sadarangani M, editors. Handbook of meningococcal disease management. Cham: Springer International Publishing; 2016. p. 25–43.
10. Brandtzaeg P. Pathogenesis and pathophysiology of invasive meningococcal disease. In: Frosch M, MCJ M, editors. Handbook of meningococcal disease: infection biology, vaccination, clinical management. Weinheim: Wiley-VCH Verlag GmbH & Co; 2006. p. 427–80.
11. Ovstebo R, Brandtzaeg P, Brusletto B, Haug KB, Lande K, Hoiby EA, Kierulf P. Use of robotized DNA isolation and real-time pcr to quantify and identify close correlation between levels of neisseria meningitidis DNA and lipopolysaccharides in plasma and cerebrospinal fluid from patients with systemic meningococcal disease. J Clin Microbiol. 2004;42(7):2980–7.
12. Stephens DS, Greenwood B, Brandtzaeg P. Epidemic meningitis, meningococcaemia, and neisseria meningitidis. Lancet (London, England). 2007;369(9580):2196–210.
13. van Deuren M, Brandtzaeg P, van der Meer JW. Update on meningococcal disease with emphasis on pathogenesis and clinical management. Clin Microbiol Rev. 2000;13(1):144–66. table of contents
14. Ferguson JH, Chapman OD. Fulminating meningococcic infections and the so-called waterhouse-friderichsen syndrome. Am J Pathol. 1948;24(4):763–95.
15. Bjerre A, Brusletto B, Ovstebo R, Joo GB, Kierulf P, Brandtzaeg P. Identification of meningococcal lps as a major monocyte activator in il-10 depleted shock plasmas and csf by blocking the cd14-tlr4 receptor complex. J Endotoxin Res. 2003;9(3):155–63.
16. Brandtzaeg P, Bryn K, Kierulf P, Ovstebo R, Namork E, Aase B, Jantzen E. Meningococcal endotoxin in lethal septic shock plasma studied by gas chromatography, mass-spectrometry, ultracentrifugation, and electron microscopy. J Clin Invest. 1992;89(3):816–23.
17. Sprong T, Stikkelbroeck N, van der Ley P, Steeghs L, van Alphen L, Klein N, Netea MG, van der Meer JW, van Deuren M. Contributions of neisseria meningitidis lps and non-lps to proinflammatory cytokine response. J Leukoc Biol. 2001;70(2):283–8.
18. Hellerud BC, Nielsen EW, Thorgersen EB, Lindstad JK, Pharo A, Tonnessen TI, Castellheim A, Mollnes TE, Brandtzaeg P. Dissecting the effects of lipopolysaccharides from nonlipopolysaccharide molecules in experimental porcine meningococcal sepsis. Crit Care Med. 2010;38(6):1467–74.
19. Guarner J, Greer PW, Whitney A, Shieh WJ, Fischer M, White EH, Carlone GM, Stephens DS, Popovic T, Zaki SR. Pathogenesis and diagnosis of human meningococcal disease using immunohistochemical and pcr assays. Am J Clin Pathol. 2004;122(5):754–64.
20. Fernandez-Rodriguez A, Alcala B, Alvarez-Lafuente R. Real-time polymerase chain reaction detection of neisseria meningitidis in formalin-fixed tissues from sudden deaths. Diagn Microbiol Infect Dis. 2008;60(4):339–46.
21. Hellerud BC, Olstad OK, Nielsen EW, Troseid AM, Skadberg O, Thorgersen EB, Vege A, Mollnes TE, Brandtzaeg P. Massive organ inflammation in experimental and in clinical meningococcal septic shock. Shock (Augusta, Ga). 2015;44(5):458–69.
22. Frosch M, Muller D, Bousset K, Muller A. Conserved outer membrane protein of neisseria meningitidis involved in capsule expression. Infect Immun. 1992; 60(3):798–803.
23. Bhatnagar J, Deleon-Carnes M, Kellar KL, Bandyopadhyay K, Antoniadou ZA, Shieh WJ, Paddock CD, Zaki SR. Rapid, simultaneous detection of clostridium sordellii and clostridium perfringens in archived tissues by a novel pcr-based microsphere assay: diagnostic implications for pregnancy-associated toxic shock syndrome cases. Infect Dis Obstet Gynecol. 2012; 2012:972845.
24. Sheikh TI, Qadri I. Expression of ebv encoded viral rna 1, 2 and anti-inflammatory cytokine (interleukin-10) in ffpe lymphoma specimens: a preliminary study for diagnostic implication in pakistan. Diagn Pathol. 2011;6:70.
25. Tucker RA, Unger ER, Holloway BP, Swan DC. Real-time pcr-based fluorescent assay for quantitation of human papillomavirus types 6, 11, 16, and 18. Molecular diagnosis: a journal devoted to the understanding of human disease through the clinical application of molecular biology. 2001;6(1):39–47.
26. Dietrich D, Uhl B, Sailer V, Holmes EE, Jung M, Meller S, Kristiansen G. Improved pcr performance using template DNA from formalin-fixed and paraffin-embedded tissues by overcoming pcr inhibition. PLoS One. 2013;8(10):e77771.

27. Brandtzaeg P, Ovstebo R, Kierulf P. Quantitative detection of bacterial lipopolysaccharides in clinical specimens. Methods in molecular medicine. 2001;67:427–39.

28. Gopinathan U, Ovstebo R, Olstad OK, Brusletto B, Dalsbotten Aass HC, Kierulf P, Brandtzaeg P, Berg JP. Global effect of interleukin-10 on the transcriptional profile induced by neisseria meningitidis in human monocytes. Infect Immun. 2012;80(11):4046–54.

29. Waage A, Halstensen A, Shalaby R, Brandtzaeg P, Kierulf P, Espevik T. Local production of tumor necrosis factor alpha, interleukin 1, and interleukin 6 in meningococcal meningitis. Relation to the inflammatory response. J Exp Med. 1989;170(6):1859–67.

30. van Deuren M, van der Ven-Jongekrijg J, Bartelink AK, van Dalen R, Sauerwein RW, van der Meer JW. Correlation between proinflammatory cytokines and antiinflammatory mediators and the severity of disease in meningococcal infections. J Infect Dis. 1995;172(2):433–9.

31. Paireder S, Werner B, Bailer J, Werther W, Schmid E, Patzak B, Cichna-Markl M. Comparison of protocols for DNA extraction from long-term preserved formalin fixed tissues. Anal Biochem. 2013;439(2):152–60.

32. Senguven B, Baris E, Oygur T, Berktas M. Comparison of methods for the extraction of DNA from formalin-fixed, paraffin-embedded archival tissues. Int J Med Sci. 2014;11(5):494–9.

33. Mairey E, Genovesio A, Donnadieu E, Bernard C, Jaubert F, Pinard E, Seylaz J, Olivo-Marin JC, Nassif X, Dumenil G. Cerebral microcirculation shear stress levels determine neisseria meningitidis attachment sites along the blood-brain barrier. J Exp Med. 2006;203(8):1939–50.

34. Witzleb E. Functions of the vascular system. In: Schmidt RF, Thews G, editors. Human physiology. Berlin: Springer; 2013. p. 397–455.

35. Grote J. Tissue respiraion. In: Schmidt RF, Thews G, editors. Human physiology. Berlin: Springer; 2013. p. 508–22.

36. Bass BP, Engel KB, Greytak SR, Moore HM. A review of preanalytical factors affecting molecular, protein, and morphological analysis of formalin-fixed, paraffin-embedded (ffpe) tissue: how well do you know your ffpe specimen? Archives of pathology & laboratory medicine. 2014; 138(11):1520–30.

37. Bonin S, Stanta G. Nucleic acid extraction methods from fixed and paraffin-embedded tissues in cancer diagnostics. Expert Rev Mol Diagn. 2013;13(3):271–82.

38. Srinivasan M, Sedmak D, Jewell S. Effect of fixatives and tissue processing on the content and integrity of nucleic acids. Am J Pathol. 2002;161(6):1961–71.

39. Turashvili G, Yang W, McKinney S, Kalloger S, Gale N, Ng Y, Chow K, Bell L, Lorette J, Carrier M, et al. Nucleic acid quantity and quality from paraffin blocks: defining optimal fixation, processing and DNA/rna extraction techniques. Exp Mol Pathol. 2012;92(1):33–43.

40. Van Ooyen S, Loeffert D, Korfhage C. Overcoming constraints of genomic DNA isolated from paraffin-embedded tissue. Qiagen GmbH. 2011;1–5. https://webcache.googleusercontent.com/search?q=cache:DLLU850h6KwJ:https://www.qiagen.com/resources/download.aspx%3Fid%3D554f8671-17ee-4bd4-bad1-db32d65a6daa%26lang%3Den+&cd=1&hl=en&ct=clnk&gl=no.

41. Ludyga N, Grunwald B, Azimzadeh O, Englert S, Hofler H, Tapio S, Aubele M. Nucleic acids from long-term preserved ffpe tissues are suitable for downstream analyses. Virchows Archiv: an international journal of pathology. 2012;460(2):131–40.

42. Alvarez-Aldana A, Martinez JW, Sepulveda-Arias JC. Comparison of five protocols to extract DNA from paraffin-embedded tissues for the detection of human papillomavirus. Pathol Res Pract. 2015;211(2):150–5.

43. Munoz-Cadavid C, Rudd S, Zaki SR, Patel M, Moser SA, Brandt ME, Gomez BL. Improving molecular detection of fungal DNA in formalin-fixed paraffin-embedded tissues: comparison of five tissue DNA extraction methods using panfungal pcr. J Clin Microbiol. 2010;48(6):2147–53.

44. Hedegaard J, Thorsen K, Lund MK, Hein AM, Hamilton-Dutoit SJ, Vang S, Nordentoft I, Birkenkamp-Demtroder K, Kruhoffer M, Hager H, et al. Next-generation sequencing of rna and DNA isolated from paired fresh-frozen and formalin-fixed paraffin-embedded samples of human cancer and normal tissue. PLoS One. 2014;9(5):e98187.

45. Greer CE, Wheeler CM, Manos MM. Sample preparation and pcr amplification from paraffin-embedded tissues. PCR methods and applications. 1994;3(6):S113–22.

46. Kokkat TJ, Patel MS, McGarvey D, LiVolsi VA, Baloch ZW. Archived formalin-fixed paraffin-embedded (ffpe) blocks: a valuable underexploited resource for extraction of DNA, rna, and protein. Biopreservation and biobanking. 2013;11(2):101–6.

47. Lin J, Kennedy SH, Svarovsky T, Rogers J, Kemnitz JW, Xu A, Zondervan KT. High-quality genomic DNA extraction from formalin-fixed and paraffin-embedded samples deparaffinized using mineral oil. Anal Biochem. 2009;395(2):265–7.

48. Wang JH, Gouda-Vossos A, Dzamko N, Halliday G, Huang Y. DNA extraction from fresh-frozen and formalin-fixed, paraffin-embedded human brain tissue. Neurosci Bull. 2013;29(5):649–54.

49. Liu X, Harada S: DNA isolation from mammalian samples. Current protocols in molecular biology / edited by Frederick M Ausubel [et al] 2013, Chapter 2:Unit2.14.

30

Nucleic acid extraction from formalin-fixed paraffin-embedded cancer cell line samples: a trade off between quantity and quality?

Caroline Seiler[1,4], Alan Sharpe[1], J. Carl Barrett[3], Elizabeth A. Harrington[2], Emma V. Jones[2] and Gayle B. Marshall[1,5*]

Abstract

Background: Advanced genomic techniques such as Next-Generation-Sequencing (NGS) and gene expression profiling, including NanoString, are vital for the development of personalised medicines, as they enable molecular disease classification. This has become increasingly important in the treatment of cancer, aiding patient selection. However, it requires efficient nucleic acid extraction often from formalin-fixed paraffin-embedded tissue (FFPE).

Methods: Here we provide a comparison of several commercially available manual and automated methods for DNA and/or RNA extraction from FFPE cancer cell line samples from Qiagen, life Technologies and Promega. Differing extraction geometric mean yields were evaluated across each of the kits tested, assessing dual DNA/RNA extraction vs. specialised single extraction, manual silica column based extraction techniques vs. automated magnetic bead based methods along with a comparison of subsequent nucleic acid purity methods, providing a full evaluation of nucleic acids isolated.

Results: Out of the four RNA extraction kits evaluated the RNeasy FFPE kit, from Qiagen, gave superior geometric mean yields, whilst the Maxwell 16 automated method, from Promega, yielded the highest quality RNA by quantitative real time RT-PCR. Of the DNA extraction kits evaluated the PicoPure DNA kit, from Life Technologies, isolated 2–14x more DNA. A miniaturised qPCR assay was developed for DNA quantification and quality assessment.

Conclusions: Careful consideration of an extraction kit is necessary dependent on quality or quantity of material required. Here we provide a flow diagram on the factors to consider when choosing an extraction kit as well as how to accurately quantify and QC the extracted material.

Keywords: FFPE, DNA, RNA, Manual, Automated, Extraction

Background

Highly multiplexed assays, capable of profiling many genetic biomarkers in a single experiment, are of rising importance in the field of life sciences, enabling mapping of entire biological pathways [1–5]. Our rapidly growing understanding of the molecular mechanisms driving disease progression enables acceleration of personalised medicines into the clinic, particularly in oncology [6–8]. Such assays require sufficient quantities of high quality DNA and RNA extracted from clinically relevant patient samples.

Formalin is the most widely used fixative, used for over a century by hospitals to preserve clinical samples for long term storage. Extensive collections of formalin fixed paraffin embedded (FFPE) clinical samples exist worldwide, representing an invaluable resource for prospective and retrospective studies on archival tissue [9, 10]. However, multiple factors influence the efficiency of formalin fixation including tissue size, fixation temperature and duration, and the amount of time that elapses before the

---

* Correspondence: GayleMarshall61@gmail.com
[1]AstraZeneca Oncology Innovative Medicines, Alderley Park, Macclesfield, UK
[5]AstraZeneca, 8AF6, Mereside, Alderley Park, Alderley Edge, Cheshire SK10 4TG, UK
Full list of author information is available at the end of the article

sample is fixed [11]. The lack of standardised procedures for collecting and processing tissue samples results in a range of FFPE qualities across different sites which can be further influenced by the age of the tissue block [10]. Scientists are constantly faced with the challenge of obtaining sufficient amounts of high quality nucleic acids from suboptimal FFPE samples containing minimal amounts of tissue. Furthermore, the fixation process leads to the cross linking of nucleic acids and proteins resulting in highly fragmented nucleic acid species with amplimers around 100 bases. This can introduce sequence alterations and mono methylol addition of nucleic acids which can impact downstream PCR based assays [12–15]. A number of companies supply off the shelf kits optimised for the extraction of DNA and/or RNA from FFPE sections using varying amounts of tissue. Therefore, we carefully selected seven commercially available FFPE extraction kits with a broad range of properties to assess nucleic acid yield and the quality and purity of the extracted material.

Differing extraction methods were assessed: dual DNA/RNA extraction vs. specialised single extraction, manual silica column based extraction techniques vs. automated magnetic bead based methods and finally a comparison between extraction kits across a range of manufacturers. A number of papers have been published previously comparing the performance of manual FFPE extractions kits from different suppliers [16–18], with more recent studies focusing on comparisons between automated extraction methods and their manual counterpart in order to reduce the hands on time of laborious extraction processes [19–22]. However, the studies use different samples and methods for quantifying and assessing the quality of the extracted material that are not always comparable, making it challenging to cross compare disparate data sets. It is for this reason that we present a comprehensive analysis of seven selected kits using a single sample set. In addition, we provide a head-to-head comparison of commonly used platforms to aid decisions around how to extract, quantify, and assess the quality of nucleic acids.

Cell blocks were used to ensure sufficient sections could be generated to enable robust analysis of each extraction method; although tissue blocks were initially used, the material was rapidly exhausted thereby preventing all extraction kits from being evaluated across all variables using tissue from a single block. Cancer cell lines were cultured, fixed in formalin and embedded in paraffin, to represent the process of preserving clinical tissue whilst achieving a homogenous cell population with known expression of genes of interest for downstream evaluation. This ensured that variability in this assessment is solely due to differences in the extraction kits and not by fixation methods, times and heterogeneity of the tissue. An additional advantage of having a large quantity of cells embedded

within a block, is that it allows each kit to be tested using optimal conditions, so significant differences between kits can be identified.

Methods

Formalin fixed paraffin embedded cancer cell line blocks

Human chronic myeloid leukaemia and breast cancer cell lines, used in this study, were obtained from the American Type Culture Collection (ATCC) and the Deutsche Sammlung von Mikroorganismen und Zellkulturen (DSMZ). Cells were grown in T225 tissue culture flasks in RPMI1640 media (phenol red free; Sigma) supplemented with 10% foetal calf serum and 1% L-Glutamine (Life Technologies Bethesda Research Laboratories Ltd) and maintained at 37 °C with 5% CO_2. Each cell line was passaged up to 3 times and at approximately 80% confluence, the cells were fixed in 10% neutral buffered formalin for 24 h at room temperature before embedding in paraffin wax. Consecutive 5 μm sections were generated from each of the FFPE cell blocks using a standard microtome blade and fixed onto glass microscope slides. All FFPE cell blocks and 5 μm sections were stored at room temperature until nucleic acid extraction was performed.

Nucleic acid extraction

Seven commercially available nucleic acid extraction kits were used in this study (Table 1). Kits were selected based on prior reviews of performance [21, 23] and their extraction properties. Four of the kits tested, rely on the selective binding of nucleic acids to silica columns, two of the kits exploit binding to paramagnetic beads allowing automation of the extraction and one kit tested did not require nucleic acid binding to a solid interphase. Another factor taken into account when selecting kits was the suitability of the extracted material for use in downstream applications including RT-qPCR, qPCR, and gene expression analysis.

A total of 30 samples from 6 FFPE cell line blocks were generated using each extraction method yielding a total of 240 samples as one method extracted both DNA and RNA. RNA extractions were performed on the following cell line blocks: KCL22, MDA-MB-468, MDA-MB-453 (fixed less than 6 months prior to this work) and MDA-MB-231, MDA-MB-468 and MDA-MB-453 (fixed 2–3 years prior to this work). DNA extractions were performed on the following cell line blocks T47D, MDA-MB-468 and MDA-MB-453 from each age group (Table 2). 15 consecutive 5 μm sections were generated from each block and processed as 5 μm, 10 μm (2 combined sections), 15 μm (3 combined sections), 20 μm (4 combined sections) and 25 μm (5 combined sections) in each extraction method. All FFPE sections were deparaffinised using an automated protocol

Table 1 Summary of the seven off the shelf nucleic extraction kits evaluated in this study, including the key differences between each method

Extraction kit	Manufacturer	Extracted Material	Input tissue amount	Elution Volume	Purification Method	Level of automation	Proteinase K digestion	DNase I digestion	Geometric mean Yield (ng)
RNeasy FFPE	Qiagen	RNA	Up to 40 μm	30 μl	Silica Column	Manual	15 min at 56 °C, 15 min at 80 °C	15 min at room temperature in the cell lysate	398.0
Arcturus Paradise plus RNA extraction and isolation	Life technologies	RNA	Up to 40 μm	12 μl	Silica Column	Manual	5 h at 37 °C	20 min at room temperature on the column	197.0
Maxwell 16 LEV RNA FFPE Kit	Promega	RNA	Up to 10 μm	50 μl	Paramagnetic beads	Automated	15 min at 56 °C, 60 min at 80 °C	15 min at room temperature in the cell lysate	231.5
AllPrep DNA/RNA FFPE	Qiagen	RNA & DNA	Up to 40 μm	RNA 30 μl DNA 50 μl	Silica Column	Manual	15 min at 56 °C	15 min at room temperature on the column	RNA 267.7 DNA 10.1
Arcturus PicoPure DNA extraction kit	Life technologies	DNA	1.5–2.0 μg tissue	150 μl	Single tube extraction	Manual	24 h at 65 °C (lyophilised before use)	N/A	172.6
QIAmp DNA FFPE tissue	Qiagen	DNA	Up to 80 μm	50 μl	Silica Column	Manual	60 min at 56 °C, 60 min at 80 °C	N/A	40.9
Maxwell 16 FFPE Tissue LEV DNA Purification Kit	Promega	DNA	Up to 50 μm	50 μl	Paramagnetic beads	Automated	Overnight at 70 °C	N/A	88.3

Table 2 Summary of the FFPE cell pellet blocks used in the study

	<6 months of age	>2 years of age
RNA extraction kits	KCL22, MDA-MB-468, MDA-MB-453	MDA-MB-231, MDA-MB-468, MDA-MB-453
DNA extraction kits	T47D, MDA-MB-453, MDA-MB-468	T47D, MDA-MB-453, MDA-MB-468

on the Leica autostainer XL, involving immersion into xylene twice followed by immersion into 100% ethanol twice then left to air dry for 15 min, with the exception of the two Promega kits where no deparaffinisation was performed. All extraction kits were used according to the manufacturer's instructions including elution volumes quoted and all optional DNase 1 steps in RNA extractions. Following deparaffinisation, the surface area of the cell line pellet was checked by eye from consecutive sections within a block to ensure they matched. All RNA samples were stored at −80 °C and all DNA and cDNA samples were stored at −20 °C throughout the study.

Quantitative and qualitative RNA assessment
Yield
RNA concentration was determined using the Qubit HS RNA assay (Life Technologies, catalogue number Q32852) on the Qubit 2.0 fluorometer. 1.0 µl of RNA in a total 200 µl volume of working solution was prepared. The fluorescence of unknown RNA samples was measured and converted to RNA concentration using a calibration curve generated from newly prepared RNA standards at 0 ng/µl and 10 ng/µl.

Integrity
The extent of RNA fragmentation was assessed via capillary chip electrophoresis. RNA samples at a concentration ≥5 ng/µl were tested using RNA 6000 nano LabChips. The chips were run on the Agilent 2100 Bioanalyser according to the manufacturer's instructions.

Purity
RNA concentration and purity were measured on the Nanodrop 2000 using 1 µl of RNA. The ratio between the absorbance at 260 nm and 280 nm was used to evaluate purity; we assumed ratios between 1.8 and 2.0 to be pure.

mRNA quality assessment
Multiplex quantitative 2-step reverse transcriptase PCR was performed to assess mRNA quality for the same sample set analysed on the Agilent. 7 µl of RNA at a concentration of 5 ng/µl (quantified using the Qubit 2.0 fluorometer) was used to generate cDNA in a 10 µl total extraction volume using the SuperScript VILO cDNA

synthesis kit (Life Technologies, Catalogue Number 11754-050) followed by incubation at 25 °C for 10 min, 42 °C for 60 min and 85 °C for 5 min.

The qPCR assay was prepared in Roche 384 well PCR plates (product no. 04729749001) in a 10 µl reaction volume fired using an ECHO 525 non-contact micro dispenser (LabCyte). Three primer probe pairs were used in each assay against the following housekeeping genes: RPLP0 (CY5), RPL19 (FAM) and ACTB (CYAN500) using three unique fluorophores compatible with the Roche LightCycler480 PCR machine. 0.5 µl of cDNA at 3.5 ng/µl (within the linear range of the assay, Additional file 1: Figure S1) was run in duplicate alongside negative controls lacking the cDNA template on the Roche LightCycler480 PCR machine with 1 pre incubation cycle at 95 °C for 10 min followed by 45 amplification cycles at 95 °C for 10 s, 60 °C for 30 s, 72 °C for 1 s before cooling to 40 °C for 30 s. Data was analysed using the LightCycler 480 software (version 1.5.1.62) under the "Abs quant/ 2nd Derivative Max analyses" programme. This software calculated the average Cq per gene for sample duplicates; this was then used to calculate the average across the 3 house keeping genes and this value was used to compare mRNA quality obtained using the different extraction kits, lower Cq values indicated higher quality mRNA.

Quantitative and qualitative DNA assessment
For DNA to be used in downstream genomic techniques, for example NGS, quality and quantity of amplifiable DNA needs to be assessed. Qubit and Nanodrop will not generate this information so Quantitative PCR was performed for DNA quantification and quality assessment, using the hgDNA Quantification and QC kit from Kapa Biosystems (KK4960) as per the manufacturer's instructions. Two amplicons from a conserved single copy DNA locus were generated, one 41 bp in length and one 129 bp in length. Amplification of the 41 bp target was used for quantitation of amplifiable DNA. This was compared to data generated using the 129 bp assay, to ensure valid conclusion for the Qiagen extraction kits that are less able to retain fragments <100 bp. The 129 bp assay was used to assess DNA quality, since poor DNA quality influences the ability to amplify longer DNA fragments. The relative quality of DNA samples was calculated by normalising the concentration obtained using the 129 bp assay against the concentration obtained from the 41 bp assay, which generates a Q-ratio value between 0 and 1 (0 represents highly fragmented DNA whilst 1 represents high quality DNA). Both assays were performed on the Roche LightCycler480 PCR machine in a 3.0 µl reaction volume. Data was analysed using the Roche LC480 software using the "Abs quant/ 2nd Derivative Max analyses" programme. This software calculated the average Cq

value of duplicates, the standard deviation and DNA concentrations were generated from a standard curve.

Statistical evaluation

Graphical representations were generated using TIBCO Spotfire software version 5.0 and Microsoft Office Excel 2007. Data was represented as the geometric mean with corresponding geometric standard error as the data was found to have an asymmetrical distribution. The statistical significance of the data was assessed using two sample unequal variance t tests as preliminary analysis was performed in the absence of an appropriate rationale as to the direction of the relationship. In the results and discussion, we refer to P-values <0.05 as significant. The coefficient of variation was calculated for correlation plots to assess the fit of simple linear regressions.

Results and discussion

Total RNA yield

All 4 methods successfully extracted RNA (determined as generating a measurable signal using the Qubit) from as little as one 5 μm section, with geometric mean RNA yields greater than 100 ng (Table 1/Fig. 1). The Qiagen RNeasy FFPE extraction kit gave a superior geometric mean RNA yield of 398 ng; however, the difference in the performance of the RNeasy single RNA extraction

and the AllPrep DNA/RNA FFPE kit was not significant (P-value 0.16).

Both Qiagen RNA extraction kits significantly outperformed the Artcturus paradise plus FFPE RNA isolation kit and the automated Maxwell 16 LEV RNA FFPE Kit. The RNeasy FFPE Kit gave geometric mean RNA yields 166 ng greater than the Maxwell 16 and 200 ng greater than the Artcturus paradise plus FFPE RNA isolation kit. The AllPrep gave geometric mean RNA yields 36 ng greater than the Maxwell 16 and 70 ng greater than the Arcturus paradise plus FFPE RNA isolation kit. Multiple factors may contribute to the lower RNA yields obtained using the Artcturus paradise plus FFPE RNA isolation kit. Firstly, the lower temperature used during tissue digestion may less efficiently reverse formaldehyde-induced cross links between nucleic acids and proteins, previous studies have reported heating tissues at higher temperatures (>50 °C) as being more efficient [13, 23]. Also the lengthy 5 h digestion time may not be necessary as previous papers have published that no more than 3 h is required [24]. Finally, this method uses less than half the elution volume of the two Qiagen kits potentially compromising the efficiency of the elution buffer to cover the silica membrane which could contribute to the lower RNA yield observed. Despite the lower yield, the Artcturus kit gave the highest RNA concentration which may be desirable for some studies (Table 1).

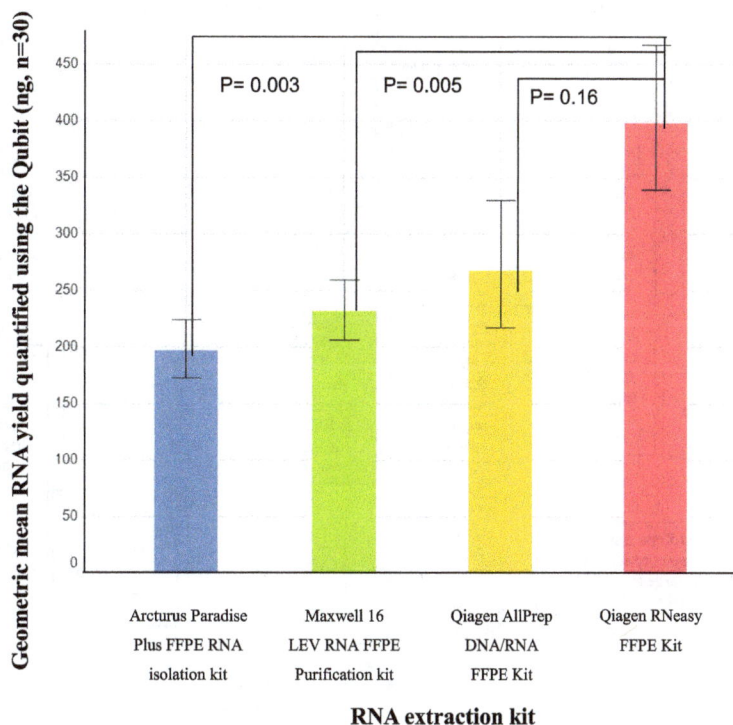

Fig. 1 Comparison of Qubit RNA yields obtained using four off the shelf extraction kits: Geometric mean RNA yield and associated geometric standard error of mean for the four extraction kits tested in this study, n = 30 for each method. P-values show the statistical significance of the difference in yield between each method

The Maxwell 16 RNA extraction is the only method that does not involve deparaffinisation; we hypothesise that excess paraffin may reduce the efficiency of cell lysis, since some studies have shown deparaffinisation to be a key pre-treatment step [25]. In addition, this protocol uses paramagnetic beads for purification as opposed to silica columns. The speed at which the beads are mixed with the cell lysate has been shown to have a strong influence on the efficiency of nucleic acid binding with faster mixing speeds being linked to higher RNA yields. Furthermore, the process of transferring the beads through a series of wash buffers can result in the loss of beads which will negatively impact yield. Although the Maxwell 16 automated the binding, washing, and elution steps, up-front sample preparation was required which took approximately 2 h before loading the lysate onto the machine. In addition, it limited the number of samples processed per run to 16 as opposed to batches of 24, which we feel can comfortably be processed using any of the manual extraction kits. This shows the automated RNA extraction on the Maxwell 16 provides no increase in throughput, and we saw no advantage in terms of yield when using this bead based purification method for RNA extraction over silica columns.

Based on this data, the Qiagen kits (AllPrep and RNeasy) demonstrated superior performance when mRNA expression and quantity of RNA is the priority. However, if quality is key and quantity of less importance, we would recommend the automated Maxwell 16 LEV FFPE kit (Fig. 2).

Fluorescence vs. absorbance for RNA quantification

Each of the extracted RNA samples were quantified using both the Qubit RNA HS fluorescence based assay and the Nanodrop 2000 spectrophotometer (for 5 samples there was insufficient sample remaining to run on the Nanodrop). The Nanodrop also generated A260/A280 ratios as a means of assessing purity. All four RNA extraction kits gave mean ratios ≥1.8 indicating good purity.

Nanodrop consistently underestimated the RNA concentration due to the lower sensitivity of the assay (Additional file 2: Figure S2). The limit of detection of the Nanodrop 2000 is 2 ng/μl whereas for the Qubit it is 0.25 ng/μl; 37% of the samples extracted using the Maxwell 16 gave RNA concentrations <2 ng/μl but greater that 0.25 ng/μl and therefore fell within the background noise of the Nanodrop assay but not the Qubit. For these reasons we chose to use RNA concentration

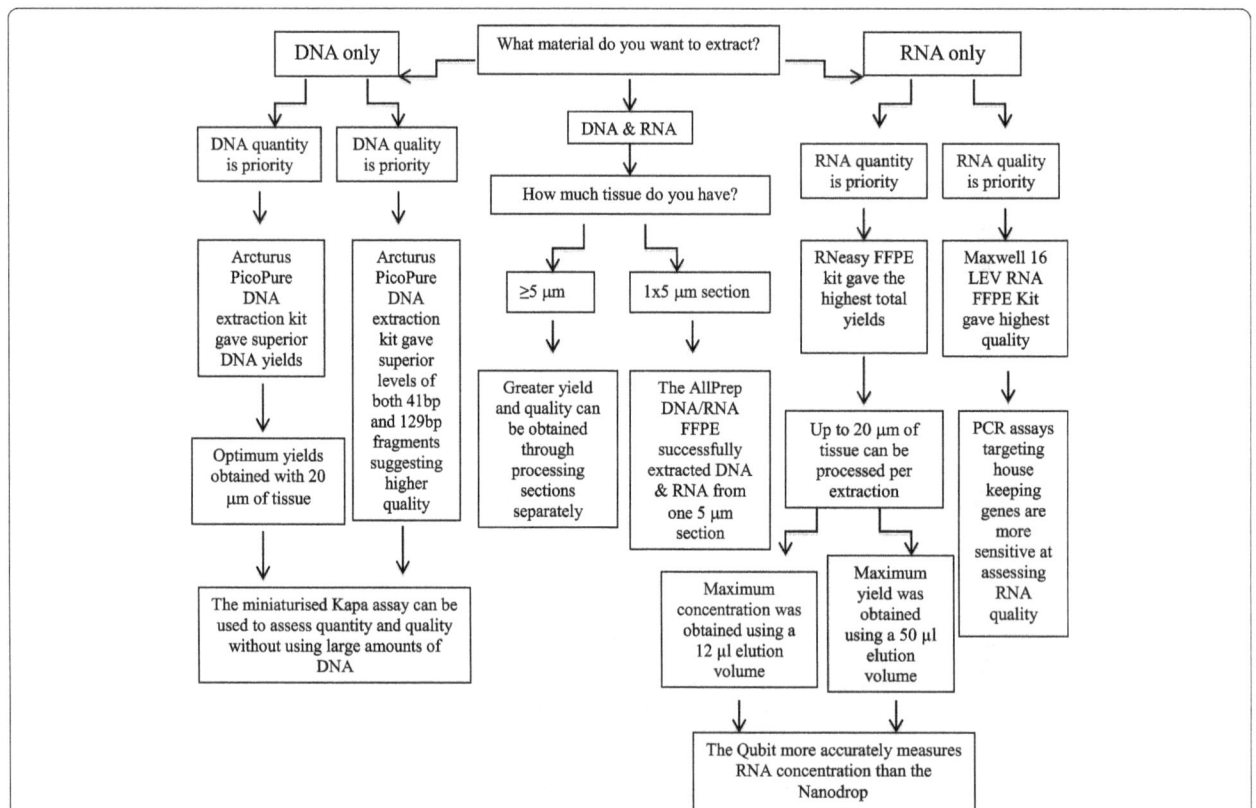

Fig. 2 Flow diagram summarising the key points from this study: Decision tree to highlight which extraction kits demonstrated superior performance in terms of nucleic acid yield and quality as well as guidance on how to quantify and QC the extracted material

readings generated from the Qubit in all subsequent analyses.

Effect of tissue input on RNA concentration/yield using a fixed elution volume

Total nucleic acid yield and concentration are influenced by the elution volume and the amount of tissue processed. We investigated the effect of varying the amount of tissue on nucleic acid concentration and yield by processing 5 μm, 10 μm, 15 μm, 20 μm and 25 μm of tissue.

The Qiagen extraction kits demonstrated a clear linear relationship in concentration with increasing tissue amount (Fig. 3). The Dual extraction kit showed extraction efficiencies of up to 87% (assuming the 5 μm section has 100% extraction efficiency) when processing ≤15 μm of tissue. The RNeasy FFPE kit gave extraction efficiencies of 86% when processing up to 20 μm of tissue, above this the efficiencies were much less. We felt these small losses in yield (~14%) were an acceptable compromise for the increase in concentration achieved through combining

tissue sections (Fig. 3a and b). However, the Arcturus Paradise plus RNA extraction kit showed extraction efficiencies between 55 and 60% when processing between 10 and 25 μm of tissue; 45% of the RNA was lost through combining the tissue sections (Fig. 3c). The Maxwell 16 automated RNA extraction method had a very narrow linear range of 5–10 μm tissue. Within this range, 80% extraction efficiency was obtained, but when >10 μm tissue was used a 50% reduction in yield was observed (Fig. 3d).

Therefore, our data shows that combining tissue sections offers no advantage in terms of yield when compared to extracting sections individually, but does provide a method of increasing RNA concentration although in a non-linear fashion.

Effect of elution volume on RNA concentration/yield using a fixed amount of tissue

In previous experiments the RNeasy FFPE kit gave superior RNA yields, therefore we investigated the relationship between RNA yield/concentration and elution volume.

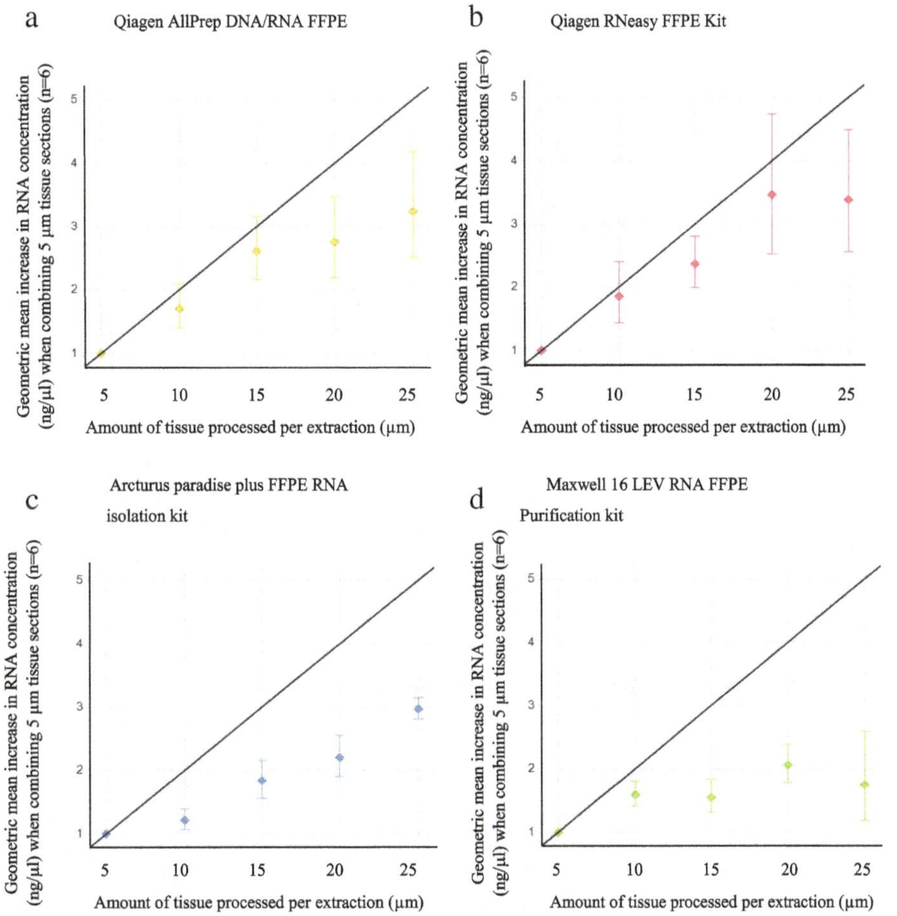

Fig. 3 Investigating the relationship between RNA concentration and the input amount of tissue: Geometric mean increase in RNA concentration (n = 6) when combining 5 μm sections in a linear fashion and associated standard error of mean, line of Y = X/5 represents a linear relationship **a** Qiagen AllPrep DNA/RNA FFPE kit, **b** Qiagen RNeasy, **c** Arcturus Paradise plus FFPE RNA isolation kit, **d** Maxwell 16 LEV RNA FFPE Purification kit

12 μl, 20 μl, 30 μl 40 μl and 50 μl elution volumes were tested using 5 μm of tissue from four different FFPE cancer cell line blocks.

Results showed a 20 μl elution volume was optimal and resulted in high RNA yields and RNA concentrations (Additional file 3: Figure S3). However, we acknowledge that the amount of RNA bound to the column will also have an impact on elution efficiency; samples with higher amounts of RNA may require larger elution volumes.

RNA quality assessment: Agilent vs RT-PCR

RNA samples with a concentration ≥5 ng/μl (limit of detection of the Agilent nano assay), obtained using four different extraction kits, were analysed for quality using the Agilent RNA 6000 nano assay. The assigned RNA integrity number (RIN) values were compared to the in house multiplex RT-PCR assay as an assessment of amplifiable RNA. The RNA samples fell into two groups, those obtained from FFPE cell line pellets generated <6 months prior to commencing the study and those obtained from FFPE cell line pellets generated >2 years prior to commencing the study.

The percentage of samples assigned a RIN value varies between the kits tested: 69% of samples were assigned a RIN value for the Arcturus Paradise Plus RNA kit, 13% for the Maxwell 16 LEV RNA FFPE kit, 64% for the AllPrep DNA/RNA FFPE kit and 71% for the Qiagen RNeasy FFPE kit. However, the assigned RIN values failed to show any significant differences in the quality of the RNA released (Fig. 4a).

To allow for a more sensitive, quantitative assessment of RNA quality isolated from FFPE samples, we developed a multiplex PCR assay in house targeting 3 housekeeping genes ActB, RPL19 and RPLP0 to asses RNA quality based on the ability to amplify targets. The multiplex PCR assay showed good concordance with single-plex PCR assays for each housekeeping gene (Additional file 4: Figure S4) and little intra-assay variation was seen, demonstrated by the strong correlation (R^2 value of 0.985) between technical replicates (Additional file 5: Figure S5). Only RNA samples that were at a concentration ≥5 ng/μl were analysed in this assay.

The multiplex PCR assay was able to demonstrate statistically significant differences in the quality of the RNA released from the different age FFPE blocks (Fig. 4b). Across all the extraction kits, lower quality RNA was obtained from the blocks fixed between 2 and 3 years ago than those fixed <6 months ago. Furthermore, differences in the quality of the RNA released from different RNA extraction kits were also found to be statistically significant. The Maxwell 16 gave significantly higher quality RNA (lowest mean Cq value) than the three other extraction methods, although only 50% of samples

were >5 ng/μl indicating a compromise in yield. The mean Cq value for the Maxwell 16 was 25.9, 2.4 Cq lower than the Arcturus Paradise Plus FFPE RNA isolation kit, 1.6 Cq lower than the RNeasy and 2.0 Cq lower than the Dual extraction kit. The Maxwell 16 is the only method which uses paramagnetic beads and the lack of mechanical force applied through centrifugation in this extraction technique may account for the higher quality of the RNA released. No significant differences in the mean Cq values between the two Qiagen extraction kits were seen. This data demonstrates the in house multiplex PCR assay is a much more sensitive approach, allowing multiple measures of RNA quality from minimal amounts of sample.

Total amplifiable DNA recovery

A total of 120 DNA samples from 6 different FFPE cell line pellets were obtained using four different DNA extraction kits. 5–25 μm of tissue from each block was processed using each method. DNA concentration was quantified based on the amplification of a 41 bp DNA target from a conserved single copy DNA locus. Due to Qiagen kits not retaining products <100 bp, the DNA concentration was also quantified using amplication of a 129 bp DNA target.

All four kits successfully extracted amplifiable DNA from all samples as judged by a Cq value <35 for amplification of the 41 bp and 129 bp targets. PicoPure generated a superior geometric mean DNA yield of 172 ng in 41 bp assay in comparison to the Maxwell 16 (88 ng), QIAmp (40.9 ng) and AllPrep (10.1 ng) (Fig. 5/Table 1). However, the difference in yield seen between the Maxwell 16 and PicoPure were not significant (P-value 0.17). Single and dual DNA extraction kits from Qiagen gave significantly lower DNA yields than the other two kits, but were not significantly different from each other. The same conclusions were drawn from the 129 bp assay (Fig. 5). The PicoPure kit from Life Technologies is a single tube extraction method, thus avoiding the need to bind DNA to a solid interphase followed by laborious wash steps prior to eluting, all potentially resulting in lower DNA yields. This method comprises solely of a 24 h Proteinase K digestion which may account for the higher yields as longer incubation periods have been linked to the increased release of amplifiable DNA through more efficient reversal of formaldehyde induced cross linking [24]. Also, in contrast to the other kits tested, Proteinase K is stored in a lyophilised form in the PicoPure kit and is only reconstituted prior to extraction thus maintaining optimal enzyme activity. Furthermore, the PicoPure kit elutes DNA in a total volume of 150 μl, three times that of the other methods, which may also contribute to the superior yields (Table 1). Although the Maxwell 16 uses a magnetic particle movement

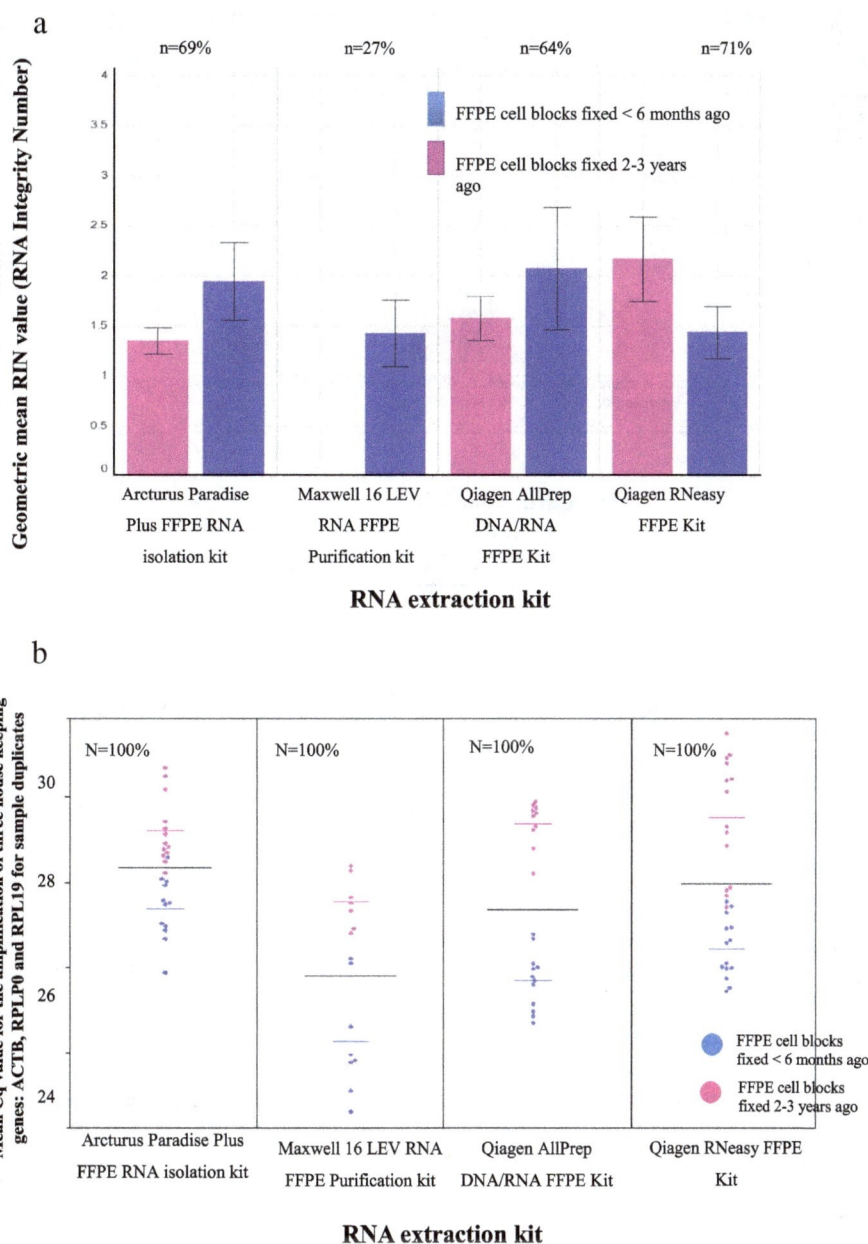

Fig. 4 Comparison of the Agilent RNA assay and our in house PCR assay for assessing RNA quality: **a** Agilent RNA assay, graph shows Geometric mean RIN values and associated standard error of mean for RNA samples extracted using four different RNA extraction kits from FFPE blocks <6 months of age or between 2 and 3 years of age. N represents the percentage of samples analysed that were assigned a RIN value. **b** In-house PCR assay, graph shows Mean Cq value for the amplification of three housekeeping genes: ACTB, RPLP0 and RPL19 for sample duplicates, for RNA samples extracted using four different RNA extraction kits from FFPE blocks either <6 months of age (*blue*) or between 2 and 3 years of age (*pink*), horizontal black lines represent the mean Cq for the entire sample population, with pink and blue lines for the two subgroups of FFPE blocks, N represents the percentage of samples analysed assigned a Cq value

automated extraction process, the total hands on time was greater than the manual PicoPure kit and therefore provided no advantage in terms of yield or efficiency.

Based on this data, the Arcturus PicoPure DNA extraction kit demonstrated superior performance in terms of DNA yield from FFPE tissue.

Effect of tissue input on DNA concentration/yield using a fixed elution volume

Each DNA extraction method was tested using 5 μm, 10 μm, 15 μm, 20 μm and 25 μm of tissue from 6 different FFPE cancer cell line pellets. The relationship between DNA concentration, quantified by qPCR as above, and amount of tissue processed was investigated.

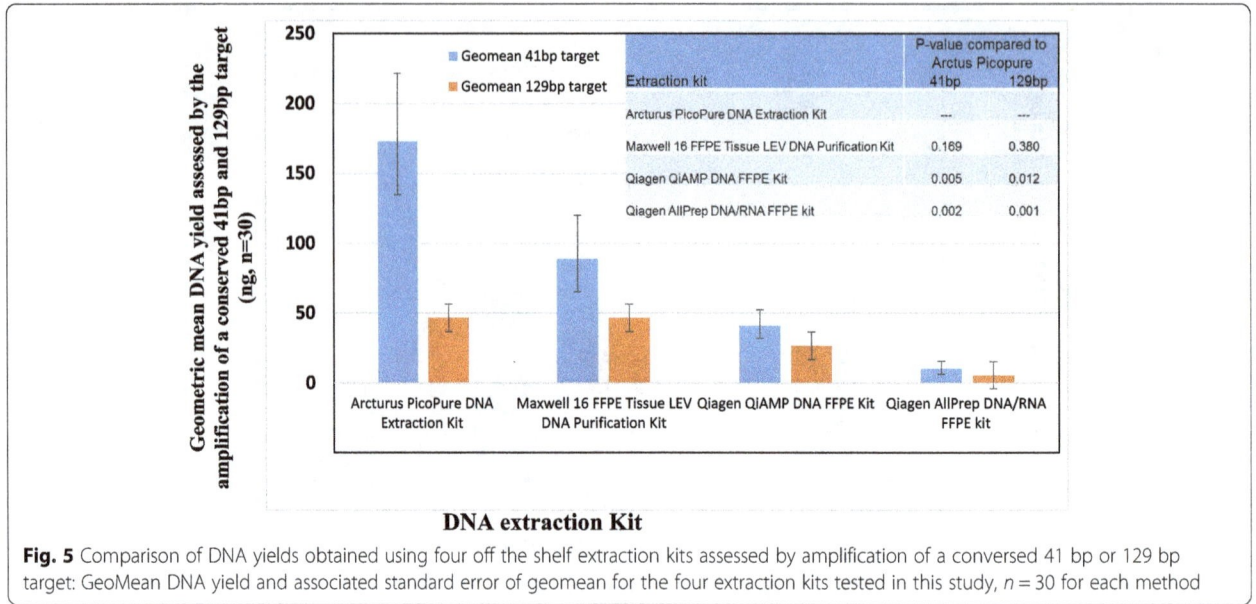

Fig. 5 Comparison of DNA yields obtained using four off the shelf extraction kits assessed by amplification of a conserved 41 bp or 129 bp target: GeoMean DNA yield and associated standard error of geomean for the four extraction kits tested in this study, $n = 30$ for each method

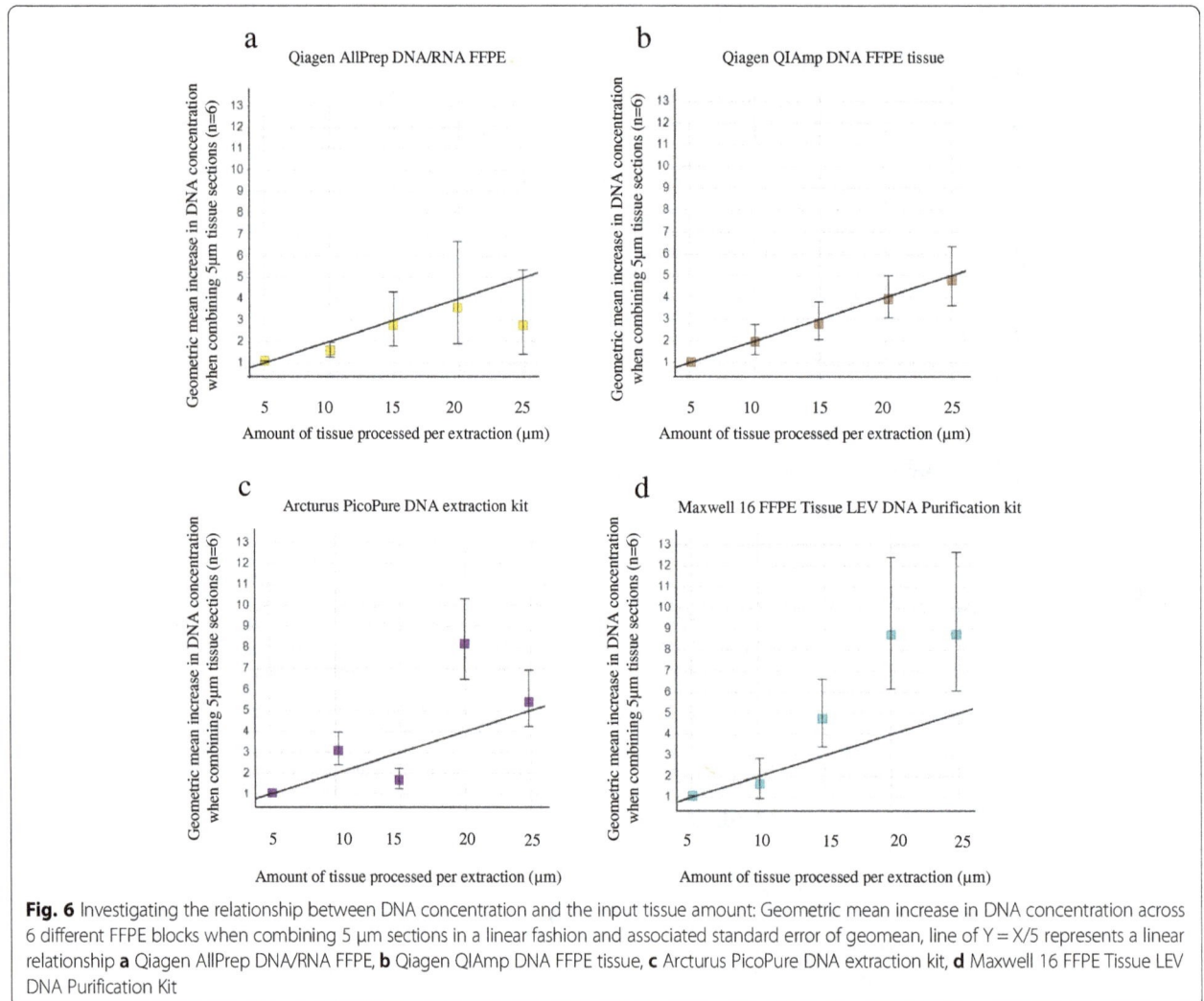

Fig. 6 Investigating the relationship between DNA concentration and the input tissue amount: Geometric mean increase in DNA concentration across 6 different FFPE blocks when combining 5 μm sections in a linear fashion and associated standard error of geomean, line of $Y = X/5$ represents a linear relationship **a** Qiagen AllPrep DNA/RNA FFPE, **b** Qiagen QIAmp DNA FFPE tissue, **c** Arcturus PicoPure DNA extraction kit, **d** Maxwell 16 FFPE Tissue LEV DNA Purification Kit

Differences in extraction efficiencies were observed across the 4 kits tested. The Dual kit showed extraction efficiencies between 79 and 90% when processing up to 20 µm of tissue. The efficiency decreased by 55% when extracting >20 µm suggesting processing >20 µm of tissue in a single extraction would not be recommended due to potential loss of DNA (Fig. 6a). The QIAmp DNA FFPE extraction kit demonstrated a linear relationship between DNA concentration and the input amount of tissue (Fig. 6b). The Arcturus PicoPure DNA kit and the Maxwell 16 FFPE Tissue LEV DNA purification kit both produced extraction efficiencies >100% when processing up to 20 µm of tissue (Fig. 6c, d) indicating that for these kits using 5 µm sections is not optimal.

Overall results showed that extraction from 20 µm tissue sections gave optimal yields across all the kits (Fig. 2).

DNA quality assessment

The quality of 120 DNA samples extracted from different age FFPE blocks using four different extraction kits was assessed using two qPCR assays targeting a 41 bp amplicon and a 129b amplicon from a conserved single copy DNA locus. The ratio between the concentration of the 129 bp amplicon and 41 bp amplicon (Q ratio)

was used as a measure of DNA quality as fragmentation will impact the amplification of the longer DNA target, resulting in a lower ratio. However, running this assay in the recommended 20 µl reaction volume with sample duplicates, limits the ability to assess the quality of scarce clinical samples, so the assay was miniaturised to a 3.0 µl reaction volume.

All DNA extraction kits released higher quality DNA from FFPE blocks <6 months old with higher Q ratios (Fig. 7). The qPCR assay did show differences in the quality of the DNA released using different extraction kits. Significantly lower mean Q ratio of 0.37 was obtained with the Arcturus PicoPure DNA extraction kit compared to the other 3 DNA extraction methods, which were not significantly different to each other. The difference in mean ratio between the single and dual DNA extraction kits from Qiagen was a mere 0.1, showing that neither yield nor quality is compromised through dual extraction procedures.

Silica column and bead based extractions rely on the DNA binding ability of a solid phase. The columns supplied in the Qiagen single and dual DNA extraction kits are only able to bind DNA molecules ≥100 base pairs in length, resulting in the loss of the 41 bp fragment and

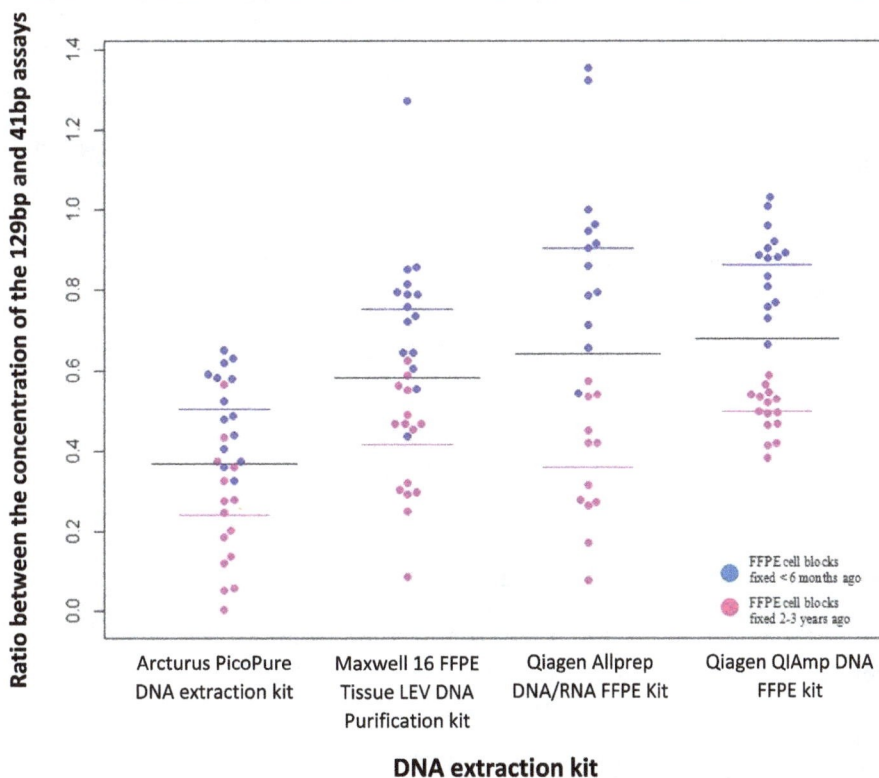

Fig. 7 Comparison of the quality of DNA released using four off the shelf extraction kits: Relative quality of DNA samples calculated by normalising the concentration of 129 bp amplicon to the 41 bp amplicon using the KAPA Biosystems kit. from 6 different FFPE blocks either <6 months of age (*blue*) or between 2 and 3 years of age (*pink*), horizontal black lines represent the mean Cq for the entire sample population, with pink and blue lines for the two equal subgroups of FFPE blocks

selective enrichment of DNA fragments ≥100 base pairs. This leads to an over estimation of the ratio between the 129 bp target and the 41 bp target, so caution when analysing this data is required. In contrast, the Picopure DNA extraction kit is not reliant on the binding of DNA molecules to a solid phase and therefore all DNA fragments are retained, giving a more realistic representation of the quality of the DNA released from FFPE samples.

Data showed the miniaturised KAPA assay can be used to assess quantity and quality of DNA extracted without sacrificing large amounts of DNA (Fig. 7).

Conclusions
Previous publications have compared the performance of manual FFPE extraction kits [16–18] and automated and manual kit counterparts [19–22], but different samples and methods for quantifying and assessing quality makes comparisons challenging. We have presented a comprehensive analysis of seven selected kits with a single sample set and compared directly platforms to assess quantity and quality of nucleic acids.

This study demonstrates that a number of factors influence the quantity and quality of nucleic acids obtained from FFPE samples, including the age of the samples, the extraction method, the amount of tissue processed and the elution volume. Following the manufacturer's instructions, the data showed that no single protocol will consistently release high yields of high quality nucleic acids across all sample types.

Perhaps not surprisingly, our data shows that superior performance in high yields will often result in a compromise in concentration and/or quality. Therefore, downstream applications and nature of the samples to be tested should be given consideration up front before choosing the extraction method to apply.

Although FFPE cell line material was used in this study to remove sample heterogeneity, and supply issues, Qiagen RNeasy FFPE kit has been successfully utilised on clinical FFPE samples following this study [26]. Indicating that conclusions from this study are applicable to clinical FFPE tissue samples.

To potentially improve the performance of the kits tested in this study a wider validation study would need to be conducted, to test variables such as; method of deparaffinisation (deparaffinisation buffers vs. xylene), lysis volume and incubation time, column vs. cell lysate DNase digestion (for RNA isolation), and testing reagents such as Proteinase K from a lyophilised stock rather than a readymade solution.

This study successfully highlighted the key benefits of each extraction method tested, following the manufacturer's protocols, with the aim to aid scientists in choosing a particular method dependent on individual goals. We provide a flow diagram to help question the properties

that are most important to the success of studies with additional information around the most accurate and efficient methods to quantify and QC the extracted material (Fig. 2).

Additional files

Additional file 1: Figure S1. Investigating the linearity of the multiplex PCR assay: relationship between cDNA concentration and mean Cq value for serial dilutions of a 10 ng/µl RNA sample ran in the multiplex PCR assay.

Additional file 2: Figure S2. Comparison of the Nanodrop and Qubit for RNA quantification: Correlation plot between RNA concentrations measured using the Nanodrop absorbance based assay and the Qubit fluorescence based assay, r^2 represents the correlation coefficient, (a) Qiagen AllPrep DNA/RNA FFPE kit $n = 30$, (b) Qiagen RNeasy FFPE kit, $n = 30$, (c) Arcturus paradise plus FFPE RNA isolation kit, $n = 25$, (d) Maxwell 16 LEV RNA FFPE Purification kit, $n = 30$.

Additional file 3: Figure S3. Investigating the relationship between elution volume, RNA concentration and yield: Geometric mean RNA yield (orange bars) and geometric mean RNA concentration (black line) across four FFPE blocks when processing 5 µm of tissue using the RNeasy FFPE kit using varied elution volumes, error bars represent the standard error of geomean.

Additional file 4: Figure S4. Validation of the in house multiplex PCR assay: Correlation between the Cq values for each housekeeping gene for samples ran in both the single and multiplex PCR assay, r^2 represents correlation coefficient

Additional file 5: Figure S5. Assessing intra assay variation of the multiplex PCR assay: Correlation between the Cq values of technical replicates for each housekeeping gene for samples ran in the multiplex PCR assay, r^2 represents the correlation coefficient.

Additional file 6: Table S1. Properties of the three primers and probes used in the in house multiplex PCR assay to asses RNA quality. Roche LightCycler480 PCR machine conditions: 1 pre incubation cycle at 95 °C for 10 min followed by 45 amplification cycles at 95 °C for 10 s, 60 °C for 30 s, 72 °C for 1 s before cooling to 40 °C for 30 s.

Abbreviations
FFPE: Formalin fixed paraffin embedded

Acknowledgements
Not applicable.

Funding
AstraZeneca funded the study and AstraZeneca employees. This experimental design, analysis and interpretation along with authorship of the manuscript was also funded by AstraZeneca.

Authors' contributions
CS generated and analysed data, and wrote manuscript. AS performed statistical analyses of the data, and contributed to writing the manuscript. GBM, JCB, LH, and EJ provided key technical and scientific input, and all were major contributors in writing the manuscript. All authors read and approved the final manuscript.

Competing interests
CS has no competing interests. GBM, AS, JCB and EAH and EVJ are employees and shareholders at AZ and have no other competing interests.

Author details
[1]AstraZeneca Oncology Innovative Medicines, Alderley Park, Macclesfield, UK. [2]AstraZeneca, Cambridge, UK. [3]AstraZeneca, Waltham, USA. [4]Leeds University-AZ Sandwich Placement, Leeds, UK. [5]AstraZeneca, 8AF6, Mereside, Alderley Park, Alderley Edge, Cheshire SK10 4TG, UK.

References
1. Kalmar A, Wichmann B, Galamb O, Spisák S, Tóth K, Leiszter K, Tulassay Z, Molnár B. Gene expression analysis of normal and colorectal cancer tissue samples from fresh frozen and matched formalin-fixed, paraffin-embedded (FFPE) specimens after manual and automated RNA isolation. Methods. 2013;59(1):S16–9.
2. Northcott P, Shih D, Remke M, Cho YJ, Kool M, Hawkins C, Eberhart C, Dubuc A, Guettouche T, Cardentey Y, Bouffet E, Pomeroy S, Marra M, Malkin D, Rutka J, Korshunov A, Pfister S, Taylor M. Rapid, reliable, and reproducible molecular sub-grouping of clinical medulloblastoma samples. Acta Neuropathol. 2012;123(4):615–26.
3. Rahimov F, King OD, Leung DG, Bibat GM, Emerson Jr CP, Kunkel LM, Wagner KR. Transcriptional profiling in facioscapulohumeral muscular dystrophy to identify candidate biomarkers. Proc Natl Acad Sci U S A. 2012; 109(40):16234–9.
4. Sun Z, Asmann YW, Kalari KR, Bot B, Eckel-Passow JE, Baker TR, Carr JM, Khrebtukova I, Luo S, Zhang L, Schroth G, Perez EA, Thompson EA. Integrated analysis of gene expression, CpG island methylation, and gene copy number in breast cancer cells by deep sequencing. PLoS One. 2011; 6(2):e17490.
5. Valleron W, Ysebaert L, Berquet L, Fataccioli V, Quelen C, Martin A, Parrens M, Lamant L, de Leval L, Gisselbrecht C, Gaulard P, Brousset P. Small nucleolar RNA expression profiling identifies potential prognostic markers in peripheral T-cell lymphoma. Blood. 2012;120(19):3997–4005.
6. Levy MA, Lovly CM, Pao W. Translating genomic information into clinical medicine: lung cancer as a paradigm. Genome Res. 2012;22(11):2101–8.
7. Mayeux R. Biomarkers: potential uses and limitations. NeuroRx. 2004;1(2):182–8.
8. Simon R. Genomic biomarkers in predictive medicine: an interim analysis. EMBO Mol Med. 2011;3(8):429–35.
9. Asslaber M, Zatloukal K. Biobanks: transnational, European and global networks. Brief Funct Genomic Proteomic. 2007;6(3):193–201.
10. Moore H, Compton C, Alper J, Vaught J. 2009 Biospecimen research network symposium: advancing cancer research through biospecimen science. Cancer Res. 2009;69(17):6770–2.
11. Srinivasan M, Sedmak D, Jewell S. Effect of fixatives and tissue processing on the content and integrity of nucleic acids. Am J Pathol. 2002;161(6):1961–71.
12. Florell SR, Coffin CM, Holden JA, Zimmermann JW, Gerwels JW, Summers BK, Jones DA, Leachman SA. Preservation of RNA for functional genomic studies: a multidisciplinary tumor bank protocol. Mod Pathol. 2001;14(2):116–28.
13. Masuda N, Ohnishi T, Kawamoto S, Monden M, Okubo K. Analysis of chemical modification of RNA from formalin-fixed samples and optimization of molecular biology applications for such samples. Nucleic Acids Res. 1999; 27(22):4436–43.
14. McGhee JD, von Hippel PH. Formaldehyde as a probe of DNA structure. r. Mechanism of the initial reaction of Formaldehyde with DNA. Biochemistry. 1977;16(15):3276–93.
15. Williams C, Pontén F, Moberg C, Söderkvist P, Uhlén M, Pontén J, Sitbon G, Lundeberg J. A high frequency of sequence alterations is due to formalin fixation of archival specimens. Am J Pathol. 1999;155(5):1467–71.
16. Dedhia P, Tarale S, Dhongde G, Khadapkar R, Das B. Evaluation of DNA extraction methods and real time PCR optimization on formalin-fixed paraffin-embedded tissues. Asian Pac J Cancer Prev. 2007;8(1):55–9.
17. Huang WY, Sheehy TM, Moore LE, Hsing AW, Purdue MP. Simultaneous recovery of DNA and RNA from formalin-fixed paraffin-embedded tissue and application in epidemiologic studies. Cancer Epidemiol Biomarkers Prev. 2010;19(4):973–7.
18. Okello JB, Zurek J, Devault AM, Kuch M, Okwi AL, Sewankambo NK, Bimenya GS, Poinar D, Poinar HN. Comparison of methods in the recovery of nucleic acids from archival formalin-fixed paraffin-embedded autopsy tissues. Anal Biochem. 2010;400(1):110–7.
19. Bohmann K, Hennig G, Rogel U, Poremba C, Mueller BM, Fritz P, Stoerkel S, Schaefer KL. RNA extraction from archival formalin-fixed paraffin-embedded tissue: a comparison of manual, semiautomated, and fully automated purification methods. Clin Chem. 2009;55(9):1719–27.
20. Hennig G, Gehrmann M, Stropp U, Brauch H, Fritz P, Eichelbaum M, Schwab M, Schroth W. Automated extraction of DNA and RNA from a single formalin-fixed paraffin-embedded tissue section for analysis of both single-nucleotide polymorphisms and mRNA expression. Clin Chem. 2010;56(12):1845–53.
21. Khokhar SK, Mitui M, Leos NK, Rogers BB, Park JY. Evaluation of Maxwell(R) 16 for automated DNA extraction from whole blood and formalin-fixed paraffin embedded (FFPE) tissue. Clin Chem Lab Med. 2012;50(2):267–72.
22. Sam SS, Lebel KA, Bissaillon CL, Tafe LJ, Tsongalis GJ, Lefferts JA. Automation of genomic DNA isolation from formalin-fixed, paraffin-embedded tissues. Pathol Res Pract. 2012;208(12):705–7.
23. Ribeiro-Silva A, Zhang H, Jeffrey SS. RNA extraction from ten year old formalin-fixed paraffin-embedded breast cancer samples: a comparison of column purification and magnetic bead-based technologies. BMC Mol Biol. 2007;8:118.
24. Gilbert MT, Haselkorn T, Bunce M, Sanchez JJ, Lucas SB, Jewell LD, Van Marck E, Worobey M. The isolation of nucleic acids from fixed, paraffin-embedded tissues-which methods are useful when? PLoS One. 2007;2(6):e537.
25. Stanta G, Schneider C. RNA extracted from paraffin-embedded human tissues is amenable to analysis by PCR amplification. Biotechniques. 1991; 11(3):304. 306, 308.
26. Veldman-Jones MH, Brant R, Rooney C, Geh C, Emery H, Harbron CG, Wappett M, Sharpe A, Dymond M, Barrett JC, Harrington EA, Marshall G. Evaluating robustness and sensitivity of the NanoString technologies nCounter platform to enable multiplexed gene expression analysis of clinical samples. Cancer Res. 2015;75(13):2587–93.

Permissions

List of Contributors

Asif Ali
Wolfson Wohl Cancer Research Centre, Institute of Cancer Sciences, College of Medical Veterinary and Life Sciences, University of Glasgow, Garscube Estate, Switchback Road, Bearsden G61 1QH, UK

Karin A Oien
Wolfson Wohl Cancer Research Centre, Institute of Cancer Sciences, College of Medical Veterinary and Life Sciences, University of Glasgow, Garscube Estate, Switchback Road, Bearsden G61 1QH, UK
Department of Pathology, Southern General Hospital, Greater Glasgow and Clyde NHS, Glasgow G51 4TF, UK

Victoria Brown
Pathology Laboratory, Forth Valley Royal Hospital, Stirling Road, Larbert FK5 4WR, UK

Simon Denley, Nigel B Jamieson, C Ross Carter and Colin J McKay
West of Scotland Pancreatic Unit and Glasgow Royal Infirmary, Alexandra Parade, Glasgow G31 2ER, UK

Jennifer P Morton, Colin Nixon and Owen J Sansom
Beatson Institute for Cancer Research, Glasgow G61 1BD, UK

Janet S Graham
Medical Oncology, Beatson West of Scotland Cancer Centre, Glasgow G12 0YN, UK

Fraser R Duthie
Department of Pathology, Southern General Hospital, Greater Glasgow and Clyde NHS, Glasgow G51 4TF, UK

William H. Bradley and Janet S. Rader
Department of Obstetrics and Gynecology, Medical College of Wisconsin, 8701 Watertown Plank Road, Milwaukee, WI 53226, USA

Christina Kendziorski
Department of Biostatistics and Medical Informatics, University of Wisconsin-Madison, Madison, WI 53792, USA

Kevin Eng
Department of Biostatistics and Medical Informatics, University of Wisconsin-Madison, Madison, WI 53792, USA

Current Address: Department of Biostatistics and Bioinformatics, Roswell Park Cancer Institute, Buffalo, NY, USA

Min Le and A. Craig Mackinnon
Department of Pathology, Medical College of Wisconsin, Milwaukee, WI 53226, USA

Sveinung W Sørbye
Department of Clinical Pathology, University Hospital of Northern Norway, N-9038 Tromsø, Norway

Kenneth Lønvik
Department of Clinical Pathology, University Hospital of Northern Norway, N-9038 Tromsø, Norway
Department of Medical Biology, Tromsø, Norway

Marit N Nilsen
Department of Medical Biology, Tromsø, Norway

Ruth H Paulssen
Department of Clinical Medicine, UiT – The Arctic University of Norway, N-9037 Tromsø, Norway

Emma Gustbée, Andrea Markkula, Maria Simonsson, Björn Nodin, Karin Jirström and Helena Jernström
Division of Oncology and Pathology, Department of Clinical Sciences, Lund, Lund University, Barngatan 2B, SE 22185 Lund, Sweden

Helga Tryggvadottir and Signe Borgquist
Division of Oncology and Pathology, Department of Clinical Sciences, Lund, Lund University, Barngatan 2B, SE 22185 Lund, Sweden
Department of Oncology, Skåne University Hospital, Lund, Sweden

Carsten Rose
CREATE Health and Department of Immunotechnology, Lund University, Medicon Village, Building 406, Lund, Sweden

Christian Ingvar
Department of Clinical Sciences, Division of Surgery, Lund, Lund University, Lund, Sweden and Skåne University Hospital, Lund, Sweden

Louis S. Nelson, Scott R. Davis, Robert M. Humble, Jeff Kulhavy and Matthew D. Krasowski
Department of Pathology, University of Iowa Hospitals and Clinics, Iowa City, IA 52242, USA

Dean R. Aman
Hospital Computing Information Services, University of Iowa Hospitals and Clinics, Iowa City, IA 52242, USA

Anna M Wirsing and Elin Hadler-Olsen
Department of Medical Biology, Faculty of Health Sciences, University of Tromsø, Tromsø 9037, Norway

Oddveig G Rikardsen
Department of Medical Biology, Faculty of Health Sciences, University of Tromsø, Tromsø 9037, Norway
Department of Otorhinolaryngology, University Hospital of North Norway, Tromsø 9038, Norway

Sonja E Steigen and Lars Uhlin-Hansen
Department of Medical Biology, Faculty of Health Sciences, University of Tromsø, Tromsø 9037, Norway
Diagnostic Clinic – Clinical Pathology, University Hospital of North Norway, Tromsø 9038, Norway

Ruza Arsenic, Denise Treue, Annika Lehmann, Michael Hummel, Manfred Dietel, Carsten Denkert and Jan Budczies
Institute of Pathology, Charité University Hospital Berlin, Berlin, Germany

Joel E. Mortensen, Cindi Ventrola and Sarah Hanna
Department of Laboratory Medicine, Cincinnati Children's Hospital, MLC1010, 3333 Burnet Ave, 45229 Cincinnati, OH, USA

Adam Walter
BD Diagnostics, Sparks, MD, USA

Xi Wang, Kirsten Woolf, David G. Hicks and Shuyuan Yeh
Department of Pathology, University of Rochester Medical Center, Rochester, NY 14642, USA

Brian Z. Ring
Institute for Genomic and Personalized Medicine, School of Life Science and Technology, Huazhong University of Science and Technology, Wuhan, China

Robert S. Seitz
Insight Genetics Inc., Nashville, TN, USA

Douglas T. Ross
CardioDx, Inc., Redwood City, CA, USA.

Rodney A. Beck
Conversant Biologics, Huntsville, AL, USA

Fierdoz Omar and Judy A King
Division of Chemical Pathology, C17 NHLS, Groote Schuur Hospital, University of Cape Town, Anzio Road Observatory, Cape Town 7925, South Africa

Tahir S Pillay
Division of Chemical Pathology, C17 NHLS, Groote Schuur Hospital, University of Cape Town, Anzio Road Observatory, Cape Town 7925, South Africa
Department of Chemical Pathology, University of Pretoria and NHLS Tshwane Academic Division/ Steve Biko Academic Hospital, Tshwane, South Africa

Joel A Dave and Naomi S Levitt
Division of Diabetic Medicine and Endocrinology, Groote Schuur Hospital and University of Cape Town, Cape Town, South Africa

Suvi Lokka and Josef Rüschoff
Institute of Pathology Nordhessen, Germaniastr. 7, 34119 Kassel, Germany

Andreas H Scheel
Institute of Pathology Nordhessen, Germaniastr. 7, 34119 Kassel, Germany
Department of Pathology, University Medical Centre Göttingen, Robert-Koch-Str. 38, 37077 Göttingen, Germany

Katja Schmitz and Hans-Ulrich Schildhaus
Department of Pathology, University Medical Centre Göttingen, Robert-Koch-Str. 38, 37077 Göttingen, Germany

Rudolf Hesterberg
Rotes Kreuz Krankenhaus, Department of Surgery, Hansteinstrasse 29, 34121 Kassel, Germany

Sebastian Dango
Rotes Kreuz Krankenhaus, Department of Surgery, Hansteinstrasse 29, 34121 Kassel, Germany
Department of General, Visceral, and Paediatric Surgery, University Medical Centre Göttingen, Robert-Koch-Str. 38, 37077 Göttingen, Germany

Imogen Ptacek, Ainslie Garrod, Sian Bullough, Nicola Bradley, Colin P. Sibley, Rebecca L. Jones, Paul Brownbill and Alexander E. P. Heazell
Institute of Human Development, Faculty of Medical and Human Sciences, University of Manchester, Oxford Rd, Manchester M13 9PL, UK
Maternal and Fetal Health Research Centre, 5th floor (Research), St Mary's Hospital, Oxford Road, Manchester M13 9WL, UK

Anna Smith and Gauri Batra
Department of Histopathology, Royal Manchester Children's Hospital, Central Manchester University Hospitals NHS Foundation Trust, Manchester Academic Health Science Centre, Manchester M13 9WL, UK

Lara Termini, Maria A Andreoli and Maria C Costa
Santa Casa de São Paulo, INCT-HPV at Santa Casa Research Institute, School of Medicine, Rua Marquês de Itú, 381, 01223-001 São Paulo, Brazil

Luisa L Villa
Santa Casa de São Paulo, INCT-HPV at Santa Casa Research Institute, School of Medicine, Rua Marquês de Itú, 381, 01223-001 São Paulo, Brazil
Department of Radiology and Oncology, School of Medicine, University of São Paulo and Cancer Institute of the State of São Paulo, ICESP, Av Dr Arnaldo 250, 01246-000 São Paulo, Brazil

José H Fregnani
Teaching and Research Institute, Barretos Cancer Hospital, Rua Antenor Duarte Vilela, 1331, 14784-006 Barretos, Brazil

Enrique Boccardo
Department of Microbiology, Institute of Biomedical Sciences, University of São Paulo, Av. Prof. Lineu Prestes, 1374 - Ed. Biomédicas II, Cidade Universitária, 05508-900 São Paulo, Brazil

Walter H da Costa, Ademar Lopes and Gustavo C Guimarães
Pelvic Surgery Department, A. C. Camargo Cancer Center, Rua Prof. Antônio Prudente 211, 01509-010 São Paulo, Brazil

Adhemar Longatto-Filho
Laboratory of Medical Investigation (LIM) 14, Department of Pathology, School of Medicine, University of São Paulo, Av. Dr. Arnaldo 455, 01246-903 São Paulo, Brazil
Life and Health Sciences Research Institute, School of Health Sciences, ICVS/3B's - PT Government Associate Laboratory, University of Minho, Braga, Guimarães, Portugal
Molecular Oncology Research Center, Barretos Cancer Hospital, Pio XII Foundation, Barretos, Rua Antenor Duarte Villela, 1331, 14784-400 Barretos, Brazil

Isabela W da Cunha and Fernando A Soares
Department of Anatomic Pathology, A. C. Camargo Cancer Center, Rua Prof. Antônio Prudente 109, 01509-900 São Paulo, Brazil

Joanna J Moser, Marvin J Fritzler and Jerome B Rattner
Department of Biochemistry and Molecular Biology, Faculty of Medicine, University of Calgary, Calgary, AB, Canada

Melkamu Getinet and Abinet Sisay
Debre Markos Referral Hospital, Debre Markos, Ethiopia

Baye Gelaw and Abate Assefa
Department of Medical Microbiology, School of Biomedical and Laboratory Sciences, College of Medicine and Health Sciences, University of Gondar, Gondar, Ethiopia

Eiman A. Mahmoud
Department of Basic Sciences, College of Osteopathic Medicine, Touro University, Vallejo, CA, USA

Roney Santos Coimbra
Biosystems Informatics, Research Center Rene Rachou, FIOCRUZ, Av. Augusto de Lima 1715, Belo Horizonte, MG Zip Code: 30190-002, Brazil

Bruno Frederico Aguilar Calegare and Vânia D'Almeida
Department of Psychobiology, Universidade Federal de São Paulo (UNIFESP/EPM), São Paulo, SP, Brazil

Talitah Michel Sanchez Candiani
Children's Hospital João Paulo II –FHEMIG, Belo Horizonte, MG, Brazil

Mouna Khmou, Karima Laadam and Nadia Cherradi
Department of Pathology, Hospital of Specialities, Rabat, Morocco
Faculty of Medicine and Pharmacy Rabat, University Mohammed V Rabat, Rabat, Morocco

Ayşe Latif, Kay M. Marshall, Kaye J. Williams and Ian J. Stratford
Division of Pharmacy and Optometry, Faculty of Biology, Medicine and Health, University of Manchester, Manchester, UK

Amy L. Chadwick
Division of Pharmacy and Optometry, Faculty of Biology, Medicine and Health, University of Manchester, Manchester, UK
Gynaecological Oncology Research Group, Division of Cancer Sciences, Faculty of Biology, Medicine and Health, University of Manchester, Level 5 – Research, St Mary's Hospital, Oxford Road, Manchester M13 9WL, UK

Sarah J. Kitson, Hannah J. Gregson and Vanitha N. Sivalingam
Gynaecological Oncology Research Group, Division of Cancer Sciences, Faculty of Biology, Medicine and Health, University of Manchester, Level 5 – Research, St Mary's Hospital, Oxford Road, Manchester M13 9WL, UK

Emma J. Crosbie
Gynaecological Oncology Research Group, Division of Cancer Sciences, Faculty of Biology, Medicine and Health, University of Manchester, Level 5 – Research, St Mary's Hospital, Oxford Road, Manchester M13 9WL, UK
Department of Obstetrics and Gynaecology, St Mary's Hospital, Central Manchester University Hospitals NHS Foundation Trust, Manchester Academic Health Science Centre, Manchester, UK

James Bolton and Rhona J. McVey
Department of Histopathology, Central Manchester University Hospitals NHS Foundation Trust, Manchester Academic Health Science Centre, Manchester, UK

Stephen A. Roberts
Division of Population Health, Health Services Research and Primary Care, Faculty of Biology, Medicine and Health, University of Manchester, Manchester, UK

Boubacar Efared, Layla Tahiri, Gabrielle Atsam-Ebang, Nawal Hammas, El Fatemi Hinde and Laila Chbani
Departement of Pathology, Hassan II Teaching Hospital, Fès, Morocco

Marou Soumana Boubacar
Departement of Parasitology, Hassan II Teaching Hospital, Fès, Morocco

Kimihiro Igari, Toshifumi Kudo, Takahiro Toyofuku and Yoshinori Inoue
Division of Vascular and Endovascular Surgery, Department of Surgery, Tokyo Medical and Dental University, 1-5-45, Yushima, Bunkyo-ku, Tokyo 113-8519, Japan

Elizabeth L. Courville, Megan Griffith and Sophia Yohe
Department of Laboratory Medicine and Pathology, University of Minnesota, 420 Delaware St SE, MMC 609, Minneapolis, MN 55455, USA

Celalettin Ustun and Erica Warlick
Division of Hematology, Oncology, and Transplantation, Department of Medicine, University of Minnesota, Minneapolis, MN, USA

Grace Mashavave and Cuthbert Musarurwa
Department of Chemical Pathology, College of Health Sciences, University of Zimbabwe, PO BOX A178, Avondale, Harare, Zimbabwe

Patience Kuona
Department of Paediatrics and Child Health, College of Health Sciences, University of Zimbabwe, Harare, Zimbabwe

Willard Tinago
Department of Community Medicine, College of Health Sciences, University of Zimbabwe, Harare, Zimbabwe

Babill Stray-Pedersen
Division of Women and Children, Oslo University Hospital and Institute of Clinical Medicine, University of Oslo, Oslo, Norway

Marshall Munjoma
Department of Obstetrics and Gynaecology, College of Health Sciences, University of Zimbabwe, Harare, Zimbabwe

Markos Negash and Beyene Moges
Department of Immunology and Molecular Biology, School of Biomedical and Laboratory Sciences, College of Medicine and Health Sciences, University of Gondar, Gondar, Ethiopia

Afework Kassu and Gizachew Yismaw
Department of Medical Microbiology, School of Biomedical and Laboratory Sciences, College of Medicine and Health Sciences, University of Gondar, Gondar, Ethiopia

Bemnet Amare
Department of Biochemistry, School of Medicine, College of Medicine and Health Sciences, University of Gondar, P.O.BOX 196, Gondar, Ethiopia

Hania Naveed, Mariam Abid and Ghazala Mudassir
Shifa Medical College, Islamabad, Pakistan

Atif Ali Hashmi
Liaquat National Hospital and Medical College, Karachi, Pakistan

Muhammad Muzammamil Edhi
Brown University, Providence, RI, USA

Ahmareen Khalid Sheikh
Pakistan Institute of Medical Sciences, Islamabad, Pakistan

Amir Khan
Kandahar University, Kandahar, Afghanistan

Atif Ali Hashmi, Samreen Naz, Zubaida Fida Hussain, Muhammad Irfan, Erum Yousuf Khan and Naveen Faridi
Liaquat National Hospital and Medical College, Karachi, Pakistan

Shumaila Kanwal Hashmi
CMH Institute of Medical Sciences, Multan, Pakistan

Amir Khan
Kandahar University, North, Kandahar 3802, Afghanistan

Muhammad Muzzammil Edhi
Brown University, Providence, RI, USA

Baongoc Nasri
Matsuzawa Hospital, Setagaya-ku, Tokyo, Japan

Mikito Inokuchi, Toshiaki Ishikawa, Hiroyuki Uetake, Sho Otsuki, Kazuyuki Kojima and Tatsuyuki Kawano
Department of Surgical Oncology, Graduate School, Tokyo Medical and Dental University, Bunkyo-ku, Tokyo, Japan

Yoko Takagi
Department of Translational Oncology, Graduate School, Tokyo Medical and Dental University, Bunkyo-ku, Tokyo, Japan

David Borg, Charlotta Hedner, Björn Nodin, Anna Larsson, Anders Johnsson, Jakob Eberhard and Karin Jirström
Department of Clinical Sciences Lund, Division of Oncology and Pathology, Lund University, Skåne University Hospital, SE-221 85 Lund, Sweden

Fernanda A. Lucena and Ricardo F. A. Costa
Faculty of Health Science of Barretos Dr. Paulo Prata, Avenida Loja Maçônica Renovadora 68, Nº 100, Barretos 14785-002, São Paulo, Brazil

Maira D. Stein
Department of Pathology, Barretos Cancer Hospital, Rua Antenor Duarte Villela, 1331 - Dr. Paulo Prata, Barretos 14784-400, São Paulo, Brazil

Carlos E. M. C. Andrade, Geórgia F. Cintra, Marcelo A. Vieira and Ricardo dos Reis
Department of Gynecologic Oncology, Barretos Cancer Hospital, Rua Antenor Duarte Villela, 1331 - Dr. Paulo Prata, Barretos 14784-400, São Paulo, Brazil

Rozany M. Dufloth and José Humberto T. G. Fregnani
Post-Graduation Program in Oncology, Barretos Cancer Hospital, Rua Antenor Duarte Villela, 1331 - Dr. Paulo Prata, Barretos 14784-400, São Paulo, Brazil

Reidun Øvstebø
Blood Cell Research Group, Section for Research, Department of Medical Biochemistry, Oslo University Hospital HF, Ullevål Hospital, PO Box 4956 Nydalen, 0424 Oslo, Norway

Berit Sletbakk Brusletto, Jens Petter Berg and Petter Brandtzaeg
Blood Cell Research Group, Section for Research, Department of Medical Biochemistry, Oslo University Hospital HF, Ullevål Hospital, PO Box 4956 Nydalen, 0424 Oslo, Norway
Institute of Clinical Medicine, University of Oslo, Oslo, Norway

Else Marit Løberg and Ingeborg Løstegaard Goverud
Department of Pathology, Oslo University Hospital, Oslo, Norway
Institute of Clinical Medicine, University of Oslo, Oslo, Norway

Bernt Christian Hellerud
Institute of Immunology, Oslo University Hospital, Oslo, Norway

Åshild Vege
Section for Forensic Pediatric Pathology, Department of Forensic Sciences, Oslo University Hospital, Oslo, Norway
Institute of Clinical Medicine, University of Oslo, Oslo, Norway

Alan Sharpe
AstraZeneca Oncology Innovative Medicines, Alderley Park, Macclesfield, UK

Caroline Seiler
AstraZeneca Oncology Innovative Medicines, Alderley Park, Macclesfield, UK
Leeds University-AZ Sandwich Placement, Leeds, UK

Gayle B. Marshall
AstraZeneca Oncology Innovative Medicines, Alderley Park, Macclesfield, UK
AstraZeneca, 8AF6, Mereside, Alderley Park, Alderley Edge, Cheshire SK10 4TG, UK

Elizabeth A. Harrington and Emma V. Jones
AstraZeneca, Cambridge, UK

J. Carl Barrett
AstraZeneca, Waltham, USA

Index

www.ingramcontent.com/pod-product-compliance
Lightning Source LLC
Chambersburg PA
CBHW080457200326
41458CB00012B/4007